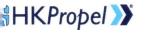 Accessing your HK*Propel* digital product is easy!

INSTRUCTORS: Use the access instructions provided by your sales rep. instead of the student access code below.

If it's your first time using HK*Propel*:
- Visit HKPropel.HumanKinetics.com.
- Click the "New user? Register here" link on the opening screen to register for an account and redeem your one-time-use access code.
- Follow the onscreen prompts to create your HK*Propel* account. Use a **valid email address** as your username to ensure you receive important system updates and to help us find your account if you ever need assistance.
- Enter the access code exactly as shown below, including hyphens. You will not need to re-enter this access code on subsequent visits, and this access code cannot be redeemed by any other user.
- After your first visit, simply log in to HKPropel.HumanKinetics.com to access your digital product.

If you already have an HK*Propel* account:
- Visit HKPropel.HumanKinetics.com and log in with your username (email address) and password.
- Once you are logged in, click the arrow next to your name in the top right corner and then click **My Account**.
- Under the "Add Access Code" heading, enter the access code exactly as shown below, including hyphens, and click the **Add** button.
- Once your code is redeemed, navigate to your Library on the Dashboard to access your digital content.

Product: Nutrition for Sport, Exercise, and Health 2nd Edition HKPropel Access

Student access code: L49Y-Y17B-KD5F-SS43

NOTE TO STUDENTS: If your instructor uses HK*Propel* to assign work to your class, you will need to enter a **class enrollment token** in HK*Propel* on the **My Account** page. This token will be provided **by your instructor at no cost to you**, but it is required **in addition** to the unique access code that is printed above.

Helpful tips:
- You may reset your password from the log in screen at any time if you forget it.
- Your license to this digital product will expire **2 years** after the date you redeem the access code. You can check the expiration dates of all your HK*Propel* products at any time in **My Account**.
- If you purchased a used book, you may purchase a new access code by visiting US.HumanKinetics.com and searching for "Nutrition for Sport, Exercise, and Health HKPropel Access".

For assistance, contact us via email at HKPropelCustSer@hkusa.com.

07-2023

NUTRITION FOR SPORT, EXERCISE, AND HEALTH

SECOND EDITION

Marie A. Spano, MS, RD, CSCS, CSSD
Spano Sports Nutrition Consulting, LLC

Laura J. Kruskall, PhD, RDN, CSSD, LD, FACSM, FAND
University of Nevada, Las Vegas

D. Travis Thomas, PhD, RDN, CSSD, LD, FAND
University of Kentucky

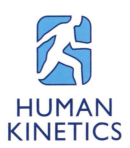

HUMAN KINETICS

Library of Congress Cataloging-in-Publication Data

Names: Spano, Marie A., 1972- author. | Kruskall, Laura J., 1967- author. | Thomas, D. Travis, 1977- author.
Title: Nutrition for sport, exercise, and health / Marie A. Spano, MS, RD, CSCS, CSSD, Spano Sports Nutrition Consulting, LLC, Laura J. Kruskall, PhD, RDN, CSSD, LD, FACSM, FAND University of Nevada, Las Vegas, D. Travis Thomas, PhD, RDN, CSSD, LD, FAND, University of Kentucky.
Description: Second edition. | Champaign : Human Kinetics, [2024] | Includes bibliographical references and index.
Identifiers: LCCN 2023004521 (print) | LCCN 2023004522 (ebook) | ISBN 9781718207783 (paperback) | ISBN 9781718223127 (loose-leaf) | ISBN 9781718207790 (epub) | ISBN 9781718207806 (pdf)
Subjects: MESH: Sports Nutritional Physiological Phenomena | Physical Fitness--physiology
Classification: LCC RA784 .S6557 2024 (print) | LCC RA784 (ebook) | DDC 613.7--dc23/eng/20230527
LC record available at https://lccn.loc.gov/2023004521
LC ebook record available at https://lccn.loc.gov/2023004522

ISBN: 978-1-7182-0778-3 (paperback)
ISBN: 978-1-7182-2312-7 (loose-leaf)

Copyright © 2024, 2018 by Spano Sports Nutrition Consulting, LLC, Laura J. Kruskall, and D. Travis Thomas

Human Kinetics supports copyright. Copyright fuels scientific and artistic endeavor, encourages authors to create new works, and promotes free speech. Thank you for buying an authorized edition of this work and for complying with copyright laws by not reproducing, scanning, or distributing any part of it in any form without written permission from the publisher. You are supporting authors and allowing Human Kinetics to continue to publish works that increase the knowledge, enhance the performance, and improve the lives of people all over the world.

The online learning content that accompanies this product is delivered on HK*Propel*, **HKPropel.HumanKinetics.com**. You agree that you will not use HK*Propel* if you do not accept the site's Privacy Policy and Terms and Conditions, which detail approved uses of the online content.

To report suspected copyright infringement of content published by Human Kinetics, contact us at **permissions@hkusa.com**. To request permission to legally reuse content published by Human Kinetics, please refer to the information at **https://US.HumanKinetics.com/pages/permissions-information**.

Permission notices for material reprinted in this book from other sources can be found on pages xi-xii.

The web addresses cited in this text were current as of March 2023, unless otherwise noted.

Acquisitions Editor: Amy N. Tocco; **Managing Editor:** Anna Lan Seaman; **Copyeditor:** Bob Replinger; **Proofreader:** Joyce H.-S. Li; **Indexer:** Nancy Ball; **Permissions Manager:** Laurel Mitchell; **Senior Graphic Designer:** Nancy Rasmus; **Cover Designer:** Keri Evans; **Cover Design Specialist:** Susan Rothermel Allen; **Photograph (cover):** Mike Kemp/Tetra images/Getty Images; **Photo Asset Manager:** Laura Fitch; **Photo Production Specialist:** Amy M. Rose; **Photo Production Manager:** Jason Allen; **Senior Art Manager:** Kelly Hendren; **Illustrations:** Human Kinetics, unless otherwise noted; **Printer:** Walsworth

Printed in the United States of America   10 9 8 7 6 5 4 3 2 1

The paper in this book was manufactured using responsible forestry methods.

Human Kinetics	*United States and International*	*Canada*
1607 N. Market Street	Website: **US.HumanKinetics.com**	Website: **Canada.HumanKinetics.com**
Champaign, IL 61820	Email: info@hkusa.com	Email: info@hkcanada.com
USA	Phone: 1-800-747-4457	

E8333 (paperback) / E9207 (loose-leaf)

Preface   vii
Photo Credits   xi

PART I   THE BIG PICTURE   1

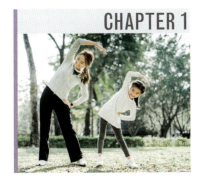

CHAPTER 1   Optimizing Health and Well-Being Throughout the Lifespan   3
Nutrients   4
General Nutrition Guidelines   6
Exercise   11
Sports Nutrition   15
Credentials and Scope of Practice   18
Summary   23

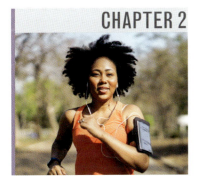

CHAPTER 2   Energy Metabolism   25
How Energy Fuels the Body   26
Human Energy Metabolism   28
Benefits of Training on Health and Athletic Performance   47
Biosynthesis and Storage Pathways in Metabolism   50
Hormonal Control of Metabolism   51
Measuring Energy Intake and Expenditure   52
Energy Availability in Sport   59
Summary   60

PART II   ROLE OF ENERGY-YIELDING MACRONUTRIENTS   61

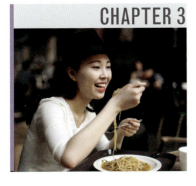

CHAPTER 3   Carbohydrate   63
Classification of Carbohydrate   64
Digestion and Absorption   68
Metabolism of Carbohydrate   70
Regulation of Glucose Metabolism   71
Glycemic Response   73
Carbohydrate as Fuel During Exercise   76
Role of Carbohydrate in Exercise Fatigue   76
Carbohydrate Recommendations   77
Carbohydrate Content of Foods   81
Carbohydrate and Health   81
Summary   90

iv　Contents

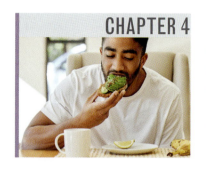

CHAPTER 4　Fat　93

Digestion and Metabolism　94
Dietary Fats and Exercise　95
Lipids and Dietary Fat　96
Triglycerides and Health　99
Dietary Recommendations　114
Summary　114

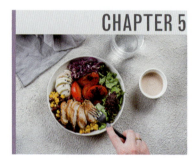

CHAPTER 5　Protein　117

Amino Acids　118
Classification and Function of Protein　121
Digestion and Absorption　130
Metabolic Fate of Protein in the Body　132
Protein in the Diet　135
Protein Quality　137
Protein in Exercise and Sport　142
Vegetarianism and Veganism　149
Protein Deficiency and Excess Protein　151
Summary　152

PART III　ROLE OF MICRONUTRIENTS, WATER, AND NUTRITIONAL SUPPLEMENTS　153

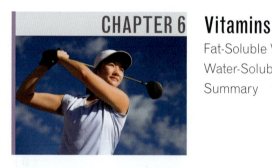

CHAPTER 6　Vitamins　155

Fat-Soluble Vitamins　156
Water-Soluble Vitamins　173
Summary　180

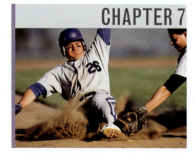

CHAPTER 7　Minerals　183

Macrominerals　184
Trace Minerals　199
Summary　208

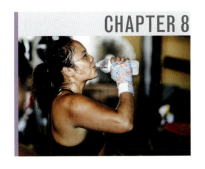

CHAPTER 8 Water and Electrolytes — 211
Water 212
Electrolytes 221
Water, Electrolytes, and Exercise Performance 222
Hydration Assessment 226
Hydration Recommendations for Exercise 232
Summary 235

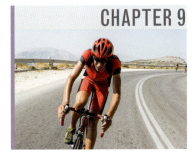

CHAPTER 9 Nutritional Supplements and Other Substances Commonly Used in Sport — 237
Popularity of Supplement Use in Sport 238
Regulation of Dietary Supplements 238
Evaluation of Dietary Supplements 241
Common Products and Supplements Used for Performance Enhancement 247
Drugs Commonly Used in Sport 259
Summary 261

PART IV APPLICATION OF NUTRITION FOR SPORT, EXERCISE, AND HEALTH 263

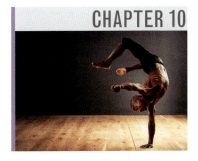

CHAPTER 10 Body Weight and Composition — 265
Factors Contributing to Body Weight and Composition 266
Body Weight and Composition Concerns in Activity and Sport 267
Estimating Body Composition 271
Summary 279

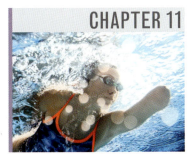

CHAPTER 11 Nutrition for Aerobic Endurance — 281
ATP Production During Endurance Activities 282
Energy-Yielding Macronutrient Requirements of Endurance Athletes 283
Food Selection to Meet Nutrient Requirements 293
Types of Carbohydrate and Performance 294
Unique Challenges Facing Endurance Athletes 295
General Recovery From Training 300
Effects of Endurance Training on Macronutrient Metabolism 301
Summary 301

vi   Contents

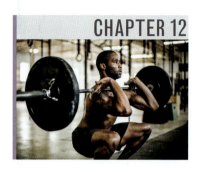

Chapter 12 Nutrition for Resistance Training   303
Nutrition Before Resistance Training 304
Nutrition During Resistance Training 306
Nutrition After Resistance Training 306
How Daily Dietary Intake Affects Muscle 311
How Dieting Affects Muscle 315
Nutrients That Support Muscle Functioning 318
Sport Supplements for Resistance Training 318
Summary 319

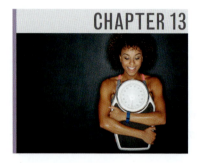

Chapter 13 Changing Weight and Body Composition   321
Understanding Body Fat 322
Decreasing Body Fat 326
Gaining Muscle Mass 338
Losing Fat and Gaining Muscle at the Same Time 340
Summary 341

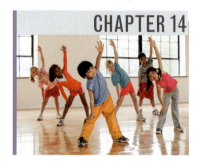

Chapter 14 Nutrition Concerns for Special Populations   343
Children and Adolescents 344
Masters Athletes 351
People With Diabetes and Metabolic Syndrome 355
Pregnant Women 363
Vegetarian Populations 368
People With Disordered Eating and Eating Disorders 373
Summary 380

Glossary 383
References 395
Index 449
About the Authors 467

PREFACE

Nutrition affects overall health and exercise performance in myriad ways. In *Nutrition for Sport, Exercise, and Health, Second Edition,* our goal is to provide readers with practical information they can use to enhance their everyday lives as well as the sports and physical activities that are part of their lives. For the student with an interest in working in the field of sports nutrition, sports medicine, or a related field, our goal is to supply the foundation of knowledge you will need to get the best start on your career path.

Given the plethora of nutrition misinformation consumers are hearing and reading from television, the Internet, magazines, coaches, trainers, parents, and their peers, this comprehensive textbook will help readers distinguish between nutrition recommendations based on quality scientific research and those that are not backed by science and have no foothold in basic biochemistry or physiology.

WHO NEEDS THIS BOOK

We have written *Nutrition for Sport, Exercise, and Health, Second Edition,* for students studying fitness, exercise science, health, nutrition, physical therapy, and closely related majors. This text is also an excellent reference for athletic trainers, strength coaches, wellness professionals, health coaches, health and physical education teachers, coaches, fitness instructors, athletic directors, exercise physiologists, registered dietitians, military personnel, and government employees working in health and human performance.

TOPICS COVERED

Our text covers the basics of nutrition for health, including the functions and daily allowances for the energy-yielding macronutrients—carbohydrate, protein, and fat—and micronutrients; nutrition in health and disease prevention; population-based nutrition considerations for training and sport; and practical information on measuring and altering body composition.

The text is organized in a logical sequence. Each chapter builds on what was learned in the previous chapter. In part I we provide an overview of the role nutrition plays in overall well-being throughout the life span. Energy metabolism is discussed, including the roles of macronutrients and micronutrients and the way exercise affects nutrient needs. The three chapters in part II focus on each of the energy-yielding macronutrients, their roles in health and disease, and dietary recommendations that support health and an active lifestyle. After learning about macronutrients, in part III readers are introduced to the roles of micronutrients in health and performance. Chapters on vitamins and minerals cover population-specific intake recommendations, consequences of excess intake or dietary shortfalls, and supplemental intake. This part of the book covers water and electrolytes as well as nutrition supplements and drugs. The role of fluid in health and human performance is discussed, and fluid and electrolyte guidelines are recommended. The chapter on nutrition supplements and drugs covers popular dietary supplements, supplement claims, third-party testing, drugs in sport, and the untoward effects of alcohol on sport performance. In part IV we provide information on the application of nutrition for health and fitness. Ideal body weight and body composition is discussed, including how to measure body composition and achieve optimal body composition and weight, and nutrition recommendations are provided for aerobic endurance and resistance training. In the final chapter we discuss nutrition concerns and recommendations for special populations and people at distinct life stages, including children, adolescents, masters athletes, people with diabetes, vegetarians, pregnant women, and people with eating disorders or disordered eating.

NEW TO THIS EDITION

The second edition of this textbook includes a web study guide with learning activities, as well as 25 checklists and forms. Quiz-based activities and interactive activities will help students learn to apply the information they have learned. In addition, the entire book has been extensively updated to include the most up-to-date research and relevant content, including updates based on *Dietary Guidelines for Americans, 2020-2025* (*DGA*). Some of the key updates with this edition include the following:

- Updated information on the dietary guidelines, food labels, related professional organizations and certifications, and scope of practice (chapter 1)
- The effect of progressive training programs on metabolism (chapter 2)
- Updated information on carbohydrate guidelines for before, during, and after exercise (chapter 3)
- Updated information on ketogenic diets, including specific information about the effect of ketogenic diets on health and muscle (chapter 4)
- New content on the Mediterranean eating pattern and cardiovascular health (chapter 4)
- Updated content on daily protein needs for athletes (chapter 5)
- Importance of protein food diversity to maintain or improve diet quality (chapter 5)
- Updated content on vitamin D status in athletes and the role of vitamin D in performance and inflammation (chapter 6)
- Updated and refined content on each mineral and its relation to disease, including a sample plan to meet mineral needs (chapter 7)
- Sample daily fluid plan for an athlete who loses a lot of fluid through sweat (chapter 8)
- Practical ideas on increasing fluid intake (chapter 8)
- A new section on omega-3 supplementation for inflammation and concussion prevention and recovery, as well as the effect of creatine taken before concussions (chapter 9)
- Ways to communicate body composition limitations to athletes and coaches (chapter 10)
- Expanded content on carbohydrate mouth rinsing for endurance athletes (chapter 11)
- Updated content on eating for concurrent training (chapter 12)
- Sample food plans (with various caloric needs) for athletes who are resistance training (chapter 12)
- New content on eating disorders or disordered eating (chapter 13)
- The latest research on why people regain weight after weight loss (chapter 13)
- Updates on the benefits of exercise for cognitive function (chapter 14)
- Further exploration of the effect of insufficient nutrient consumption on health and performance during the adolescent life stage (chapter 14)

UNIQUE FEATURES THAT ENHANCE LEARNING

The book includes a number of features that help highlight key concepts and provide practical examples to enhance understanding. Each chapter includes the following elements:

- Chapter objectives

  Included at the start of each chapter, these points give you an overview of what lies ahead.

- Putting It Into Perspective sidebars

  These elements help engage college readers by providing information that is relevant to them, including practical case studies; tips on improving health, enhancing sport performance, or achieving a desired physique; and other helpful material that can be applied in everyday living.

- Do You Know? sidebars

  These brief information nuggets provide key insights, little-known details, and evidence-based facts that might surprise you.

- Reflection Time sidebars

  These elements prompt readers to dig deeper and consider how certain concepts presented in the book relate to their everyday lives.

- Nutrition Tip sidebars

  Intriguing, real-world tips related to nutrition for the college student.

- Review questions

    Questions to evoke further thought and ensure that readers have digested the key points in each chapter.

- Glossary

    A handy listing of key terms to help you fill your memory bank—or for your future reference.

INSTRUCTOR RESOURCES

Instructor resources include an instructor guide, presentation package, test package, and chapter quizzes. The instructor guide includes chapter outlines and chapter summaries, objectives, and review questions from the book. The presentation package includes PowerPoint slides and an image bank of most of the art and tables from the book that instructors may use to create customized lecture presentations. The test package and chapter quizzes provide questions in various formats that can be used to create customized tests. Ancillary products supporting this are available online on HK*Propel*.

STUDENT RESOURCES

Student resources include 25 downloadable checklists and forms, flash cards to review key terms, and supplemental chapter activities to assess student learning and engagement. The student resource can be accessed online at HK*Propel*. If you purchased a new print book, follow the directions included on the orange-framed page at the front of your book. That page includes access steps and the unique key code that you'll need the first time you visit the *Nutrition for Sport, Exercise, and Health* website. If you purchased an ebook from HumanKinetics.com, follow the access instructions that were emailed to you following your purchase.

PHOTO CREDITS

Table of contents photos in chronological order: Images By Tang Ming Tung/Digital Vision/Getty Images; wera Rodsawang/Moment/Getty Images; RUNSTUDIO/Moment/Getty Images; PeopleImages/iStock/Getty Images; Anikona/iStock/Getty Images; nycshooter/E+/Getty Images; David Madison/Photographer's Choice RF/Getty Images; Thomas Barwick/Stone/Getty Images; Image Source/Digital Vision/Getty Images; PeopleImages/iStock/Getty Images; Tempura/E+/Getty Images; MoMo Productions/Stone/Getty Images; laflor/E+/Getty Images; Ariel Skelley/DigitalVision/Getty Images

Page 1: Patrik Giardino/Stone/Getty Images

Page 2: Images By Tang Ming Tung/Digital Vision/Getty Images

Page 10: skynesher/E+/Getty Images

Page 24: wera Rodsawang/Moment/Getty Images

Page 61: Edwin Tan/E+/Getty Images

Page 62: RUNSTUDIO/Moment/Getty Images

Page 77: ©Drazen Lovric/Getty Images

Page 81 (from top to bottom): xxmmxx/iStock/Getty Image; tanuha2001/iStock/Getty Images; SharonDay/iStock/Getty Image; Ekaterina_Lin/iStock/Getty Images; Magone/iStock/Getty Images; KMNPhoto/iStock/Getty Images

Page 85: Mark Hatfield/Getty Images

Page 92: PeopleImages/iStock/Getty Images

Page 95: © Human Kinetics

Page 103: Srdjan Stefanovic/iStockphoto/Getty Images

Page 113: FG Trade/E+/Getty Images

Page 116: Anikona/iStock/Getty Images

Page 140: © Human Kinetics

Page 150 (from top to bottom): loops7/Getty Images; Magone/Getty Images/iStockphoto; Kaan Ates/Getty Images

Page 153: Isitsharp/E+/Getty Images

Page 154: nycshooter/E+/Getty Images

Page 158 (clockwise from top): Creativeye99/iStockphoto/Getty Images; DeeNida/iStockphoto/Getty Images; OLEKSANDR PEREPELYTSIA/iStockphoto/Getty Images; popovaphoto/iStockphoto/Getty Images; ValentynVolkov/iStockphoto/Getty Images

Page 161 (clockwise from top): bdspn/iStockphoto/Getty Images; Burke/Triolo Productions/The Image Bank RF/Getty Images; Dominik Pabis/Getty Images; gbh007/iStockphoto/Getty Images

Page 170 (clockwise from top): IgorDutina/iStockphoto/Getty Images; Srdjan Stefanovic/iStockphoto/Getty Images; Kaan Ates/Getty Images; Image Source/Getty Images; Kaan Ates/Getty Images; Srdjan Stefanovic/iStockphoto/Getty Images

Page 172 (clockwise from top left): Lee Rogers/iStockphoto/Getty Images; Selektor/Getty Images; Kaan Ates/Getty Images; getsaraporn/iStockphoto/Getty Images; li jingwang/Getty Images; naran/iStockphoto/Getty Images; bhofack2/iStockphoto/Getty Images; Huw Jones/The Image Bank RF/Getty Images; retales botijero/Moment RF/Getty Images; papkin/iStockphoto/Getty Images

Page 176 (clockwise from top): Picsfive/iStockphoto/Getty Images; Kateryna Maksimenko/iStockphoto/Getty Images; popovaphoto/iStockphoto/Getty Images; bhofack2/iStockphoto/Getty Images; AlasdairJames/Getty Images; Kaan Ates/Getty Images

Page 177 (clockwise from top): Ekaterina_Lin/iStock/Getty Images; Kaan Ates/iStockphoto/Getty Images; Antonio Scarpi/iStockphoto/Getty Images; IgorDutina/iStockphoto/Getty Images; ithinksky/iStockphoto/Getty Images; milanfoto/Getty Images

Page 178: © Human Kinetics

Page 182: David Madison/Photographer's Choice RF/Getty Images

Page 185 (from top to bottom): Praiwun/

xi

iStockphoto/Getty Image; Kaan Ates/Getty Images; Kaan Ates/Getty Images; bhofack2/iStockphoto/Getty Images

Page 186 (clockwise from top): © Human Kinetics; Creativeye99/iStockphoto/Getty Images; Ekaterina_Lin/iStock/Getty Images; Sjoerd van der Wal/Getty Images/iStockphoto; Maris Zemgalietis/Getty Images/iStockphoto; margouillatphotos/Getty Images/iStockphoto; vitalssss/Getty Images/iStockphoto

Page 188 (from top to bottom): nezabudka123/Getty Images/iStockphoto; AlinaMD/Getty Images/iStockphoto; Carlos Gawronski/Getty Images

Page 192 (clockwise from top left): vikif/iStockphoto/Getty Images; Ekaterina_Lin/iStock/Getty Images; Kaan Ates/Getty Images; SharonDay/iStock/Getty Images; getsaraporn/iStockphoto/Getty Images; John Lawson/Moment RF/Getty Images; AlasdairJames/E+/Getty Images

Page 196: © Human Kinetics

Page 202 (clockwise from top left): Mizina/Getty Images/iStockphoto; vertmedia/Getty Images/iStockphoto; Anna Pustynnikova/Getty Images/iStockphoto; Lauri Patterson/Getty Images

Page 210: Thomas Barwick/Stone/Getty Images

Page 227: Peter Dazeley/The Image Bank/Getty Images

Page 228: © Human Kinetics

Page 233: © Human Kinetics

Page 234: © Human Kinetics

Page 236: Image Source/Digital Vision/Getty Images

Page 263: fancy.yan/Moment/Getty Images

Page 264: PeopleImages/iStock/Getty Images

Page 275: Courtesy of GE Healthcare

Page 276: © Human Kinetics; © Human Kinetics; © Human Kinetics

Page 280: Tempura/E+/Getty Images

Page 284: monkeybusinessimages/Getty Images/iStockphoto

Page 294 (from top to bottom): xxmmxx/iStock/Getty Images; getsaraporn/iStockphoto/Getty Images; bhofack2/Getty Images/iStockphoto; Magone/iStock/Getty Images

Page 297: © Stephen Mally/Icon Sportswire

Page 302: MoMo Productions/Stone/Getty Images

Page 314 (from top to bottom): gbh007/iStockphoto/Getty Images; Carlos Gawronski/Getty Images; Kaan Ates/Getty Images; ansonsaw/Getty Images/iStockphoto; Magone/iStock/Getty Images

Page 317: PeopleImages/Getty Images

Page 320: laflor/E+/Getty Images

Page 334: ©Anton/fotolia.com

Page 342: Ariel Skelley/DigitalVision/Getty Images

Page 345: © Human Kinetics

Page 351: © Human Kinetics

Page 369 (from left to right): Elena Schweitzer/Getty Images/iStockphoto; gbh007/iStockphoto/Getty Images; AlinaMD/Getty Images/iStockphoto; nezabudka123/Getty Images/iStockphoto

Page 371 (clockwise from top left): Elena Schweitzer/Getty Images/iStockphoto; popovaphoto/Getty Images/iStockphoto; egal/Getty Images/iStockphoto; AlinaMD/Getty Images/iStockphoto

Page 372: ©Elenathewise/fotolia.com

Page 378: simonkr/Getty Images/iStockphoto; © Human Kinetics

Page 379: simonkr/Getty Images/iStockphoto; © Human Kinetics

Page 467 (from left to right): Photo courtesy of Marie A. Spano; Photo courtesy of Laura J. Kruskall

PART I

THE BIG PICTURE

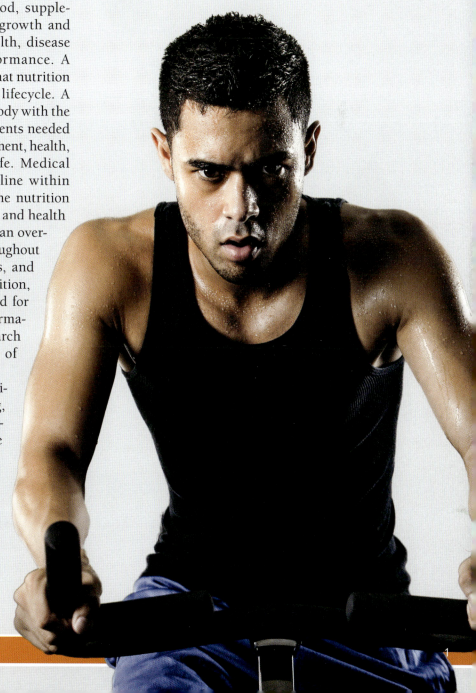

Nutrition is a complex and vast science that covers the role of food, supplementation, and hydration for growth and development, metabolism, health, disease prevention, and sports performance. A look at the big picture reveals that nutrition needs change throughout the lifecycle. A nutrient-rich diet supplies the body with the macronutrients and micronutrients needed for optimal growth and development, health, and well-being throughout life. Medical nutrition therapy, a subdiscipline within the field of nutrition, covers the nutrition needs for specific disease states and health conditions. Chapter 1 provides an overview of nutrition for health throughout the lifecycle, for disease states, and for athletic performance. In addition, food guidance systems intended for the public are covered, and information is provided about the research process and reliable sources of nutrition information.

Following an overview of nutrition for health and well-being, chapter 2 explores energy metabolism. Before delving into the specific role of nutrition in exercise and athletic performance, you will learn about the different energy systems that the body can use to generate fuel during various types of exercise at both high and low intensity.

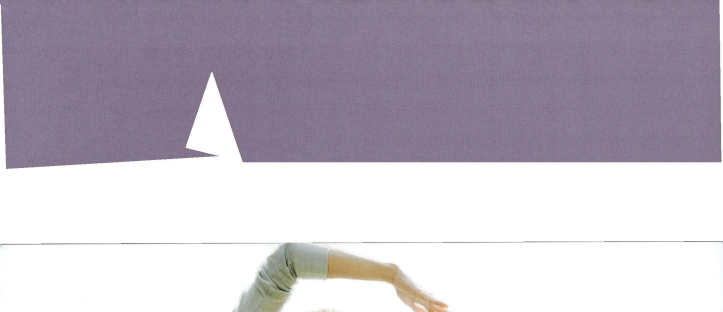
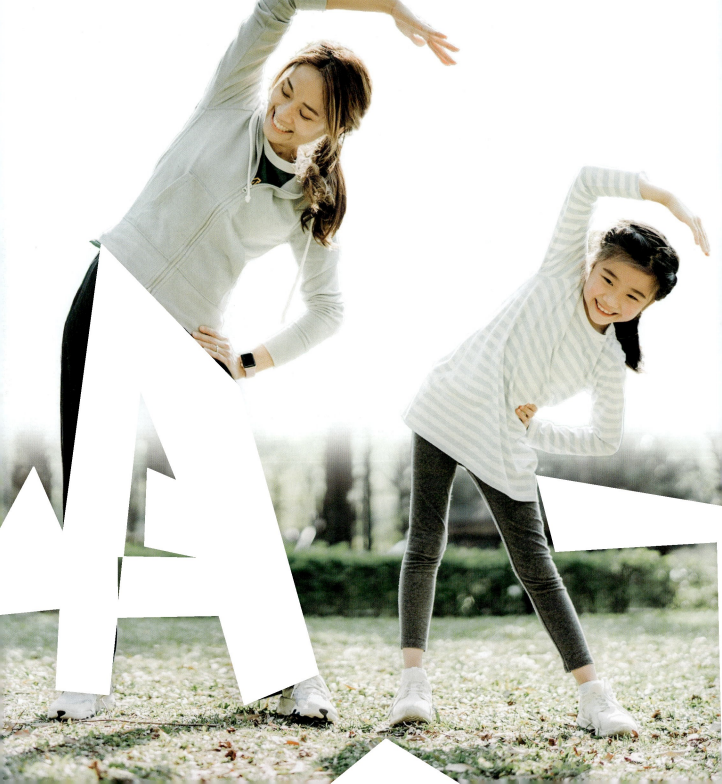

Optimizing Health and Well-Being Throughout the Lifespan

> ### ▶ CHAPTER OBJECTIVES
>
> After completing this chapter, you will be able to do the following:
>
> - Explain functions of nutrients and their roles in health.
> - Describe the differences between macronutrients and micronutrients.
> - Explain the difference between general nutrition information and medical nutrition therapy.
> - Identify and understand the major food guidance systems in the United States (*Dietary Guidelines*, food labels, dietary reference intakes, and MyPlate).
> - Describe the basic principles of exercise and training.
> - Discuss the role of nutrition in optimizing athletic performance.
> - Summarize the scientific research process and types of research designs, as well as how to evaluate reputable sources for sports nutrition information.
> - Understand credentials available in exercise science and the scope of practice between nutrition and exercise professionals.

Nutrition, as a scientific discipline, is the study of how food and its components affect growth and development, metabolism, health, and disease as well as mental and physical performance. Food refers to anything people eat or drink that supports life and growth. **Nutrients** are substances that elicit a biochemical or physiological function in the body. The science of nutrition involves the processes of consumption or ingestion, digestion, absorption, metabolism, transport, storage, and elimination. In addition to the science behind it, nutrition is an extremely broad field that encompasses everything from the food supply and food safety to eating behavior and nutrient recommendations for optimal health (1, 2). **Sports nutrition** is a specialty discipline that merges nutrition and sports science research, resulting in nutrition guidelines for physique changes as well as optimal training, performance, and recovery from exercise and competition (3).

NUTRIENTS

There are six groups of nutrients: carbohydrate, lipids, protein, vitamins, minerals, and water. Alcohol is not a nutrient, but it does contain energy. Carbohydrate, fat (including fatty acids and cholesterol), protein (including amino acids), fiber, and water are **macronutrients**, which are required in the diet in larger amounts. Carbohydrate, fat, and protein are also referred to as **energy-yielding macronutrients** because they supply the body with energy. Vitamins and minerals are **micronutrients**, which are required in the body in smaller amounts in comparison with macronutrients. A common misconception is that vitamins and minerals are energy nutrients. These do not contain energy, although they play essential roles in the production of energy. Deficiencies of certain vitamins and minerals can lead to fatigue. Macronutrients and micronutrients work together for optimal physiological function. The unit of energy in food is called a **kilocalorie**, commonly referred to as a calorie or kcal. To achieve consistency, throughout the book we will use the term *calorie* and, when the term is coupled with a number, the abbreviation *kcal*. A calorie is the amount of heat it takes to raise the temperature of one kilogram of water by one degree Celsius. A person's energy requirement refers to the number of calories needed each day. Food labels list calories per serving of the item. Both carbohydrate and protein contain 4 kcal per gram, whereas lipids provide 9 kcal per gram, making lipids more **energy dense**—that is, they contain more calories per mass or volume than does carbohydrate or protein (2).

Dietary Reference Intakes

The Institute of Medicine (IOM) of the United States Department of Agriculture (USDA) developed the dietary reference intakes (DRIs) (4), a set of recommendations based on the latest "scientific knowledge of the nutrient needs of healthy populations" (figure 1.1). The DRIs include the following:

> **Estimated average requirement (EAR).** The EAR is the estimated mean daily requirement for a nutrient as determined to meet the requirements of 50 percent of healthy people in each age range, life stage, and gender group (different amounts are provided based on age ranges, whether a person is male or female, and based on life stages, such as pregnancy and lactation). The EAR is based on the reduction of disease and overall health promotion. It does not reflect the daily needs of individuals but is used to set the RDA and for research purposes.

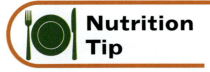

Counting your grams of carbohydrate? Note that although all vegetables contain primarily carbohydrate, their content per serving is not the same. Vegetables can be categorized as starchy or nonstarchy. Starchy vegetables, such as potatoes, corn, and peas, have approximately 15 grams of carbohydrate in a half-cup serving. Nonstarchy vegetables, such as broccoli, beets, and asparagus, have considerably less carbohydrate—about 5 grams per half-cup serving. If you want to reduce your intake of carbohydrate, choose more nonstarchy versus starchy vegetables.

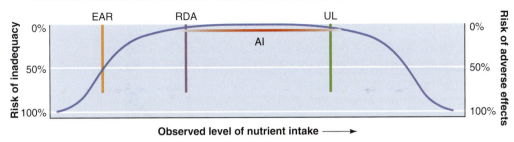

Figure 1.1 Dietary reference intakes. The AI or RDA describes the recommended daily amount of a nutrient, whereas the UL describes the amount not to exceed. Too little or too much of a nutrient can increase the risk of undesirable effects.

› **Recommended dietary allowance (RDA).** The RDA is set to meet the needs of nearly all (97-98%) healthy people in each age range, gender group, and life stage. This amount should be consumed daily. The RDA is two standard deviations above the EAR based on variability in requirements, or if the standard deviation is not known, the RDA is 1.2 times the EAR.

› **Adequate intake (AI).** The AI is the recommended average daily nutrient level assumed to be adequate for all healthy people. The AI is based on estimates—observed or experimentally determined approximations—and used when the RDA cannot be established because of insufficient data.

› **Tolerable upper intake level (UL).** The UL is the highest average daily intake considered safe for almost all people. The UL represents average daily intake from all sources, including food, water, and supplements. Lack of a published UL does not indicate that high levels of the nutrient are safe. Instead, it means that sufficient research is not currently available to establish a UL.

› **Acceptable macronutrient distribution range (AMDR).** The AMDR is a range given as a percentage of total energy intake—including carbohydrate, protein, and fat—and is associated with a reduced risk of chronic disease and adequate intake of essential nutrients.

› **Estimated energy requirement (EER).** The EER is the average daily energy intake that should maintain energy balance in a healthy person. Factors such as gender, age, height, weight, and activity level are all considerations when calculating this value.

Energy-Yielding Macronutrients

The primary function of carbohydrate is to provide energy. Carbohydrate becomes increasingly important when exercising at a high intensity. High-intensity exercise increases energy (calorie) demands, and carbohydrate is a fast source of energy—the body can quickly access it—whereas fat, another source of energy, is much slower in meeting the body's demand for energy during high-intensity exercise. Carbohydrate can be stored, to an extent, in the human body as an energy reserve in the form of glycogen in the liver and muscle. The AMDR for carbohydrate is 45 to 65 percent of totally daily calories for both males and females ages 19 and older (4, 5). Common sources of carbohydrate are rice, pasta, wheat products, corn, beans, legumes, fruits, vegetables, and milk. Some carbohydrates are considered nutrient dense because they contain nutrients important for good health, including vitamins, minerals, and dietary fiber. A type of carbohydrate, fiber, is discussed in detail in chapter 3.

Dietary fats and oils are examples of lipids. Dietary fats and oils provide energy and aid in the absorption of fat-soluble vitamins and food components. Fat can be stored in limitless quantities in the body, serving as an energy reserve. Fat can be an important energy source during long-duration activities, such as an ultraendurance race. The AMDR for fat is 20 to 35 percent of total daily calories for both males and females ages 19 years and older (4, 5). Common sources of fat include meat, nuts, seeds, oils, dairy products, and vegetable spreads (2).

Protein can be used for energy, but its primary function is to support cell and tissue growth, maintenance, and repair. Therefore, people need to consume an adequate amount daily. The RDA for protein is 56 grams per day for males aged 19 and over, and 46 grams per day for females aged 14 and over. The RDA for pregnant and lactating women of all ages is 71 grams per day. Despite these recommendations, considerable evidence suggests that the RDA for protein is too low to support muscle growth and maintenance, particularly for athletes and older adults. The AMDR for protein is 10 to 35 percent of total daily calories for both males and females ages 19 and older (4, 5). Common sources of protein include poultry, beef, fish, eggs, dairy foods, and some plant foods, particularly soy foods, nuts, and seeds (2).

Micronutrients

Vitamins are essential nutrients, necessary for releasing and using energy during the metabolism of carbohydrates, lipids, and proteins. Vitamins also support proper growth and development, vision, organ and immune functioning, muscle contraction and relaxation, oxygen transport, building and maintaining bone and cartilage, building and repairing muscle tissue, and protecting the body's cells from damage. Vitamins are classified as fat soluble or water soluble depending on how they are absorbed, transported, and stored in the body. Most water-soluble vitamins (e.g., some B vitamins, vitamin C) are not stored in the body, and any excess is excreted in urine; fat-soluble vitamins (e.g., vitamins A, D, E, K) are stored in the liver and adipose (fat) tissue. Tolerable upper limits have been established for many of the micronutrients. Daily vitamin requirements depend on many factors, including health status, gender, life stage, and age (4). Vitamin deficiencies or insufficiencies may negatively affect training gains and athletic performance, although there is no evidence to suggest those who exercise or train for competition need greater intakes beyond their requirements for general health (6).

Minerals are structural components of many body tissues, including bones, nails, and teeth. They also help regulate fluid balance, muscle pH, muscle contraction (including heartbeat), nerve impulses, oxygen transport, immune functioning, and muscle building and repair and are part of enzymes that facilitate several metabolic functions (4, 7, 8).

Macrominerals are required in higher amounts (i.e., grams and milligrams) than are trace minerals (i.e., micrograms). Mineral deficiencies can impair health as well as exercise and athletic performance, though research does not indicate that excess intake, beyond the DRIs, will improve results from an exercise program or improve athletic performance (4, 8-11).

Water

Water plays a role in nutrient transport, waste removal, biochemical reactions, blood pressure, and regulation of body temperature. Water needs depend on many factors, including age, body size, health status, medication use, environment (heat), altitude, and physical activity, particularly sweat losses. Daily water requirements can be met through a combination of fluids and the water found in food. In particular, soups, fruits, and vegetables contain a considerable amount of water (9, 12-14).

GENERAL NUTRITION GUIDELINES

Nutrition plays a significant role in health and **wellness**. Nutrition guidelines exist for healthy persons as well as those with specific diseases or conditions. Medical nutrition therapy includes diet interventions to treat or prevent health conditions and diseases (15). Other guidelines exist for athletes and active people specific to the activity or sport (16). In some respects, general nutrition guidelines for health overlap with those for activity or sports. Understanding both is important to recognize when general versus sport-specific guidelines should be considered.

> **PUTTING IT INTO PERSPECTIVE**
>
> ### GENERAL NUTRITION INFORMATION VERSUS MEDICAL NUTRITION THERAPY
>
> General, nonmedical nutrition information is designed to provide healthy people with food and nutrition guidelines for health promotion and disease prevention. Many of these guidelines come from government agencies, including the United States Department of Agriculture (USDA). If a person has a health condition or disease for which food and nutrition play a role in prevention or management, they are receiving **medical nutrition therapy (MNT)**. MNT is most often provided by a registered dietitian nutritionist (RD or RDN), and in many states providing MNT is limited to practitioners who are RDs or RDNs and hold a license (15).

Dietary Guidelines

Although the rate of many infectious diseases has dropped over the years, largely because of immunizations (17), an increase has occurred in chronic diseases and conditions related to poor nutrition habits and physical inactivity. Examples include cardiovascular disease, high blood pressure, type 2 diabetes, some types of cancer, and osteoporosis. In addition, more than two-thirds of adults and almost one-third of children and adolescents are overweight or obese (18). *2020–2025 Dietary Guidelines for Americans* includes evidence-based recommendations and guidelines designed for professionals to help guide Americans toward healthier eating patterns and **physical activity levels (PALs)** to improve and maintain good health and reduce risk of chronic disease (19).

Dietary Guidelines is used to develop federal food, nutrition, and health policies and programs. *Dietary Guidelines* is evidence based and is intended for policymakers and nutrition and health professionals, not the public. Educational materials and programs for the public are developed based on *Dietary Guidelines*. The current *Dietary Guidelines* translates nutrition science and physical activity research into food-based guidance as well as physical activity recommendations that people can use to choose foods and incorporate physical activity patterns into their lives to promote optimal health and reduce risk of chronic disease. The guidelines are too extensive to discuss fully in this text, but they can be obtained free of charge by visiting the USDA website. Resources and toolkits for both health professionals and consumers are also being developed from *Dietary Guidelines* (19).

Food Labels

The **U.S. Food and Drug Administration (FDA)** requires nutrition labeling on most foods, and any nutrient content claims and health messages must comply with agency regulations. Some foods are exempt from nutrition labeling. For example, foods that do not supply significant nutrition value, including coffee and most spices, are exempt. Fresh produce is also exempt. For those foods requiring a label, five key components must be listed (20, 21):

1. Name of the product or something to identify what it is
2. The net weight, volume, or numerical count of the package contents
3. Ingredients by common name and in descending order by weight
4. The name and address of the manufacturer, packer, or distributor
5. The Nutrition Facts label (figure 1.2)

Fortunately, government agencies help make the process of translating nutrition requirements into food choices a fairly straightforward process. The FDA regulates the contents of most food labels affixed to packaged products in the United States, whereas meat and poultry product labels are governed by the United States Department of Agriculture (USDA) Food Safety and Inspection Service (FSIS). Food labels display, among other nutrients, the amount of carbohydrate, fiber, fat, and protein included in each serving of the product. Serving sizes are somewhat standardized among products but, more importantly, are in familiar household measurements such as cups, tablespoons, and whole units (pieces).

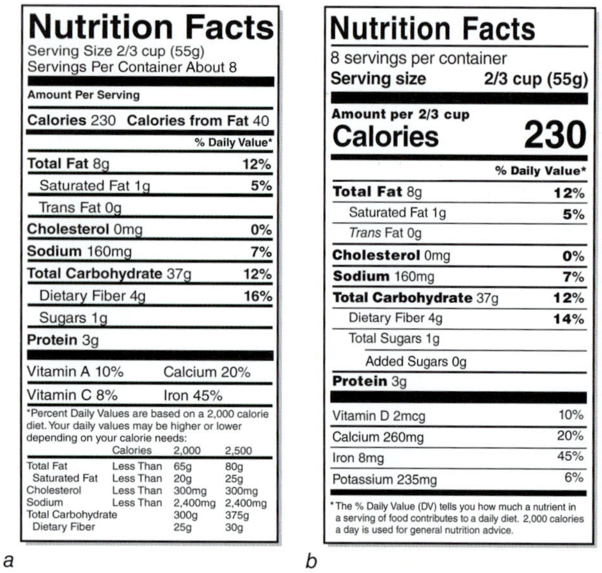

Figure 1.2 The Nutrition Facts label has been updated for easy understanding of the information provided. (*a*) This label is what you have been seeing for several years. (*b*) This is the current label. Recently the FDA published a variety of consumer education materials and social media toolkits for use when educating patients and clients (20, 21).

> **DO YOU KNOW?**
>
> Vitamin D, calcium, iron, and potassium are listed on the Nutrition Facts label because many Americans are not meeting recommendations for these nutrients (20, 21).

Serving size is an important consideration. For example, a sports drink may have three servings per bottle, yet the nutrition information is listed per serving—that is, for one-third of the bottle. Servings must be listed in common household measures and grams. The quantity of energy-yielding nutrients—carbohydrate, fat, and protein—are provided in grams, which can be useful for nutrition guidelines presented in grams per day or grams per kilograms of body weight, as commonly used in sports nutrition guidelines. Macronutrients and micronutrients are also expressed in terms of percent of **daily value (DV)**. DV is an indicator of how much of one serving of a food item contributes to a person's nutrition needs, based on a 2,000 kcal diet. The percent DV puts nutrition information in context of overall daily diet. Less than 5 percent of the DV is low for a nutrient; greater than 20 percent is high (21). Finally, a footnote at the bottom of the Nutrition Facts label describes %DV: "The % Daily Value tells you how much a nutrient in a serving of food contributes to a daily diet. 2,000 kcals a day is used for general nutrition advice" (20, 21).

Food products and dietary supplements are allowed to make **nutrient content claims** and **health claims**, as regulated by the FDA. Nutrient content claims describe the level of a nutrient in a food product. For instance, a claim may say "no salt added," "fat free," or "reduced-fat cheesecake." Examples of terms defined by the FDA include "light," "lite," "sodium free," "trivial source of sodium," "reduced," "less," "low-fat," "sugar free," "low calorie," "good source," "high," "more," and "high potency." Some of the terms compare the level of the nutrient in a product with the DV for that nutrient (e.g., "excellent source"), whereas others compare the level of the nutrient in a product with that in a reference food. A reference food is defined as a food within the same category (potato chips and pretzels, for instance) or similar food (comparing two brands of potato chips, for example). Detailed descriptions of FDA-approved nutrient content claims can be found on the FDA's website (22).

Health claims can be used on food as well as dietary supplements to describe a relationship between a substance and a health-related condition or disease. Several requirements must be met before FDA approval of a health claim, including significant scientific agreement supporting the

---

PUTTING IT INTO PERSPECTIVE

PORTION DISTORTION

A product's serving size, shown in large bold font on the Nutrition Facts label, reflects what people normally eat. You may, however, eat more or less than the serving size listed. Use measuring cups to pour a serving onto your plate or into a bowl so that you can see what a serving looks like.

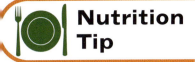

Nutrition Tip The terms "light" or "lite" can have several meanings when used on a food product. These terms are regulated by the FDA yet remain confusing to consumers. When one of these terms is used it can mean the product contains one-third fewer calories, or no more than half the fat of the original version of the product. The term can also refer to sodium, meaning that the food has no more than half the sodium compared with the comparable product. Examples include "light" salad dressing, referring to calories and fat, and "light" soy sauce, meaning that the product has half the sodium of a typical soy sauce. Here is the tricky part: These terms can also refer to color and texture, and in such cases the terms have no relation to nutrition value. For example, "light" brown sugar is a description of the color, and something described as "light and fluffy" refers to food texture.

proposed claim. Only a limited number of health claims are approved for use; the complete list can be found on the FDA's website (22).

MyPlate

The general website for MyPlate can be found at www.myplate.gov, and a downloadable app is available for smartphones. MyPlate has an extensive resource library on nutrition, as well as online tools that can be used for both knowledge-based education and practical application. Numerous printable materials on several nutrition education topics are available, as are toolkits for professionals to use when providing education in various settings. The MyPlate resources are evidence based and fall under the category of nutrition information available to the public. Health professionals can use these resources to guide clients with scientifically supported nutritional guidelines while staying within their individual scope of practice. Check the site periodically for updates (23).

In addition, MyPlate outlines healthy dietary patterns based on *Dietary Guidelines* and focuses on variety, amount, and nutrition. The website shares information in multiple languages based on life stages. In addition to focusing on food groups and portion sizes, the website includes recipes, printable infographics to share on social media, seasonal food suggestions, and videos. MyPlate also encourages more nutritious food choices from the five food groups: fruits, vegetables, grains, protein, and dairy. For example, whole grains are a better choice than refined white bread or pasta. See figure 1.3 for more details. Finally, MyPlate encourages people to stay within their daily energy limits (23).

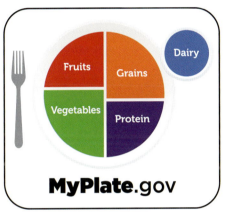

Figure 1.3 MyPlate provides a reminder that all food groups are important. Half of the plate should be filled with fruits and vegetables, one-quarter with lean protein, and one-quarter with quality grain. Dairy is represented as a side dish or a beverage, as commonly consumed.

U.S. Department of Agriculture (2022).

In addition to all the useful resources that it offers, MyPlate has an interactive online tool and an app that encourages users to "build healthy eating habits one goal at a time." The interactive system, called MyPlate Plan (www.myplate.gov/myplate-plan), can create a meal plan based on age, gender, height, weight, and current level of physical activity. The system creates a meal plan with the recommended number of servings from each of the five food groups. The user can explore each food group in detail to determine the healthiest choices and the guidelines for serving sizes. Though other, more sophisticated, programs are on the market for diet and physical activity tracking, www.myplate.gov is free of charge (24). When assessing any diet analysis program, accuracy and ease of use are both important. Accurate programs use the USDA database (25) for the energy and nutrient content of foods in addition to information from food labels on packaged foods.

The MyPlate plan and the various other MyPlate resources can teach athletes about portion sizes and accompanying nutrient content. For example, a half-cup of cooked rice is a serving size of grains and provides about 20 to 25 grams of carbohydrate, depending on the variety. A serving of protein is one ounce of meat or one egg, each containing 7 grams of protein per serving.

The MyPlate Plan and educational materials based on MyPlate provide energy intake guidelines and portions for people who get less than 30 minutes of moderate physical activity most days of the week, so their guidelines are not fit for athletes because they are too low in calories, protein, and carbohydrate and therefore need to be adjusted (23, 24).

Guidelines for Athletes

Because the DRIs do not take exercise into account, the AMDRs are not the primary consideration for athletes; rather, specific guidelines for carbohydrate, lipids, and protein for athletes are expressed in grams or in grams per kilogram body weight. These energy-yielding macronutrients are discussed in detail in chapters 3, 4, and 5. Although athletes might benefit from slightly greater intake of certain micronutrients to keep levels in the body within normal limits, many can meet these needs with a well-planned diet that meets their energy demands. Greater energy intake provides the opportunity to consume more food and therefore more nutrients. Micronutrients of greater concern for athletes are discussed in chapters 6 and 7. The ULs apply to athletes and active people. When considering the UL for vitamins and minerals, people must consider total intake of nutrients from all sources, including food, beverages, sports nutrition products (e.g., bars, protein powders), and supplements.

> Nutritional requirements for athletes may vary by sport. Water polo, for example, is a high-intensity activity. If you are an athlete, consider what aspects of your sport may require specialized nutrition to replenish your body and improve performance.

Learning to read food labels can help athletes plan their diets. Most energy-yielding macronutrient guidelines for athletes are expressed in grams, as listed on food labels. Grams per serving for carbohydrate, fat, and protein are clearly listed on the Nutrition Facts label.

EXERCISE

Exercise includes any activity that enhances physical fitness and health. Exercise is a type of physical activity that is planned and repetitive. Exercise is important throughout the lifespan, because it can help prevent or delay the development of many diseases and health conditions, including certain types of cancer, cardiovascular disease, osteoporosis, and sarcopenia (age-related loss of muscle mass). Sport-specific training results in physiological adaptations to improve performance.

> **DO YOU KNOW?**
>
> Some people think they are too old to reap the benefits of exercise. In reality, it is never too late. Although muscle mass declines with age, older adults can improve strength through resistance training. This activity can lead to improved health and enhanced mobility and daily functioning (26, 27).

Health Benefits of Exercise

Physical Activity Guidelines for Americans (28, 29) is a public document that summarizes the research findings on the health benefits of physical activity. This document provides numerous resources that can be used to disseminate the key points of the guidelines. Some of the major findings include the following:

- All adults should avoid physical inactivity; some physical activity is better than none. Regular physical activity reduces the risk of many adverse health outcomes.
- Most health outcomes have a dose-response relationship. As the amount of physical activity increases through higher intensity, greater frequency, or longer duration, many health outcomes improve.
- Most health benefits occur with at least 150 minutes (2 hours and 30 minutes) a week of moderate-intensity **aerobic physical activity**, or 75 minutes (1 hour and 15 minutes) a week of vigorous-intensity aerobic physical activity, or an equivalent combination of the two intensities.
- For more extensive health benefits, adults should aim to achieve 300 minutes (5 hours) a week of moderate-intensity aerobic physical activity, or 150 minutes a week of vigorous-intensity aerobic physical activity, or an equivalent combination of the two intensities. Additional health benefits may be gained by engaging in physical activity beyond this amount.
- Both endurance (aerobic) and resistance training are beneficial. Resistance training should be moderate or high intensity and involve all major muscle groups 2 or more days per week.
- Health benefits occur for children and adolescents, young and middle-aged adults, older adults, those in every studied racial and ethnic group, and for people with disabilities.
- The benefits of physical activity far outweigh the possibility of adverse outcomes stemming from exercise.

Many competitive athletes far exceed these general recommendations for health.

Components of Fitness

Physical fitness involves many systems of the body working together to produce a desired outcome. The key components of fitness include cardiovascular or cardiorespiratory endurance, muscular strength and endurance, flexibility, and body composition. Aerobic power (aerobic capacity) is dependent on a continuous supply of oxygen and is determined by measuring maximal oxygen uptake, also referred to as maximal oxygen consumption ($\dot{V}O_2$max). **$\dot{V}O_2$max** measures the maximum volume ($\dot{V}$) of oxygen (O_2) taken in, transported, and used by muscles to produce energy. $\dot{V}O_2$max is measured using an incremental (increases in speed, incline, or both) exercise test on a cycle ergometer or treadmill (30). A higher $\dot{V}O_2$max means that the athlete can consume more oxygen and deliver it to hard-working muscles. $\dot{V}O_2$max declines with age, yet aerobic training can increase $\dot{V}O_2$max in people of all ages, including older adults (31, 32). High-intensity, low-duration training and low-intensity, high-duration training increase $\dot{V}O_2$max to a similar extent (32, 33).

Anaerobic means "without oxygen." **Anaerobic activity** is intense activity performed without sufficient oxygen over a short period (figure 1.4). Sprinting is an example. Increasing anaerobic power or capacity depends on the anaerobic energy systems, the adenosine triphosphate-phosphocreatine system (ATP-PC), and anaerobic glycolysis (see chapter 2 for more details). Optimizing anaerobic power means the body has trained these systems to maximally produce **ATP**, a high-energy molecule used in all cells of the body and during exercise (32, 34).

Muscular strength is the maximal force that a skeletal muscle or group of muscles can produce, whereas **muscular power** is the rate at which the work (contraction) is performed. Muscular power is the product of strength and velocity or speed of the contraction. **Muscular endurance** is the ability to perform repeated skeletal muscle contractions or to hold a contraction over a period of time. Both skeletal muscle strength and endurance can be increased with training. **Muscular flexibility** is the ability to move through a joint's range of motion. Like other components of fitness, flexibility can be improved through exercise (28, 29, 32).

Body composition describes the makeup of tissues in the body. Percent body fat is the percentage of body weight that is fat, rather than fat-free mass such as muscle, organs, water, connective tissue, and bone. Ranges of body fat associated with both health and athletic performance are discussed in chapter 13. Although excess body fat is a risk factor for developing several chronic diseases, too little body fat is also detrimental to health. In some sports, athletes require a high level of muscle mass and strength, whereas other sports require leanness and optimal muscle endurance. More details on body composition are provided in chapters 10 and 13.

Both genetics and environmental factors, including physical activity, activities of daily living, and nutrition, influence body composition. Although genetics can influence tendency for overweight and obesity, as well as where fat is deposited on the body (hips, buttocks, breasts, etc.), many people with obesity genes never become overweight or obese (35). Environment plays a tremendous role, and there is also a link between genetics and the environment. Making good nutrition choices, decreasing energy intake to lose weight or consuming enough energy to maintain yet not gain weight, and being physically active all have a profound influence on genetic predisposition to overweight or obesity (36-41).

Principles of Exercise Training

Exercise training describes the body's response to consistent exercise, resulting in physiological adaptations (32). A well-designed training program combined with proper nutrition and adequate sleep and recovery generally leads to

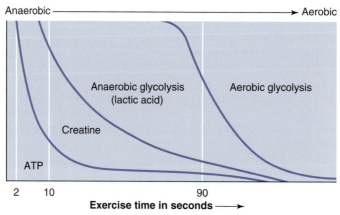

Figure 1.4 Anaerobic activities do not require oxygen for ATP generation. Training results in optimization of this system for enhanced ATP production and greater performance.

Based on Rice University, WebMed. Available: http://www.rice.edu/~jenky/images/creatine_reviewPCT11.JPG.

performance improvements, whereas overtraining or undertraining can result in a performance decrement.

Specificity

The **principle of specificity** dictates that training adaptations and performance improvements are specific to the type, intensity, and duration of training. Training must induce a physical stress specific to the system needed for performance enhancements. For example, a triathlete must perform endurance activities that are long in duration and include the activities in competition: swimming, cycling, and running. Weightlifting promotes increased muscle strength and hypertrophy (growth), which are beneficial adaptations for power lifters. Endurance training alone will not promote the increased muscular strength and hypertrophy necessary for power lifting. In simplest terms, for the principle to apply, the training program must be specific to the sport or activity and support the physiological adaptations needed to succeed at the desired sport or activity (28, 29, 32).

> **? DO YOU KNOW?**
>
> Training-induced muscle fatigue is important for increased skeletal muscle hypertrophy and gains in strength. Whether fatigue is induced with heavier weights and fewer repetitions or lighter weights with more repetitions, the skeletal muscle motor units are recruited and hypertrophy occurs. Alternating styles can also be used to give the body a break from heavy use (42).

Overload

To see improvements in performance, a person must **overload** the system (e.g., cardiovascular, muscular) being trained with a load greater than normal. For example, if you bench press 150 pounds (68 kg) for a maximum of eight repetitions, at which time your muscles become fatigued and you cannot lift one more repetition, 150 pounds is your eight-repetition max, or 8RM. With regular training over time, you will be able to lift the same 150 pounds more than eight times before your muscles fatigue and you must stop. If you wish to become stronger, you must add more weight to your press to establish a new 8RM or experience complete muscle fatigue after eight repetitions. Adjusting weight and number of repetitions while focusing on **eccentric contractions** (lengthening of the muscle, such as lowering your arm during a biceps curl) can improve muscle hypertrophy and strength. For endurance performance improvement, you must increase total training volume through intensity, duration, or a combination of the two (28, 29, 32).

> **? DO YOU KNOW?**
>
> When you begin a resistance-training program, you may fatigue quickly. When you become stronger, resistance training becomes easier. If you do not increase the weight to make it harder to lift again, you will not experience any additional strength gains.

Periodization

The **principle of periodization** schedules training for a particular sport or event into smaller blocks of time (figure 1.5). Proper periodization allows for the intensity of training required for the desired performance outcome while also allowing adequate rest and recovery. Traditional periodization plans are usually mapped over a long duration, such as a year to 4 years. Within that period are various cycles of months (macrocycles), weeks (mesocycles), days (microcycles), and individual training sessions. Such a plan might work well for people training for a single competition like a marathon, in which the focus is on one system (the cardiovascular system). Training blocks can also be customized to a particular sport or activity to emphasize a smaller number of performance outcomes at once or to design a smaller number of blocks at one time. These blocks might be a shorter duration than in single-sport training (e.g., a few weeks). The number, sequence, and outcomes can be highly customized for the sport or event (43-45).

Detraining

Regular resistance or endurance training produces physiological training responses beneficial for both athletes and other people. Unfortunately, when you discontinue training, you no longer

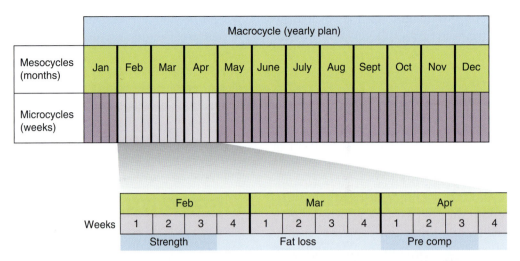

Figure 1.5 Periodization is a concept that simplifies training regimens and goals into smaller blocks of time. Intensity and duration of training may vary depending on the desired performance outcome. The actual length of time in each block or period will depend on the sport or activity.

make gains and you will gradually return to your pretrained physiological state. This process is called the **principle of detraining**. Maintenance-level training programs are needed to prevent physiological declines from the trained state. Physiological reductions with detraining can be partial or full, and cardiorespiratory endurance decrements appear to be greater than loss of muscular strength and power. Data vary regarding muscle strength, power, and endurance, but some research suggests just 2 weeks of inactivity can lead to declines in muscular endurance. Fortunately, resuming training can result in restoration of both cardiorespiratory endurance and skeletal muscle performance (43, 45-49).

Overtraining

It is well established that appropriate training and adequate recovery and rest leads to enhanced performance, but unfortunately, many athletes believe that more is better. Excessive training usually results in a performance decrement, often followed by the compensatory behavior of even more physical effort. The American College of Sports Medicine and the European College of Sports Science have a Joint Consensus Statement on this topic (16). The two terms to describe the condition of excessive training are overreaching and overtraining. **Overreaching** describes excessive training volume that results in short-term performance decrements and usually occurs during periods of competition. These declines can be reversed in several days to several weeks through proper training, nutrition intervention, and rest. Key nutrients include adequate fluid to restore hydration, carbohydrate to replenish glycogen stores, and protein to optimize protein synthesis (particularly in muscle) and healing. The symptoms accompanying overreaching include overall fatigue, muscular fatigue, chronic muscle tenderness and soreness, lack of concentration, and disrupted eating habits or loss of interest in food. **Overtraining** results in a compendium of symptoms referred to as the overtraining syndrome (OTS) (figure 1.6). This condition is more

PUTTING IT INTO PERSPECTIVE

YOU CAN COME BACK FROM DETRAINING

Have you ever worked hard in an exercise program and then, for whatever reason, taken an unexpected long break? Although your body will become detrained during your down time, you can bounce back. For most people, after exercise resumes, physiological gains occur faster than the initial changes did.

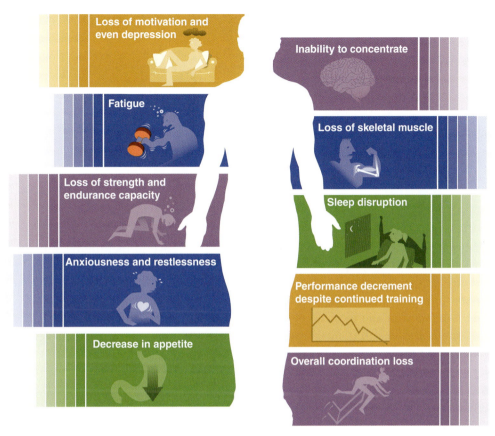

Figure 1.6 Common signs and symptoms characteristic of overtraining syndrome (OTS).

serious than overreaching, often causing long-term performance impairment that takes several weeks or months to recover from. OTS is complex because there are both physiological abnormalities and often psychological challenges stemming from the stress of competition, family and social relationships, and other life demands. There are no set diagnostic criteria for OTS, because symptoms vary from athlete to athlete and are highly individualized. Athletes with suspected OTS should seek medical attention to rule out other confounding conditions and to develop a sound plan for recovery (16, 49).

SPORTS NUTRITION

Exercise physiology is the study of the body's response to exercise, from acute bouts to chronic adaptations with repeated activity and long-term training (32). Nutrition includes the science of the ingestion, digestion, absorption, and metabolism of nutrients and the accompanying physiological and biochemical functions of those nutrients. Sports nutrition integrates exercise physiology and nutrition. Athletes and active people will benefit from adhering to the principles of sound nutrition for optimal health, but they also need to address the appropriate nutrition intake to support training, performance, and recovery from exercise. Nutrition guidelines have been established to support the unique needs of various sports and physical activities (6, 16).

General Principles

The goal for most athletes is to optimize performance in their sport or activity. Training is required for the metabolic adaptations that lead to improved performance, and nutrition strategies are important to providing adequate fuel and nutrients to support training. Sports nutrition strategies encompass food and beverage intake on a regular or daily basis and then specifically before, during, and after competition or activity. **Nutrient absorption** and utilization are also considered. Nutrition goals need to be individualized for each athlete within and between sports. For example, although general carbohydrate guidelines exist for the endurance athlete, the actual

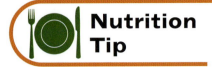

Nutrition Tip: Because nutrition guidelines exist for many sports and training regimens, you might think that athletes must be extremely rigid to achieve success. Although you need adequate fuel and nutrients to support training and recovery from exercise, in some people eating with extreme rigidity can lead to the development of compulsive behaviors or disordered eating patterns. If left unaddressed, such behavior can cause development of an eating disorder, requiring specialized psychological treatment. Varying your food choices and eating patterns, within the nutrition guidelines you are following, should provide a good balance (48, 50).

amounts that should be consumed are far different for a small female athlete versus a large male athlete. In addition, endurance athletes may have different carbohydrate and protein needs than strength athletes. Individualization should also consider the training cycle and goals, food preferences, food intolerances or allergies, blood work if available, diseases and health issues, desire to cook or rely on restaurant food, finances, and any other special needs that help the athlete maintain compliance.

In addition to individualized needs that vary from person to person, sports nutrition guidelines are dynamic and change depending on exercise training cycles. In **nutrition periodization**, nutrition guidelines are adjusted depending on the cycle of training or individual training sessions. For example, nutrition needs will differ depending on whether a person is in training, precompetition, competition, or the off-season. Many protocols for nutrition periodization can be individualized to meet the needs of any athlete. A common periodization program is broken into the same cycles as exercise training: macrocycles, mesocycles, and microcycles. During the off-season, if athletes are not in training, their macronutrient needs will decrease significantly (16).

Optimal body composition for performance is a goal for many athletes. An athlete who wishes to lose body weight or fat should usually do this during the off-season, or very early in training, to avoid any performance declines caused by an energy deficit (16, 48).

Evidence-Based Practice

Most reputable professional organizations related to health care have a code of ethics. Although codes of ethics vary across disciplines, a common element is evidence-based practice. Evidence-based practice requires the use of a systematic process for identifying, assessing, analyzing, and synthesizing the available evidence; using the best evidence in making recommendations; and promoting the use of professional expertise when evidence is weak or lacking. All evidence-based practice is founded on well-established, scientific guidelines and never relies on anecdotal information (50).

Scientific Evidence

In large part because of the media, conflicting information regarding nutrition abounds. When trying to determine if information is accurate and complete, one approach to employ is the scientific method (figure 1.7). The scientific method is a standardized process that scientists and other professionals use to answer research questions. The process begins with an observation of a relation between two or more elements. The scientist (or other professional) then develops a hypothesis, or educated guess, regarding the basis for the observation. The hypothesis is similar to the research question. For instance, hypotheses may be developed based on the effect of a dietary intervention on performance, the effect of a sports supplement on body composition, or a relation between two variables (e.g., is vitamin D deficiency related to bone fracture risk?). After a hypothesis is established, the scientist develops a study design including an appropriate number of subjects to answer the research question with valid statistics, methodology, and statistical control. Data are then collected and analyzed, and decisions, and sometimes conclusions, are made from the experiment. The study design and statistical analyses must be appropriate to answer the research questions, and the experiment must be repeatable for other scientists to see if they obtain similar results. After many repeated experiments demonstrate similar results, a theory can be proposed.

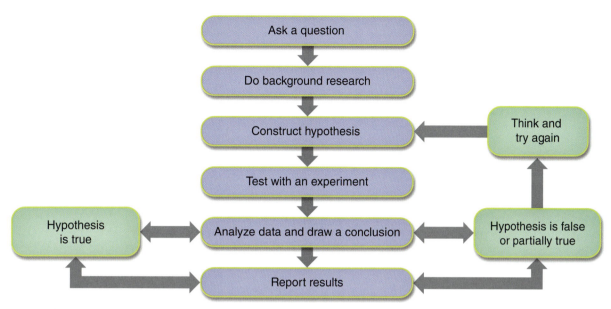

Figure 1.7 The scientific method is a way of ensuring that a standardized process is used when examining scientific evidence and evaluating claims.

DO YOU KNOW?

A crossover study is a type of longitudinal study (people are studied over time rather than at one point in time) in which all study subjects go through each type of treatment. If treatment options are a high-fat diet, moderate-fat diet, or low-fat diet, for instance, each subject rotates through all three diets, adhering to one diet for a set period, followed by a "washout period" during which they are not on any of the treatment diets, before progressing to the next diet.

Reputable Sources of Nutrition Information

In the nutrition world, there is a lot of **quackery**—misleading, unproven, or unsupported information—driven by marketing rather than science and often promoted for the purpose of financial gain. Thus, distinguishing misinformation from sound scientific evidence may be difficult. Several factors should be considered when evaluating a nutrition or dietary supplement claim:

> Who is making the claim or report? What is their training and what credentials do they have? Anyone can claim to be an expert in a subject and publish in popular print or on the Internet (and even credentialed people can misinterpret scientific research).

> Where is the information published? Although quality information can be published in popular outlets, some material offered by these channels is substandard. Popular websites and print publications may have incorrect and misleading information. Scientific evidence is published in peer-reviewed journals. Before publication this research is critiqued by other experts in the field in a blinded manner.

> Is the report based on credible research? Has the research been interpreted correctly? To convince consumers, some websites for dietary supplements cite research that was not conducted on their product or stretch the truth regarding the research on their product.

> Is the report founded on personal observation, testimony, or small, unpublished research findings?

> Are the claims being made too good to be true? Does the report criticize the scientific community? Companies who manufacture "breakthrough" products sometimes criticize scientific experts.

Because of the abundance of available nutrition information, it is important to ensure that sound scientific principles are being considered. Some research studies are difficult to understand, and access to some studies may be limited. Although typing questions into a search engine or skimming

> **PUTTING IT INTO PERSPECTIVE**
>
> ## EVALUATING WEBSITES
>
> The Internet is loaded with nutrition misinformation. Here are some tips to help find credible websites:
>
> - Who is sponsoring the site? Individual people, private companies, nonprofit organizations, or government agencies all create websites. Look for the credentials and training of people who contribute to the content on the site as well as who is sponsoring it. If a food or supplement manufacturer or trade organization is sponsoring the site, the information may be credible but biased. Be sure to evaluate the content carefully.
> - When was the website last updated? The nutrition field is constantly developing, so information should be current.
> - Check the three letters following the "dot" in the web address. Dot gov (.gov) is for a government website, dot edu (.edu) is an educational institution, dot org (.org) is for nonprofit or professional organizations, and dot com (.com) is for commercial and business sites. The first two are usually more reputable (though some dot-edu sites are the personal websites of faculty members, who might have their own agenda or post their own opinions to sound like facts). Dot org may or may not be credible, because these organizations often have sponsors they must please or promote.
> - Does the site distrust credible organizations? Do the authors of the site appear to benefit from financial gain?

through popular magazines or websites is easy, it is worth taking the time to evaluate nutrition claims critically before considering a dietary supplement or diet change.

CREDENTIALS AND SCOPE OF PRACTICE

Credentials and certifications vary tremendously among the professions of nutrition and dietetics and exercise science. Nutrition and dietetics have one uniform credential, recognized by all 50 states in the United States, the registered dietitian nutritionist (RDN) (51) credential, whereas exercise professionals have many different certification options with varying degrees of credibility. Dietitians of Canada is an organization that issues and regulates the profession of nutrition and dietetics in Canada. The credentials may vary slightly by province, but most use the credential registered dietitian (RD). Dietitians in both countries require education and skills to provide proper care for members of the public.

Exercise Science and Fitness Certifications

No single accrediting body governing academic programs in the exercise sciences leads to a nationally recognized practice credential. Titles for exercise professionals—personal trainer, fitness professional, exercise physiologist, and so on—can be used by anyone. Further, the term *certified* can be meaningless, depending on where the certification came from. Some certifications come from reputable exercise and fitness professional organizations; others can be obtained over the Internet. The public can therefore be confused when seeking professional exercise advice. Making matters more confusing, many people who call themselves nutrition experts may have taken a weekend nutrition or nutrition and fitness certification class but have no formal training or education in nutrition. Further, some exercise science degree programs may require one or two nutrition courses, whereas others may have no requirement for nutrition classes. Limited nutrition education does not provide the training and skills necessary to perform an individualized nutrition assessment and intervention, especially for those who have health conditions or diseases.

Not all exercise certifications are equal in curriculum and rigor. Before choosing a certification, the candidate should investigate the expertise of the individuals developing the curriculum, the evidence used, the rigor of the exam, and the continuing education requirements. The area of exercise science is ever evolving, and new research-based information becomes available regularly. Professionals should hold a certification where they will receive credible continuing education for the safety of patients and clients. The American College of Sports Medicine (ACSM) (52), the National Strength and Conditioning Association (NSCA) (53), and the American Council on Exercise (ACE) (54) are examples of leading, reputable exercise certifications that understand the scope of practice of exercise professionals and encourage

SUMMARY OF SOME REPUTABLE EXERCISE CERTIFICATIONS

American College of Sports Medicine (ACSM) (56)

Whether training one on one or instructing groups, these certifications lead to the development and implementation of safe, effective exercise programs and modifications to meet the specific needs of clients.

- Certified Personal Trainer (ACSM-CPT)
- Certified Group Exercise Instructor (ACSM-CEI)
- Certified Exercise Physiologist (ACSM-EP)

A clinical certification leads to being part of the health care team. Clinical exercise physiologists use primary and secondary prevention strategies to improve patient outcomes.

- Certified Clinical Exercise Physiologist (ACSM-CEP)

ACSM provides specialty options as well. These are geared toward practitioners who are dedicated to increasing the inclusiveness and accessibility to exercise for everyone.

- The Exercise Is Medicine Credential
- ACSM/ACS Certified Cancer Exercise Trainer (CET),
- ACSM/NCHPAD Certified Inclusive Fitness Trainer (CIFT)
- ACSM/NPAS Physical Activity in Public Health Specialist (PAPHS)

National Strength and Conditioning Association (NSCA) (57)

These certifications are for exercise professionals who use an individualized or team approach to assess, motivate, educate, and train clients regarding their personal health and fitness or their strength and conditioning needs.

- Certified Personal Trainer (NSCA-CPT)
- Certified Special Population Specialist
- Certified Strength and Conditioning Specialist

American Council on Exercise (ACE) (58)

These certifications help exercise professionals lead clients to sustainable, healthy behavior change by applying knowledge of physical activity and nutrition.

- Personal Trainer Certification
- Group Fitness Instructor Certification
- Health Coach Certification
- Specialty Certifications
  - Mind Body
  - Fitness Nutrition
  - Weight Management

their patrons to discuss nutrition, while staying within that scope. Furthermore, these certifications are evidence based and have curriculums designed by appropriate experts in the field. The National Commission for Certifying Agencies (NCCA) (55) accredits these and other fitness and exercise certifications. The NCCA provides a standardized, independent, and objective third-party evaluation of the certification programs and subsequent examinations (55).

Credentials in Nutrition and Dietetics

The Academy of Nutrition and Dietetics (known simply as the academy) (61) governs the practice credential **registered dietitian nutritionist** (**RD or RDN**, which are interchangeable; we will use RDN in this text). This credential is granted and governed by the Commission on Dietetic Registration (CDR) (51) of the academy. To be eligible to take the National Registration Examination for Dietitians (to obtain the RDN credential) as of January 1, 2024, the candidate must obtain a minimum of a master's degree and complete an ACEND (62)-accredited supervised practice experience that provides at least 1,000 hours of supervised practice experience in various health care and community settings. Additional board certifications beyond the RDN credential (51) include the certified specialist in sports dietetics

REPUTABLE SPORTS NUTRITION ORGANIZATIONS

You might consider spending some time learning about the following organizations to see which interest you most.

> - Sports and Human Performance Nutrition (SHPN) (www.shpndpg.org/home) (59). SHPN is a dietetic practice group of the Academy of Nutrition and Dietetics (3). It is a sound source of sports nutrition information and can be used to find a certified specialist in sports dietetics (CSSD). Although this organization reserves most of its resources for members, it offers links to some publicly available position papers, sports nutrition fact sheets for consumers, and useful websites with sports nutrition–related information. Other resources are available for purchase. SHPN holds an annual symposium where current sports nutrition–related information is presented to attendees.

> - Professionals in Nutrition for Exercise and Sport (PINES) (60). PINES is an international nonprofit organization that promotes sports nutrition practice and research. Associate membership is available to those who hold current employment in a health sciences field that requires ongoing continuing education. Students enrolled in a sports nutrition, sport science, or sports medicine program are also eligible for membership. PINES provides a variety of sports nutrition resources and links to other organizations and documents related to the field.

> - American College of Sports Medicine (ACSM) (52). ACSM is a nonprofit organization providing resource for the exercise sciences as well as sports nutrition. There is a nutrition interest group within ACSM. ACSM offers several levels of membership, from student members to degreed professionals. The organization provides access to information related to sports medicine, position papers, and, for members, journals. ACSM also provides numerous exercise-related certifications.

> - American Council on Exercise (ACE) (54). ACE is a nonprofit organization catering to health coaches and exercise professionals. The organization offers many levels and a variety of certifications. In addition, ACE offer evidence-based nutrition information specifically designed for health professionals who do not hold the RDN credential.

> - National Strength and Conditioning Association (NSCA) (53). The NSCA is a professional membership organization for thousands of strength coaches, personal trainers, and people conducting research and providing education.

(CSSD). The person holding the CSSD credential has specialized experience in sports dietetics. The CSSD translates that information to specific dietary guidance when working with athletes of all levels participating in different sports and activities. The CSSD conducts a thorough nutrition assessment and uses the data to provide safe and effective nutrition interventions aimed at promoting health and optimizing performance (3, 51).

Currently, 48 states, the District of Columbia, and Puerto Rico have enacted statutory provisions regulating the practice of nutrition and dietetics either through state licensure or statutory certification. Two states, Arizona and Michigan, have no licensure of practice of nutrition and dietetics or title. The categories of regulation regarding the practice of nutrition and dietetics in the United States and its territories include the following (63):

> "Practice exclusivity" means that a license is required to practice nutrition and dietetics, which generally encompasses the nutrition care process (64) (nutrition assessment, nutrition diagnosis, nutrition intervention, and nutrition monitoring and evaluation). Medical nutrition therapy (MNT) is part of the intervention step.

> "Licensure of title only or certification of RDNs" means that the state holds a license over the title "licensed dietitian" (or a similar title) or provides an optional certification if required by a health care employer. In these states, a board exists to enforce the law, but no license is required to practice MNT or dietetics.

> "Title protection without formal state regulation" means that the state restricts use of the title only. In other words, you cannot call yourself an RDN or dietitian of any kind, but no board exists, and no license is required to use the title.

The states with practice exclusivity require RDNs be licensed to practice nutrition and dietetics where the scope of practice of the RDN is defined by each state. In these cases, violating the state licensure law is a criminal offense, subject to misdemeanor or felony penalties ranging from a cease-and-desist order to fines and imprisonment. Because nutrition and dietetics is regulated at the level of the state and state statutes can change with time, the practitioner needs to understand the regulations where they live and practice. The Academy of Nutrition and Dietetics provides current information for each state and territory, so checking for updates regularly is important (61, 63).

Some people might hold a master's or doctoral degree in nutrition but might not hold the credential RDN. Depending on the state, these individuals may not be able to practice dietetics (e.g., complete a nutrition assessment, an intervention, or a provision of medical nutrition therapy). They may, however, have extensive training in nutrition sciences and can be a reliable resource for sound nutrition information (65).

Scope of Practice

State licensure supersedes both registration and certification. Thus, in states with licensure, only those with a license can practice nutrition and dietetics. Does this mean that only RDNs can provide education? The answer is no. Other health, fitness, and wellness professionals may discuss nutrition as long as it is general, nonmedical nutrition information. For instance, these people may say, "Dietary fiber is important for gut health and promoting regular bowel movements." This

---

PUTTING IT INTO PERSPECTIVE

CERTIFICATES AND CERTIFICATIONS

Many organizations offer certificates of training or a certification related to nutrition. Earning a certificate usually means that a person attended and completed a course (in person or online). The course could be a single class or a series of educational sessions. Certificates usually do not expire and do not require continuing education. A certification also involves attending and completing a program of study but usually requires recertification with continuing education. The quality of these can vary tremendously and may or may not provide credible information. If you live in a state that licenses the nutrition and dietetics profession, be aware that licensure trumps any certificates or certifications related to nutrition (61, 63, 65).

> **REFLECTION TIME**
>
> ## NUTRITION PROFESSIONALS WHO WORK WITH ATHLETES
>
> Are you interested in a profession in which you will work with athletes? A certified specialist in sports dietetics (CSSD) is a specialty credential that can be earned by RDNs. People holding the CSSD credential have specialized knowledge in performance nutrition. In addition to providing general sports nutrition guidelines, the CSSD can provide individualized nutrition plans for optimizing performance and, as an RDN, can work with athletes who have (or might have) a disease or nutrition-related condition. This credential can be earned after an RDN has at least 1,500 practice hours in sports dietetics. For more information on earning this credential, visit the Sports and Human Performance Nutrition website (www.shpndpg.org/home) (3).

statement is an example of general nutrition information. Education should be directed only to healthy people and should be based on sound scientific nutrition principles. Conducting a nutrition assessment and providing a nutrition intervention is considered dietetics, and licensure is required for this activity in certain states. Further, if working with a person with a disease or a health-related condition, the assessment of nutrition status and any nutrition intervention is considered medical nutrition therapy and should be reserved for the RDN (63, 66).

General, nonmedical nutrition therapy includes any public guidance systems such as *2020-2025 Dietary Guidelines* (19), food labels as guided by the FDA (20, 21), the DRIs (4), and interactive systems such as MyPlate (23). Topics may also include the functions of nutrients in the body and principles of healthy food preparation. For a more detailed list, refer to table 1.1. Providing nutrition education within the scope of practice and taking actions that are permitted by the professional license are encouraged and beneficial to the public. Professionals should understand the laws

Table 1.1 Samples of General, Nonmedical Nutrition Information

Nutrition principle	Example application of the principle
Principles of healthy food preparation	Baking fish or chicken is healthier than batter dipping and deep frying.
Foods to be included in the normal daily diet of healthy people	Fruits, vegetables, quality grains, lean proteins, low-fat dairy, and healthy fats are all part of a healthy, balanced diet.
The functions of nutrients in the body	Carbohydrate is a fuel source for skeletal muscle and organs; iron is a component of hemoglobin.
Recommended amounts of the essential nutrients (DRIs) for healthy people	Share the USDA DRI tables.
The effects of deficiencies or excesses of nutrients	Excess energy leads to obesity; iron deficiency leads to the medical condition iron-deficiency anemia.
Food sources of essential nutrients	Orange juice is an excellent source of vitamin C; whole grains contain dietary fiber.
Providing information about food guidance systems (e.g., *Dietary Guidelines*, food labels, and MyPlate)	Showing the actual food label or MyPlate system.
The basic roles of carbohydrates, proteins, fats, vitamins, minerals, water	Protein is important for tissue growth and repair; calcium is an important mineral for bone health; water plays an important role in body temperature regulation.
Giving statistical information about the relationship between chronic disease and the excesses or deficiencies of certain nutrients	Obesity is a leading cause of type 2 diabetes mellitus.
Proper hydration in healthy individuals	Use the current position stand on this topic (16).

where they live and their own level of nutrition knowledge and skills before they communicate information to the public (63, 65).

SUMMARY

Nutrition is a scientific discipline that examines how food and nutrients affect physiological functioning and health. The science of nutrition is rapidly evolving, and new information is published regularly. These scientific findings are translated into the nutrition guidelines that are used to determine which foods and nutrients to consume for health. The energy-yielding macronutrients—carbohydrate, fat, and protein—play a significant role in fueling, and in the case of protein, repairing the body. The micronutrients—vitamins and minerals—have numerous roles in physiological functions within the body. Water is an essential macronutrient for survival and is critical for several physiological processes, including regulation of body temperature. The nutrients work together to keep the body systems running smoothly.

Look for evidence-based nutrition guidelines; these have been compiled and designed to translate the science into food and nutrient choices for all individuals. Food labels, DRIs, and MyPlate are some of the food guidance systems that can be used for healthy people of all ages. Although these systems and tools are not specifically designed for athletes, they can be useful when making food choices based on a desired nutrient content.

Physical activity and health are strongly related. Athletes usually exceed the general physical activity guidelines because training is essential for performance in their activity or sport. Athletes must understand the basic principles of training that can lead to the physical gains they need for effective performance in their sport. Although adequate training is required for sport performance, overtraining can disrupt normal physiological function and impair performance.

Sports nutrition is a relatively young subdiscipline that integrates the disciplines of nutrition sciences and exercise physiology. It is a dynamic field in which new research is constantly evolving. Many of the principles of nutrition for health promotion and disease prevention apply to all athletes and active people. Defined guidelines, however, have been set for various nutrients that are sport and activity specific. Nutrition and sports nutrition are disciplines surrounded by a lot of misinformation and quackery, so sound scientific information must be identified before decisions are made and implemented. Nutrition and dietetics are regulated in many states; those who provide nutrition education must take care to do so within their scope of practice.

FOR REVIEW

1. What is the percent of daily value, and why is it used?
2. Explain the difference between a nutrient content claim and health claim.
3. What are the general physical activity guidelines for adults for both aerobic training and resistance training?
4. List the factors that influence body composition.
5. Describe the differences between overreaching and overtraining.
6. How do you go about finding accurate nutrition information?
7. Should athletes follow the DRIs and MyPlate? Why or why not?
8. List the benefits associated with regular exercise.

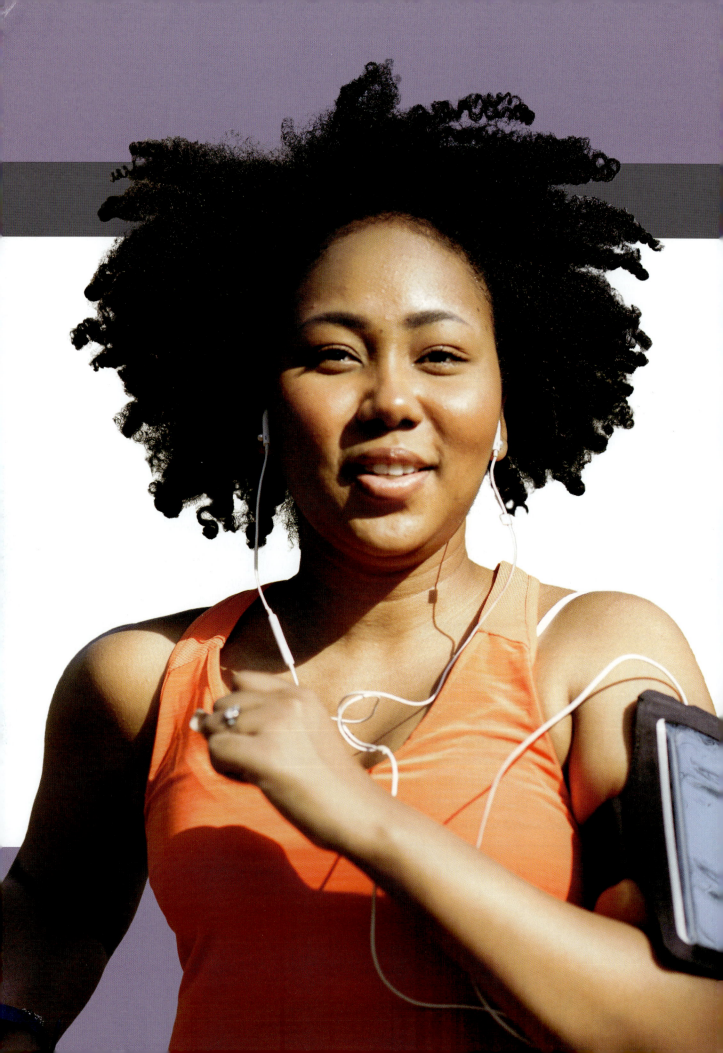

Energy Metabolism

> **CHAPTER OBJECTIVES**
>
> After completing this chapter, you will be able to do the following:
> - Summarize the principles of energy metabolism and the production of ATP.
> - Describe how energy expenditure is measured and estimated.
> - Identify the energy systems.
> - Explain which fuels are used in the different energy systems.
> - Explain why the fuels used in energy metabolism are used during different exercise intensities.
> - Discuss other metabolic systems: gluconeogenesis, Cori cycle, glucose-alanine cycle.
> - Describe how energy content of food is measured.

Appropriate energy (calorie) intake is the cornerstone of the athlete's diet. Proper energy intake supports optimal body functioning, determines the capacity for intake of macro- and micronutrients, and assists in manipulating body composition. Fortunately, the human body works hard as an efficient factory by transferring the chemical energy derived from food through digestion, absorption, and metabolism to generate power that fuels muscle contraction. The body can also use this chemical energy to synthesize new products in the body, such as chemical messengers or structural proteins (including muscle), to direct some energy for storage in glycogen and fat tissue, and to help discard waste. Muscle uses a significant amount of energy. The metabolic factory analogy of energy metabolism in muscle tissue includes the cellular enzymes, organelles, and metabolic pathways responsible for converting and using chemical energy to support muscle contraction. The muscle metabolic factory is always on. The body relies on these metabolic pathways to maintain healthy muscle function. Depending on whether chemical energy from food is either scarce or plentiful and if muscle is active or at rest, different metabolic pathways in the muscle may take center stage.

HOW ENERGY FUELS THE BODY

Collectively, the use of energy for bodily processes, including all chemical changes, is known as **metabolism**. Metabolic processes involving thousands of chemical reactions can be further categorized as anabolism and catabolism. **Anabolism**, sometimes referred to as "growth," involves metabolic processes that use energy to synthesize building blocks to produce new molecules. **Catabolism** is characterized by the breakdown of molecules to generate usable energy or to break down molecules to create building blocks for anabolism. Catabolism is often referred to as "breakdown."

> **? DO YOU KNOW?**
>
> Although all cell types in the human body require energy to function, the most active metabolic sites in the body during physical activity include muscle and liver cells, which use fuel derived from energy-yielding macronutrients (carbohydrate, protein, and fat).

The phrase *metabolic pathway* describes a series of chemical reactions that can result in catabolic or anabolic outcomes. These metabolic pathways are never completely inactive and constantly adapt to external stimuli that the body experiences (figure 2.1). For example, let's say someone schedules a challenging workout with friends before afternoon classes. On these days, the carbohydrate consumed for lunch is broken down into glucose units. The muscle cells can further catabolize (break down) these glucose units in metabolic pathways occurring in the **cytosol** and **mitochondria** of the cell to produce **adenosine triphosphate (ATP)** to fuel muscle contraction. After the workout is over and the group is sitting in class eating bananas as a recovery snack, their bodies take the carbohydrate consumed and make glycogen, the storage form of carbohydrate in skeletal muscle and the liver.

The law of energy conservation states that energy can be neither created nor destroyed; rather, it transforms from one form to another. The total amount of energy in the universe is constant. Although it can change from one form to another and can move from one location to another, the system never gains or loses energy. The conservation of energy law is a principle component of the first law of thermodynamics. So how does this apply to the human body? Where does the energy come from to power the body? Although the universe includes several forms of energy, including heat, mechanical, and electrical, it is the **chemical energy** derived from food that fuels the body. This form of energy is essential to human life and is responsible for much more than skeletal muscle work. Chemical energy provides energy needs for many processes, including breathing, pumping blood, maintaining body temperature, delivering oxygen to tissues, removing waste products, synthesizing new tissue for growth or adaptation to exercise and stress, and repairing damaged or worn-out tissues. Energy demands never cease and continue even when you are sleeping. When awake, the body needs energy not only to support the aforementioned processes but also to support physical movement as well as digestion and absorption of food.

Chemical energy is derived from the molecular bonds that make up carbohydrate, fat, and protein that are consumed or broken down (catabolized) from stored forms of these nutrients in our body

Energy Metabolism   27

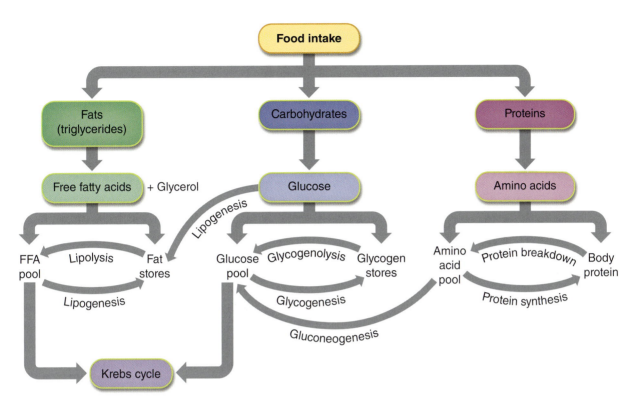

Figure 2.1 Metabolic pathways. Food intake sparks anabolism through the various biosynthetic pathways.

Reprinted by permission from L.W. Kenney, J.H. Wilmore, and D.L. Costill, *Physiology of Sport and Exercise*, 6th ed. (Champaign, IL: Human Kinetics, 2015), 51.

(glycogen, fat tissue, and skeletal muscle—although skeletal muscle is dense with protein, as mentioned in chapter 1, it isn't intended to serve as a backup source of amino acids). As discussed in chapter 5, energy can also be derived from the breakdown of alcohol. The next step in the process is for our bodies to harness and transfer this energy from food into cellular energy to perform physiological tasks. We extract energy from food in three stages. Stage 1 is digestion, absorption, and transportation of energy-yielding nutrients, which are simple sugars from carbohydrate, amino acids from protein, **fatty acids** from lipids, and alcohol. Stage 2 consists of a more in-depth breakdown of small food-derived molecules to key energy-producing metabolites. For example, the simple sugar glucose derived from carbohydrate foods can be converted to the metabolite pyruvate. Two three-carbon pyruvate metabolites are formed from the breakdown of one six-carbon glucose molecule. These important molecules serve as metabolic intermediates. This process of breaking down glucose to pyruvate releases usable energy for the body to harness but, more important, serves as a precursor for the final stage. During stage 3, the body's cells can use energy-producing metabolites (such as **acetyl-CoA** derived from pyruvate) to completely break down ("burn") these compounds to a converted form of energy that the body can use. Although this process releases some energy as heat, unfortunately, the human body is not good at using heat to power cellular functions. Instead, cells transfer this energy into ATP as the form of chemical energy that the body can use. This transfer of energy is not entirely efficient, and a significant portion of the food energy consumed is lost as heat (1). But the energy we use from food and the energy we store in glycogen and fat tissue allows the continuous synthesis of ATP from energy stores that are comparable to an energy bank account, where energy consumed from food can be used as needed and the leftover excess can be saved for future use.

? DO YOU KNOW?

In survival situations, such as when stranded, food consumption, particularly protein, helps the body stay warm because of the metabolic production of heat. During digestion, protein produces more heat than either carbohydrate or fat.

HUMAN ENERGY METABOLISM

To fully comprehend and appreciate how our bodies use and transfer energy into ATP, we need to understand the centers within the cells that do the work. Although the body is made up of many types of cells, the cells share many of the same basic structures to facilitate metabolism. The two major compartments of the cell are its **cytoplasm** and **nucleus**. The cytoplasm is enclosed within the cell membrane and consists of a semifluid called cytosol. This cytosol is the site of a catabolic process known as **glycolysis** and anabolic processes such as fatty acid synthesis and glycogen synthesis. Also found within the cytoplasm are tiny, specialized factories, known as **organelles**, which have unique metabolic functions. When discussing energy, arguably the most important organelle is known as the **mitochondria**, the powerhouse of the cell (figure 2.2). Liver, brain, kidney, and muscle cells all have similar organelle structure and multiple mitochondria. This is because several metabolic pathways exist in this organelle, and it is the final stop in the energy-transfer journey, where in the presence of oxygen, metabolites originating from carbohydrate, protein, fat, and alcohol produce ATP, carbon dioxide, and small amounts of water. The structure of the mitochondrion consists of two highly specialized membranes: an outer membrane and a highly folded inner membrane that surrounds the mitochondrial matrix. In conjunction with important metabolic processes that occur in the cytoplasm, key metabolic pathways occur in specific locations within the mitochondrion. In the matrix, the **tricarboxylic acid cycle (TCA cycle)**, also known as the Krebs cycle or the citric acid cycle, can accept various metabolites that enter from the cytosol as pyruvate, fatty acids, and amino acids. This process is illustrated in figure 2.3. The catabolism of acetyl-CoA in the TCA cycle breaks carbon bonds through a process known as **oxidative decarboxylation** and produces free electrons that bind with coenzymes, which carry the electrons to the **electron transport chain (ETC)**. The ETC is made up of a series of complex protein channels that accept the electrons from the coenzymes. This process harnesses energy to fuel the final step in ATP formation, known as **oxidative phosphorylation (OP)**. ATP is often called the molecular unit of currency for our bodies to perform work. ATP is the fundamental

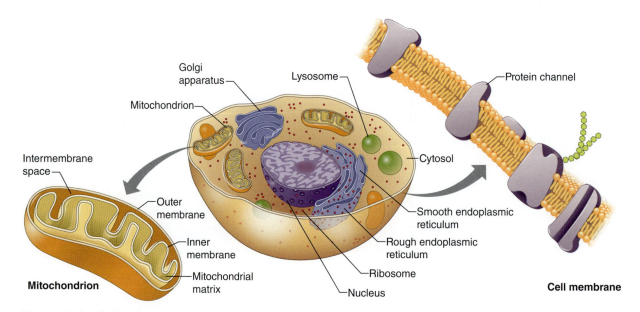

Figure 2.2 Cell structure and organelles necessary for ATP production.

Energy Metabolism 29

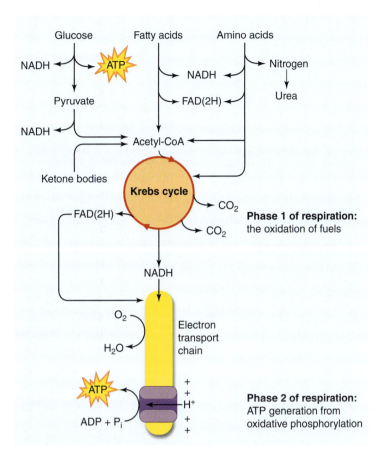

Figure 2.3 Metabolic phases of respiration necessary to produce ATP.

energy molecule to power cellular functions. To make ATP, catalytic enzymes play key roles in the cell by speeding up chemical reactions in the ATP biosynthesis pathway. These enzymes bind with smaller molecules called coenzymes. The coenzyme molecules nicotinamide adenine dinucleotide (NAD⁺) and flavin adenine dinucleotide (**FADH$_2$**), serve as important couriers that carry liberated electrons as a form of energy from fuel catabolism to the ETC for the synthesis of ATP. When breaking down energy-producing nutrients with oxidative decarboxylation, carbohydrate, fat, and protein, the carbon chains are broken by catabolic enzymes. This process frees high-energy electrons that must be harnessed to reach the site of ATP production, the ETC. To do this, these electrons ride on special electron acceptor molecules NAD⁺ and FAD. These molecules are derivatives of the B vitamins niacin and riboflavin, respectively, and have several energy-transfer points where NAD⁺ and FAD accept two high-energy electrons and two protons (2H⁺) to form the reduced coenzymes NADH and FADH$_2$.

PUTTING IT INTO PERSPECTIVE

LEO THE LION SAYS, "GER"

During the synthesis of ATP, electrons are transferred when carbon-carbon bonds are split during the formation of pyruvate, acetyl-CoA, and metabolites found within the TCA cycle. A mnemonic can help you remember the process of electron movement and molecule charge. When a molecule Loses an Electron, the molecule is Oxidized (LEO); when a molecule Gains an Electron, the molecule is Reduced (GER).

Energy Metabolism: Transforming Energy to a Usable Form in the Body

The use of ATP in the body is constant and never-ending—it exists if life exists. ATP also powers energy-consuming processes, such as making new glucose for the body when a meal is missed. ATP's role in biosynthesis is synonymous with building construction. To make larger molecules from smaller molecules, energy is required to form the chemical bonds as well as the physical structure, just as construction workers are necessary to lay the bricks of a new building foundation.

The production of ATP is the fundamental goal of energy-producing pathways in metabolism. The ATP molecule has three phosphate groups attached to the organic molecule adenosine. When the phosphate bonds break, a tremendous amount of energy is released, and cells can use this to power biological work. When the first phosphate-adenosine bond breaks from ATP, the reaction leaves the still energy-rich compound **adenosine diphosphate (ADP)** and a free molecule of **pyrophosphate**, inorganic phosphate (P_i). Breaking the remaining phosphate bond releases a lesser amount of energy and breaks down ADP to **adenosine monophosphate (AMP)** and P_i. Under normal conditions, concentrations of AMP are very low in the cell, as ADP is constantly re-phosphorylated into ATP. As energy demands rise, however, physiological processes increasingly rely on conversion from ADP to AMP, although this process is less energy efficient. As seen in figure 2.4, AMP is interconvertible with both ADP and ATP, and because it contains only one phosphate, it does not contain any high-energy phosphate-to-phosphate bonds. These reactions are considered interconvertible because P_i can break free from adenosine to release energy or can be bound to adenosine from the extraction of energy from carbohydrate, protein, and fat. This process most commonly occurs with ADP binding with P_i, forming a phosphate bond and capturing energy in a new ATP molecule. Because energy is required, the reaction then goes in the opposite direction, breaking the phosphate bond and liberating energy while re-forming ADP. This energy is used to power activities such as muscle contraction, transporting substances across cell membranes, making new molecules, and jump-starting other biological pathways. ATP is not considered an energy-storage molecule; in fact, the body's pool of ATP is a very small (about 100 g),

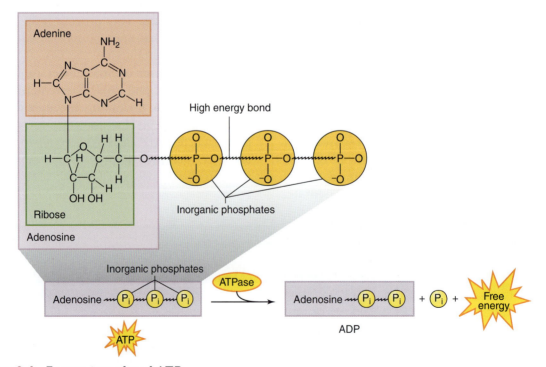

Figure 2.4 Energy transfer of ATP.

immediately accessible energy reservoir capable of providing energy for only a few seconds. ATP production rate is directly related to muscle mass and the changing energy demands of the body. For example, at rest, the body breaks down approximately 90 pounds (40 kg) of ATP over 24 hours. At the immediate onset of strenuous exercise or physical activity, however, it is possible to break down over a pound (0.45 kg) of ATP per minute, while the production of ATP skyrockets to keep up with the energy demand of quickly contracting muscles.

Energy Systems Used by the Human Body

Before discussing the specifics of ATP production and how each energy-yielding macronutrient is used to generate ATP using both unique and commonly used metabolic pathways, it is helpful to categorize ATP production from a systems approach. This approach not only aids in understanding the integrated nature of ATP production but also helps with real-life application of how different systems are used to meet our ever-changing ATP demand. As discussed earlier, the body readily uses carbohydrate and fat from the diet or from body stores to make ATP. Protein also contributes but to a much lower extent. In energy metabolism, carbohydrate, fat, and protein are all considered biological substrates. A substrate is a molecule upon which an enzyme acts to create different metabolite products along its journey to make ATP. Although carbohydrate, fat, and protein are the three major fuel substrates, there is a fourth called **phosphocreatine (PCr)**. You may have heard of a similar compound in the gym as a popular dietary supplement called creatine (much more on supplements in chapter 9).

In muscle tissue, phosphocreatine can be split into a creatine component and a phosphate (P_i) component. It is the presence of this additional P_i from the phosphocreatine compound that can be used to resynthesize ADP into ATP. This general process describes the **phosphagen system (ATP-PC system)**. This system uses exclusively phosphocreatine to regenerate ATP in muscle tissue. In addition to the phosphagen system, the body has two other energy systems that use energy-yielding macronutrients to make ATP. These energy systems are known as the **anaerobic system** and the **aerobic system**. Each of these energy systems can be described by the complexity of their metabolic pathways, rate or speed of ATP production, capacity to produce ATP, and the lag time required to contribute significant amounts of ATP when ATP is in increased demand. The relative significance and contribution of each energy system to ATP production in various exercise or sporting activities is described in table 2.1 and figure 2.5. In brief, the phosphagen system uses small stores of ATP and PC to support short bursts of energy, the anaerobic system burns only carbohydrate and produces lactic acid for bouts of exercise up to a couple minutes, and the aerobic system uses a variety of substrates in conjunction with oxygen to support exercise lasting tens of minutes to many hours. At any given point in time, ATP is being produced by these energy systems to some degree, even if only in a minute amount. No energy system is *ever* turned off. Figure 2.5 illustrates the constant change in the relative proportion of ATP produced from different body tissues at any one point in time. In the world of exercise and sport, we think about how these energy systems are integrated in muscle tissue to produce ATP along a wide spectrum of intensity, ranging from sleep,

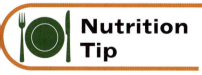

Nutrition Tip

About half of the creatine in our bodies is from the consumption of meat and fish. The other half is made from amino acids in the liver, kidney, and pancreas. Taken together, depending on how much meat and fish is consumed, these processes can account for roughly 1 to 3 grams of creatine per day that can be converted into phosphocreatine to store in our muscle to help with ATP generation. Vegetarians, including vegans, who do not consume creatine supplements have been shown to have lower muscle stores of phosphocreatine than their meat-eating or supplementing peers (2) and may have a compromised ability to generate ATP when high-intensity, short-duration efforts are important for competition.

Table 2.1 Relative Significance of Each Energy System to ATP Production

	Phosphagen	Anaerobic	Aerobic
Neighborhood walk	Tertiary	Secondary	Primary
100-yard (meter) sprint	Primary	Secondary	Tertiary
Soccer game	Tertiary	Primary	Primary
Marathon	Tertiary	Secondary	Primary

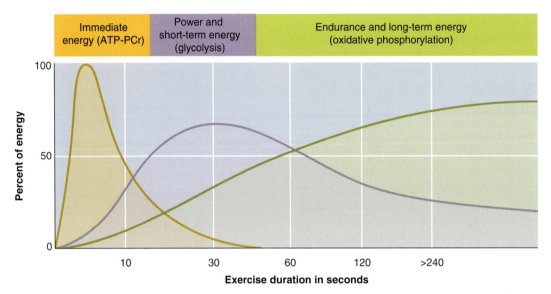

Figure 2.5 The three systems of energy transfer and the percentage contribution to total energy output during all-out exercise of different durations.

to playing sedentary video games, to steady-state exercise, to high-intensity, stop-and-go sports.

Before exploring each energy system in detail, let's review the chemical energy sources that can be used by the three energy systems to produce ATP. As mentioned, phosphocreatine is specific to the phosphagen system. The carbohydrate family contributes serum glucose, also known as blood sugar, liver glycogen, and muscle glycogen. Fat contributes serum-free fatty acids (FFAs), serum triglycerides (TG), muscle TG, and adipose TG. Finally, protein contributes muscle protein, mostly in small amounts. If we think about each of these sources of stored energy as total calories available to the body to burn, stored adipose TG have the highest caloric value, theoretically providing tens of thousands of calories, followed by muscle protein at no more than half of the calories that could potentially be supplied by **adipose tissue** (fat tissue).

> **? DO YOU KNOW?**
>
> We certainly do not want to make a habit of digging into our muscle tissue (protein) to supply our energy needs, because that process can decrease muscle mass and strength. Fortunately, stored fat tissue and any available carbohydrate largely meet the body's energy demands.

Although it might seem that we have near endless amounts of stored energy in our body to use for exercise and sport, several variables come into play that limit our ability to access this energy. Some barriers relate to the practical aspects of exercise, when the onset of fatigue limits the ability to continue exercise, which, in turn, limits the ability to use stored energy. Other variables involve limitations of the energy systems to produce ATP because they have reached their capacity to make it. With regard to stored lipid in the body, the amount of energy derived from fat stores to support exercise or training is a small fraction of the thousands of calories of stored energy in adipose, making it evident that we cannot completely exhaust this stored fuel source. Further, of the described energy-yielding macronutrients found in the body that are fed into the energy systems for ATP production, a key point is that the anaerobic system can use only carbohydrate. In contrast, the aerobic system can use and completely break down all energy-yielding macronutrient fuel sources. Although on the surface it seems that the aerobic system should pick up the slack to tap into our stored fuel sources, it is not that simple. Consistent with all energy systems, the aerobic system also faces barriers to producing ATP. The most significant of these barriers is oxygen availability. Without adequate oxygen delivery to the muscle, ATP production through the aerobic system is severely compromised. Unless other energy systems step up to meet ATP needs, exercise cannot continue.

Phosphagen System

The phosphagen system relies only on the P_i that is liberated from phosphocreatine to produce ATP, so by nature it is not a highly complex energy system (figure 2.6). The minimal lag time and the rapid rate of ATP production are this system's most impressive attributes. The rate of ATP generation is the fastest of all energy systems. Because it is such a simple chemical reaction (not defined as a metabolic pathway), ATP is produced virtually instantaneously. Despite these impressive characteristics, this system's capacity to produce ATP is severely limited by the amount of phosphocreatine substrate found in muscle tissue. This energy system can produce significant amounts of ATP for no longer than a few seconds.

The precise number of seconds of significant ATP production depends on phosphocreatine concentrations in the muscle tissue and the intensity of the physical movement or exercise required that will have a direct effect on ATP demand. Maximal physical efforts tap into this energy system, immediately stimulating the simple metabolic reaction to occur continuously until phosphocreatine substrate is depleted in the engaged muscle groups. The best examples of this energy system at play are when you must move your body or another heavy object quickly. "Heavy" implies a certain level of elevated intensity that produces an immediate, exponential increase in ATP demand that can be met with the phosphagen system. These examples are clearly different from, say, moving your hand quickly from the keyboard to the computer mouse, an exertion for which negligible ATP is required. In athletes, heavy weightlifting and sprinting are examples of activities requiring an increase in rate of ATP production. Although the phosphagen system in these examples can certainly affect performance, any athlete who must give an all-out effort by intensely moving an object or their body relies on the phosphagen system until phosphocreatine is depleted. This can be for the duration of the event (if only seconds in duration) or, if intensity decreases, can serve as a bridge until other energy systems can help out and pick up the slack.

> **? DO YOU KNOW?**
>
> As you move abruptly out of your chair after class to hurry to your next class, the ATP you require to move quickly comes primarily from the phosphagen system. Now consider which athletes rely most on the phosphagen system. Maneuvers by offensive and defensive linemen in American football, field events in track, and sprint swimming all depend primarily on this energy system, but remember that all energy systems are always active in muscle tissue somewhere and are never turned off completely.

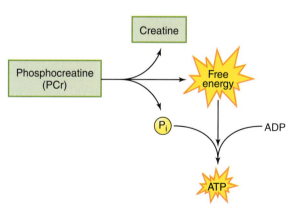

Figure 2.6 The phosphagen system.

CREATINE SUPPLEMENTATION: POINTS TO PONDER

Many athletes consume a dietary supplement containing phosphocreatine to gain strength and muscle mass. This strategy can be effective for some when it is combined with a well-rounded diet and exercise plan. Creatine supplementation effectiveness is related to many mechanisms including the bolstering of phosphocreatine concentrations in muscle that create a larger P_i pool, which takes a longer time to be depleted in short-lived, high-intensity efforts. Supplementation of creatine (usually 3 to 20 g per day) is much higher than what is naturally synthesized by the body and consumed in the diet. For many people in an exercise program that engages the phosphagen system, creatine supplementation can augment this system to allow athletes to lift slightly heavier weights and complete more repetitions of an exercise. This process helps create more contractile protein breakdown to stimulate the muscle to grow larger and become stronger. Although this approach sounds great and in many cases is effective in helping athletes meet strength goals, there are caveats. For instance, not everyone responds to creatine supplements (a nonresponder is a person who doesn't benefit from the supplement), and dietary supplement manufacturers are not required to prove safety to the U.S. Food and Drug Administration (FDA), meaning that the product is not guaranteed to have the amount of creatine listed on the label or to be safe and free from banned substances. Still, many dietary supplement companies ensure a greater level of safety.

Despite anecdotal reports, most available evidence suggests that creatine consumption for up to 5 consecutive years in healthy people is safe (3-5). In fact, many studies continue to examine the health benefits of creatine supplementation in cardiovascular disease, Parkinson's disease, and in patients who experienced mild traumatic brain injury (concussion). Although interest in creatine use and its growing safety profile is expanding, we should all stay up to date on studies on creatine, particularly its use by adult athletes with disease processes or conditions in which creatine may be contraindicated, and its use by young adults and preadolescents. Although creatine use in young athletes is not recommended by the American Academy of Pediatrics (6), the International Society of Sports Nutrition provides prudent guidelines for adolescent use (5). For further discussion of creatine, see chapter 9.

Anaerobic System

The anaerobic system is much more complex than the phosphagen system. This system features a 12-step process known as glycolysis. The rate of ATP production in the anaerobic system is fast and runs a close second to the phosphagen system. The speed of the anaerobic system allows it to be ready to receive the handoff from the phosphagen system as the primary ATP producer when all-out exercise efforts continue beyond 10 seconds. A great example of this occurs in the 200-meter sprint. Within seconds of exploding off the starting block, phosphocreatine stores rapidly plummet in the leg muscles, while the anaerobic system begins to skyrocket its ATP production. Although ATP production in the anaerobic system lags seconds behind ATP production in the phosphagen system, the capacity of this system to make ATP is significantly greater because more substrate, in the form of carbohydrate, is available. Still, in this aspect, the anaerobic system is limited when compared with the aerobic system.

Glycolysis, a key metabolic pathway, occurs in the cytoplasm of the cell and is associated with both the anaerobic and aerobic energy systems. Glycolysis takes a six-carbon molecule of glucose and breaks it down into two three-carbon molecules of pyruvate along with electron carriers NAD^+H and $FADH_2$. Glycolysis ends with the synthesis of pyruvate and the production of a minimal amount of ATP. Although aerobic glycolysis utilizes oxygen, anaerobic glycolysis takes place without adequate oxygen delivery to the mitochondria. This process results in a large portion of pyruvate being converted to **lactic acid**, also known as **lactate** (the chemical suffix *–ate* means "acid"). Alternatively, if oxygen is present, pyruvate is metabolized in other metabolic pathways involving the aerobic energy system in the mitochondria to produce more ATP.

In the anaerobic system, two molecules of lactic acid form from the oxidation (donating electrons) of pyruvate. The basic reason for this is that, in an anaerobic environment, the participation of mitochondria in ATP production is drastically reduced, so calling exercise "anaerobic" or "without oxygen" is about the same as saying "without mitochondria." In this example, then, anaerobic glycolysis is the only efficient way to make ATP to fuel intense muscle contractions, and for this energy system to be self-functioning, it must also produce lactic acid from pyruvate through the acceptance of hydrogen ions (H+). The NADH that is also produced from glycolysis (a carrier of H+) is oxidized and recycled to NAD+ through the enzyme **lactate dehydrogenase (LDH)**. This process allows for the continuous breakdown of glucose to pyruvate to make ATP.

LDH accomplishes this process by recycling NAD+ from NADH to allow the anaerobic system to continue. At high concentrations of lactate (the conjugate base of lactic acid after the H+ is donated), LDH exhibits **feedback inhibition**, and the rate of conversion of pyruvate to lactic acid is decreased. The eventual fate of cytosolic NADH that has not yet donated its H+ ultimately depends on mitochondrial oxygen availability. If oxygen is limited, NADH is oxidized by LDH, and LDH then reduces (donates electrons) to pyruvate to form lactic acid. If mitochondrial oxygen is adequate, NADH is able to be shuttled to the ETC within the mitochondria for the aerobic energy system to proceed. See figure 2.7 for a summary of the basic processes of the anaerobic energy system.

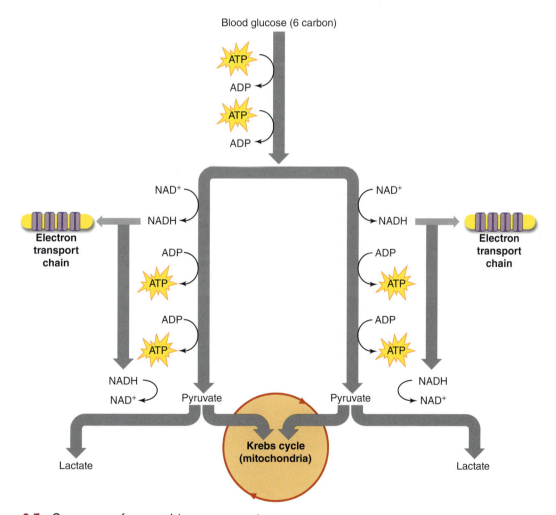

Figure 2.7 Summary of anaerobic energy system.

Reprinted by permission from T.J. Herda and J.T. Cramer, "Bioenergetics of Exercise and Training," in *Essentials of Strength Training and Conditioning*, 4th ed., edited for the National Strength and Conditioning Association by G.G. Haff and N.T. Triplett (Champaign, IL; Human Kinetics, 2015), 47.

The muscle oxygen deficit associated with the anaerobic energy system that leads to this cascade of events does not imply that someone is holding their breath to limit oxygen consumption. Instead, it means that oxygen *uptake and delivery* to the active muscle cell with high ATP demands is compromised to some degree. In the highly trained sprint athlete, this diminution occurs in a 100-meter or 200-meter running event. The ATP demand at maximal physical exertion to move the body at competitive speeds is so great that it is not physiologically possible to deliver enough oxygen by increasing respiration rate. After oxygen is consumed through inhalation, it still must be processed by the lungs and delivered to the active muscle cell by the end of the race. This process is not feasible, so the anaerobic system is in place to meet ATP needs where the phosphagen system left off. For a sedentary person just starting a running program, the anaerobic energy system is also important because oxygen insufficiency in untrained muscle is much more prevalent, even during low-intensity exercise, than in a trained athlete. As the sedentary person begins running the first mile on the first training day, the phosphagen system is immediately activated. Quickly thereafter the anaerobic energy system starts up or, to some degree, the aerobic system may launch, depending on oxygen availability in the mitochondria. If this formerly sedentary individual continues to push to maintain a running pace faster than they are used to, they will have to rely heavily on the anaerobic system. Although the anaerobic energy system is extremely important for supporting the energy needs of high-intensity efforts, it is limited by the hydrogen ions it produces that lower the pH, increasing the acidity of the muscle tissue. This factor contributes to muscular fatigue. The anaerobic energy system is also limited by substrate availability, because carbohydrate is the only substrate that this system can used. Over time, with repeated training, muscles can make physiological adaptations to improve the buffering mechanisms that can limit the drop in tissue pH caused by hydrogen ions. Other physiological adaptations include improved muscle handling of lactic acid, improvements in the capacity of the phosphagen system, and many mechanisms associated with improved oxygen delivery to working muscle. Arguably the most important physiological adaptation resulting from intense anaerobic training is the increased capacity for the muscle to store and use carbohydrate in the anaerobic energy system. Because carbohydrate is the only fuel source that can be used when training and competing at the highest intensity (90%–100% of $\dot{V}O_2$max, resulting in an anaerobic muscle environment), adequate carbohydrate consumption is vital to optimal high-intensity performance. If a suboptimal amount of carbohydrate is consumed, carbohydrate becomes a limited fuel, and the intensity of the exercise effort will inevitably decrease.

Aerobic System

The aerobic energy system is the most complex of the three energy systems. As illustrated in figure 2.8, this system incorporates many pathways to process each energy-yielding macronutrient for ATP production. These pathways include beta-oxidation (7), glycolysis (carbohydrate), deamination (protein), and the TCA cycle and the ETC (all energy-yielding macronutrients). The aerobic energy system requires adequate oxygen availability for the mitochondria. The available oxygen is used in the final set of metabolic reactions that occur in the ETC, where oxygen serves as the final electron acceptor. Because the aerobic energy system requires oxygen, the maximal rate of ATP production is considered relatively slow in comparison with the phosphagen and anaerobic system. Time is needed to deliver oxygen from the air we breathe to the mitochondrial matrix, contributing to the longest lag time to increase ATP production of any energy system. The aerobic energy system can take minutes to produce enough ATP to fuel a physical workload that is within a person's **aerobic capacity**. The aerobic capacity is the maximal amount of oxygen (measured in milliliters) that an athlete can use in 1 minute per kilogram (kg) of body weight (ml · kg^{-1} · min^{-1}). For the purposes of fuel metabolism to produce ATP by the aerobic system, this measure is used to estimate the maximal amount of oxygen the muscle can use aerobically. It is tightly connected to aerobic fitness and how long a person can rely on the aerobic system as exercise intensity increases (figure 2.9). This measure is called aerobic capacity, or $\dot{V}O_2$max, the maximal amount of oxygen someone can use. As exercise

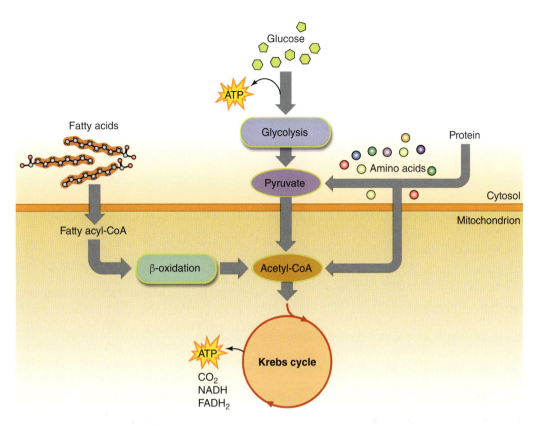

Figure 2.8 The aerobic energy system allows entry points of fat, carbohydrate, and protein in the oxidative pathway.

Reprinted by permission from A. Jeukendrup and M. Gleeson, "Fuel Sources for Muscle and Exercise Metabolism," in *Sport Nutrition* (Champaign, IL; Human Kinetics, 2010), 52.

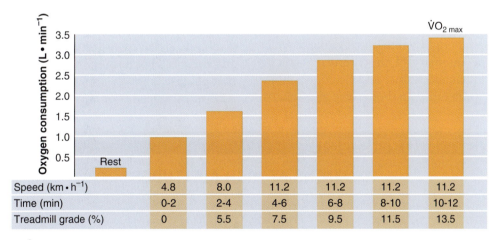

Figure 2.9 $\dot{V}O_2$max is reached when oxygen consumption fails to increase by the expected amount or decreases slightly with increased exercise intensity.

intensity increases, everyone approaches their $\dot{V}O_2$max. After the maximum peak of oxygen consumption (by the muscle) is met, any additional intensity that requires additional ATP must be met by the anaerobic system. With repeated aerobic training that tests the limits of the $\dot{V}O_2$max, a person can increase their $\dot{V}O_2$max, within their age and genetic potential, to improve the ability of the muscle to make ATP from all energy-yielding macronutrient substrates aerobically.

This reference to aerobic capacity is different from the aerobic system's capacity to make ATP. In theory, the capacity of the aerobic system to make ATP is practically unlimited when adequate oxygen is available, which is why the aerobic system is the ATP production system of choice when the body is at rest, when it can easily tap into carbohydrate and access seemingly unlimited fat stores to meet the body's energy needs. For the well-trained athlete who has benefited from cardiovascular, skeletal muscle, and metabolic adaptations that allow more efficient oxygen uptake and delivery to muscle tissue, the use of the aerobic system is much more robust than what is observed in a sedentary, untrained person. The trained athlete can tap into their aerobic system for meeting a significant portion of their ATP needs earlier in the exercise bout, for a much longer duration during the exercise bout, and at higher exercise intensities than their untrained counterparts. Ultimately, a person's capacity to make ATP aerobically is hindered by two things: (a) having some carbohydrate available for the TCA cycle to run smoothly and (b) muscle fatigue that may lead them to stop the exercise. But these barriers do not prevent some elite endurance athletes, such as triathletes and ultramarathoners, from maintaining aerobic exercise for more than 8 hours!

In summary, the three energy systems that the body uses are tightly integrated to make ATP based on the intensity of the exercise, which dictates ATP demand to fuel muscle contraction and oxygen availability. In the aerobic and anaerobic systems, the glycolysis pathway does not change; only the fate of pyruvate is different. For energy-yielding macronutrient oxidation to make ATP aerobically, each macronutrient starts the breakdown process with a metabolic pathway specific to that nutrient. Carbohydrate participates in glycolysis, protein in deamination, and fat in beta-oxidation. After this initial catabolic process is complete, metabolites from each individual breakdown source enter the TCA cycle at different entry points to yield high-energy electrons from oxidative decarboxylation and complete the ATP production cycle in the ETC.

Breakdown and Release of Energy

During the first steps of the complete breakdown of carbohydrate, fat, and protein, several metabolic pathways are involved. As breakdown of each energy-yielding macronutrient proceeds, however, all eventually converge along two shared metabolic pathways: the TCA cycle and the ETC. In this section we start with an overview of carbohydrate breakdown and then discuss the steps involved in protein and fat breakdown.

Chemical Energy Derived From Carbohydrate

Most of the cells in the body extract energy from carbohydrate through four metabolic processes: glycolysis, pyruvate to acetyl-CoA, the TCA cycle, and the ETC. For each of the metabolic pathways that glucose is involved in, a different amount of ATP is produced. For instance, glycolysis pro-

---

PUTTING IT INTO PERSPECTIVE

TRAINING AT HIGH ALTITUDES

We have all heard of athletes who travel to high-altitude locations (higher than 2,000 meters, or 6,600 feet) to train and prepare for future competition. They do so to produce metabolic changes to adapt to breathing air that contains less oxygen. Although several metabolic reasons explain why this can be advantageous for the athlete, one of the fundamental concerns that athletes should be aware of is how reduced oxygen availability affects the ability to oxidize metabolic fuels. Limited oxygen availability will impair the ability of the aerobic system to perform. Although over time, as athletes train in this environment, their bodies will begin to make metabolic adaptations to improve aerobic system efficiency, their immediate concern is ensuring that their anaerobic system has the energy substrate it needs to pick up the slack in ATP production. Because oxygen is already limited in the air, mitochondrial oxygen deficits will occur much sooner as exercise intensity increases. Adequate carbohydrate ingestion during the acute 3- to 6-week adaptation phase is critical because it is the only fuel that can be used anaerobically.

duces a small amount of ATP (+ 2 ATP) for each glucose molecule, but the complete aerobic breakdown of glucose that ends at the ETC produces roughly 16 times more ATP (+ 30–32 ATP).

Glycolysis occurs in the cytosol of the cell and does not require oxygen to proceed. The sequence of reactions involves splitting a six-carbon glucose molecule into *two* three-carbon pyruvate molecules. This catabolic process requires 2 ATP per glucose molecule and yields a gain of 4 ATP for a net gain of 2 ATP + 2 NADH + 2 pyruvates. The ATP required for this reaction serves to prime the pump to start the series of enzymatic reactions.

In the muscle cell, glucose is the only carbohydrate that can be absorbed, and after it is absorbed the muscle will not let it go. The muscle does this by adding a phosphorous group to glucose, turning it into glucose-6-phosphate (G-6-P). The structure of G-6-P will not allow it to leave the muscle cell and seals the fate of glucose to participate in either the catabolic pathway of glycolysis (when energy is needed) or the anabolic process of **glycogenesis** (when energy demands are low) to store carbohydrate as a future energy source in the form of glycogen. What about the other simple sugars, fructose and galactose? These sugars from our diet are absorbed by the liver for further metabolic processing to glucose that can be stored as liver glycogen or released into the bloodstream as glucose.

> **? DO YOU KNOW?**
>
> Muscle is the primary disposal organ of glucose (i.e., muscle uses glucose). For this fundamental reason, exercise is important for diabetes prevention and treatment. Exercise uses glucose for muscle contraction, which helps decrease the amount of glucose in the blood (blood sugar). If you have a genetic history of type 2 diabetes, maintaining fitness through exercise is extremely important. With regular exercise, your chances of getting diabetes are significantly reduced.

The next step in the aerobic energy system process is to convert pyruvate into acetyl-CoA. This highly regulated process considers the energy demands of the cell (i.e., how much ATP is needed to maintain muscle work) and oxygen availability within the cell. The **pyruvate dehydrogenase complex (PDC)**, which converts pyruvate into acetyl-CoA for the TCA cycle, helps regulate this step by receiving feedback from the cell from the available concentrations of ADP versus ATP as well as the availability of NAD^+ and FAD to accept electrons and protons for energy transfer. For example, high levels of ATP within the cell suggests energy adequacy that will slow down additional conversion of pyruvate to acetyl-CoA. Conversely, high ADP concentrations suggest an energy deficit and the need to speed up the rate in which pyruvate is converted to acetyl-CoA. The most important factor that affects this conversion pathway is the availability of oxygen. When a cell requires energy, and oxygen is readily available, aerobic reactions in the mitochondria convert each pyruvate molecule to an acetyl-CoA molecule. This reaction produces a pair of electrons to form NADH while also producing carbon dioxide. The NADH then shuttles the electrons to the ETC. The term *oxygen availability* is best conceptualized when thinking about the pyruvate-to-acetyl-CoA pathway in muscle cells. At rest, in healthy people, the body can easily deliver inhaled oxygen to muscle cells. This process gets tricky, however, when someone begins to exercise. How well oxygen remains available to exercising muscle depends on two things: a person's aerobic fitness and the relative intensity of the exercise session. Oxygen will become less available sooner in an unfit person as exercise intensity increases. Fit individuals have created physiological adaptations to deliver oxygen much more efficiently in exercising muscle and can maintain oxygen availability at higher intensities. From a metabolic perspective, everyone has an intensity limit, even fit athletes, at which oxygen becomes unavailable, and the conversion of pyruvate to acetyl-CoA then ceases.

Although many metabolic pathways can proceed either forward or backward, the formation of acetyl-CoA is an irreversible process after it is initiated in the presence of oxygen. To form acetyl-CoA, metabolic reactions remove one carbon from the three-carbon pyruvate and add the **coenzyme A** that is derived from the B vitamin, pantothenic acid. After combining with oxygen, the carbon is released to generate carbon dioxide. The end products from this process are two NADH and two acetyl-CoA molecules. The acetyl-CoA molecules produced from pyruvate are trapped inside the mitochondria and ready to enter the TCA cycle.

The oxygen-dependent reactions of the TCA cycle and the ETC liberate large amounts of energy in the form of ATP. The TCA cycle occurs in the mitochondria and serves to take the acetyl portion (CH_3COO^-) of acetyl-CoA through oxidative processes (i.e., breaking carbon-carbon bonds to liberate electrons) to yield three molecules of NADH, two molecules of carbon dioxide, and one molecule each of $FADH_2$ and GTP (guanosine triphosphate, an energy carrier similar to ATP). The TCA cycle process begins with acetyl-CoA combining with **oxaloacetate**, freeing coenzyme A and yielding a six-carbon compound called citrate. The coenzyme A can then be recycled to form another acetyl-CoA by binding with a new pyruvate molecule. Subsequent reactions in the TCA cycle convert citrate into a series of intermediate compounds, removing two additional carbons (freeing high-energy electrons) and releasing two molecules of carbon dioxide. The final step in the TCA cycle regenerates oxaloacetate (figure 2.10), which in turn reacts with pyruvate to create citric acid and start the cycle anew. The primary purpose of the TCA cycle for energy-generation purposes is to extract most of the energy from oxidative decarboxylation to harness high-energy electrons and protons to be shuttled to the ETC. For each acetyl-CoA entering the cycle, one complete cycle, or "turn," produces one GTP and transfers pairs of high-energy electrons to three NADH and one $FADH_2$. Recall that the anaerobic breakdown of one glucose molecule yields two molecules of acetyl-CoA and that the TCA cycle turns, or cycles, with each acetyl-CoA molecule provided. This process produces twice the amount of high-energy electron carriers (i.e., six NADH, two $FADH_2$, and two GTP). In addition to providing electron substrate for coenzyme energy transfer to the ETC, the TCA cycle is also an important source of building blocks for the biosynthesis of

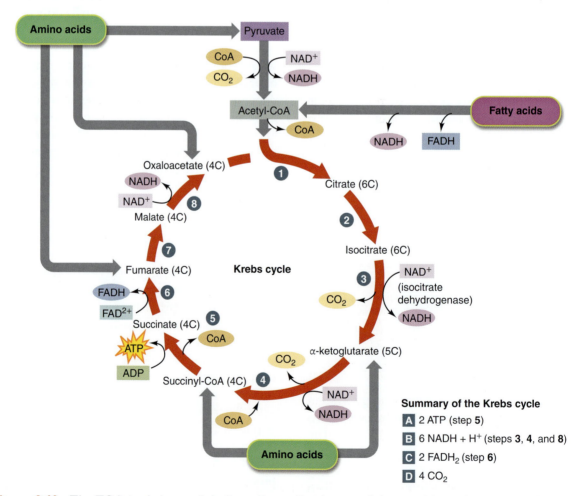

Figure 2.10 The TCA cycle is a metabolic pathway that is part of the aerobic pathway to produce ATP.

amino acids and fatty acids. When plenty of ATP is available to meet the energy demand of the cell, the TCA cycle's intermediate molecules can leave the cycle and join biosynthetic metabolic pathways. For example, during times of energy excess (i.e., consuming more calories than are burned with activity), citrate can leave the cycle to provide substrate for fatty acid synthesis and subsequent fat storage.

The ETC produces most of the ATP available from glucose and serves as the final step in glucose oxidation by accepting the high-energy electrons from the TCA cycle. The ETC consists of a sequence of linked reactions that take place on what visually appears to be a chain of linked protein channels found on the inner mitochondrial membrane (figure 2.11). Most ATP is produced here, and if mitochondrial oxygen supply is adequate, it can maintain ATP production to fuel exercise for hours. The site of the ETC is where NADH and $FADH_2$ deliver their pair of high-energy electrons to the chain. In the inner mitochondrial membrane, these electrons are passed along a chain of linked reactions, giving up energy along the way to power the final production of ATP. At the end of the ETC, oxygen accepts the energy-depleted electrons and reacts with hydrogen to form water (this is where most of the oxygen we breathe goes!). This series of oxidation-reduction reactions along the ETC (i.e., losing and gaining electrons) is known as oxidative phosphorylation and is characterized by the flow of electrons down the chain and the phosphorylation of ADP molecules to form significant amounts of ATP.

As electrons are donated and passed down the ETC, they create an electrochemical gradient that causes a pressure change between the inner mitochondrial space and the mitochondrial matrix. This creates a phenomenon known as **proton motive force** that forces protons (H+) through the ETC proton channels from the matrix into the inner mitochondrial space. The pressure that starts to build in the inner mitochondrial space provides the force to push hydrogen ions back through to the matrix through a complex protein channel called **ATP synthase**. This protein complex has been described as an energy turbine that turns and manufactures ATP by serving as the physical tool that binds P_i to ADP. This process is analogous to blowing up a balloon—the opening of the balloon serves as the pressure release valve that drives the ATP synthase machinery to form ATP. Collectively, this entire process has been termed **chemiosmotic coupling** and is illustrated in figure 2.12. The difference in NADH and $FADH_2$ contribution to ATP production is where on the

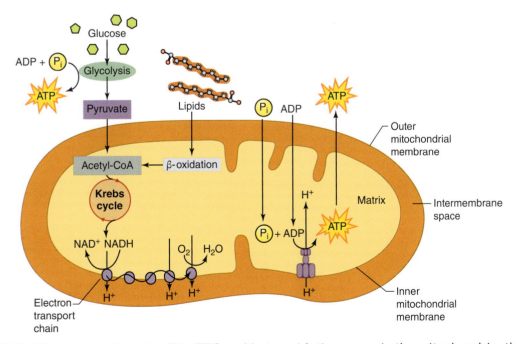

Figure 2.11 Mitochondrial matrix. The ETC and beta-oxidation occur in the mitochondria, the powerhouse of the cell.

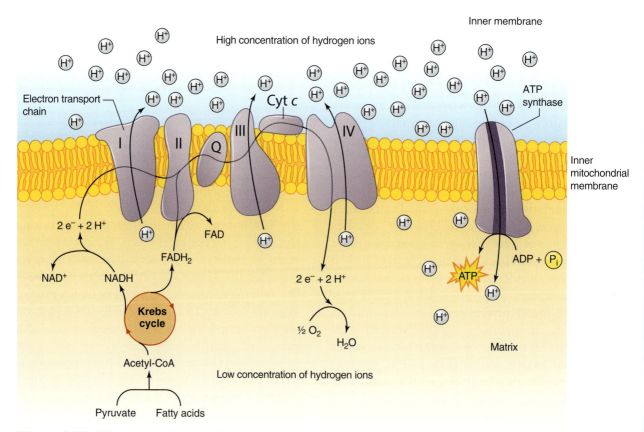

Figure 2.12 Chemiosmotic coupling. An electrochemical gradient is formed from electrons passing through the electron transport chain, causing hydrogen ions (protons) to move across from the mitochondrial matrix, producing proton motive force that activates the protein complex ATP synthase to regenerate ATP.

ETC they donate their electrons. NADH donates electrons at the beginning of the chain, whereas FADH$_2$ electrons enter the ETC at a later point. Because they travel through fewer reactions, the electrons from FADH$_2$ generate fewer ATP molecules from less proton motive force. As illustrated in table 2.2, the total amount of ATP molecules produced from one glucose molecule is currently estimated at 30 to 32 ATP (8).

Chemical Energy Derived From Fat

To generate chemical energy from fat, the body must first break down triglycerides into their

Table 2.2 Net ATP From the Complete Aerobic Oxidation of One Molecule of Glucose

Step	Coenzyme electron carriers	ATP yield
Glycolysis		2
TCA	GTP	2
Oxidative phosphorylation	2 NADH × 1.5 (G–3PO)	3
	2 NADH (oxidative decarboxylation of pyruvate) × 2.5	5
	2 FADH × 1.5	3
	6 NADH × 2.5	15
	Total yield	**30 (32) ATP**

component glycerol and fatty acids. Different hormones and metabolic processes are involved to take on this task from both fats (technically termed triglycerides) derived from the diet and fatty acids stored in fat cells. Glycerol, a small three-carbon molecule, carries a small amount of energy within its carbon-carbon bonds, and the liver readily accepts it to convert it to pyruvate or glucose. The fatty acids derived from triglycerides provide nearly all the energy found in this compound. All fatty acid breakdown and oxidation occurs within the mitochondria. But before a fatty acid can cross into mitochondria, it must be linked to coenzyme A. This activation step of fatty acid delivery into the mitochondria requires one molecule of ATP to launch the process. Figure 2.13 provides an overview of how fat is transported and used for ATP production.

The next step of fatty acid delivery into the mitochondria involves activated fatty acid interaction with the **carnitine shuttle**. Carnitine is a compound formed from the amino acid lysine and has the unique task of shepherding the activated fatty acid across the outer mitochondrial membrane from the cytosol to the mitochondrion matrix.

? DO YOU KNOW?

Although some supplement manufacturers claim the supplement carnitine can enhance "fat burning," the bulk of the scientific literature remains equivocal (9-11). Despite these findings, carnitine research continues to grow; new research questions address dose efficacy, glycogen preservation, and recovery. Some of this movement, however, has been dampened by data suggesting that carnitine supplementation may be harmful due to the need for high dosing and potential for increasing the risk of cardiovascular disease (11, 12). The highly respected Australian Institute of Sports has classified carnitine as a group B supplement that is "deserving of further research and could be considered for provision to athletes under a research protocol or case-managed monitoring situation."

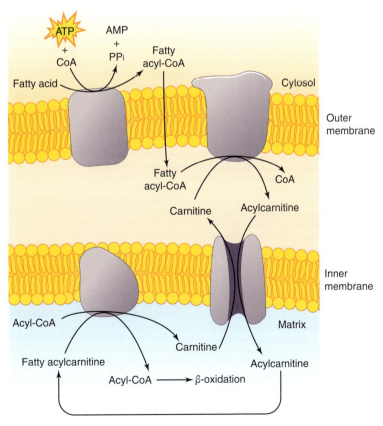

Figure 2.13 Fatty acid transport. These steps are essential for fatty acids to be oxidized in the mitochondria.

After fatty acids enter the mitochondria matrix, a process known as beta-oxidation breaks the fatty acids down into multiple molecules of acetyl-CoA for entry into the TCA cycle. After fatty acids become individual acetyl-CoA units, the remaining metabolic pathways to make ATP are the same as glucose and involve both the TCA cycle and the ETC, as previously described. But fatty acids must be activated for degradation by coenzyme A by forming a fatty acyl-CoA bond. Starting from the second carbon from the acidic end of the fatty acid chain, called the beta carbon, fat enzymes clip a two-carbon "link" off the end of the chain. Every time this happens, other reactions take place to convert this link to one acetyl-CoA, while also transferring one pair of electrons to form $FADH_2$ and another pair to form NADH. This process always occurs in a stepwise fashion, in which only two carbons are clipped at a time to generate a molecule of acetyl-CoA until only one two-carbon segment remains. The final acetyl-CoA formed does not produce an $FADH_2$ or NADH, because the final step does not generate high-energy electrons without additional carbon-carbon bonds being split.

Almost all fatty acids originating from food have an even number of carbons and vary in length from 4 to 26 carbons. Although most fatty acids are 16 to 18 carbons long, if the mitochondria encounter an odd-numbered fatty acid, it will break down the chain in the same way until it reaches a final three-carbon link. Instead of continued breakdown, the final three-carbon molecule will join with coenzyme A and enter the TCA cycle as one of the downstream intermediates (i.e., not as acetyl-CoA). Because this process skips some of the early TCA reactions, it has a shorter journey than acetyl-CoA and produces fewer high-energy electrons and thus fewer NADH molecules.

Because beta-oxidation produces many acetyl-CoA molecules from just one fatty acid (figure 2.14), it is easy to see why dietary fat is so energy dense and contributes a high calorie load for our bodies. The ETC end products of fatty acid oxidation are the same as with glucose: carbon dioxide, water, and ATP. But a few metabolic nuances are important to understand when considering the way that fat is used to produce ATP. First, the exact amount of ATP produced from fatty acid

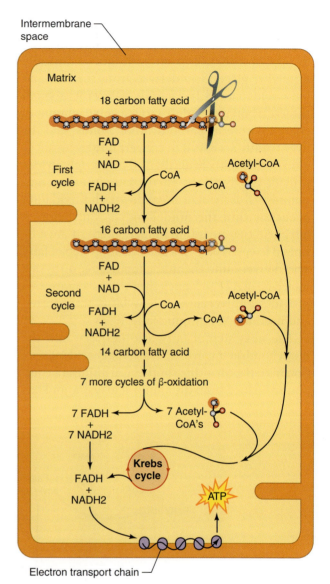

Figure 2.14 Beta-oxidation is specific to fat metabolism and provides substrate to the aerobic energy system.

oxidation depends on the length of the fatty acid chain. Longer chains have more carbon bonds and hence produce more chemical energy in the form of ATP. The complete breakdown of an 18-carbon fatty acid produces 120 ATP. This amount is substantially more ATP than is produced from one molecule of glucose. To take this a step further, a *single* triglyceride with three 18-carbon fatty acids that are completely oxidized will produce 360 ATP, a value more than 10 times the ATP produced from the complete oxidation of a single glucose molecule.

Fat metabolism is also tightly synchronized with aerobic carbohydrate metabolism. Acetyl-CoA from beta-oxidation can enter the TCA cycle only when fat and carbohydrate metabolism occur in concert. When carbohydrate availability to normal human metabolism is low, such as with very low-carbohydrate diets, uncontrolled type 1 diabetes, or during fasting and starvation, the intermediate oxaloacetate readily leaves the TCA cycle to travel to the liver and help the body make more blood glucose to prevent hypoglycemia. This metabolic pathway, known as **gluconeogenesis**, takes precedence under these circumstances because we cannot function properly or, in some cases, even survive if our blood glucose gets too low. Because of this metabolic shift, oxaloacetate is much less available to combine with acetyl-CoA, from beta-oxidation, to form citrate and continue the TCA process. Moreover, to assist in keeping up with ATP demand, the body employs another strategy to compensate for low glucose availability by increasing fat breakdown, and therefore the amount of acetyl-CoA derived from beta-oxidation. Due to the reduced availability of oxaloacetate, however, this influx of acetyl-CoAs is blocked from entry into the TCA cycle and rerouted to form a family of compounds called ketone bodies (ketones). Thus, a high rate of ketone production in the mitochondrial matrix from incomplete fat oxidation is a by-product of both low glucose availability and an excessive rate of acetyl-CoA production from beta-oxidation.

Although the body makes and uses small amounts of ketone bodies at all times, ketogenesis can be ramped up to meet ATP demand when glucose is low and normal fatty acid oxidation is compromised. Excessive acetyl-CoA molecules (from fat metabolism) are used to produce the ketones acetoacetate and beta-hydroxybutyrate in the liver (figure 2.15). These acidic and water-soluble ketones are easily transported in the bloodstream to nonhepatic tissues for utilization as fuel, an energy source for the brain, intestinal mucosa, heart, skeletal muscle, and kidneys. The principal fate of ketones involves conversion back to acetyl-CoA and oxidation in the TCA cycle (figure 2.15) (13). Because ketones can be used as an energy source and are primarily produced by fat breakdown in low glucose states, many athletes are interested in ketogenic diets in

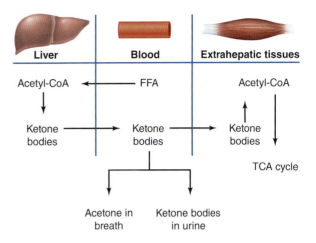

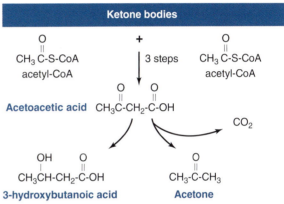

Figure 2.15 Ketogenesis and utilization of ketone bodies.

an attempt to lose body fat and improve performance. The utility, practicality, and concerns of this approach are discussed in greater detail in chapters 10 through 12.

As with the aerobic oxidation of glucose, adequate oxygen must be available in the mitochondria to oxidize fatty acids completely. Unlike carbohydrate, fatty acids cannot produce ATP anaerobically and must follow mitochondrial pathways leading up to the ETC with oxygen serving as the final electron acceptor. Take, for example, a foot race between a trained athlete and an unfit couch potato. Just as there are differences in carbohydrate metabolism between the two race participants, differences also exist in their ability to use fat as a fuel source to generate ATP. At rest, both the athlete and the couch potato have no problems burning fat as a fuel source. ATP demand is low, and oxygen is available to all mitochondria. This circumstance drastically changes at the onset of exercise. Athletes have adapted to be able to deliver more oxygen to working muscles and can do so at higher exercise intensities than the untrained. The couch potato will experience an oxygen deficit much sooner as intensity increases. The oxygen deficit will put the brakes on fat oxidation, because ATP will be generated with anaerobic glycolysis (relying on the breakdown of carbohydrate) with much less capacity than with fat oxidation.

Chemical Energy Derived From Protein

As previously discussed, the human body's preference is to use protein in structural and functional roles, such as remodeling muscle tissue. Protein is not considered a major resource for ATP production. That said, recall that no metabolic pathway involving carbohydrate, fat, or protein is ever "turned off." Some tissues will always be using protein as an ATP source, but its contribution is relatively small compared with that of carbohydrate and fat to meet chemical energy needs. But if for some reason our energy production falters, such as in starvation or when inadequate amounts of calories are available, energy production from body protein stores will increase. During starvation, blood glucose is vital to sustaining the carbons that make up amino acids as TCA intermediates.

To make ATP from protein, amino acids must first be stripped of their nitrogen component ($-NH_2$) in a process called deamination. The remaining carbon structure, often referred to as the carbon skeleton, can be used by the TCA cycle, whereas the nitrogen component is converted to ammonia and then to urea (essentially, a waste product) by the liver. The carbon skeletons from amino acid catabolism can enter the breakdown pathways of the TCA cycle at many different points. This is a key distinction from carbohydrate and fat breakdown that must enter the TCA cycle as acetyl-CoA (see figure 2.10). The carbon skeleton from each amino acid has a unique structure and number of carbon atoms. These differences determine the fate of the carbon skeleton. Some carbon skeletons are similar to pyruvate (alanine) or enter the TCA as acetyl-CoA (leucine), whereas others can enter as one of the many intermediates of the TCA cycle (asparagine, tyrosine, methionine, glutamate). The complete breakdown of an amino acid yields urea, carbon dioxide, water, and ATP. How much ATP the amino acid produces depends on where the carbon skeleton enters the TCA cycle. For example, alanine enters the TCA cycle early and can produce 12.5 ATP. In contrast, methionine enters the TCA cycle following deamination approximately halfway through the cycle, producing only five ATPs. When compared with carbohydrate and fat fuel sources, amino acids produce relatively low amounts of ATP.

Chemical Energy Derived From Alcohol

Alcohol in human nutrition usually refers to beer, wine, and distilled spirits. The technical name for alcohol is ethanol and, when consumed, the energy value is 7 kcal per gram (kcal/g), providing a chemical energy source that the body can use to make ATP. Because alcohol provides energy, it has been classified as a food, but alcohol performs no essential functions in the body and is therefore not a nutrient.

The body works extremely hard to get rid of alcohol to prevent it from accumulating and destroying cells and organs. For example, the liver selectively metabolizes alcohol before other compounds and can use alternative metabolic pathways in the liver to handle and clear excessive (i.e., binge) consumption. Generally, when small to moderate amounts of alcohol are consumed, it is first converted to acetaldehyde and rapidly converted to acetate and then acetyl-CoA (figure 2.16). Generally, very little acetyl-CoA enters the TCA cycle, and instead it is shuttled to anabolic pathways to form fat. This mechanism occurs because the metabolic reactions that convert alcohol to acetate rapidly consume the available NAD^+ that is normally available to receive high-energy electrons from the oxidation of carbohydrate and fat. The limited availability of NAD^+ restricts the rate of the TCA cycle. Because alcohol detoxification is the body's priority, accumulating acetyl-CoAs are rerouted to fatty acid synthesis. Fat accumulation in the liver can be seen after a single bout of heavy drinking. This fatty acid synthesis adapts and accelerates with chronic heavy alcohol consumption, leading to a fatty liver—the first stage of liver destruction that occurs with chronic alcohol abuse.

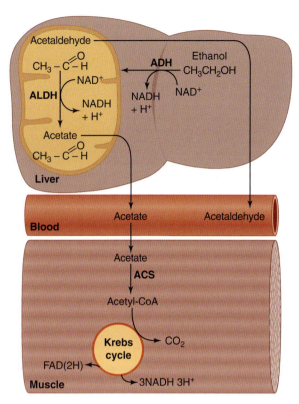

Figure 2.16 The process of ethanol metabolism.

For athletes and others who want to maintain a high level of exercise and performance, misuse of alcohol can interfere with athletic goals in a variety of ways related to the negative effects of acute intake of alcohol on the performance of, or recovery from, exercise (10). Negative effects of chronic binge drinking can also manifest as poor health and higher body fat (14). Besides loading on calories, alcohol suppresses fat oxidation, increases the likelihood of unplanned and excessive food consumption, and might compromise the achievement of a lean body composition (10).

The available evidence warns against intake of significant amounts of alcohol in the preexercise period and during training because of the direct negative effects of alcohol on exercise metabolism, thermoregulation, physical skills, and concentration (15). Any negative effects of alcohol on strength and performance may persist for several hours, even after signs and symptoms of intoxication or hangover are no longer present (10). In the postexercise phase, alcohol may interfere with recovery by impairing glycogen resynthesis and storage (16). Alcohol consumption postexercise can also slow rates of rehydration through its suppressive effect on antidiuretic hormone (17) and impair the muscle protein synthesis response that is desired for muscle adaptation and repair (18, 19). For some athletes, other effects on body function are likely, such as mild disturbances in acid-base balance, increased inflammation, and compromised glucose metabolism and cardiovascular function (20). Finally, binge drinking can indirectly affect athlete recovery goals through inattention to following proper guidelines for training recovery, such as dealing with a hangover, missing meals, overeating, and getting excessive sleep. In general, athletes are advised to consider both public health guidelines and team rules regarding use of alcohol and are encouraged to minimize or avoid alcohol consumption in the postexercise period when issues of recovery and injury repair are a priority (10). Further discussion of the effects of alcohol on athletic performance appears in chapter 9.

BENEFITS OF TRAINING ON HEALTH AND ATHLETIC PERFORMANCE

Whether you train to increase strength or endurance, your body will adapt to accommodate or get used to the repeated stimulus, which ultimately will improve performance. The concept of training to improve performance encompasses the three key principles outlined in chapter 1. Although the magnitude and specificity of these changes depend on the individual and the characteristics of the training program, any program that improves aerobic capacity will have a significant effect on fuel utilization and the energy systems. Because many athletes adopt a training regimen that promotes improvements in strength, power, and endurance, metabolic adaptations geared toward improving mitochondrial oxygen availability are prominent.

Figure 2.17 describes some key metabolic adaptations. Structural and biochemical adaptations to endurance training include increased mitochondrial number and size and increased concentration of oxidative enzymes involved in beta-oxidation, the TCA cycle, and the ETC. These changes improve aerobic energy system efficiency in the muscle. The NADH shuttling

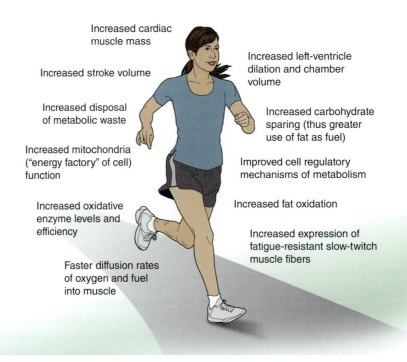

Figure 2.17 Advantages of training on metabolism.

system and a change in LDH protein structure are also observed. These adaptations improve electron delivery to the ETC and increase the ability of the muscle to oxidize lactic acid. A host of cardiovascular changes also take place to support adaptation. The most significant changes are related to improvements in the heart's **stroke volume** and **angiogenesis**, which increases capillary density and capacity to transport fatty acids from the plasma to the muscle cell. Again, these adaptations are important in promoting aerobic system efficiency and, in this case, improving oxygen delivery to working muscle. Unfortunately, the principle of **reversibility** still holds true when training ceases. Most of these adaptations are lost after approximately 5 weeks of detraining, and about half of the increase in muscle mitochondrial content is lost after just 1 week of detraining. Even more troubling to consider is that it takes about 4 weeks of retraining to regain many positive endurance-related skeletal muscle adaptations lost in the first week of detraining (21). The rapid rate of reversibility is one of the fundamental reasons why exercise is recommended as part of a healthy lifestyle that is done daily, in some form, as a key strategy to promote health, longevity, and chronic disease prevention.

Exercise training stimulus is undoubtedly instrumental in promoting a multitude of cardiovascular system, muscle tissue, and cellular changes to improve energy system efficiency. Although these adaptations have a clear benefit to metabolic health that should not be understated, other outcomes related to fuel substrate utilization offer key benefits to the competitive athlete and anyone else starting an exercise program to improve health. These benefits are best described by understanding the **crossover concept** of carbohydrate and fat utilization during exercise. By definition, the crossover is the point on the graph (see chapter 11) at which the body starts using more carbohydrate than fat as its energy source. Recall that exercise intensity is directly proportional to carbohydrate use because of the anaerobic environment created at high exercise intensities. Also recall that a person's ability to oxidize fat during exercise with increasing intensity depends on their aerobic capacity. If someone were to draw a simple figure to represent the crossover concept for a sedentary friend and compare it with an athlete friend, the figure, especially where the crossover occurs on the percent $\dot{V}O_2$max axis, would look very different. Consistent with the cardiovascular, muscle tissue, and cellular changes that occur with training, the crossover point also shifts to the right with training. This phenomenon has huge metabolic significance, for both athletes and people trying to become healthier through exercise. For those starting an exercise program, the shift to the right that occurs with chronic training adaption means they will be able to work out longer and harder using a more efficient aerobic energy system to primarily oxidize fatty acids. Although this finding may be initially interpreted as a direct strategy to lose body fat by directly oxidizing fat, this result is not the key outcome of this adaptation and is not the key player that promotes loss of body fat. The key benefit is that this adaptation allows for higher-intensity exercise capacity, an acquired advantage to training that is of primary importance for increasing energy (calorie) expenditure and thus promoting weight loss and weight maintenance. Think of trading in your four-cylinder car for a car with a V-8 engine. Although in the car world, this trade is clearly not advantageous for fuel economy, the shift in the crossover with training allows you to aerobically burn fuels more efficiently and burn more calories using large muscle groups with a reduced reliance on the lactic acid–producing anaerobic system. By continuing to push yourself with repeated training, you can further augment this adaption and increase muscle mass, which will burn more fuel (calories) at rest. Consider how long it takes someone to run a mile before training compared with how long it takes after training. Regardless of the time difference in running the mile, the number of calories burned will be similar. The major difference is the energy-yielding macronutrient distribution of fuels oxidized, the energy systems used, and the calories burned divided by the amount of time to run the mile. The trained person will oxidize more fat, feel better during the run because of less lactic acid production, and burn more calories per unit of time. The result is usually an enjoyable experience during which mileage and calorie expenditure is increased, thus improving metabolic health and assisting in the maintenance of a healthy body weight.

When continued training promotes metabolic adaptation that shifts the crossover point to the right, the athlete benefits from the same metabolic advantages as the nonathlete but to a greater degree. These adaptations support the athlete's high-intensity efforts and allow fat, as an endless fuel source, to be used earlier in the activity and at much greater intensities and power outputs than in the nonathlete. But the most important metabolic benefit of the crossover adaptation for the athlete is not weight and body composition management—the most important benefit is the ability to preserve and protect limited carbohydrate stores until the highest-intensity effort is required to compete in an athletic event. Because carbohydrate stores in the body are limited in muscle tissue, and occur in a relatively small amount in the liver, the preservation of this fuel source for anaerobic system activity to fuel ATP generation is crucial to high-intensity performance. Think of a trained distance runner metabolically capable of tapping primarily into fat stores to fuel much of the ATP demand for most of a race. When it is important for the runner to run up hills or overtake other runners in the final portion of the race, the increased intensity (and increased ATP demand) will need to be met anaerobically with the only fuel that the anaerobic system can use—

PUTTING IT INTO PERSPECTIVE

METABOLIC EFFECT OF DIETARY NITRATE

Consuming nitrate-rich vegetables such as spinach, arugula, and beetroot juice or beetroot supplements may enhance athletic performance. Several studies have documented performance enhancement and mechanisms related to metabolism. For some athletes, nitrate significantly improves skeletal muscle oxygen uptake and mitochondrial use of oxygen. Nitrate may also reduce the amount of oxygen needed to generate ATP during submaximal aerobic exercise and reduce ATP demand for muscles to produce force (11). Because these benefits may improve exercise tolerance and aerobic system efficiency, dietary nitrate supplementation may be beneficial for both trained athletes and novice athletes who do not have a highly adapted aerobic energy system (22). To learn more about the dietary nitrate supplementation, refer to chapter 9.

carbohydrate. If this runner did not adequately prepare for the race by consuming enough carbohydrate leading up to the race, their capacity to produce ATP anaerobically will be compromised and will negatively affect performance.

BIOSYNTHESIS AND STORAGE PATHWAYS IN METABOLISM

From an evolutionary perspective, the human body does not like to get rid of unexpended energy. Referring back to the first law of thermodynamics, recall that energy cannot be destroyed. So what happens in our bodies when we have excess energy remaining from the food we consume? Consider how your clothes fit after visiting home for the holidays—a little tighter than before, right? Your biosynthetic metabolic pathways work hard to capture excess energy to create heat and store ATP for future energy needs. Some of the excess energy can also be used to synthesize new proteins or to store glycogen, but a significant portion of the excess goes to fat storage.

Now fast-forward to the New Year when waistline growth and resolutions often result in new gym memberships. After several workouts, the cumulative result of increased energy expenditure and reduced calorie intake creates weight loss—and the observation that your clothes are fitting different because of muscle gain. A different biosynthetic pathway is now working hard to assemble new proteins. Other pathways are at work synthesizing and storing carbohydrate, protein, and fat. While some cells are breaking down carbohydrate, fat, and protein to extract energy, other cells are busy synthesizing and storing glycogen, building proteins, and storing fat. Depending on the energy needs of the body and the amount of energy available, either breakdown pathways or biosynthetic pathways will dominate.

Gluconeogenesis

Gluconeogenesis (figure 2.18) is a biosynthetic pathway that creates glucose for the body from carbohydrate-producing precursors, such as oxaloacetate, lactic acid, glycerol, and alanine (23). Note, however, that gluconeogenesis is not simply the reverse of glycolysis. When someone is not taking in enough carbohydrate, the body can make glucose in the gluconeogenic pathway. About 90 percent of this pathway takes place in the liver, and the kidneys pick up the rest (24). The liver and kidney cells make glucose from pyruvate by way of oxaloacetate by detouring around some of the irreversible metabolic steps found in glycolysis. These detours require the use of some ATP to bypass the glycolysis pathways that are flowing in the opposite direction. In times of glucose need, some glucose can also be synthesized from lactic acid. Although some lactic acid is continuously formed and degraded, lactic acid generation accelerates in exercising muscle dictated by the anaerobic condition of the muscle (muscle fatigue). Circulating lactic acid can be absorbed by the liver, where gluconeogenesis converts some of the lactic acid back to glucose through the **Cori cycle** (figure 2.19). In this metabolic pathway, the enzyme LDH catalyzes the conversion of lactic acid to pyruvic acid (pyruvate). Glycerol and alanine also work as gluconeogenic precursors. Although fatty acids cannot be converted to glucose, the glycerol liberated from triglyceride breakdown travels to the liver to be converted into glucose. Finally, in scenarios where muscle protein breakdown increases, the amino acid alanine can leave skeletal muscle tissue and be converted to pyruvate, and then glucose, in the liver. This process is known as the glucose-alanine cycle and serves as a form of gluconeogenesis.

Glycogenesis

Glycogenesis is a biosynthetic pathway that assembles glucose molecules into branched chains for storage as glycogen. Glycogen is a branched-chain **polysaccharide** made of glucose units (25). Liver glycogen serves as a glucose reserve for the blood, and muscle glycogen provides a glucose reserve for exercising muscle tissue. As discussed earlier, glycogen stores are limited and can be depleted after an overnight fast (in the liver) or after repeated high-intensity exercise or long endurance bouts (in the muscle). When glucose is needed, a breakdown reaction called **glycogenolysis** liberates glucose molecules from glycogen chains. In the liver, this process produces glucose that can freely enter the blood stream. In the muscle, glucose is trapped and is often shuttled to glycolysis to produce ATP.

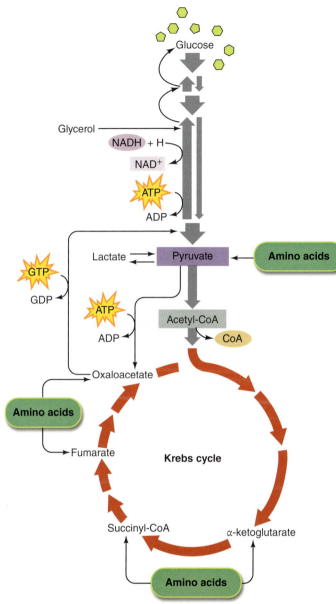

Figure 2.18 Gluconeogenesis.

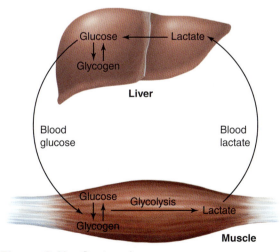

Figure 2.19 Cori cycle.

Lipogenesis

The biosynthetic pathway involving **lipogenesis** is accelerated during times of excess calorie consumption and often leads to the gain of fat tissue. When ATP supply exceeds the body's energy demand excess, acetyl-CoA is available to make long-chain fatty acids. Accumulating acetyl Co-A molecules are assembled within this biosynthetic pathway as links to form fatty acid chains in the cytosol. Fatty acid synthesis through the lipogenesis pathway also requires energy in the form of **nicotinamide adenine dinucleotide phosphate (NADPH)** to drive the synthetic reaction (note that NADH and NADPH, although similar molecules, have very different biological roles) (26). As the final step, the **endoplasmic reticulum** will then take the surplus of fatty acids formed and combine them with glycerol to form triglycerides, the body's primary storage form of fat.

Because only acetyl-CoA molecules feed the lipogenesis synthetic pathway, note that any precursor substrates involved in acetyl-CoA synthesis can feed fatty acid synthesis. This concept is important to grasp because carbohydrate, many amino acids, alcohol, and fatty acids can all contribute to acetyl-CoA production. Therefore, when energy intake exceeds ATP demands, additional intake from any of these precursor sources may efficiently activate lipogenesis to store additional body fat. From a practical standpoint, excess energy consumption in any form—sugar-sweetened beverages, meat, protein supplements, fat, alcohol—can contribute to fat storage. The key point here is that overeating is the primary driving force behind increasing body fat storage.

HORMONAL CONTROL OF METABOLISM

How are these breakdown and synthetic biological pathways regulated? What triggers the shift in the dominant pathway from one to the other after consuming food (fed state) or after a night of sleeping (fasted state)? The answer is hormonal control of

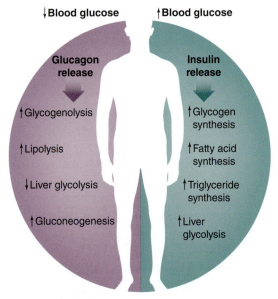

Figure 2.20 Glucagon and insulin are major players in the metabolic pathway control.

Based on McCarthy et al. (2022).

metabolism. The body can tightly regulate and control the reactions of metabolic pathways. In many ways, hormones circulating through the body act as traffic police, ensuring that each metabolic pathway proceeds at just the right speed. Although the body has many strategies to help control metabolism simultaneously, hormones serve as the master regulators. The key players are illustrated in figure 2.20.

MEASURING ENERGY INTAKE AND EXPENDITURE

By definition, energy is the capacity to do work. Without energy, our bodies cannot function. The energy in the food we eat is considered chemical energy, which our bodies convert from potential energy to mechanical, electrical, or heat energy. For an energy boost, we must eat food, which is then converted to ATP by the process described earlier. Every muscle movement, every nerve impulse, every cellular reaction requires ATP, and carbohydrate, triglycerides, and protein are the vehicles through which this energy is supplied.

Estimating Energy Content of Food

In the field of nutrition science, we discuss the potential energy in food, or the body's use of energy (i.e., using ATP), in units of heat called calories. One calorie (1 kcal) is the amount of energy (in the form of heat) required to raise the temperature of 1 kilogram (2.2 lb) of water by 1 degree Celsius (1.8 degrees Fahrenheit). Although this statement might sound like an abstract concept, it makes more sense when thinking about how a bomb calorimeter (i.e., a meter for measuring calories) works to liberate chemical energy from food that is placed in it to heat energy. As shown in figure 2.21, food is placed within a sealed chamber, and the food is completely burned while sensors placed outside the chamber in a water bath measure the amount of heat produced by combustion within the inner chamber. The difference in water temperature from the heat energy produced is a measure of the sample's energy output and provides an accurate assessment of the total energy content of the particular food. Because this method is a direct method of measuring heat production, the use of the bomb calorimeter is often categorized as direct calorimetry. Although the human body is not as efficient as the bomb calorimeter in energy transfer from one form to another, following a few metabolic adjustments, the same basic principle applies and can be used to determine the amount of food energy we consume from our diet. Thus, the number of calories from complete combustion in a bomb calorimeter is adjusted downward:

> 4 kcal per gram pure carbohydrate
> 4 kcal per gram pure protein

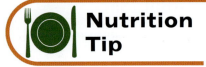

Nutrition Tip

Need an energy boost? You won't find it in your coffee cup. You might think that coffee, or a caffeinated alternative, increases your energy, but based on the first law of thermodynamics, this idea makes no sense. Caffeine is not an energy source; it is a central nervous system stimulant. For an energy boost, try eating nutrient-dense carbohydrate foods.

Energy Metabolism 53

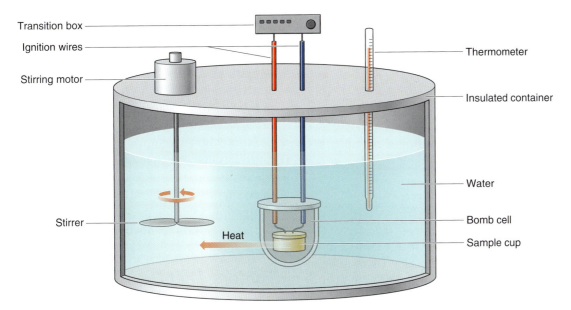

Figure 2.21 A bomb calorimeter determines the total energy content of food.

> 9 kcal per gram pure fat
> 7 kcal per gram pure alcohol

The number of calories derived from the complete combustion of these energy-yielding macronutrients and alcohol in a bomb calorimeter is slightly higher than what is listed here. This discrepancy occurs primarily because the human body does not completely digest all food and therefore does not extract all calories from the food. As discussed earlier, nitrogen from protein foods cannot be oxidized to produce ATP. These adjustments let us know the calorie content of each energy-producing food component, and we can use these numbers to estimate its calorie content, as long as we know the weight of each component.

Assessing an Athlete's Energy Intake

Some athletes may have an idea of how much energy they consume at different stages of their training regimen, both to support athletic performance and to promote health and injury prevention. Because an athlete's energy requirements vary from day to day throughout the yearly training plan, relative to changes in training volume and intensity, reliable estimates of energy intake (EI) can be helpful in developing an individualized nutrition plan. An athlete's energy intake from food, fluids, and supplements can be estimated from measured food records, a multipass 24-hour dietary recall, or from food frequency questionnaires (27). For athletes and nonathletes alike, all these methods have limitations, with a bias to the underreporting of intakes (10). Extensive education regarding the purpose and protocols of documenting calorie intake may assist with compliance to the measurement techniques and enhance the accuracy and validity of self-reported information.

Factors that can increase energy needs in athletes (28)
> Exposure to cold or heat
> Fear
> Stress
> High altitude
> Some physical injuries, wound healing
> Stimulant drugs (caffeine, nicotine)
> Increases in **fat-free mass (FFM)**

Factors that can decrease energy needs in athletes (29)
> Aging-related declines in movement and therefore energy expenditure
> Decreases in FFM
> Sedentary behavior between training sessions
> Decreased training volume

Estimating Energy Expenditure

Energy expenditure (EE), or the amount of calories burned by the body, can be measured and estimated using several methods. The body uses energy (expends calories) for three primary reasons.

1. To maintain basic physiological function, such as pumping blood and breathing
2. To process the food we eat
3. To power muscles for all movements—called the **thermic effect of activity (TEA)**

These are examples of the major contributors to energy expenditure, but in fact the body can also use additional fuel to support growth during childhood, adolescence, and pregnancy. In times of stress, such as exposure to cold environments, fever, trauma, and psychological stress, energy expenditure is also increased. The sum of all energy expended over a set period (usually 24 hours) is called the **total energy expenditure (TEE)**. The TEE calculation has several energy expenditure variables that can be measured independently to help estimate TEE.

$$TEE = BMR + TEF + NEAT + TEA$$

Energy Expenditure During Rest

People who are not normally physically active and consider themselves sedentary expend most of their energy at rest to maintain the basic body functions to sustain life. This type of estimated energy expenditure is called **resting energy expenditure (REE)** and is required to maintain body temperature, heartbeat, and other functions. Just like TEE, REE is an absolute measure over a period of time, such as a day. When REE measures are expressed as a rate, or as the number of calories expended per hour, energy expenditure is measured as either the **basal metabolic rate (BMR)** or the **resting metabolic rate (RMR)**. Resting metabolic rate may account for up to 60 to 80 percent of TEE (10).

In research, measuring RMR and BMR involves different procedures that produce slightly different values. The measurement of BMR is more stringent and requires the subject to be lying at rest for an extended period or to have just woken up from a normal overnight sleep and remaining in bed. BMR measures also require a 10- to 12-hour fast and no physical activity for at least 12 hours before measurement. Because these ideal conditions are difficult to meet when studying large groups of human subjects, RMR is often preferred. In measuring RMR, the subject must be in a resting position for several minutes and be 3 to 4 hours removed from a meal or strenuous activity. Because of the differences in the protocols for these measures, RMR values tend to be slightly higher, but most researchers prefer estimating RMR for its practicality. We will use the terms *resting metabolic rate* and *resting energy expenditure* throughout this book.

Factors That Can Alter RMR

We have all heard that exercise can increase your metabolism. The increase is a direct effect of exercise on RMR. Although the absolute change that a person can experience in their RMR is at most around 5 percent, these changes can be meaningful to long-term health. In examinations of large groups of people, variations in RMR can be as much as 25 percent. Large differences in muscle and organ mass account for most of the variation, which helps explain why muscle-building exercise can have a meaningful effect on RMR. Resting muscle tissue and organ tissue make up most of the contribution to RMR because they require more fuel to support metabolic activities. These two tissue compartments, along with the bone tissue and fluids that make up the human body, are collectively known as **lean body mass (LBM)**. Differences in LBM explain 60 to 80 percent of the variation seen in RMR calorie values among individuals (30).

> **? DO YOU KNOW?**
> Two people of approximately the same body weight can have far different RMR values. A person with more LBM will have a significantly higher RMR than someone with lower LBM and higher fat mass.

Several other factors can also create small but meaningful changes in RMR values. First, anything that can change LBM will affect RMR. Age, gender, exercise, and body size are primary influences on LBM. Increasing body size and regular exercise will increase or maintain LBM.

Males typically have more LBM per pound of body weight than females, and LBM steadily falls with increasing age. As we age, RMR falls by about 2 to 3 percent per decade (31). Most of this decrease is attributed to declining LBM, but declining organ function might also contribute. Regular exercise becomes even more valuable as we age because it is a strong stimulus to slowing the loss of LBM, while limiting the gain of fat mass. Body size has a strong influence on metabolic rate because more energy is needed to move a larger mass. A large person will expend more energy (calories) per unit of time doing the same activity than a smaller person. Fitness level and sport experience also influence energy expenditure. Athletes who train for a specific task tend to have stronger muscles with greater endurance that are trained for the specific movements of the competitive task, making them more efficient with energy utilization and conservation.

Thermic Effect of Activity

The energy expenditure required to move our bodies is broadly defined as any movement—not only exercise and sport but also everyday activities and movements required at work. Along with **nonexercise activity thermogenesis (NEAT)**, any type of activity, even fidgeting, is included in this category. Energy expenditure in this category typically accounts for about 15 to 30 percent of TEE (32) but can vary significantly based on duration, mode (walking, running, eating, dancing, etc.), and intensity. Therefore, elite athletes who are committed to training several hours a day can have a thermic effect of activity (TEA) that easily exceeds 50 percent of the TEE for a given day. As a component of TEA, energy expenditure from exercise (EEE) can be estimated in several ways, including activity logs (1–7 days duration), using subjective estimates of exercise intensity; activity codes; and metabolic equivalents (MET) (33-35).

Although RMR represents 60 to 80 percent of TEE for most people, it may be as little as 38 to 47 percent of TEE for elite endurance athletes, who might have a TEA as high as 50 percent of TEE (28).

Energy Expenditure to Process the Food We Consume

Energy expenditure is also required to digest, absorb, and metabolize the food we eat. The metabolic processes involved generate heat, and the energy output is collectively called the **thermic effect of feeding (TEF)**. This phenomenon generally peaks about 1 hour after the consumption of food and usually dissipates within 4 to 5 hours after eating, depending on the amount and composition of the meal. TEF values vary for each of the energy-yielding macronutrients and are highest for protein and lowest for fat. This means that the body is more efficient at storing excess dietary fat as body fat than at converting excess protein and carbohydrate to fat stores. TEF typically accounts for approximately 10 percent of total energy expenditure (36). Although changes in energy-yielding macronutrient distribution of the diet can alter the contribution of TEF to total energy expenditure, the changes are considered to have marginal impact.

Measuring Energy Expenditure

The general measurement of energy expenditure is referred to as **calorimetry** and is further broken down by methodological differences as **direct calorimetry** (mentioned earlier in the chapter) and **indirect calorimetry**. Health care professionals and nutrition and exercise scientists can use these measurements to examine individual differences in energy expenditure and to help understand the effects of age, gender, and exercise on total energy expenditure (table 2.3). Despite

Table 2.3 Thermic Effect of Food Percentage of Energy Expended to Process Food Intake

Energy-yielding macronutrient	% of calories used for digestion, metabolism, and absorption
Protein	20–25
Carbohydrate	5–15
Fat	0–5

improvements in technology, however, measuring energy expenditure is generally not practical. As a result, many energy expenditure equations have been developed and are commonly used for making predictions.

Direct Calorimetry

As you recall from our earlier example of the bomb calorimeter, direct calorimetry measures heat production by the body. When the body breaks down food, it captures some of the energy in ATP production, while losing the rest as heat. When this heat loss is measured, the measure is proportional to the body's total energy expenditure and can be measured directly within a sealed chamber (figure 2.22). With this method, a research subject is typically asked to stay in the chamber for 24 hours. The chambers are typically furnished with a bed and a television and in some cases equipment for exercising. While the person is in the chamber, changes in temperature and oxygen and carbon dioxide gas exchange can be measured to calculate the total calories expended. Although highly accurate, this method is not considered practical for most research studies. The equipment is complex, expensive, and takes up a lot of space. In addition, the chamber must comfortably accommodate people of various sizes while maintaining the precision to measure small changes in temperature. Given the alternative methods available to estimate energy expenditure, direct calorimetry is used primarily in large research universities and institutions with a heavy interest in human research studies investigating changes in metabolism.

Indirect Calorimetry

Indirect calorimetry is a method to determine energy expenditure without directly measuring the production of heat. Methods include measuring oxygen consumption and carbon dioxide production, collectively referred to as gas exchange, and the doubly labeled water technique. Overall, indirect techniques are less expensive than direct calorimetry. These methods are defined as indirect because energy expenditure as heat is not measured. The gas exchange method is based on the principle that our metabolized fuels (i.e., carbohydrate, protein, fat) require oxygen to be completely burned (oxidized). One of the by-products of burning these fuels is carbon dioxide. What is fascinating is that the consumed oxygen and carbon dioxide release is in direct proportion to the amount of fuel burned and the amount of energy (measured as calories) released. During the process, a technician can collect respiratory gases from a volunteer during rest or short bouts of exercise. This task is accomplished by attaching a face mask, using a mouthpiece with the nose closed shut, or by using a canopy system. Although these methods are commonly used in research settings, they are considered cumbersome by

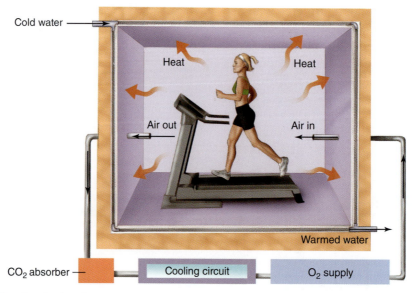

Figure 2.22 Direct calorimeter.

many researchers and research volunteers and thus carry limitations on how effectively they can be used in various living situations (figure 2.23).

The doubly labeled water technique is highly effective at measuring daily energy expenditure over extended periods while subjects are living in their usual environment. This method relies on measuring the stable isotopes of hydrogen and oxygen in excreted water and carbon dioxide. Isotopes are defined as different forms of an element in which the atoms have the same number of protons but different number of neutrons. These isotopes are nonradioactive and safe for human consumption and retain the same characteristics of the usual element, with the only difference being a higher than usual atomic mass. Small amounts of water that are isotopically labeled with deuterium and oxygen-18 (^2H_2O and $H_2{}^{18}O$) are ingested, and the difference between the rates at which the body loses each isotope can be measured to determine energy expenditure. This method is unique and practical because it avoids the need to measure heat and gas exchange. Two types of water are consumed, one with the hydrogen isotope deuterium and the other with an isotope of oxygen. Following consumption, researchers can measure isotope appearance in excreted urine (as ^2H_2O) and examine the difference between the rate of deuterium loss and ^{18}O loss to calculate the output of carbon dioxide and determine TEE. The doubly labeled water method is often considered the gold standard for determining energy expenditure and has been used alongside measuring weight change and diet assessment methods to help determine the validity of energy intake assessment techniques. This method is noninvasive and unobtrusive and allows subjects to act normally in their typical environment. On the other hand, testing protocols are recommended to last at least 14 days for the best accuracy, the technique is not widely available, and it is expensive. Isotopes and equipment to analyze isotope appearance in urine can cost thousands of dollars and are often too costly for many research budgets. Further, this technique is best at giving a summary of energy expenditure over the 14-day protocol period and cannot give information about individual days or day-to-day variability.

Estimating TEE With Prediction Equations

Because the direct measurement of a person's TEE requires costly equipment and training that is not easily accessible outside research settings, energy expenditure is widely estimated by nutrition professionals using a range of equations. Calculated estimates use many variables that are known to have a strong influence on energy expenditure, such as age, height, weight, gender, and fat-free mass. To use various equations effectively, it is important to understand their limitations, recognize the population they are intended for, know

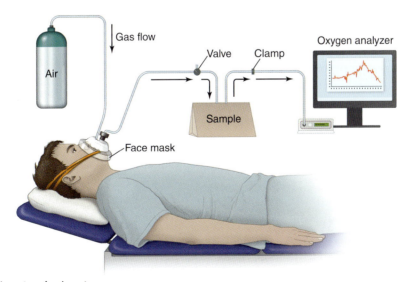

Figure 2.23 Indirect calorimeter.

> ### PUTTING IT INTO PERSPECTIVE
> ## ESTIMATING TOTAL ENERGY EXPENDITURE
>
> Estimate of the total energy expenditure of an 18-year-old college freshman with a height of 183 centimeters (6 ft) and a weight of 73 kilograms (161 lb).
>
> $$TEE = BMR + TEF + NEAT + TEA$$
>
> BMR can be estimated using the Harris-Benedict equation.
> For men, the equation looks like this:
>
> $$BMR = 66.4730 + (13.7516 \times \text{weight in kg}) + (5.0033 \times \text{height in cm}) (6.7550 \times \text{age in yr})$$
>
> Therefore, BMR for this individual is the following:
>
> $$= 66.4730 + (13.7516 \times 73 \text{ kg}) + (5.0033 \times 183 \text{ cm}) (6.7550 \times 18 \text{ yr})$$
>
> $$= 66.4730 + (1{,}003.8668) + (915.6039) (121.59)$$
>
> $$= 1{,}864.35$$
>
> $$\sim 1{,}850\text{--}1{,}900 \text{ kcal}$$
>
> TEF = thermic effect of food; TEA = planned exercise expenditure + spontaneous physical activity + non-exercise activity thermogenesis

what the calculated calorie values mean (i.e., BMR vs. RMR vs. TEE), and, most important, remember that these values are indeed estimates. When predictive equations result in an RMR or BMR value, the next step to determining TEE is to add energy expended from physical activity and the energy expenditure of exercise (EEE).

These are two components of TEA that must be added to RMR and BMR values. Energy expended from physical activity and exercise can be accounted for by using a multiple of the REE based on the level of activity intensity and duration. For example, the activity level for most of the U.S. population is considered light or moderate, and the TEF is about 10 percent of the sum of REE plus the energy expenditure of physical activity. The sum of these three components provides the estimated TEE.

For example, using the Cunningham equation to estimate RMR:

$$RMR = 500 + 22 \text{ (fat-free mass in kg)}$$

A 22-year-old collegiate female swimmer is 5 feet 10 inches (178 cm) tall and weighs 160 pounds (72.6 kg). At 20 percent body fat, she has approximately 58 kilograms of fat-free mass (160 lb × 0.2 = 32 lb; 160 lb − 32 lb = 128; 128 lb/2.2 lb/kg = 58.2 kg).

$$RMR = 500 + 22(58.2 \text{ kg})$$

$$RMR = 500 + 1{,}280$$

$$RMR = 1{,}780 \text{ kcal/d}$$

Techniques used to measure or estimate components of TEE in sedentary and moderately active populations can also be applied to athletes. But this approach has some limitations, particularly in highly competitive athletes (10). As previously discussed, it is more practical to measure resting metabolic rate (RMR), but a reasonable estimate of BMR can be obtained using either the Cunningham (37) or the Harris-Benedict (38) equations, applying an appropriate activity factor to estimate TEE.

The perfect energy expenditure prediction equation does not currently exist. Practitioners often use a combination of methods when working with athletes and refine their intervention over time based on new data becoming available, such as changes in weight, a new body composition assessment, changing training volume, and so on. They must use caution in applying these methods because RMR may over- or underestimate requirements by 10 to 20 percent. Remember that RMR is only one factor that accounts for TEE and should not be overemphasized without careful consideration of the other variables that make up TEE.

PUTTING IT INTO PERSPECTIVE

WEARABLE ACTIVITY MONITORS AND DEVICES

If you observe exercisers in a gym, you will see many people wearing a physical activity tracker or exercise monitor. These accelerometry-based devices allow us to estimate physical activity and energy expenditure (EE), as well as track data over time using the Internet or on a cell phone. Improvements in technology and reduced costs have resulted in a flood of various brands of physical activity monitors, making these devices highly accessible (39). The monitors are valuable in that they can provide a stimulus to promote behavioral change to increase physical activity and manage energy intake, leading to long-term metabolic health and reduced risk for diabetes, cardiovascular disease, and other conditions (39).

Do you question the accuracy of these devices? Their limitations? The wide variety of brands available suggests a wide range in quality. Some devices are more accurate than others. Accelerometer-based devices provide measures of body movement with validity derived from studies using doubly labeled water. Generally, commercially available monitors score lower in measures of step count and energy expenditure accuracy than more sophisticated activity monitors used for health research. A recent study examined the validity of eight consumer-based, activity-monitoring technologies using estimates of EE from a portable metabolic analyzer as a comparison. Absolute percent error ranged from approximately 9 to 23.5 percent. Overall, the performance and overall accuracy of these monitors is impressive (40).

The most important feature of these devices is that they promote increased physical activity (40). Meanwhile, companies are trying to entice more consumers by making monitors that provide goal-setting features, tracking tools, and social networking links, which could have implications for behaviorally focused research applications (41).

ENERGY AVAILABILITY IN SPORT

Energy availability (EA) is a relatively new topic in the field of sports nutrition. EA extends beyond the study of energy balance (EB) by considering the energy requirements needed to promote optimal health and function during periods of high EEE. Energy availability is defined as dietary intake minus exercise energy expenditure normalized to FFM. The resulting number from this calculation is the amount of energy available to the body to perform all other functions after the cost of exercise is subtracted (42).

The concept of EA emerged from the study of the **female athlete triad (triad)**, which started as a recognition of the interrelatedness of clinical issues with disordered eating, menstrual dysfunction, and low bone mineral density in female athletes (42). The concept then evolved into a broader understanding of the concerns associated with any movement along the spectra away from optimal energy availability, menstrual status, and bone health (43). Low EA can occur from insufficient energy intake, high TEE, or a combination of the two. It might also be associated with disordered eating, a misguided or excessively rapid program for loss of body mass, or inadvertent failure to meet energy requirements during a period of high-volume training or competition (42). It is now thought that additional physiological consequences may occur beyond that found in the female athlete triad and may also affect male athletes. Potential complications may contribute to endocrine, gastrointestinal, renal, neuropsychiatric, musculoskeletal, and cardiovascular dysfunction (43).

To capture the negative effects of low EA in both male and female athletes, an extension of the triad has been proposed, called **relative energy deficiency in sport (RED-S)**. RED-S is as an inclusive description of the entire cluster of physiological complications observed in male and female athletes who consume energy intakes insufficient to meet the needs for optimal body function after the energy cost of exercise has been removed (44). Regardless of the terminology used to describe low EA, this phenomenon may compromise athletic performance in the short and long term for both male and female athletes.

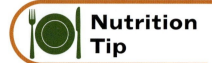

Nutrition Tip: Low EA is not synonymous with negative EB or weight loss. If reduction in EA is associated with a reduction in RMR, it may produce a new steady state of energy balance or weight stability at a lowered energy intake that is insufficient to provide for healthy body function.

Screening and treatment guidelines have been established for management of low EA (43, 44).

Potential performance effects of RED-S might include decreased endurance, increased injury risk, decreased training response, impaired judgment, decreased coordination, decreased concentration, irritability, depression, decreased glycogen stores, and decreased muscle strength (44). In terms of health, RED-S can negatively affect menstrual function, bone health, endocrine, metabolic, hematological, growth and development, psychological, cardiovascular, gastrointestinal, and immunological systems (10). It is now recognized that impairments of health and function occur across the continuum of reductions in EA, rather than occurring uniformly at an EA threshold, and require further research (44).

SUMMARY

The understanding of energy metabolism is essential to building a solid foundation for understanding the nutrition needs to support all forms of physical activity and exercise. Energy from the foods we consume is converted into a usable chemical form of energy that our bodies can use (ATP). ATP is generated by three distinct energy systems that work together in concert using several metabolic pathways to fuel muscle contraction. Several substrates are used by the energy systems to meet our ATP demands, including phosphocreatine, carbohydrate, protein, fat, and alcohol. We use calories as our universal energy currency to estimate the amount of energy we consume and expend. Several methods are available to measure both energy intake and expenditure that vary in their practicality, accuracy, time commitment, and cost. Collectively, these methods provide a mechanism to assess important aspects of energy metabolism in athletes, including energy balance and energy availability.

FOR REVIEW

1. What is energy? What are the various forms of energy? Which form of energy is most important to human physiology?
2. List the energy systems used by the body to make ATP. How do they differ in complexity, lag time, and capacity to make ATP?
3. Describe the crossover concept and explain the most important physiological adaptations that occur because of training.
4. Describe the fuel substrates that the body uses to make ATP. What is the only substrate that can be used to make ATP anaerobically?
5. Differentiate between BMR, RMR, TEA, TEE, and TEF, as defined in this chapter.
6. Several metabolic pathways were described in this chapter. List the metabolic pathways used by each energy system and where in the cell these pathways occur.
7. From the food that we eat, describe some of the metabolic fates of glucose, lipid, and amino acids that are digested and absorbed.
8. Explain how mitochondria generate ATP aerobically. How is oxygen used? How are hydrogen ions and electrons delivered to the mitochondria?

PART II

ROLE OF ENERGY-YIELDING MACRONUTRIENTS

Energy-yielding macronutrients are covered in chapters 3, 4, and 5. Foods providing carbohydrate, protein, and fat provide an array of vitamins, minerals, and, in the case of plant-based foods, plant compounds that support good health. Therefore, carbohydrate, protein, and fat can have different effects on long-term health and disease risk factors.

Slower digesting high-fiber carbohydrate-rich foods are beneficial for health and reducing chronic disease risk. A faster digesting low-fiber carbohydrate-rich food is helpful before, during, and after exercise because it is a quick, easy-to-digest source of energy. Proteins vary based on their digestibility and amino acid profile. Protein helps make up structures in the body. Dietary fat is energy dense, has many metabolic roles, and some fats affect disease risk factors. Within the body, fat also has essential roles in structure and function.

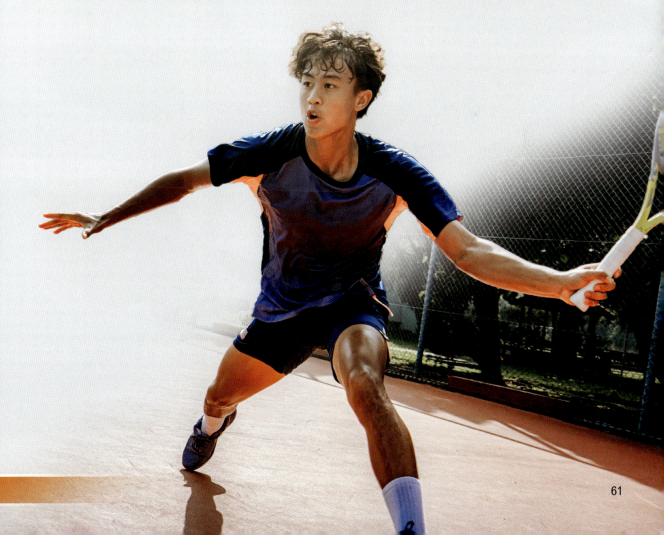

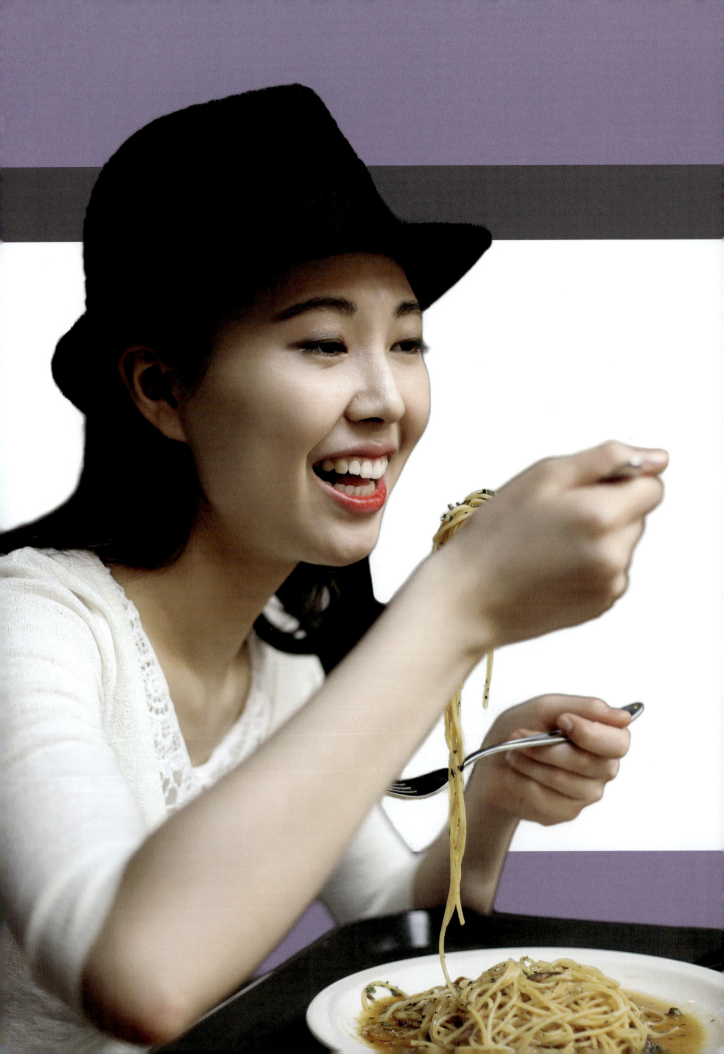

3

Carbohydrate

> **CHAPTER OBJECTIVES**
>
> After completing this chapter, you will be able to do the following:
> - Identify the classification of carbohydrate.
> - Describe the digestion and absorption of carbohydrate.
> - Discuss the metabolic fate of glucose once inside the body.
> - Describe how glucose is regulated in the body.
> - Explain the relationship between carbohydrate and exercise performance.
> - Discuss the role of carbohydrate in fatigue during exercise.
> - Identify carbohydrate recommendations for the general population, active people, and athletes.
> - Identify the carbohydrate content of common foods.
> - Discuss the role of carbohydrate in health.

Carbohydrate is an organic compound derived from plants and contains the elements carbon, hydrogen, and oxygen. Through **photosynthesis** (figure 3.1), plants use energy from the sun, which interacts with water and minerals in the soil and carbon dioxide in the air to produce glucose, the simplest form of carbohydrate. The primary purpose of carbohydrate in the human body, both at rest and during physical activity, is as a fuel source (1). Carbohydrate is an energy source for most cells in the body, a preferred fuel source for nerve and brain cells, and the required fuel for red blood cells. During physical activity, the biologically usable form of energy for the skeletal muscle, ATP, can be generated from both dietary and stored carbohydrate. The amount and source of carbohydrate that the skeletal muscle uses depends on the length and intensity of exercise and the amount of carbohydrate available (2).

In this chapter, we provide an overview of the types of carbohydrate and how they are digested, absorbed, metabolized, and stored in the human body during rest and exercise. Dietary recommendations, food sources, and the role of carbohydrate in health and disease are also discussed.

CLASSIFICATION OF CARBOHYDRATE

Carbohydrate is often classified into one of two primary classes that describe the physical structure of the nutrient: **simple carbohydrates** are relatively small compounds composed of either one or two sugar molecules, whereas **complex carbohydrates** are larger compounds that contain more than three sugar molecules joined together (1).

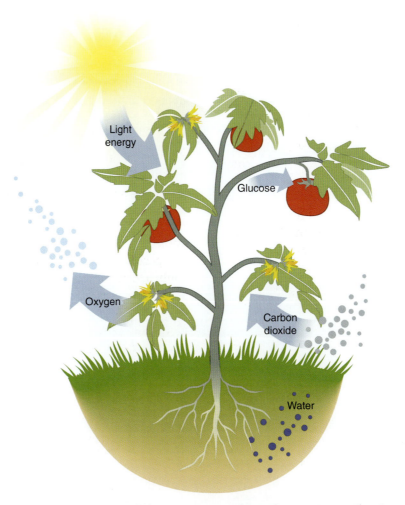

Figure 3.1 During photosynthesis, plants use energy from the sun to synthesize glucose.

Simple Carbohydrates

Monosaccharides and disaccharides are commonly referred to as simple carbohydrates, or **simple sugars**. The simplest unit of a carbohydrate is a monosaccharide—*mono* meaning "one" and *saccharide* meaning "sugar" (figure 3.2). Three common monosaccharides are present in the human diet: glucose, fructose, and galactose. All contain the elements carbon, hydrogen, and oxygen, but they differ slightly in their structure and in their level of sweetness. **Glucose** is an abundant sugar molecule in the human diet. **Fructose** is the sweetest of the monosaccharides and is sometimes referred to as fruit sugar. Although fructose is naturally found in fruits, it can also be found in processed foods, most commonly in the form of high-fructose corn syrup or sucrose. **Galactose** is not usually found alone in foods; rather, it is most commonly bound to glucose to form the disaccharide lactose (1, 3).

Two monosaccharides joined together are called **disaccharides**—*di* meaning "two" (figure 3.3). The chemical bond holding these together can be broken (digested) by the action of enzymes in the human digestive tract, thereby releasing the component monosaccharides from one another. The common natural disaccharides in the human diet are sucrose, lactose, and maltose. **Sucrose** is the sweetest and most common of the disaccharides and is composed of one glucose molecule and one fructose molecule. Sucrose can be found naturally in sugar cane, sugar beets, honey, and to some extent fruits and vegetables, but it is more commonly processed into "table sugar" and added

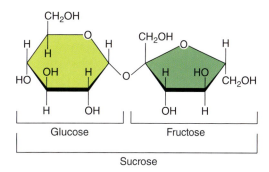

Figure 3.3 Disaccharide.

to a variety of foods during processing. **Lactose** is composed of one glucose molecule and one galactose molecule and is called "milk sugar" because it is found naturally in dairy products. **Maltose** is composed of two glucose molecules joined together. It is not commonly found in foods but rather as a by-product of the breakdown of larger carbohydrate compounds, such as starch. Maltose also forms as a result of the fermentation process during production of some alcoholic beverages. But the complete fermentation reaction results in a final low maltose concentration, so these alcoholic beverages are not a good source of dietary carbohydrate (1, 4).

Complex Carbohydrates

Complex carbohydrates are assemblies of at least three and as many as thousands of monosaccharide molecules. The term *complex carbohydrate* was once used to describe a slower digestive process compared with sugars, but now the term refers only to the chemical structure of the molecule, not digestive speed. Relatively shorter assemblies of only 3 to 10 monosaccharides are referred to as **oligosaccharides**, and larger assemblies are called polysaccharides. Oligosaccharides are commonly found in beans, legumes, some cruciferous vegetables, whole grains, and some manufactured products such as sports drinks. These usually appear on a food label as fructooligosaccharides, maltodextrins, or polydextrose. Polysaccharides have more than 10 monosaccharides and are primarily found in the form of starch and fiber. **Starch** is the primary form of carbohydrate polysaccharide found in plants and consists of simple chains of glucose molecules joined together by **alpha bonds**, which are breakable by human digestive enzymes. The most common forms of starch are

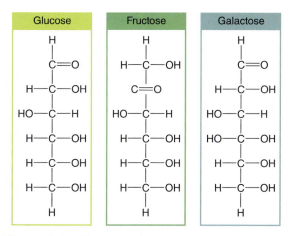

Figure 3.2 Monosaccharides.

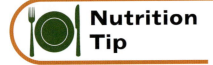

Glucose is the form of fuel the brain depends on for functioning. Research studies have demonstrated that reduced glucose availability can negatively alter attention, memory, and learning in people who regularly consume carbohydrate in their diet (as opposed to those who have adapted to a lower-carbohydrate diet). Consuming adequate dietary carbohydrate throughout the day can reverse these dips in glucose levels. The brain also has increased glucose demands as mental tasks become more challenging. Studying for exams and completing assignments require higher cognitive function, so a steady glucose supply to the brain is critical. Do not skip meals and snacks during times of mental stress, when cognition is important for success (1, 3).

amylose, which is a straight chain of glucose molecules, and **amylopectin**, which is a branched chain of the same molecules. Once consumed and digested into its component monosaccharides, the glucose molecules from starch are absorbed into the bloodstream and become indistinguishable from all other glucose molecules in the body (1, 4).

❓ DO YOU KNOW?

Companies are not required to enrich their food products, but enriched white flour has thiamin, riboflavin, niacin, iron, and folic acid, all nutrients lost during processing and added back through enrichment (5).

Fiber is another type of carbohydrate polysaccharide found in plants. It is similar to starch; both contain long chains of glucose molecules joined by bonds, except that the bonds in fiber are **beta bonds** that cannot be broken by human enzymes. Thus, fiber is not absorbed and metabolized in the human body. Nonetheless, fiber does possess health benefits, which are discussed later in this chapter. From a structural standpoint, fiber can be classified as soluble or insoluble. **Soluble fibers** are generally found in and around plant tissue cells, are dissolvable in water, have a gel-like consistency when wet, and are digested by gut bacteria (**fermentation**). Common sources include citrus fruit, berries, oats, and beans. **Insoluble fibers** are the structural component of plant cell walls, are not dissolvable in water, and are usually not fermentable. They are commonly found in the outer husks of whole grains, fruits, vegetables, and legumes. The structural classification of fiber does not adequately describe how insoluble and soluble fibers behave once inside the human body, so another way of viewing fiber is from the standpoint of how it affects physiological processes. For example, different fibers have varying effects on gastric emptying, postmeal blood glucose levels, and the absorption of dietary fat and cholesterol from the gut. In other words, some fibers are better than others at improving **satiety**, making a person feel fuller for a longer time, blunting the rise in blood sugar after eating, and improving serum lipid levels (total and LDL cholesterol). The Institute of Medicine uses the terms *dietary fiber* and *functional fiber* for those isolated, nondigestible food or commercially produced carbohydrates (6) to describe the different effects that fibers have on physiological processes within the human body.

The third category of carbohydrate polysaccharide is called **glycogen**. Glycogen is the storage form of carbohydrates (glucose) in humans and animals, where it is stored primarily in the liver and skeletal muscle. Glycogen and starch are similar in that they are chains of glucose molecules; they differ in that glycogen is much more highly branched and contains greater surface area for enzymatic action (figure 3.4). In addition, glycogen stored in the liver and muscle in its hydrated form contains three to four parts water (2, 7). Approximately three-quarters of the glycogen in the body is stored in skeletal muscle; the remaining quarter is stored in the liver.

❓ DO YOU KNOW?

When animals are prepared for sale as meat or poultry, most of their glycogen is lost through enzymatic action in the tissue. Glycogen is converted to lactic acid, which contributes to a desirable texture and tenderness of the meat (8). As a result, animal meat and poultry are rich sources of protein and fat (depending on the cut—some cuts are low in fat), but they lack appreciable amounts of carbohydrate.

PUTTING IT INTO PERSPECTIVE

WHAT IS MULTIGRAIN?

Terms like "multigrain" or "seven grain" are not synonymous with *whole grain*. Whole grains contain the bran, germ, and endosperm of the grain kernel and are rich in nutrients. *Multigrain* means only that the product contains more than one type of grain. These grains may or not be whole grains and might not be healthier choices. In general, when checking food labels, if you don't see the term "whole grain" or "whole wheat," you should assume that the product has lost nutrients during processing and has been enriched (9).

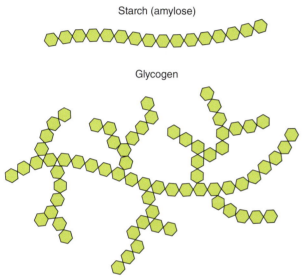

Figure 3.4 Structure of starch and glycogen.

Complex carbohydrates vary extensively in quality from the standpoint of the level of processing they undergo from farm to table. Some carbohydrates have been minimally processed and are made of **whole grains**. Refined grains have been extensively processed, to the point that some components of the whole grain have been removed or added back to make the product more palatable. Whole grains contain all the nutrients and fiber that nature intended, but processed grains have much less fiber and fewer naturally occurring vitamins and minerals (though some vitamins and minerals are added back through a process called **enrichment**). Enriched products may have lower or higher levels of some nutrients than their unprocessed counterparts (1, 3, 4, 9).

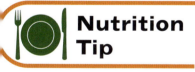 **Nutrition Tip**
When choosing food products, quality carbohydrates are those made from whole-grain flour and usually have the term "whole grain" on the label. A Whole Grain Stamp has been introduced in an attempt to simplify the shopping process for consumers. There are two varieties of the Whole Grain Stamp: the "basic stamp" and the "100% stamp." If a product displays the 100% stamp, all of its grain ingredients are whole grains and contain a minimum of 16 grams (a full serving) of whole grain. A product with the basic stamp has a minimum of 8 grams of whole grain but may also contain some refined grain. The stamps can be helpful but might also be misleading because not all products that display the stamps are the best choices for health. This caution is especially true in the cereal aisle, where products may contain whole grains but also have significant levels of added sugars. When checking food labels, beware of terms such as "wheat" and "wheat flour" (rather than "whole wheat") because these indicate that parts of the grain, along with the vitamins and minerals within the grain, are likely missing. The term "whole grain" usually indicates the product contains at least one type of whole grain; "whole wheat" indicates the specific type of grain used. Either term may identify a food rich in fiber, vitamins, and minerals. Many nutrition professionals recommend looking for a "whole food" label in addition to the term "whole grain." A **rule of five** can be used to find whole-grain products that are generally better for health. A good choice will have 5 grams or more of fiber per serving of the food and less than 5 grams of sugar per serving (10).

DIGESTION AND ABSORPTION

The **digestive tract** is essentially a long tube within the body extending from the **mouth** to the anus and whose purpose is to facilitate the digestion of food and subsequent absorption of nutrients into the body. Any food contained in the digestive tract is not considered to be part of the body until it is broken down into smaller components (**digestion**) and moved across the wall of the digestive tract into the bloodstream (absorption). A critical feature of digestion is excretion of undesirable or indigestible material from the diet (elimination). The digestive tract contains multiple segments, some of which contribute to breaking food down into smaller components that can move across the wall of the digestive tract and into the body. The primary segments of the digestive tract where carbohydrate digestion and absorption occur are the mouth and the small intestine (figure 3.5) (1, 3).

Carbohydrate in the diet is in the form of sugars, starches, and fibers, most of which are too large to be absorbed in their consumed form and must be broken down along the digestive tract. Digestion of carbohydrate begins in the mouth. Chewing food causes **mechanical digestion**. Chewing physically breaks large polysaccharides into smaller ones, and the salivary glands in the mouth secrete an enzyme called **salivary amylase** that begins the **chemical digestion** of polysaccharides. Digestion of carbohydrate in the mouth is not complete; the broken-down polysaccharides are still not small enough to cross the walls of the digestive tract. The amount of digestion occurring in the mouth depends primarily on the extent of chewing and the length of time food stays in the mouth before swallowing. Once swallowed, the carbohydrate exits the mouth and does not receive further significant digestion until it reaches the **small intestine**, which is the segment of the digestive tract where most of the carbohydrate digestion and absorption occurs (figure 3.6). The intestinal wall is composed of numerous folds called **villi** that increase the surface area for absorption. The villi contain an abundance of absorptive cells

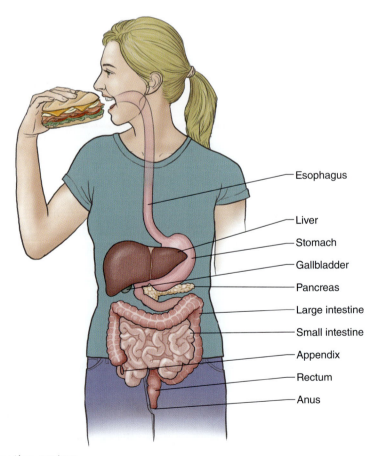

Figure 3.5 The digestive system.

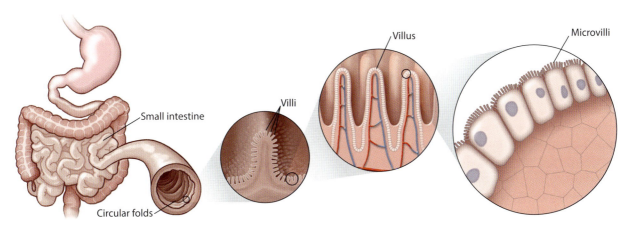

Figure 3.6 Villi and microvilli of the small intestine.

called **enterocytes**, each of which has brushlike projections called **microvilli** that further increase the surface area for absorption (1, 3).

> **? DO YOU KNOW?**
>
> Virtually all chemical carbohydrate digestion ceases in the stomach because of its extremely acidic environment, which destroys salivary amylase. But some digestion of carbohydrate does continue, particularly mechanical digestion caused by the churning of the stomach.

The primary forms of carbohydrate upon entering the small intestine are oligosaccharides, polysaccharides, and some disaccharides but very few monosaccharides. Because only monosaccharides can be absorbed into the bloodstream, a great deal of processing is still needed to convert carbohydrates into monosaccharides in the small intestine. Unlike in the mouth, where mechanical digestion by chewing is significant, no such events occur in the small intestine. In fact, virtually all carbohydrate digestion in the small intestine is chemical digestion involving enzymes released by the pancreas. The **pancreas** is an accessory organ that helps facilitate digestion by secreting many enzymes into the small intestine. One such enzyme is **pancreatic amylase**, which helps further break down polysaccharides into disaccharides, primarily maltose. Additional enzymes, namely, **maltase**, **sucrase**, and **lactase**, are secreted by cells in the intestinal wall to aid in the terminal digestion of disaccharides into their component monosaccharides (1, 3) (table 3.1).

The monosaccharides can then cross the intestinal wall and be absorbed into the body. Monosaccharides in the small intestine enter the enterocytes and move into the bloodstream through capillaries adjacent to the villi on enterocytes. An active transport process requiring ATP absorbs both glucose and galactose, but fructose relies on a more passive diffusion process that does not require ATP. This difference in the manner in which the monosaccharides are absorbed results in a slower absorption of fructose than that of glucose and galactose, which means that fructose tends to remain in the small intestine longer (3, 11).

Table 3.1 Enzymes Involved in the Digestion of Carbohydrates

Organ	Enzyme	Action
Mouth	Salivary amylase	Breaks down starch in the mouth
Pancreas	Pancreatic amylase	Breaks down starch in the small intestine
Small intestine	Maltase	Breaks down maltose to two glucose monosaccharides
Small intestine	Sucrase	Breaks down sucrose to the monosaccharides glucose and fructose
Small intestine	Lactase	Breaks down lactose to glucose and galactose

METABOLISM OF CARBOHYDRATE

After the monosaccharides are absorbed by the small intestine and enter the bloodstream, they are transported to the **liver**, where fructose and galactose undergo significant transformations. Most of fructose and galactose monosaccharides are converted to glucose in the liver, although there are other relatively insignificant fates for these monosaccharides. The key point here is that glucose is the primary usable form of carbohydrate in the body, and virtually all ingested carbohydrates are ultimately converted to glucose for use or storage.

Assuming glucose as the definitive starting point, there are several *metabolic fates* for glucose, depending primarily on the energy needs of the body cells (figure 3.7). If cells of the body need energy, they use glucose to generate ATP; otherwise, glucose is stored in a different form (primarily glycogen in the liver and muscle) for later use as a reserve or is converted to fatty acids and stored in adipose tissue (1, 3).

Glycogen storage is favored after an energy-depleting workout and when glucose and the hormone insulin are present after the consumption or ingestion of carbohydrate. On average, the liver can store approximately 70 to 110 grams of glycogen (280 to 440 kcal) and the skeletal muscle 120 to 500 grams (480 to 2,000 kcal) (table 3.2). These values can vary greatly depending on habitual dietary intake, dietary manipulation for training and competition, muscle mass, and physiological adaptations to training (1, 2, 12-14).

Because the liver and skeletal muscle have limited storage capacity for glycogen, excess glucose is typically metabolized into an alternate form of energy storage that is virtually limitless—that is, adipose tissue. Liver cells, and to a lesser extent fat cells (**adipocytes**), can convert glucose into fatty acids through a process called lipogenesis. Fatty acids combine with glycerol to form triglycerides and are stored in adipose tissue. Note that this process is only appreciable when carbohydrate is consumed in *excess of need* or amount expended during physical activity. If an excessive amount of blood glucose is not being metabolized properly or quickly enough, the glucose can be excreted in the urine. This condition is most commonly seen in a person with uncontrolled diabetes mellitus (1, 3).

> **? DO YOU KNOW?**
> The amount of glucose circulating in your blood is small and, unless replenished by reserves in your muscle and liver, can provide only enough energy for you to walk about one mile (1, 3).

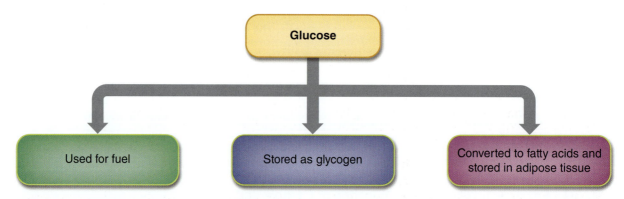

Figure 3.7 Metabolic fates of glucose.

Table 3.2 Typical Glucose and Glycogen Content in the Human Body

Source	Amount (g)	Amount (kcal)
Blood glucose	5–25	20–100
Liver glycogen	70–110	280–440
Muscle glycogen	120–500	480–2,000

Based on Ivy (1991); Jensen et al. (2011); Karpinski and Rosenbloom (2017); Kenney, Wilmore, and Costill (2015); Thompson, Manore, and Vaughan (2017).

> ### PUTTING IT INTO PERSPECTIVE
> #### GLYCOGEN STORAGE IS LIMITED
> Although dietary strategies are used to maximize the amount of glycogen stored in the liver and skeletal muscle, the amount is limited because of the size of the liver and muscles. You cannot simply grow new muscle tissue in response to excess dietary carbohydrate. If that were true, you would not need resistance train to increase muscle mass. Instead, you could eat an abundant amount of carbohydrate without exercise, and your skeletal muscle would expand to accommodate (1, 3).

REGULATION OF GLUCOSE METABOLISM

Because glucose is an important biological substrate required by almost every cell in the body, the process of managing the various fates of glucose is tightly controlled to ensure sufficient glucose availability and delivery to cells that need it. The term *glucose metabolism* encompasses all the activities that, among other functions, regulate the amount of glucose (*a*) circulating in blood, (*b*) used to produce ATP by cells, (*c*) stored as glycogen in skeletal muscle and the liver, (*d*) converted to fatty acids and stored in adipose tissue, and (*e*) synthesized from noncarbohydrate precursors to glucose whenever glucose is in short supply in the body.

Blood glucose is normally maintained within the range of 70 to 100 mg/dl under fasting conditions. This range of blood glucose under normal conditions in a healthy person is widely accepted to be sufficient to provide nourishment to the body's cells under normal resting conditions. Blood glucose values below this range are considered hypoglycemic, within the range **euglycemic** and above the range **hyperglycemic** (see chapter 14). Having acute fluctuations after and between carbohydrate-containing meals is normal, but depending on the amount of carbohydrate consumed, blood glucose levels usually return to resting levels between 30 minutes and 2 hours after eating. A person who has chronic hypoglycemia (low blood sugar) or hyperglycemia (high blood sugar) may have a condition such as diabetes mellitus or impaired carbohydrate metabolism. Diabetes mellitus is characterized by chronic hyperglycemia caused by the cells' inability to uptake glucose sufficiently and metabolize it for fuel. Diabetes mellitus is a potentially dangerous medical condition, often suspected when fasting blood glucose levels exceed 126 mg/dl, but looming dangers are associated with fasting blood glucose levels that are only moderately elevated (between 100 and 125 mg/dl), because these levels might indicate impaired glucose tolerance, a type of prediabetes (1, 3).

> ### ? DO YOU KNOW?
> Although fasting blood glucose levels may indicate diabetes mellitus, many physicians won't diagnose this disease unless a patient fails an **oral glucose tolerance test (OGTT)**. During this test, the patient consumes 75 grams of glucose, and blood samples are drawn every 30 to 60 minutes over the next 3 hours. At the end of the test period, blood glucose values between 140 and 200 mg/dl indicate impaired glucose tolerance, and a value of 200 mg/dl or higher suggests diabetes.

What causes fasting blood glucose levels to rise in people with impaired glucose metabolism? The answer lies in the inability of body cells to import glucose into the cell. For cells to use glucose for energy or storage, the glucose molecules must first enter the cell by crossing its **cell membrane** (figure 3.8).

Glucose molecules are too large to cross cell membranes and usually require assistance from transport proteins located in the cell membrane, which physically move glucose from the space outside the cell into the cell's cytoplasm. These transport proteins tend to remain inside the cytoplasm and move to the cell membrane only when needed to carry glucose into the cell. How does the cell know that glucose needs to be transported? For most cells, the mechanism involves the hormone **insulin**, which is secreted into the bloodstream by the **beta cells** of the pancreas

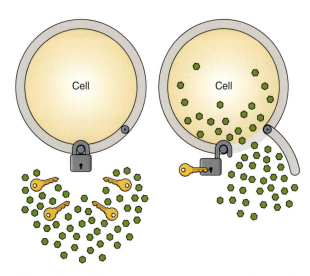

Figure 3.8 Glucose transport into a cell. Insulin is like a key that opens the lock on a door, allowing glucose to enter the cell.

in response to elevated blood glucose. Insulin binds to receptors on the cell membranes and triggers the glucose transport proteins (primarily **GLUT4**) to move from the cytoplasm to the cell membrane and begin shuttling glucose across the cell membrane back into the cytoplasm. This process is known as **insulin-dependent glucose transport (IDGT)** and is often described as a lock-and-key mechanism in which insulin is the key that unlocks the membrane and allows glucose to enter. When IDGT fails to work properly, glucose does not enter the cell and tends to build up outside the cell and in the blood, resulting in elevated blood glucose levels. IDGT may fail because the pancreas cannot produce insulin, so no insulin is available to trigger glucose uptake. This is the cause of type 1 diabetes mellitus. IDGT may also fail because the cell becomes insensitive to insulin (the key does not fit), and even though insulin is available it does not have the normal effect of signaling glucose transport proteins to the cell membrane, which is what causes type 2 diabetes mellitus. Not all glucose imported into a cell requires an insulin trigger. In fact, all brain cells and some liver cells use an insulin-independent process, and exercising skeletal muscle can also take up glucose without requiring insulin when glucose demand is high in order to generate ATP for that activity, a situation that can be quite opportune (1, 3).

What happens when blood glucose levels temporarily drop, such as when carbohydrate is not eaten for a period of time? Transient hypoglycemia triggers the pancreas to secrete the hormone **glucagon**, which has an action opposite that of insulin. Whereas insulin is released as blood glucose concentration increases, glucagon is secreted during hypoglycemia. This dual function underscores how important the pancreas is in the regulation of glucose homeostasis in the body. Glucagon stimulates the liver to break down stored glycogen to glucose (glycogenolysis), which is then released into the bloodstream. In addition, glucagon also stimulates the intrinsic (naturally occurring within the body) synthesis of glucose from noncarbohydrate precursors (gluconeogenesis). Two gluconeogenic pathways commonly convert different noncarbohydrate precursors to glucose—namely, the glucose-alanine cycle (amino acids) and the Cori cycle (lactate). Refer to chapter 2 for a review of these pathways. The combined effect of the two glucagon-stimulated processes, glycogenolysis and gluconeogenesis, is to increase the quantity of glucose circulating in blood (figure 3.9) (1-3).

In addition to insulin and glucagon, other hormones contribute to the regulation of blood glucose levels, especially during periods of increased physical activity (table 3.3). Epinephrine and norepinephrine released into the bloodstream increase significantly with the onset of exercise and work together to stimulate glycogenolysis to make glucose readily available to working skeletal muscle. Cortisol also plays a role in raising blood glucose during exercise through its stimulatory effects on gluconeogenesis (1-3).

Preventing hypoglycemia during physical activity is a unique challenge for the body that is far different from what is required when at rest. Exercise creates an internal body environment that allows skeletal muscles to take up glucose from blood through non-insulin-dependent glucose transport. As glucose is taken up by the muscle, blood glucose concentrations fall, and glucagon rises and stimulates both glycogenolysis and gluconeogenesis to help restore blood glucose levels to normal. Exercising muscle appears to prefer stored glycogen as its carbohydrate source; gluconeogenesis is a secondary system, providing a small amount of glucose to muscle in the later

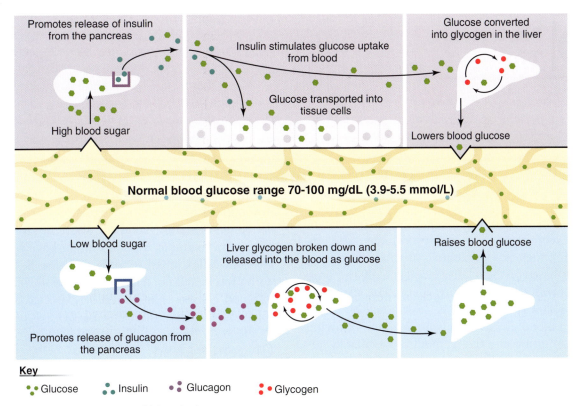

Figure 3.9 Regulation of blood glucose.

Table 3.3 Hormones Involved in Blood Glucose Regulation

Hormone	Secreting organ	Action
Epinephrine	Adrenal gland	Activates glycogenolysis
Norepinephrine	Adrenal gland	Activates glycogenolysis
Cortisol	Adrenal gland	Activates gluconeogenesis
Glucagon	Pancreas	Activates gluconeogenesis and glycogenolysis
Insulin	Pancreas	Activates glycogen synthesis Decreases gluconeogenesis

Data from Ross et al. (2014); Thompson, Manore, and Vaughan (2017).

stages of prolonged exercise but ultimately cannot keep up with energy demands. This process is finite, because eventually the glucose production through these mechanisms cannot keep up with energy needs (1-3).

GLYCEMIC RESPONSE

It is well established that eating carbohydrates causes insulin and blood glucose levels to rise for a time after consumption before returning to baseline values. But the rapidity, magnitude, and duration of this rise, better known as the **glycemic response**, is not easily predicted because many variables influence it. For many years, it was assumed that simple sugars caused a greater glycemic response than complex carbohydrates, but this simplistic theory has since been discarded. The chemical classification of carbohydrates does not fully describe the effects on digestion and metabolism. Newer theories based on the glycemic index and glycemic load of foods more accurately explain the glycemic response observed after consuming various foods (15).

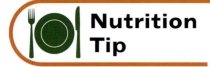

Nutrition Tip Many people choose foods low in glycemic index (GI) to help them lose weight; the research studies, however, are mixed, and some report no significant differences in energy intake or body weight as a result of eating a low-GI diet. One study did report that a low GI diet in combination with high protein enhanced weight loss and prevented weight regain (16). Until more research is available to support the use of low GI diets for weight loss, a combination of an overall healthy, energy-restricted diet and regular exercise remains the most common recommendation for losing weight.

Glycemic Index

Glycemic index, a concept first introduced in 1981, continues to be employed today. The glycemic index is a qualitative method of ranking foods based on the relative blood glucose response observed after ingesting them. The glycemic index of a specific food is determined by measuring blood glucose levels for 2 hours following consumption of a fixed amount of available carbohydrate (e.g., 50 g) and then comparing these results with the blood glucose response observed following consumption of the same amount of a reference food, such as pure glucose. Foods that cause a large blood glucose response compared with the reference food have a high glycemic index, and foods causing a relatively low blood glucose response have a low glycemic index. The reference food is usually assumed to have a glycemic index of 100, meaning that all foods causing a lower blood glucose response than the reference food have a glycemic index below 100 and vice versa. This system has a few limitations. Published glycemic index values of the same foods may vary considerably because of differences in ingredients used, ripeness, method of food processing, cooking methods, and food storage (17-19).

Also, people rarely consume a single food item in isolation, and addition of other foods to a carbohydrate-containing food will affect the glycemic index. For example, a potato might have a high glycemic index in isolation, but when consumed with protein and fat, it causes a much slower rise in blood glucose than would be expected based solely on glycemic index (15, 20, 21).

Glycemic Load

In 1997 the concept of **glycemic load** was introduced in an attempt to quantify the overall glycemic response of a portion of food, not just the amount of available carbohydrate. The glycemic load is an indicator of the blood glucose response that results from total carbohydrate ingestion. The formula for determining glycemic load is the following:

$$\text{Glycemic load} = \text{glycemic index of the food} \times \text{g CHO per portion} \div 100$$

It is possible for a food to have a high glycemic index and low glycemic load if consumed in a small quantity, and vice versa when a larger portion size is consumed. Glycemic index should never be the sole factor considered when con-

PUTTING IT INTO PERSPECTIVE

GLYCEMIC INDEX IS A TOOL, NOT A RULE

Glycemic index is an empirical measurement that can never truly be duplicated because it is impossible to repeat the test on exactly the same person under the exact same conditions (i.e., time of day) and using the exact same food (i.e., same cooking time, same cooking method, same state of maturation or ripening, etc.). Moreover, the glycemic response to a specific food in one person can be quite different from that observed in another. Furthermore, glycemic index is based on a set amount of carbohydrate, not necessarily a typical portion of the food. For example, carrots might have a high glycemic index, but a large portion is needed for a significant blood glucose response. All considered, it is most practical to think of glycemic index as simply an indicator of how high and how fast blood glucose tends to rise after eating the food, but it should never be used to predict the magnitude of the glycemic response to food with great accuracy.

suming carbohydrate. Factors such as energy density, other macronutrients, micronutrients, phytochemicals, and enjoyment of the food or beverage are additional considerations.

Table 3.4 includes some examples of the glycemic index and glycemic load of common foods. The scientific literature offers more comprehensive tables on glycemic index and glycemic load of a wide variety of foods.

Glycemic Index and Glycemic Load in Sport and Exercise

Athletes need to use caution when selecting foods based solely on glycemic index or glycemic load.

Simply choosing or avoiding a food classified as low, medium, or high glycemic index or load is not always warranted. For example, some athletes experience **reactive hypoglycemia**, or **postprandial hypoglycemia**, a condition in which blood sugar drops below normal after consuming certain foods. This circumstance can be problematic if the drop occurs at the start of exercise. Experimentation with pretraining foods would be beneficial to see if this is a potential concern. Otherwise, research to suggest that high- or low-glycemic foods are more advantageous before exercise is insufficient (22, 23). Although carbohydrates that rapidly increase insulin, such as glucose, will lead to an initial drop in blood sugar at the beginning

Table 3.4 Glycemic Index and Load of Common Foods

Food	Serving size	Serving size (g)	Glycemic index	Available carbohydrate (g/serving)	Glycemic load
Wheat bread	1 slice	30	53	20	11
Oatmeal	2/3 cup	50	69	35	24
English muffin	One-half	30	77	14	11
White bagel	Diameter 3 in.	70	72	35	25
White rice	1 cup	150	51	42	21
Brown rice	3/4 cup	150	50	33	16
Cheese pizza	1 slice	100	36	24	9
Mashed potatoes	3/4 cup	150	74	20	18
Baked potato	5.3 oz	150	60	30	18
Corn	3/4 cup	150	53	32	17
Kidney beans	0.5 cup	150	52	17	9
Apple	Diameter 2-3/4 in.	120	38	15	6
Apple juice	8 fl oz	250 ml	40	29	12
Soda	8.5 fl oz	250 ml	53	26	14
Chocolate milk	1 cup	50	43	28	12
Low-fat yogurt	7 oz	200	31	30	9
Chocolate pudding	3.5 oz	100	47	16	7
Chocolate ice cream	3/4 cup	50	87	13	8
Angel food cake	2 oz	50	67	29	19
Vanilla wafers	4 cookies	25	77	18	14
Ripe banana	7 in.	120	51	25	13
Grapes	25	120	46	18	8
Strawberries	3/4 cup	120	40	3	1
Raisins	2 oz	60	64	44	28

Adapted from K. Foster-Powell, S.H. Holt, and J.C. Brand-Miller, "International Table of Glycemic Index and Glycemic Load Values: 2002," *American Journal of Clinical Nutrition* 76 (2002): 5-56.

of exercise, blood sugar levels typically return to normal within approximately 20 minutes, and the initial drop has no negative effect on performance (24).

CARBOHYDRATE AS FUEL DURING EXERCISE

Exercise requires the ability to generate a continuous supply of energy (ATP) in order for skeletal muscle to contract and activity to continue. Because muscle can store only small amounts of ATP, other fuel sources are required, namely, glucose, fatty acids, and to a limited extent, amino acids. Glucose can be used to produce ATP for skeletal muscle contraction through partial oxidation of the glucose molecule (glycolysis) or complete oxidation of the glucose molecule (aerobic metabolism). Remember that complete glucose oxidation includes three steps that occur in the following order: glycolysis, TCA cycle, and the electron transport chain (see chapter 2). The source of glucose for exercising muscle primarily comes from stored muscle glycogen but can also come from blood glucose and gluconeogenesis. Exercise intensity plays a key role in determining how much and when glucose is used for a given activity (table 3.5). In general, glucose use is increased whenever exercise intensity increases beyond a steady state (e.g., includes the onset of exercise) and whenever steady-state exercise intensity increases (2).

? DO YOU KNOW?

The average male marathon runner stores 400 to 500 grams of skeletal muscle glycogen, which is long enough to run for 80 minutes at his normal running pace, assuming no other substrate is used to make ATP (1, 2, 12-14).

Table 3.5 Percent of Total Skeletal Muscle ATP Produced From Glucose During Exercise at Varying Intensities

Exercise intensity	% of ATP produced
Rest	35
Light to moderate	40
High and short duration	95
High and long duration	70

Data from McArdle, Katch, and Katch (2013).

ROLE OF CARBOHYDRATE IN EXERCISE FATIGUE

Muscle fatigue during exercise typically occurs as a result of three far-different circumstances: (1) muscle cannot produce enough force to meet the demands of the activity, (2) high ATP demand (high-intensity exercise) prevents the complete oxidation of glucose, causing lactate accumulation, or (3) energy reserves in muscle become depleted. The first situation does not involve carbohydrate. The second situation, known as **metabolic fatigue**, occurs when exercise intensity rises to a level that prevents glucose from being aerobically oxidized, thereby causing lactate to accumulate in the cell. Lactate gets converted to lactic acid, and the hydrogen ions produced in the process create an acidic environment in the muscle cell that disrupts ATP production and muscle contraction, thus producing symptoms of fatigue. Once metabolic fatigue has occurred, the exerciser will have to slow down or stop so that the body can work to clear the excess hydrogen ions from the muscle. Lactate is not only a metabolic by-product but also a fuel source for many cells throughout the body, so clearing excess lactate and subsequent hydrogen ions is simply a matter of time. After these metabolic products are cleared, which occurs fairly rapidly, the fatigue dissipates and the skeletal muscle can again contract and perform. Note that endurance-trained people are better able than sedentary people to use lactate for energy (1, 2, 14, 25, 26).

? DO YOU KNOW?

When you first start an exercise program or engage in a tough bout of exercise, the muscle soreness you feel 1 to 3 days later is not caused by lactic acid. The soreness you experience is caused by overexerting your muscles, resulting in microtrauma and inflammation, which causes pain. After healing takes place, soreness should subside after a few days. During this time, it is usually best to perform only light activities. If the soreness or pain persists, seek the advice of a physician before resuming your normal routine.

The third situation is called **substrate fatigue**, which occurs when skeletal muscles essentially run out of substrate (i.e., glucose). When glycogen reserves in the skeletal muscles become significantly reduced, no glucose is available to produce ATP to any meaningful extent; exercise must slow down or stop entirely and cannot recommence until more glucose is introduced into the system through consumption or gluconeogenesis (1, 2, 14, 25, 26). Substrate fatigue is a real concern for endurance athletes. See a detailed discussion in chapter 11.

CARBOHYDRATE RECOMMENDATIONS

The Food and Nutrition Board of the Institute of Medicine **dietary reference intakes (DRIs)** (27) serve as a recommendation of carbohydrate intake for healthy people. The DRIs include recommendations for women who are pregnant and breastfeeding, infants, children, and adults. DRIs are not designed to replace medical nutrition therapy for persons with certain nutrition-related diseases and conditions. These values take into consideration age and gender but do not account for activity or disease states. Special recommendations exist for these unique populations.

Recommendations for the General Population

The acceptable macronutrient distribution range (AMDR) for carbohydrate is 45 to 65 percent of total energy intake; this range applies to males and females in all age brackets and life stages (pregnancy and lactation are life stages) (4, 27). The recommended dietary allowance (RDA) for carbohydrate is based on the minimum requirement needed for brain function and is currently set at 130 grams per day for toddlers, children, adolescents, and adults of all ages. For more information on low-carbohydrate diets and brain function, turn to *Dietary Guidelines for Americans, 2020-2025* (28). This value does not reflect the amount needed for daily activities and purposeful exercise. Women who are pregnant need at least 175 grams per day, and women who are breastfeeding need at least 210 grams per day. The RDA is lower for infants; those under 6 months of age need at least 60 grams per day, and those between 7 and 12 months need at least 95 grams per day. Most of the daily carbohydrate intake should come from high-quality food sources such as whole grains, fruits, vegetables, beans, and legumes, and added sugar intake should be limited to 10 percent of energy consumption or less (28).

Fiber is a type of carbohydrate with its own set of recommendations because fiber can have unique health benefits different from the other types of carbohydrate. The DRI for fiber is 38 grams per day for males aged 14 to 50, and 25 grams per day for females aged 19 to 50. Pregnant and lactating women need more—28 and 29 grams per day, respectively (29). Average intake in the United States is approximately 15 grams per day. The DRIs for fiber are currently set based on the available data examining the relation between

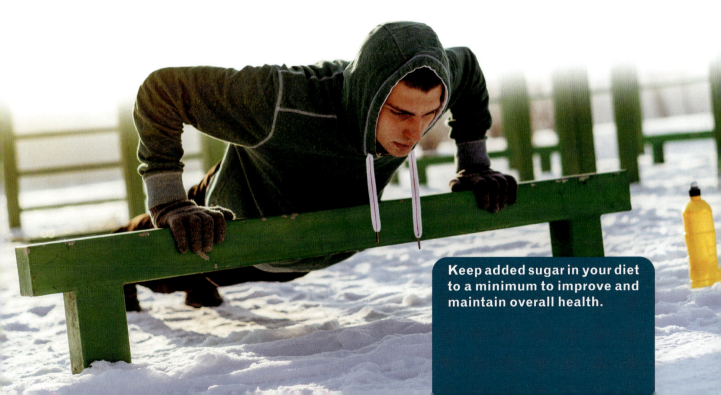

Keep added sugar in your diet to a minimum to improve and maintain overall health.

fiber and cardiovascular disease, but research examining fiber's relation to other aspects of health is emerging. Until that research progresses, the current DRIs are the best guidelines we have for daily fiber intake. If an individual chooses to increase fiber intake to improve health, it is recommended that they do this gradually and with a concomitant increase in fluid. Increased fiber intake without adequate fluid could result in constipation.

Recommendations for Active People and Athletes

For athletes, the absolute quantity of carbohydrate in grams and g/kg body weight consumed is more important than considering total carbohydrate intake as a percentage of total calories. As an example, because of their high calorie intake, some endurance athletes may consume up to 70 percent of their total energy intake in the form of carbohydrate while still meeting their total protein and fat requirements. In general, athletes should consume from 3 to 12 g/kg carbohydrate per day (table 3.6) (30). This is a large range intended to accommodate athletes with ever-changing training volume and intensity.

> The low end of the range, 3 to 5 g/kg, is usually best for athletes undergoing a light training regimen, playing a skill-based sport, having a large body mass, or attempting to lose body fat through an energy-restricted diet (30).

> The middle range of 5 to 7 g/kg should be used by athletes exercising at a moderate intensity for approximately an hour per day or those participating in high-intensity, short-duration types of sports (30).

> The range of 6 to 10 g/kg is recommended for those engaged in high-intensity exercise between 1 to 3 hours per day (30).

> The upper end of the range, 8 to 12 g/kg, is usually reserved for extremely committed athletes exercising at the highest intensity or for greater than 4 to 5 hours per day (30).

These general recommendations are not meant as prescriptions for individuals. Values will vary depending on total energy expenditure, specific training regimens, and personal experience with strategies that optimize performance. Athletes tend to know their physiological responses to diet and training, and their practice may deviate from these general recommendations. These guidelines should serve as a starting point for *healthy* athletes and be fine-tuned to meet the specific needs of each athlete. If these guidelines are not working, or if an athlete has a nutrition-related medical condition, the athlete may need to obtain sport- and training-specific carbohydrate recommendations from a certified specialist in sports dietetics (CSSD) (31). The CSSD can tailor meal planning to the individual and consider any issues that warrant a balance in carbohydrate need and medical nutrition therapy (e.g., celiac disease, lactose intolerance, and irritable bowel syndrome).

Table 3.6 Daily Carbohydrate Recommendations for Trained Athletes

Carbohydrate recommendation	Exercise intensity and duration	Daily amount for 59 kg (130 lb) athlete (g)	Daily amount for 79 kg (175 lb) athlete (g)
3–5 g/kg	Low-intensity training	177–295	237–395
5–7 g/kg	• More than 60 minutes per day of low-intensity training • 60 minutes per day of moderate-intensity training • Up to 30 minutes per day of high-intensity training	295–413	395–553
6–10 g/kg	1–3 hours per day of moderate- to high-intensity training	354–590	474–790
8–12 g/kg	4–5 hours per day of moderate- to high-intensity training	472–708	632–948

Assumes adequate total calorie intake and that carbohydrate is spread throughout the day, depending on training schedule.
Data from Thomas, Erdman, and Burke (2016).

Table 3.7 provides the estimated number of grams of daily carbohydrate needed to maintain glycogen stores for athletes of varying body weights. Athletes should time the intake of carbohydrate at appropriate intervals throughout the day, considering when practice and competition occur during the day.

Percentages of total energy do not always align with absolute quantity of carbohydrate. For example, large people with more muscle mass often have a higher energy requirement and might be able to meet carbohydrate needs with a lower total percentage of energy. An athlete consuming 4,000 kcal per day, 50 percent of that from carbohydrate, would be eating 500 grams of carbohydrate. This amount would be equivalent to 7.4 g/kg for a 150-pound (68 kg) man—well within the recommendation. On the contrary, a 120-pound (54.5 kg) woman consuming 1,400 kcal per day, 65 percent from carbohydrate, would be eating 4.2 g/kg, which may or may not be adequate for her training (figure 3.10). From these examples you can see that a lower percentage of carbohydrate, 50 percent, could be adequate, whereas a higher percentage, 65 percent, might not be ideal for a person who is endurance training at moderate to high intensity.

Table 3.7 Daily Carbohydrate Needs by Target Intake Level and Body Weight

Weight (lb)	Weight (kg)	3 g/kg	4 g/kg	5 g/kg	6 g/kg	7 g/kg	8 g/kg	9 g/kg	10 g/kg	11 g/kg	12 g/kg
100	45	136	182	227	273	318	364	409	455	500	545
105	48	143	191	239	286	334	382	430	477	525	573
110	50	150	200	250	300	350	400	450	500	550	600
115	52	157	209	261	314	366	418	470	523	575	627
120	55	164	218	273	327	382	436	491	545	600	655
125	57	170	227	28	341	398	455	511	568	625	682
130	59	177	236	295	355	414	473	532	591	650	709
135	61	184	245	307	368	430	491	552	614	675	736
140	64	191	255	318	382	445	509	573	636	700	764
145	66	198	264	330	395	461	527	593	659	725	791
150	68	205	273	341	409	477	545	614	682	750	818
155	70	211	282	352	423	493	564	634	705	775	845
160	73	218	291	364	436	509	582	655	727	800	873
165	75	225	300	375	450	525	600	675	750	825	900
170	77	232	309	386	464	541	618	695	773	850	927
175	80	239	318	398	477	557	636	716	795	875	955
180	82	245	327	409	491	573	655	736	818	900	982
185	84	252	336	420	505	589	673	757	841	925	1,009
190	86	259	345	432	518	605	691	777	864	950	1,036
195	89	266	355	443	532	620	709	798	886	975	1,064
200	91	273	364	455	545	636	727	818	909	1,000	1,091

Formulas were used to complete this table, but whole numbers are written. For example, 100 lb ÷ 2.2 = 45.45 kg. 45.45 kg × 3 g/kg = 136.35 g carbohydrate. The numbers 45 and 136 are represented in the table.

Data from Thomas, Erdman, and Burke (2016).

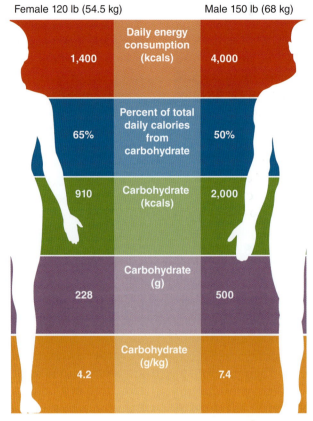

Figure 3.10 Example of percentage of energy from carbohydrate versus amount of carbohydrate.

Carbohydrate Recommendations Before, During, and After Training and Competition

Because carbohydrate becomes the predominate fuel source as exercise intensity increases and because depletion of the body's limited glycogen stores will lead to performance decrements, it is important to implement strategies to maximize glycogen stores going into an event (often spanning days before the event), to provide a source of carbohydrate as fuel during an event, and to replenish those depleted stores after an event. Table 3.8 summarizes the before, during, and after strategies for carbohydrate intake. More details on this topic are discussed in later chapters; most content is addressed in chapter 11.

Table 3.8 Summary of Carbohydrate Recommendations Before, During, and After Exercise

Activity type	Amount of carbohydrate recommended
Carbohydrate loading—useful for >90 minutes of sustained activity	10-12 g/kg body weight daily for 26–48 hours before activity
During activity lasting 45–75 minutes	Mouth rinsing or small amounts (15–60 g total)
Preactivity fuel for >60 minutes of sustained activity	1–4 g/kg body weight consumed 1–4 hours before activity
During endurance activity and stop-and-go sports lasting 60–150 minutes	30–60 total g per hour
During long endurance activities lasting >150 minutes	Up to 90 g per hour
Glycogen replenishment following activity	1.0–1.2 g/kg body weight per hour for first 4 hours and then resume daily carbohydrate targets

Data from Thomas, Erdman, and Burke (2016).

CARBOHYDRATE CONTENT OF FOODS

Figure 3.11 lists some popular foods and their associated carbohydrate content. When reading Nutrition Facts labels, keep in mind that a package may contain more than one serving (32).

CARBOHYDRATE AND HEALTH

Much of this chapter has focused on carbohydrate as an energy source for athletes, but carbohydrate can also have an important role in overall health and well-being. Although athletes might have an immediate need of performance optimization for a specific event or competitive season, long-term health is also of concern. Some types of carbohydrate, such as whole grains that contain fiber, might promote health and prevent disease. Other types, such as simple sugars and processed flours, might contribute negatively to health. Some of these topics have been investigated for years, but others have more limited data. In either case, more research is needed in these areas to understand the relation of carbohydrate consumption to health.

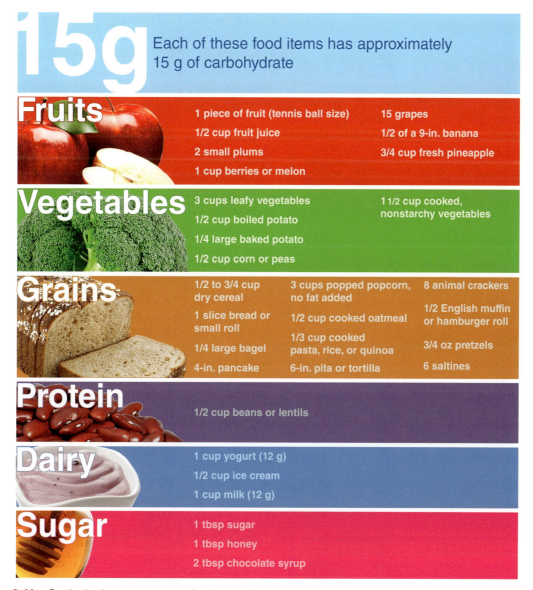

Figure 3.11 Carbohydrate content of selected foods.
Data from American Diabetes Association (2014).

The Nutrition Facts label is an easy way to check the fiber content of foods. The label discloses the amount of dietary fiber in each serving, as well as the percent daily value (%DV). In general, a low-fiber food is one that has 5 percent or less of the DV, and a high-fiber food is one with 20 percent or more of the DV (figure 3.12) (32).

Health Benefits of Fiber

Although **dietary fiber** is not digested, it might be beneficial in the fight against diseases of the digestive tract, cardiovascular disease, and diabetes mellitus. Through its action binding toxins in the **colon** and facilitating their elimination from the body, fiber might reduce the risk of developing colon and rectal cancer. Other cancers with a possible healthy relation to fiber include cancer of the mouth, pharynx, larynx, esophagus, and stomach (32). Fiber also increases stool bulk, and with adequate fluid intake, keeps stool smooth and easy to eliminate. This ease of elimination may reduce the chance of developing the painful condition known as **diverticulosis**, which occurs when small pockets form in the intestinal walls caused by the high pressure required to eliminate small, hard stools from the colon. These pockets become inflamed and infected, causing transition to **diverticulitis** (1, 6).

Fiber might also play a role in the prevention of cardiovascular disease, by reducing serum total and LDL cholesterol levels. One theory suggests that fiber binds to the cholesterol eaten in the same meal and eliminates it in the stool. Another theory assumes that fiber binds with and eliminates **bile** from the gut, which stimulates the liver to synthesize new bile to replace what is lost in stool. Bile itself contains cholesterol, so synthesizing new bile requires cholesterol to be removed from the blood and incorporated into newly produced bile, thereby reducing serum cholesterol levels over time. Without this function of fiber, bile is recycled and not eliminated from the body. New emerging research suggests that fiber might also reduce inflammatory markers for heart disease and blood pressure. Given this promising body of evidence, increasing fiber intake from whole grains, fruits, vegetables, or supplements likely helps reduce the risk of developing certain diseases (1, 6).

Diseases and Conditions Related to Carbohydrate

Lactose intolerance and celiac disease are two conditions that usually require afflicted persons to modify their dietary intakes, and possibly their lifestyle habits, to compensate for the disease.

Lactose Intolerance

Recall that carbohydrates must be digested into their simplest form, monosaccharides, to be absorbed into the small intestine. **Lactose intolerance** is a condition in which the small intestine does not produce enough of the enzyme lactase,

Nutrition Facts

8 servings per container
Serving size 2/3 cup (55g)

Amount per 2/3 cup
Calories 230

	% Daily Value*
Total Fat 8g	10%
Saturated Fat 1g	5%
Trans Fat 0g	
Cholesterol 0mg	0%
Sodium 160mg	7%
Total Carbohydrate 37g	13%
Dietary Fiber 7g	20%
Total Sugars 12g	
Added Sugars 10g	20%
Protein 3g	
Vitamin D 2mcg	10%
Calcium 260mg	20%
Iron 8mg	45%
Potassium 235mg	6%

*The % Daily Value (DV) tells you how much a nutrient in a serving of food contributes to a daily diet. 2,000 calories a day is used for general nutrition advice.

Figure 3.12 The Nutrition Facts label indicates the amount of dietary fiber in a serving of food.

Carbohydrate 83

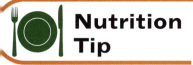

Nutrition Tip

High-fiber diets might reduce the risk of developing type 2 diabetes mellitus or may help manage marked fluctuations in blood glucose. Fiber absorbs fluid and expands in the intestine, slowing digestion. Fiber also stimulates the release of hormones that increase satiety (33). All these factors have been cited as explanations for the association between diets higher in fiber and whole grains and both lower body weight and prevention of weight gain (34, 35). A systematic review of the research examining 38 types of fiber, however, found that the majority of short-term fiber treatments did not enhance satiety or reduce food intake (35).

Despite the conflicting evidence regarding the role of dietary fiber in weight control, research suggests that the type of fiber matters and that the form of food might matter as well (i.e., liquid vs. solid food). Beta-glucan (from oats and barley), lupin kernel fiber, whole-grain rye, rye bran, and a mixed diet of specific fiber-containing foods (five to eight grains, legumes, vegetables, and fruits) have all been shown to enhance satiety. Increases in satiety, however, do not necessarily correspond to a decrease in food intake, total calories, and weight loss. Oat and barley beta-glucan might be superior to other types of fiber for reducing total calorie intake (34).

---

so the disaccharide lactose present in dairy foods cannot be digested (1, 36). Because lactose cannot cross the intestinal cell wall, it progresses to the large intestine, where gut bacteria act on it. This leads to gas, abdominal distension and watery stools or diarrhea. The condition can be uncomfortable but generally does not require medical attention (1, 36).

Not all those with lactose intolerance experience the same level of symptoms. Some people are mildly intolerant and can consume milk, yogurt, cheese, and related foods in small quantities. Others might not tolerate milk but can consume yogurt and cheese; because these products have already been fermented, they contain less lactose than milk. Aged, hard cheeses have very little lactose. Still others are severely intolerant and cannot consume any dairy products at all without having side effects. This possibility is important to understand, because milk is often recommended for athletes as a recovery beverage because of its composition of carbohydrate and protein. Milk contains 13 essential nutrients and is an excellent source of calcium and good source of vitamin D. Fortunately, over-the-counter products are available that contain the enzyme lactase that can be consumed along with dairy foods to reduce the amount of lactose ultimately delivered to gut bacteria. In addition, some brands of milk are lactose free. For those who prefer no dairy, many dairy alternatives are on the market that have varying levels of carbohydrate, protein, and calcium (1, 3). Many of these drinks are not equivalent to dairy in terms of nutrient composition. According to *Dietary Guidelines for Americans*, only soy milk is considered a suitable replacement for dairy milk. Figure 3.13 presents a list of foods that contain lactose.

❓ DO YOU KNOW?

Don't confuse lactose intolerance with a milk allergy, which is an allergy to the protein in milk. Lactose intolerance involves symptoms of the gastrointestinal tract, whereas milk allergies involve an immune response.

Celiac Disease and Other Gastrointestinal Disturbances

Celiac disease is an autoimmune disease that involves an interaction between genetics (a person must have the gene) and environment (exposure to the protein gluten). Gluten contains a specific sequence of amino acids located in the prolamin fraction of wheat. Barley and rye contain proteins related to gluten (though all these proteins are typically referred to as gluten). Prolamins are storage proteins found in many grains, but it is the amino acid sequence in those grains that is harmful to those with celiac disease. When gluten is consumed, an immune response is triggered, result-

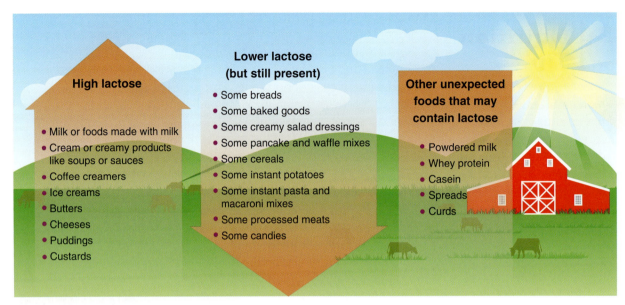

Figure 3.13 Lactose-containing foods.
Data from Cleveland Clinic (2016).

ing in damage to the small intestinal mucosa, which alters the absorptive surface area and compromises the absorption of nutrients in the small intestine. Over time, this issue can progress to the malabsorption of both macronutrients and micronutrients. This condition is different from a wheat allergy, which is an immediate immune system allergic reaction to wheat proteins. Some food allergy reactions, such as anaphylactic shock, require immediate medical attention (1).

People with celiac disease require medical nutrition therapy and should seek the advice of a registered dietitian nutritionist (RDN) (37). Treatment for celiac disease involves following a gluten-free diet by avoiding wheat, barley, and rye in any form, as well as other grains, such as triticale. Some other grains and flours can be tolerated, such as corn, potato, rice, amaranth, quinoa, and buckwheat (buckwheat is a vegetable). Fortunately, gluten-free products are becoming easy to find, although many of them are higher in calories and sugar than their counterparts with gluten.

Many people now prefer a gluten-free diet even in the absence of a wheat allergy or celiac disease. Some people suffer from gluten sensitivity, which is not the same autoimmune disease as celiac disease and is not a protein allergy. These individuals report feeling better when they avoid gluten. Although evidence is not sufficient to support the gluten-free approach for athletes or others without celiac disease, gluten sensitivity, or wheat allergy, eating a balanced diet without gluten is certainly possible (1, 3).

More recent research has confirmed that foods containing gluten often also contain compounds called fermentable oligo-, di-, and monosaccharides and polyols (FODMAPs). For some, these compounds cause gastrointestinal distress even without being in the presence of gluten. Therefore, the issue may be not gluten but instead FODMAPs. These molecules are most commonly found in fructose (e.g., apples, pears, honey), lactose (e.g., milk, cottage cheese), fructans (e.g., wheat, garlic, onions), galactans (e.g., beans, lentils, soy), and polyols (e.g., sweeteners). These may have an osmotic effect, pulling water into the small intestine, which can result in bloating, abdominal pain, and diarrhea. Fortunately, these effects do not happen to everyone, and it is an individual tolerance If they go undigested and travel to the large intestine, gas is usually another side effect. People have different tolerances to different foods high in FODMAPs. Other potential symptoms from FODMAP intake in those who are sensitive to FODMAPs include constipation or alternating constipation and diarrhea. A person who has chronic gastrointestinal issues should seek medical attention before trying to self-diagnose or treat the problem. Low FODMAPs diets are therapeutic for irritable bowel syndrome (IBS) and small bacterial intestinal overgrowth (SIBO). People without a specific disease may also follow this diet if undesirable side effects are a consequence of eating a diet rich in FODMAPs (38). Because foods containing FODMAPS offer important nutrients and prebiotic fiber to the diet, they are not intended to be taken out of the diet entirely for a prolonged period. Anyone who suspects they are having issues with FODMAPs should work with an RDN experienced in FODMAPs.

Health Effects of Nutritive Sweeteners

Nutritive sweeteners contain carbohydrate, usually sugar, and provide energy. They may be monosaccharides, disaccharides, or sugar alcohols (e.g., mannitol, sorbitol). Nutritive sweeteners can be found naturally in foods such as fruits, vegetables, and dairy; can be added to foods such as baked goods, salad dressings, and peanut butter; or can be consumed by themselves.

Sugar

The most common nutritive sweeteners, or "sugars," are glucose (found in food such as dextrose or glucose syrup), fructose, galactose, sucrose, maltose, and corn-based sweeteners such as high-fructose corn syrup. Although providing sweetness is a key function of these products, sugars also play a role in supplying texture and volume, supporting yeast growth, balancing acidity, and enhancing crystallization. The Food and Nutrition Board of the Institute of Medicine recommends that no more than 10 percent of total energy intake should come from added sugars (4, 27, 28). Foods high in sugar tend to be processed, and although they are calorie dense, they are often not nutrient dense. Consuming a large percentage of energy from sugar without exceeding total energy needs would be difficult because it would displace protein and sacrifice micronutrient needs. The most common source of sugar in the U.S. diet is from sweetened beverages (4, 27, 28, 39). On average, one 12-ounce (360 ml) can of soda contains almost 10 teaspoons of sugar. When you consider that many servings of soda available

> Careful monitoring of blood sugar along with regular exercise and a healthy diet can help people with diabetes.

at fast-food restaurants, theaters, amusement parks, and other venues are 16 or 24 ounces (480 or 720 ml), or even larger, you can see how the amounts of sugar really add up. Even moderate sugar consumption may contribute to a significant number of adverse health conditions, including cardiovascular disease, inflammation, diabetes, and obesity (1, 40). Independent of the potential contribution of excess energy, excess sugar may promote inflammation leading to disease formation and progression. Note that most research studies support a relationship between sugar consumption and health issues, and more data are needed to distinguish between added sugars, excess calories, and many other dietary factors.

Dyslipidemia Some evidence indicates that overconsumption of sugar and other processed carbohydrates are associated with increased levels of low-density lipoprotein (LDL) cholesterol and triglycerides (blood fats), both risk factors for cardiovascular disease, and a reduced level of high-density lipoprotein (HDL) cholesterol—the kind that removes LDL from the arteries. This pattern, called **dyslipidemia**, is thought to increase the risk of developing cardiovascular disease. Although there is not enough evidence to say with certainty that sugar or processed carbohydrates promote heart disease, those who have dyslipidemia are prudent to be concerned (1, 3). Note that dyslipidemia is primarily a concern for people who are overconsuming sugar and carbohydrates and also overconsuming calories. The concern might not apply (at least not to the same degree) to normal-weight athletes who consume large quantities to fuel a sport or activity.

Inflammation Although much of the research on diet and **inflammation** has focused on fats, it appears that carbohydrates play a role as well. High consumption of highly **refined carbohydrates**—that is, those made from white flour and sugar—are associated with increased blood glucose levels and accompanying inflammatory messengers called cytokines. On the other hand, it also appears that replacing refined carbohydrates in the diet by consuming larger quantities of plants in the form of whole fruits and vegetables may help limit these inflammatory markers (1, 41, 42).

Diabetes No indisputable scientific evidence implicates sugar consumption as a direct cause of diabetes mellitus, but people who already have diabetes must learn to modify their carbohydrate intake and balance it with insulin or oral medications and physical activity to keep their blood glucose levels under control. Some athletes who participate in rigorous sports also have diabetes, yet they still require large amounts of carbohydrates and have the unique challenge of eating enough carbohydrates to fuel their activity while maintaining blood glucose balance (1).

Obesity Although more data are needed to establish a cause-and-effect relationship (43), some observational and controlled research studies report weight loss with reduced intake of sugars and weight gain with increased intake. Similarly, sugar consumption may also play a role in obesity development in children; those consuming one or more sugar-sweetened beverages a day are at higher risk of becoming overweight (39). Many of the studies agree that it is the excess energy from the sugar that contributes to the weight gain rather than the chemistry of the sugar molecules themselves (44). Excess energy in any form can contribute to weight gain, so if a person is consistently consuming more sugar than they are using as fuel or storing as glycogen, they will gain fat over time.

> **? DO YOU KNOW?**
>
> Data from the United States Department of Agriculture suggest that consumption of high-fructose corn syrup (HFCS) has been declining over the years, but obesity and diabetes rates continue to rise. In other parts of the world, HFCS is limited in the food supply, yet obesity rates are still rising in those areas (40).

High-Fructose Corn Syrup

High-fructose corn syrup (HFCS) is a synthesized product derived from cornstarch. HFCS is inexpensive to produce and results in a stable, concentrated, sweet product with a long shelf life. Currently, the FDA does not have a formal definition for the term "natural," but when it comes to food labeling, the FDA considers "natural" to mean that nothing artificial or synthetic has been included in, or added to, the food item in question (45). HFCS does not contain artificial ingredients or color additives, and thus meets the FDA's requirements for use of the term *natural*. HFCS also makes food more palatable and is currently found in a seemingly endless number of food and beverage products, although this trend is reversing because of the negative publicity associated with HFCS (1, 40).

Much attention has been given to HFCS and the development of diabetes and obesity, but evidence is insufficient to support the notion that HFCS is less healthy than any of the other nutritive sweeteners. Some evidence strongly suggests that consumption of excess sugar, in any form, can contribute to excess energy intake and fat gain, which, in turn, increases the risk of developing type 2 diabetes, metabolic syndrome, and cardiovascular disease. But obesity is a multifactorial disease affected by overall lifestyle, and sugar intake is only one contributor (1, 40, 46).

> **? DO YOU KNOW?**
>
> Contrary to its name, high-fructose corn syrup is not extremely high in fructose, at least not relative to other ingredients. HFCS is between 42 and 55 percent fructose, depending on the processing, and the remainder is glucose. This composition is nearly identical to sucrose and honey and is apparently metabolized the same way in the body (1, 40, 46).

Sugar Alcohols

Sugar alcohols are carbohydrates present naturally in some fruits and vegetables, and made in laboratories. These alcohols are less sweet than sugar, contain 2 kcal per gram (kcal/g) instead of the 4 kcal/g found in sugar, and do not promote tooth decay. They are not readily available as isolated products on supermarket shelves, but they are abundant in manufactured products such as candy (especially sugar-free candy), frozen desserts, gum, toothpaste, mouthwash, and baked goods. They are often combined with nonnutritive sweeteners to enhance the sweet taste in a food product. Sugar alcohols, also called polyols (these are FODMAPs), are called by many names on food labels, but the most common are xylitol, maltitol, mannitol, sorbitol, or simply "sugar alcohol." Sugar alcohols are incompletely absorbed in the gut. Polyols not absorbed in the small intestine enter the large intestine where they are fermented by bacteria, which leads to gas and bloating. Cramping and diarrhea are additional side effects noted from polyol intake. Side effects are generally noted when polyols are consumed in amounts exceeding 20 grams per day. Everyone's tolerance is different, however, so a trial-and-error approach might be best. When comparing sweet products made with sugar alcohols to those made with glucose or sucrose, the sugar-alcohol products produce a lower glycemic response and so are often promoted for people with diabetes (1, 40, 47).

Health Effects of Nonnutritive Sweeteners

Because they are generally not digested, **nonnutritive sweeteners (NNS)** such as saccharin and sucralose contain little or no energy. They are considered high-intensity sweeteners because their sweetness-to-energy ratio is much greater than that of sugar. In addition, they generally do not cause a significant rise in blood glucose. They can be used alone as a tabletop sweetener or added to foods and beverages that traditionally contain sugar. Although sweet in taste, they often do not offer the same desirable food science properties as sugar. Some nonnutritive sweeteners do not contribute the bulk that sugar contributes to a recipe and do not aid in browning or crystallization, so they might not be ideal for baking (40, 48, 49).

Nonnutritive sweeteners are often a topic of public opinion, although the scientific evidence is ongoing and inconclusive. It appears that NNS can be used effectively in blood glucose management in people with diabetes, because their consumption does not negatively affect glycemic or insulinemic responses (50). Other studies,

> ### PUTTING IT INTO PERSPECTIVE
>
> #### DOES ASPARTAME AFFECT ENERGY BALANCE OR APPETITE?
>
> Significant evidence suggests that using food items and products sweetened with aspartame as part of a comprehensive weight-management program might assist people with weight loss and weight maintenance over time by helping them lower total calorie intake. Evidence also suggests that aspartame does not increase appetite or total food intake in adults, but evidence in children is limited. Use of any nonnutritive sweetener may be useful in improving energy balance only if it is replacing a more energy-dense choice and the consumer is not compensating for the lower-energy product consumption with overindulgence of other items in the same meal or at another time in the day (40, 52).

however, suggest that regular use of NNS does not cause metabolic syndrome but also may not play a role in preventing it (51). Although research is not conclusive, it appears that use of NNS is not associated with higher body weight (51, 52). But some evidence in both animals and humans indicates that some NNS can lead to imbalances in the gut microbiota that may play a role in obesity (51, 53). Current data indicate that aspartame and acesulfame potassium (acesulfame-K) have lesser effects, whereas saccharin and sucralose induce some gut microbial shifts. Steviol glycosides may be metabolized by gut bacteria, so there is potential for an altered environment. With all the research being conducted, it appears that the alterations in the gut microbiome have not led to either beneficial or negative health outcomes (50-53). More research is needed before concrete conclusions can be made. Practitioners need to keep abreast of any changes in the FDA guidelines and the current literature regarding the use of NNS in specific populations.

Most nonnutritive sweeteners are regulated as food additives by the FDA. An exception is made for substances **generally recognized as safe (GRAS)** because these substances are recognized by qualified scientists as safe for consumption for their intended use. This classification makes them exempt from the food-additive approval process. Companies wishing to manufacture and market a new nonnutritive sweetener must conduct significant research on the product and present all the required safety data to the FDA in consideration of approval. Research includes the extent of the absorption of the substance, any distribution in tissues, mechanisms and rates of metabolism, and rates of elimination of the substance or any metabolites. The FDA examines probable intake of the population, cumulative effects from using the product, and toxicology data. The FDA sets an acceptable daily intake (ADI) for a human, which is defined as the amount considered safe for daily consumption over the course of a lifetime without adverse health effects. This value considers even the estimated intake of a "high consumer." The FDA may request additional consumption or safety data during the postapproval period. Note that FDA approval holds only in the United States. Consumers may be able purchase other, sometimes unapproved, products from other countries. Currently, six high-intensity sweeteners are FDA approved as food additives: saccharin, aspartame, acesulfame potassium (Ace-K), sucralose, neotame, and advantame. Two other types of high-intensity sweeteners have been submitted to the FDA as GRAS: Stevia rebaudiana (Bertoni) and luo han guo (monk fruit). See table 3.9 for a summary of the most common nonnutritive sweeteners approved for use in the United States. Allulose is a sweetener found in fruits such as jackfruit, raisins, and figs, and it can also be made by enzymatic conversion of fructose from corn. Allulose is 70 percent less sweet than sugar, but it is not absorbed in the body and is excreted intact in the urine. It has been reviewed by the FDA and is GRAS (49, 54-56).

Table 3.9 Common Nonnutritive Sweeteners in the United States

Name of NNS	Description	Sweetness (number of times sweeter than sucrose)	ADI (mg/kg body weight) per day	Number of tabletop packets equivalent to ADI*	Common uses
Saccharin	• Oldest NNS on the market • Not metabolized and heat stable • Some experience a bitter aftertaste	200–700	15	45	Beverages, juice drinks, bases, mixes, sugar substitute for cooking, table use, processed foods
Aspartame	• Dipeptide of phenylalanine and aspartate • Provides 4 kcal/g but need such small quantity for sweet taste • Metabolized to aspartic acid, phenylalanine, and methanol • Persons with phenylketonuria (PKU) should not consume, • Degrades and loses sweetness during heating	200	50	75	Tabletop sweetener, chewing gum, cold cereals, beverages, syrups, puddings or fillings, and general flavor enhancer
Acesulfame potassium	• Approximately 95% is excreted unchanged in the urine and therefore does not provide significant energy • Stable for cooking and baking • Usually combined with another NNS	200	15	23	• General flavor enhancer, frozen desserts, candy, beverages, baked goods • Not approved for meat and poultry
Sucralose	• Often marketed as "made from sugar" • Three chloride molecules replace OH groups on sucrose • Approximately 85% is not absorbed and excreted in the feces unchanged. The 15% absorbed is excreted unchanged in the urine • Heat stable for cooking and baking	600	5	23	General purpose sweetener, general flavor enhancer, baked goods, beverages, chewing gum, gelatins, frozen desserts
Neotame	Heat stable for cooking and baking	7,000–13,000	0.3	23	General sweetener, general flavor enhancer, baked goods, not approved for meat and poultry

>continued

Table 3.9 >continued

Name of NNS	Description	Sweetness (number of times sweeter than sucrose)	ADI (mg/kg body weight) per day	Number of tabletop packets equivalent to ADI*	Common uses
Stevia (steviol glycosides)	• Extract from the leaves of the *Stevia rebaudiana* (Bertoni) plant • Different from whole stevia leaves • May be bitter in large quantities • Stable in dry form; may be more stable than others in liquid form	200–400	4	9	• GRAS** • General sweetener
Luo han guo	• Marketed as powdered "monk fruit extract" • Heat stable for cooking and baking	100–250	NS***	Not determined	• GRAS** • General sweetener
Advantame	• Does not yet have a brand name • Chemically related to aspartame but much sweeter • Does not carry the PKU warning	20,000	32.8	4,920	General sweetener, general flavor enhancer, baked goods, not approved for meat and poultry

*The number of common tabletop packets that a 132-pound (60 kg) person would need to ingest for equivalence to the ADI.
**GRAS = generally recognized as safe. There must be "a reasonable certainty of no harm" to earn this category.
***NS = not specified. An ADI may not be necessary at this point because safety levels are well above that used in food.

SUMMARY

Carbohydrate is an important fuel source for the human body and abundant in many foods. Virtually all ingested carbohydrates absorbed in the small intestine are ultimately converted to glucose, which is the form of carbohydrate used by the body's cells. Blood glucose level is normally tightly regulated by hormones that work by modulating glycogenolysis and gluconeogenesis as needed. Glucose reserves in the body are stored in the form of glycogen primarily in skeletal muscle and to a lesser extent in the liver.

Although everyone needs a minimal amount of carbohydrate for normal physiological function, it is a particularly important fuel source for the exercising skeletal muscle. Many athletes need more dietary carbohydrate than a sedentary person to meet the physical demands of training. The AMDR for carbohydrate is 45 to 65 percent of total energy intake from high-quality sources and with minimal added sugar. Carbohydrate recommendations for athletes are better expressed in absolute terms ranging from 3 g/kg to 12 g/kg body weight depending on the day-to-day training volume and intensity.

The quantity of sugar, refined starch, and fiber consumed in the diet may affect overall health and well-being. Certain diseases and conditions are related to carbohydrate consumption, and managing those conditions may require the help of an RDN or CSSD. Nutritive and nonnutritive sweeteners are widely used in manufactured food and beverage products and may have effects on overall health.

Remember that sports nutrition is a young science and that new research is emerging on a regular basis. Principles and guidelines presented in the chapter are based on current available evidence and may change or expand as new information becomes available. These guidelines are designed for healthy people. Those with a disease or nutrition-related condition may need to seek specific medical nutrition therapy from an RDN or CSSD.

FOR REVIEW

1. Describe the classification of carbohydrate.
2. How is carbohydrate absorbed?
3. After carbohydrate gets to the liver as glucose, what are its possible metabolic fates?
4. Describe how blood glucose is regulated. Include the organs and hormones involved.
5. Describe the fuel used at rest and at high-intensity exercise.
6. What is the cause of metabolic fatigue?
7. What are the dietary carbohydrate recommendations for the general population?
8. What are the dietary carbohydrate recommendations for athletes? How do these differ from recommendations for the general population?
9. List the sources of dietary carbohydrate (food groups that contain carbohydrate). How much carbohydrate is in a serving size of these groups?
10. Describe the differences in carbohydrate quality.
11. How does carbohydrate quality affect health?
12. Does sugar intake cause obesity and chronic diseases?
13. What is the difference between nutritive and nonnutritive sweeteners?
14. How are nonnutritive sweeteners regulated?

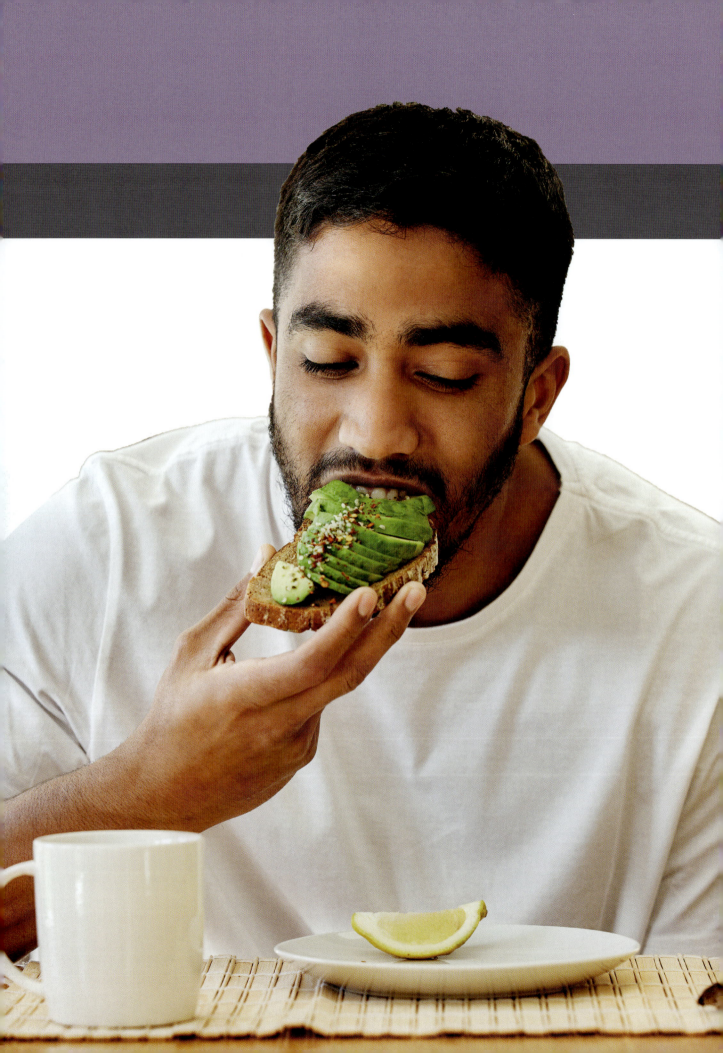

4

Fat

> ### ▶ CHAPTER OBJECTIVES
>
> After completing this chapter, you will be able to do the following:
> - Discuss the main types of dietary fats and their health implications.
> - Distinguish between dictary fats and dietary fatty acids within each category.
> - Discuss the importance of dietary cholesterol in the body.
> - Summarize the health implications of excess blood cholesterol and the effects of various dietary fats and dietary cholesterol on blood cholesterol levels.
> - List dietary fat recommendations for the prevention of cardiovascular disease.

DIGESTION AND METABOLISM

Dietary fat digestion starts in the mouth with the enzyme lingual lipase, but this part of the digestion process is minor. When dietary fat enters the small intestine, the gallbladder releases bile, and the pancreas releases lipases. Bile mixes partially digested fat so that enzymes can further hydrolyze (break down) the fat into free fatty acids, glycerol, cholesterol, and phospholipids, all of which are almost completely absorbed into the intestinal lining.

After absorption, free fatty acids, glycerol, cholesterol, and phospholipids are packaged into chylomicrons. Chylomicrons are a type of lipoprotein composed of 85 to 92 percent triglycerides, 6 to 12 percent phospholipids, 1 to 3 percent cholesterol, and 1 to 2 percent protein. Chylomicrons are triglyceride-transport vehicles (1). Chylomicrons leave the small intestine and eventually enter the blood, where the enzyme lipoprotein lipase takes them apart. The fatty acids are delivered to fat cells for storage or muscle cells for energy. Some fat and cholesterol are held by fiber and exit the body through feces.

Because of their shorter carbon chain length, short-chain fatty acids and medium-chain saturated fatty acids (referred to as **medium-chain triglycerides, or MCTs**) are not packaged into chylomicrons. Medium-chain triglycerides are absorbed in the blood and transported to the liver, where they are quickly broken down into fatty acids and glycerol. Supplemental medium-chain triglycerides can cause gastrointestinal side effects, including abdominal cramps, diarrhea, and nausea (2, 3).

Storing Fat in Adipose Tissue

All energy-yielding macronutrients—carbohydrate, protein, and fat—can be stored as body fat. When more calories are consumed than are burned, excess is stored in adipose tissue (body fat) for later use. The enzyme lipoprotein lipase breaks down triglycerides from lipoproteins in the bloodstream. Fatty acids, diglycerides, and monoglycerides are delivered to adipose cells, where enzymes reassemble these parts into triglycerides for storage (4). Although most excess fat is stored in adipose tissue (fat tissue), relatively small amounts are stored in skeletal muscle (5).

? DO YOU KNOW?

Consuming more calories than needed drives the storage of fat in adipose cells. But the acute (i.e., short term, such as after a large meal) storage of fat is not as important as calorie balance over time. Even if more calories are consumed than needed over the course of a few hours or a day, the body will pull fat from adipose tissue for energy during periods when fewer calories are consumed than needed.

Using Body Fat

Skeletal muscle and adipose tissue, as well as the heart, lungs, kidney, and liver, break down stored body fat. Stored triglycerides are degraded into free fatty acids and glycerol by the enzyme lipoprotein lipase. The fatty acids are transported in the blood and taken up by cells. Most of the cells in the human body can oxidize fatty acids to

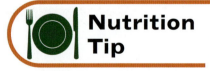

Nutrition Tip

Although excess calories lead to weight gain, the composition of energy-yielding macronutrients in the diet determines whether excess calories contribute to greater increases in fat storage or lean body mass. When a greater amount of excess calories consumed comes from fat, more energy is stored as body fat, when compared with consuming a greater amount of excess calories from carbohydrate. Carbohydrate overfeeding increases total calories burned, whereas overfeeding fat does not (6, 7). Overfeeding protein appears to support greater increases in lean body mass, as opposed to fat mass, in comparison with overfeeding carbohydrate or fat (8). Without training, however, most of the lean body mass gains come from water (remember that muscle is largely composed of water) (9).

produce energy, but the brain and nervous tissue cannot use fatty acids for fuel. The fatty acids can also be repackaged into triglyceride molecules and stored until needed. The glycerol released from the breakdown of body fat is transported to the liver, where a phosphate is added. The resulting compound can be used as triglyceride by the liver or be converted into a compound that enters glycolysis or gluconeogenesis (4).

DIETARY FATS AND EXERCISE

Although the human body has a limited capacity to store carbohydrate, fat stores are vast, even in lean athletes, providing enough energy to fuel several back-to-back marathons (10). For instance, a 160-pound (73 kg) athlete with 4 percent body fat has approximately 22,400 kcal stored in fat tissue (11). Although the human body contains significant fat reserves, fat is a slow source of fuel; it takes time to use it, and therefore when relying on fat, a person cannot keep up with the energy demands of high-intensity exercise. At rest and during low-intensity exercise (walking for instance), fat is the primary source of energy used (12). Low-intensity exercise is not calorically demanding; the body does not need as many calories to walk as it does to run. Thus, the rate of fat breakdown can easily meet energy needs during low-intensity exercise. As exercise intensity increases from low to moderate, the amount of fat released from adipose tissue into the bloodstream decreases, while intramuscular triglyceride use increases (13). Increasing intensity from moderate to high decreases the percentage of fat used as energy, while carbohydrate (from glycogen and glucose) use increases.

Although higher-intensity exercise shifts relative fuel use from fat to carbohydrate as the preferred source of energy, training and diet also influence the type of energy used. Consistent aerobic training increases the muscle's capacity to use fat as a source of energy (14). Besides adapting to training, the body will adapt to greater reliance on fat for energy when a higher-fat, lower-carbohydrate diet is consumed consistently over time (14, 15). Adapting to a higher-fat, lower-carbohydrate diet, however, does not necessarily translate to improved performance (16-19). Therefore, prudent athletes should stick to a dietary fat intake within the AMDR of 20 to 35 percent of total daily calories. In addition, training with low glycogen stores can suppress immune and central nervous system functioning (15, 20).

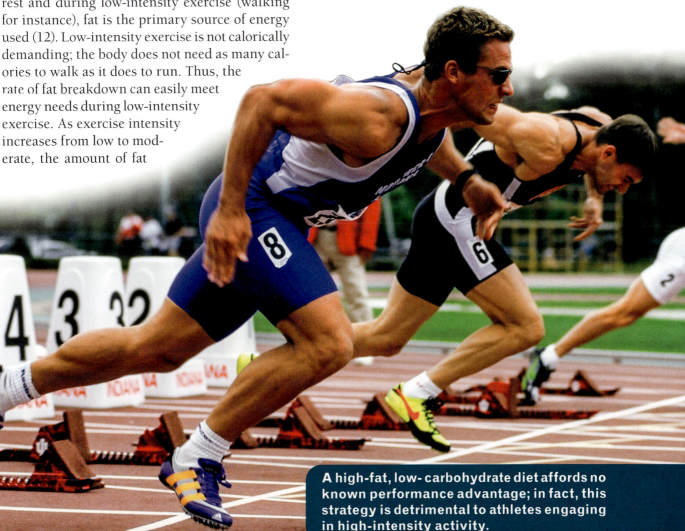

A high-fat, low-carbohydrate diet affords no known performance advantage; in fact, this strategy is detrimental to athletes engaging in high-intensity activity.

DO YOU KNOW?

Excess dietary fat should be avoided before workouts and competition. Fat slows the rate of digestion. The combination of digestion and exercise can lead to stomach cramps (21, 22).

Dietary fats are composed of a mixture of saturated, monounsaturated, and polyunsaturated fatty acids. Some fatty acids have positive or negative effects on various aspects of health, including risk factors for developing cardiovascular disease. Only two dietary fatty acids are essential to be consumed in the diet. The human body can make all other fats from the carbon skeletons of carbohydrate and protein. In the body, fat serves as a source of energy, helps with the absorption of fat-soluble vitamins and certain plant-based compounds, and plays an important structural and functional role in cell membranes, the brain, and myelin, the protective layer covering nerve cells. Though some athletes prefer a high-fat diet or believe it improves performance, no clear performance advantage is evident from following that approach. Ultraendurance athletes, who train and compete at a relatively slow pace, rely on more fat as a percentage of energy (calories) used during activity and might be able to get away with a diet higher in fat, but research has yet to show that this approach is advantageous for performance. This topic is covered in more detail in chapter 11. A high-fat, low-carbohydrate diet will likely have deleterious effects on training and performance for athletes participating in high-intensity training programs or competing in high-intensity sports such as football, tennis, basketball, or rugby.

LIPIDS AND DIETARY FAT

Lipids are a category of macronutrients that are insoluble in water. Collectively, lipids have various biological functions in the body. The three main categories of lipids are triglycerides, sterols, and phospholipids; each has different functions in the body (figure 4.1). Dietary fat is composed primarily of triglycerides, with smaller amounts of phospholipids and sterols. Cooking oils, butter, animal fat, nuts, seeds, avocados, and olives are

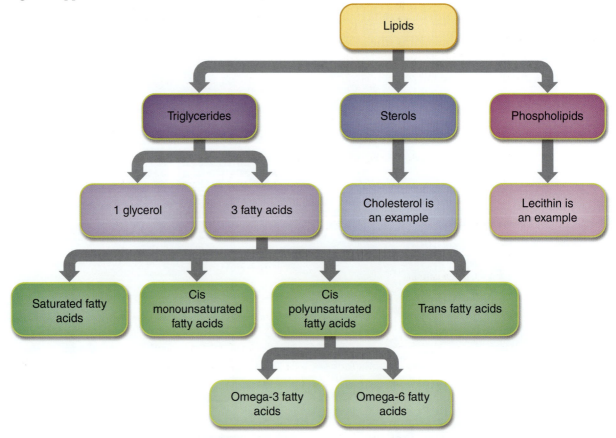

Figure 4.1 The classification of lipids.

all significant sources of triglycerides in the diet (23). Dietary fats and oils provide energy and aid in the absorption of fat-soluble vitamins A, D, E, and K, as well as certain food components such as carotenoids (24). Dietary fats and oils also have a textural role in foods, increasing palatability (25).

Triglycerides

Triglycerides are composed of one glycerol molecule and three fatty acid molecules. Fatty acids are either saturated, containing no double bonds, or unsaturated, containing one or more double bonds. Saturated fatty acids are the building blocks of saturated fat. **Saturated fatty acids** can stack together, making them solid at room temperature. **Unsaturated fatty acids** are the building blocks of unsaturated fat. Because of the kinks at double bonds (figure 4.2), unsaturated fatty acids do not stack neatly on top of one another and are therefore liquid at room temperature. **Monounsaturated fatty acids (MUFA)** contain one double bond, and **polyunsaturated fatty acids (PUFA)** contain more than one double bond and are identified based on the location of their first double bond. So, for instance, omega-3 fatty acids have their first double bond at the third carbon from the methyl end of the FA structure, whereas omega-6 fatty acids have their first double bond at the sixth carbon (figure 4.3). Most animal fats are high in saturated fat and therefore solid at room temperature, whereas plant-based fats (such as nut and fruit-based oils, including walnut oil and olive oil) tend to be liquid at room temperature because of their higher unsaturated fatty acid content. Coconut oil and palm kernel oil, however, are plant-based fats that are more solid, yet soft (due to their shorter carbon chains) at room temperature and have a high content of saturated fat (25). Regardless of the source, 1 gram of fat contains approximately 9 kcal.

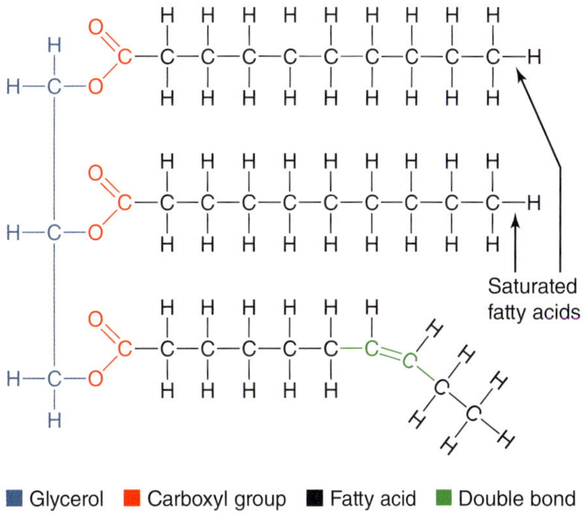

■ Glycerol ■ Carboxyl group ■ Fatty acid ■ Double bond

Figure 4.2 Triglycerides contain one glycerol molecule and three fatty acids.

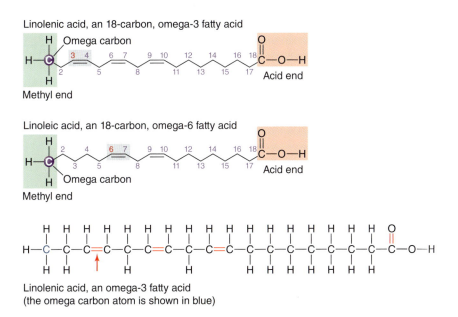

Figure 4.3 Chemical structure of omega-3 and omega-6 fatty acids. Polyunsaturated fatty acids are identified by the location of their first double bond from CH_3 (methyl group).

Fatty acids vary in the number of double bonds they contain, the structure or configuration of the double bonds, and carbon chain length (25, 26). Although fatty acids are often referenced by their saturation status—saturated, monounsaturated (containing one double bond), or polyunsaturated (containing more than one double bond)—individual fatty acids that are members of the same category can have vastly different effects on health. The carbon chain length and structure of a fatty acid determines its function in food and cooking, its role in the body, and its effect on health and disease (26).

In addition to differences in location and number of double bonds, unsaturated fatty acids have two chemical configurations. Those in the **cis configuration** have hydrogen ions on the same side of the double bond, whereas unsaturated fatty acids in the trans configuration have hydrogen ions on the opposite side of the double bond (25) (figure 4.4). The carbon chain can range from 2 to 40 carbons in length, though most dietary fatty acids contain 12 to 20 carbons (27). Short-chain fatty acids contain up to 6 carbons, medium-chain contain from 8 to 12 carbons, and long-chain fatty acids contain more than 12 carbons (26).

Fatty acids are necessary for cell signaling and the expression of genes involved in carbohydrate and fat metabolism. Fatty acids also influence inflammation, insulin action, cell signaling, and neurological functioning. The body can produce all necessary fatty acids in the liver from dietary fat, carbohydrate, and protein with the exception of **linoleic acid (LA)** and **alpha-linolenic acid (ALA)**, which are "essential" fatty acids, meaning they must be consumed in the diet (24).

Glycerol is the backbone of triglycerides. In the human body, glycerol is released in the bloodstream from the breakdown of stored body fat. Like fatty acids, glycerol can be used to build molecules necessary for membranes or stored in body fat for later use. Glycerol can also be converted to carbohydrate through glycolysis or gluconeogenesis (28). Glycerol (glycerin) is produced synthetically or derived from plants and is used as an ingredient in food and pharmaceuticals (29). Glycerol is a colorless, thick liquid with a mild odor and sweet, warm taste. It is a sugar alcohol (sugar alcohols are not completely absorbed in the body and so provide fewer calories than sugar) (30).

Sterols

Sterols are compounds with a multiple-ring structure found in both plants and animals. **Cholesterol**, the most well-recognized sterol in food (figure 4.5), is a component of all animal tissues and is found only in animal-based foods such as eggs, meat, poultry, cheese, and milk (23). Humans absorb 20 to 80 percent of cholesterol from food. Genetic variations in cholesterol absorption can influence blood cholesterol levels (31). For most people, however, dietary cholesterol is not the main factor that raises serum cholesterol. Instead, higher intakes of saturated fat raise serum cholesterol in the body (32, 33). In the body, cholesterol is essential for all cells; it is a structural component of cell membranes, helps repair and form new cells, and is necessary for synthesizing steroid hormones (such as testosterone, androgen, and estrogen) and bile acids (which facilitate lipid digestion and absorption and are important for regulating cholesterol in the body) (34). Although cholesterol is absolutely necessary, high levels of LDL (low-density lipoprotein) cholesterol

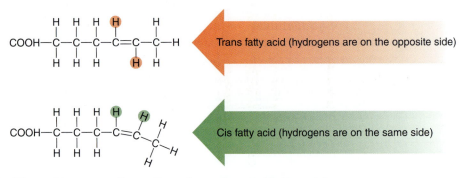

Figure 4.4 Cis and trans configuration of unsaturated fatty acids.

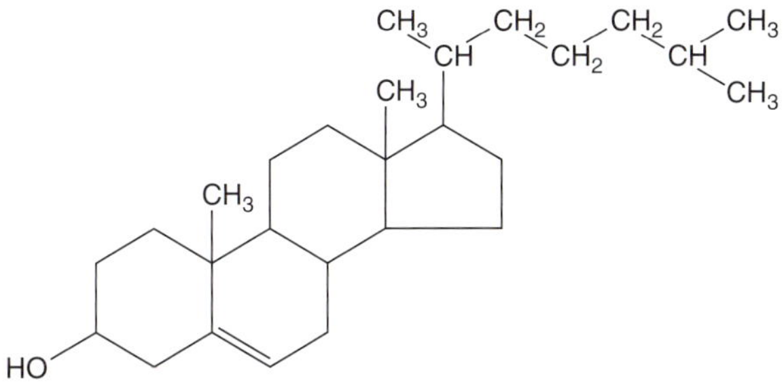

Figure 4.5 Chemical structure of cholesterol.

and total cholesterol (which includes LDL and HDL, high-density lipoprotein) in the blood are considered risk factors for developing cardiovascular disease because they contribute to plaque formation in arteries (32, 33, 35).

> **? DO YOU KNOW?**
>
> Humans do not need to consume cholesterol in food because the body makes enough to meet physiological requirements (34).

Plant sterols, compounds naturally found in plants, are similar in structure to cholesterol and interfere with the body's absorption of cholesterol (36). Plant sterols are not consumed in high enough doses through food to have an appreciable effect on blood cholesterol levels. Supplemental doses of at least 1 gram per day of plant sterols, however, can help lower blood cholesterol levels, yet these supplements also decrease the bioavailability of fat-soluble vitamins and carotenoids including beta-carotene, lycopene, zeaxanthin, and more (36, 37).

Phospholipids

Phospholipids are composed of glycerol, fatty acids, phosphate, and inositol, choline, serine, or ethanolamine (38). Phospholipids are naturally found in some foods and added to others as emulsifiers (helping liquids stay mixed, such as oil and vinegar as a salad dressing). Lecithin (phosphatidylcholine) is a naturally occurring phospholipid found in several foods, including egg yolks, liver, soybeans, wheat germ, and peanuts. In the body, phospholipids are structural components of cell membranes and lipoproteins (*lipo* means "lipid"; lipoproteins, including LDL and HDL, contain both proteins and lipids and are transporters of cholesterol and fats in blood) (38). Phospholipids are necessary for the absorption, transport, and storage of lipids and aid in the digestion and absorption of dietary fat (39).

TRIGLYCERIDES AND HEALTH

Most fats found in food, including oils, contain triglycerides with a mixture of fatty acids (figure 4.6). Although many studies have focused on the

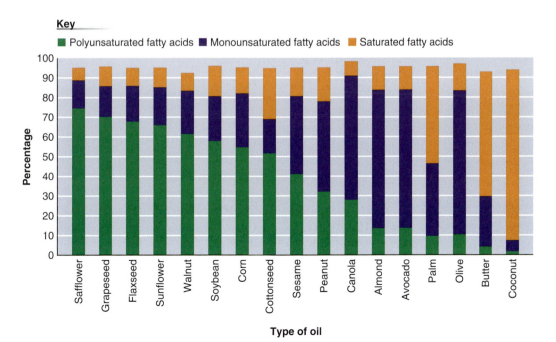

Figure 4.6 Fatty acid content of oils.

health effects of fatty acids based on their saturation status (saturated, monounsaturated, or polyunsaturated), fatty acids within a particular group can have different actions in the body, much as athletes on the same team can have different roles in a game. In addition, determining the health effects stemming from intake of a specific fatty acid can be difficult. A effect of a fatty acid on health may be influenced by the food matrix (the combination of nutrient and nonnutrient compounds found in food and their chemical bonds to each other), the way in which the fat is processed and cooked, and a person's health status and overall dietary intake (26, 40, 41). More recent research is teasing out the effects of individual fatty acids from the category of fats they belong to while also emphasizing the effect that certain fat-containing foods, versus just the fat within the food, have on health parameters, including serum cholesterol levels.

Saturated Fatty Acids

Saturated fatty acids are a source of energy and a structural component of cell membranes; some saturated fatty acids are necessary for normal protein functioning. Saturated fatty acids can be made in the body; there is no dietary requirement for them (25, 41). Most saturated fatty acids contain 14 or more carbon atoms.

The main sources of saturated fat in the U.S. diet are mixed dishes containing cheese or meat, such as burgers, sandwiches, tacos, and pizza; rice, pasta, and grain dishes; and meat, poultry, and seafood dishes (41). Saturated fats are typically more resistant to oxidation and therefore less likely to spoil.

There is no indication at this time that saturated fats prevent chronic disease. Higher intake of saturated fats are associated with higher total and LDL cholesterol and increased risk of developing coronary heart disease (CHD) (25). Dyslipidemia, high total or LDL cholesterol, or low levels of HDL cholesterol, is an important risk factor for coronary heart disease and stroke. Yet the association between greater dietary intake of saturated fat, higher levels of blood cholesterol, and cardiovascular disease has become controversial for several reasons. For one thing, some population-based studies, in which dietary intake was accessed through 24-hour recalls and food frequency questionnaires, found no relation between saturated fat intake and fatal heart attacks and stroke (42). Also, two meta-analyses found no significant relationship between total saturated fat intake and risk of coronary heart disease (32, 43). Confusing matters more, some studies show that patients hospitalized with coronary artery disease had LDL levels within normal limits. But relying only on population-based studies for data is problematic. In many of these studies, a single 24-hour dietary recall, taken at one point in time, was used, which does not reflect long-term dietary intake (44). Also, 24-hour dietary recalls and food frequency questionnaires (a series of questions asking how often standard serving sizes of common foods and beverages are consumed) depend on a subject's memory of their dietary intake, including the method of food preparation and portion sizes (44). In addition, all saturated fatty acids are grouped together, yet the effect that saturated fat has on cholesterol depends on the type of saturated fatty acids and the food that fat is incorporated into.

Each saturated fatty acid affects blood cholesterol differently (some have little to no effect on blood cholesterol, whereas others raise total and LDL cholesterol). The atherogenic (artery-clogging) potential of specific saturated fatty acids varies depending on carbon chain length (table 4.1), fats eaten concurrently, overall diet, carbohydrate intake, and overall health (45). Also, the food matrix, the combination of fatty acids, nutrients, and bioactive compounds found in a food, can modify the effect that saturated fat has on blood cholesterol and CHD. For instance, several studies show aged cheese appears to have a relatively minor effect on LDL cholesterol or no effect at all. This outcome could be due to the calcium content, which leads to the excretion of some fat, or fermentation may have an effect (46, 47). Also, yogurt appears to have less of a cholesterol-raising effect than expected. This research is inconsistent, however, possibly due to differences in the type of bacteria in the yogurt (48). Finally, population studies cannot be used to determine cause and effect because they aren't designed to answer the question "Do higher levels of intake of saturated fatty acids increase risk of coronary heart disease?" (43). Taken together, these factors are sufficient to make some researchers dubious

Table 4.1 Types of Fatty Acids Found in Common Foods

Fatty acid	Common food sources (not all inclusive)
CIS POLYUNSATURATED FATTY ACIDS (PUFA)	
Omega-3 PUFAs	
Alpha-linolenic acid (ALA)	Flaxseeds, chia seeds, walnuts, canola oil, soybean oil, flaxseed oil
Stearidonic acid (SDA)	Sardines, herring, algae, GMO soybean oil
Eicosapentaenoic acid (EPA)	Seafood, especially fatty fish such as salmon, mackerel, herring, and halibut
Docosapentaenoic acid (DPA)	Seafood, especially fatty fish such as salmon, mackerel, herring, and halibut
Docosahexaenoic acid (DHA)	Seafood, especially fatty fish such as salmon, mackerel, herring, and halibut
Omega-6 PUFAs	
Linoleic acid (LA)	Soybean oil, corn oil, meat, sunflower oil, safflower oil
Gamma linolenic acid (GLA)	Black currant seed oil, evening primrose oil
Arachidonic acid (ARA)	Meat, poultry, eggs
CIS MONOUNSATURATED FATTY ACIDS (MUFA)	
Palmitoleic acid	Macadamia nuts, sea buckthorn oil, some blue-green algae (26)
Oleic acid*	Olive oil, canola oil, beef tallow, lard, avocado
Erucic acid	Available in low quantities in food, including rapeseed, kale, and broccoli (26)
TRANS FATTY ACIDS (UNSATURATED)	
Elaidic acid**	Partially hydrogenated vegetable oils
Vaccenic acid**	Butterfat, meat
Conjugated linoleic acid (CLA)**	Ruminant meat, dairy, CLA supplements; food typically contains more cis 9, trans 11 18:2, whereas supplements often contain an equal mix of both isomers (26)
SATURATED FATTY ACIDS (SFAs)	
Caprylic acid (MCT)	Coconut oil, palm kernel oil
Capric acid (MCT)	Coconut oil, palm kernel oil
Lauric acid (MCT)	Coconut oil, palm kernel oil
Myristic acid	Several types of cheese, coconut meat, coconut oil, beef fat
Palmitic acid	Beef, pork, and bacon fat; butter; several types of cheese; whipped cream; whole milk; egg yolks; palm oil; palm kernel oil; most fats and oils contain some palmitic acid
Stearic acid	Beef and pork fat; Brazil nuts; lamb; cashew nuts; chocolate

GMO = genetically modified organism; MCT = medium-chain triglycerides.
*Oleic acid is the most common monounsaturated fatty acid, accounting for approximately 92% of MUFAs found in the diet.
**In high doses (3.7% of calorie intake), trans fatty acids from industrial sources and naturally occurring trans fatty acids both increase LDL cholesterol and decrease HDL cholesterol.
(73).
Based on Vannice (2014); U.S. Department of Agriculture (2013); U.S. Institute of Medicine (2002).

about the efficacy of population-based studies, particularly when the results of such studies are not supported by clinical trials. As an example, clinical trials show replacing saturated fat and polyunsaturated fat leads to a decrease in LDL cholesterol coronary artery disease in men (49).

In the two meta-analyses that found no significant relationship between total saturated fat intake and risk of coronary heart disease (32, 43), only total saturated fat intake was taken into account. These studies did not take into consideration the substitution pattern—how substituting saturated fat with other macronutrients affects cardiovascular disease risk. In particular, substituting saturated fat with refined higher-sugar carbohydrates does not reduce risk of cardiovascular disease. Instead, replacing saturated fat with polyunsaturated fat is the most beneficial strategy for reducing cardiovascular disease risk (see figures 4.7 and 4.8 for more information) (32). Interestingly, in the Nurses' Health Study and Health Professional Follow-up Study, substituting unsaturated fats for saturated fats (5% of energy) reduced total mortality, mortality from coronary heart disease, and mortality from cancer and neurodegenerative diseases (35).

The replacement strategy (see figure 4.8) might make a difference. The strategy presented is a generalization. On the right-hand side of the figure, note that replacing saturated fat with high-fiber carbohydrate-rich foods such as whole grains may help reduce CHD risk by reducing total cholesterol. Replacing saturated fat with refined carbohydrate or added sugar, however, is not associated with improved cholesterol or a reduction in CHD.

Also muddling the understanding of the relationship between LDL and cardiovascular disease are the studies showing that many patients hospitalized with coronary artery disease did not have high LDL cholesterol upon admission. For instance, in one study, almost half of patients hospitalized with coronary artery disease had LDL levels within normal limits. But when examining their blood work in greater detail, more than half of the patients had low HDL (high-density lipoprotein) and only about 2 percent of patients had ideal levels of both HDL and LDL. Additionally, the study authors suggest that "normal" LDL guidelines should be lowered even further to prevent cardiovascular events (50). This study highlights how important it is to look at the total picture and not a single value as a predictor for cardiovascular disease.

When substituting other energy-yielding macronutrients for saturated fat in the diet, clinical trials show that replacement strategy matters. When saturated fat is taken out of the diet, the specific macronutrient used to replace

Instead of:	Choose:
White pasta	Whole grain, lentil, or bean pasta
Butter	Avocado oil (which has a slight buttery taste)
Coconut oil	Corn oil
Beef ribeye	Sirloin
55% ground beef	90% ground beef
85% ground turkey	93% or 97% ground turkey
Pork ribs	Pork loin
Sausage	Lower-fat sausage
Lard	Cooking oil
Cream	2% milk or full-fat oat milk (if more fat is needed for thickness)
Whole-fat dairy products	Low-fat or skim dairy products
Coconut cream	Coconut beverage (lower fat)
Pastries, pies	Fresh fruit with granola
Biscuits	Oat bran muffins
Ice cream	Smoothie bowl made with frozen fruit and 1% or 2% milk
Fried food	Baked food
Cookies	Granola bars made with nuts, seeds, or nut butter

Figure 4.7 Food replacement strategies to lower blood cholesterol.

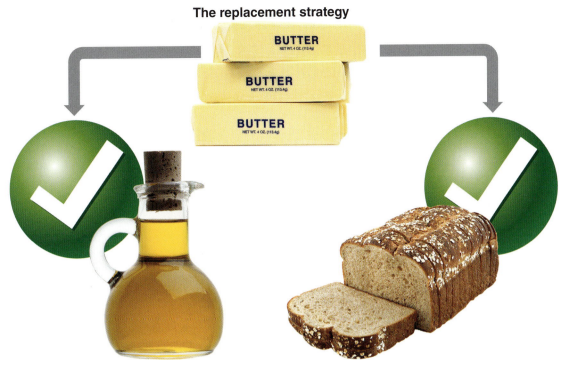

Some research suggests replacing fats high in saturated fatty acids with fats high in polyunsaturated fatty acids can decrease LDL cholesterol and reduce the risk of CHD.

Some research suggests replacing foods high in saturated fatty acids with foods naturally higher in fiber and lower in refined carbohydrates can decrease total cholesterol and reduce the risk of CHD.

Figure 4.8 Replacement strategy.

saturated fat determines changes in serum cholesterol levels, triglycerides, and risk of coronary heart disease (42). Replacing saturated fats with unsaturated fats, particularly PUFAs, is associated with a reduction in total and LDL cholesterol (41). Replacing saturated fat with PUFAs is also associated with a reduction in heart attacks and death from heart attacks (41) (figure 4.8). In addition, randomized controlled trials show that replacing saturated fat with PUFAs decreases coronary heart disease events (57). Additional benefits might also be associated with this strategy. A crossover study in adults with type 2 diabetes as well as healthy obese and nonobese adults found that PUFAs improved insulin sensitivity and LDL levels compared to diets high in saturated fats (58). Also, a study in healthy non-overweight and nonobese adults found overeating saturated fat, as opposed to overeating polyunsaturated fat, increased liver and visceral fat storage. (Visceral fat wraps around organs like a blanket and is associated with insulin resistance and increased risk of type 2 diabetes and cardiovascular disease.) Overeating polyunsaturated fat, and not saturated fat, led to greater gains in muscle, as opposed to body fat (59). Note that considerable differences exist among people in their response to saturated fat intake (60, 61). In addition to the potential for intrinsic genetic differences in lipid metabolism among individuals (62), higher body weight and insulin resistance may reduce the beneficial effects of a reduction in saturated fat intake on LDL cholesterol.

> **? DO YOU KNOW?**
>
> Several factors affect cardiovascular disease risk including total, LDL, and HDL cholesterol; high blood pressure, smoking, diabetes, overweight, and obesity.

Replacing saturated fats with carbohydrates can reduce total and LDL cholesterol, yet also decrease HDL cholesterol and increase triglycerides—this strategy will not decrease risk of cardiovascular disease. Studies examining the association (these studies cannot determine cause and effect) between different types of carbohydrate and

PUTTING IT INTO PERSPECTIVE

THE FOOD MATRIX AND HOW FOODS HIGH IN SATURATED FAT AFFECT BLOOD CHOLESTEROL

In addition to varying physiological effects from different saturated fatty acids, the food matrix influences how saturated fat affects blood cholesterol levels. Dairy foods are a good example. Although all full-fat dairy products have a high percentage of saturated fat, they have differing effects on blood cholesterol. Several studies show that aged cheeses have a relatively minor effect on LDL cholesterol or no effect at all (51-53). By way of explanation, some scientists point to the calcium content of the cheese or the fermentation of aged cheeses (46). Full-fat yogurt also appears to affect cholesterol levels less than would be expected. The research on yogurt is inconsistent, however, possibly because of differences in yogurt used in studies (54, 55). The live and active cultures may be responsible for the positive research results (56).

Whole milk raises LDL to the same extent as butter, but milk contributes substantially less fat per amount consumed compared with butter. Butter raises LDL cholesterol and should be replaced with oils rich in polyunsaturated fat, such as olive oil.

In addition to considering the entire picture (LDL, total, and HDL cholesterol, overall diet, weight, etc.), making food-based suggestions that are practical is often more helpful than suggesting that people "lower their saturated fat intake" (33). See figure 4.7.

---

cardiovascular disease risk show higher intakes of whole grains are associated with lower risk of coronary heart disease, whereas refined starches and added sugars are positively associated with coronary heart disease risk. Given the state of the current evidence, whenever possible, foods high in saturated fats should be replaced with foods higher in polyunsaturated fats or whole grains (41, 63).

> **DO YOU KNOW?**
>
> For better cholesterol, limit foods high in saturated fat as well as foods rich in refined carbohydrate and sugars. Eat more fruits, vegetables including legumes, and fiber-rich whole grains.

Ketogenic diets are high in fat, moderate in protein, and contain very little carbohydrate. Although the specific percentages of fat, protein, and carbohydrate vary, ketogenic diets generally contain about 75 to 90 percent fat, 5 to 20 percent protein, and 5 to 10 percent carbohydrate (64). Carbohydrate intake is kept low enough that the body goes into a state of nutritional ketosis, as determined by circulating ketone levels reaching more than 0.5 mmol/L as measured through urine, blood, or breath tests. Ketones are used as a source of energy when the body has insufficient glucose.

Ketogenic diets were originally designed to decrease the incidence and severity of seizures in epileptic patients, and they are extremely effective for this purpose (65). They have also been studied as a potential therapy for minimizing the damaging effects resulting from traumatic brain injury. But some athletes and active gym goers are going "keto" to lose weight or try to improve athletic performance (this is covered in more detail in chapters 11 and 12). Proponents of ketogenic diets suggest an increased reliance on body fat as a source of fuel will lead to greater overall fat loss, fewer hunger pangs, and a decrease in mental and physical fatigue. Additionally, some suggest that the likelihood of gastric distress is minimized because the athlete will not have to rely on carbohydrate during exercise and will consume fewer calories, which will decrease the likelihood of stomach upset (66). The effects of a ketogenic diet on body composition is covered in more detail in chapter 13.

> **DO YOU KNOW?**
>
> Nutritional ketosis should not be confused with ketoacidosis—the rapid production of specific ketone bodies leading to a life-threatening change in the body's acid-base buffering system in uncontrolled diabetics.

Ketogenic diets have variable effects on cardiovascular disease risk factors including cholesterol, blood pressure, and arterial stiffness. The differences seen in study results are likely due to differences in the types of fat consumed, changes in body weight, and populations studied. Research in children following a ketogenic diet as treatment for epileptic seizures consistently reports an increase in total and LDL cholesterol as well as triglycerides (67-69). But one longer-term study found that blood cholesterol levels returned to baseline after 24 months on the diet (68). Some research has shown an increase in artery stiffness in children with epilepsy following a ketogenic diet, but other research has shown no change in artery stiffness. This result could be due, in part, to the composition of the diet. An olive oil–based ketogenic diet resulted in no change in artery stiffness after 12 months on the diet (67). Yet in a study spanning 24 months, artery stiffness increased after 12 months and then returned to baseline when measured 24 months into the study (68).

In adults without epilepsy, some studies showed that the ketogenic diet increases HDL cholesterol and decreases LDL cholesterol and triglycerides. Other studies found that this diet increases LDL cholesterol. These differences in results seem to be due to the composition of the diet and changes in body weight. Those consuming more saturated fat tended to increase LDL (70). Additionally, weight loss in those who are overweight or obese can independently lower total and LDL cholesterol and triglycerides (71, 72).

Monounsaturated Fatty Acids

There is no known requirement or health benefit associated with the consumption of monounsaturated fatty acids. Monounsaturated fats can be synthesized by the body (24). As noted in the previous section, some research shows replacing saturated fat with monounsaturated fats lowers total and LDL cholesterol (75, 76). Monounsaturated fat can also increase HDL and lower triglycerides compared with carbohydrate (77). The average American diet contains more monounsaturated fat than saturated or polyunsaturated fat. The monounsaturated fatty acid oleic acid is the most abundant fatty acid in the American diet (78).

❓ DO YOU KNOW?

Monounsaturated fat supplements are available alone and in mixtures with omega-3 and omega-6 fatty acids. There is no reason to take these supplements (26).

Polyunsaturated Fatty Acids

The omega-6 polyunsaturated fatty acid LA and omega-3 polyunsaturated fatty acid ALA are required in small amounts for structural integrity and fluidity of membrane lipids, synthesis of **eicosanoids** (hormone-like agents), and as substrates for biological pathways that produce metabolic products necessary for structural and functional roles within the human body (figure 4.9) (4, 79-81).

PUTTING IT INTO PERSPECTIVE

THE MEDITERRANEAN DIET, BLOOD CHOLESTEROL, AND CARDIOVASCULAR HEALTH

The Mediterranean diet is named after the dietary pattern of people who live in the Mediterranean region including Italy, Greece, and Spain. Several decades ago research showed that people in the Mediterranean region experience lower incidence of death from coronary heart disease. Later, observational studies suggested that their dietary pattern may be an underlying factor (74). This diet is based on fresh fruits and vegetables including legumes, nuts, seeds, whole grains, herbs, spices, fish and other seafood, and olive oil as a source of fat for food preparation. Poultry, eggs, cheese, and yogurt are consumed in moderation, whereas red meat is consumed sparingly. There is some evidence, although this is not consistent in the research, that a Mediterranean-style diet may improve some cardiovascular disease risk factors, including a possible small reduction in both total and LDL cholesterol in those without a history of cardiovascular disease (74).

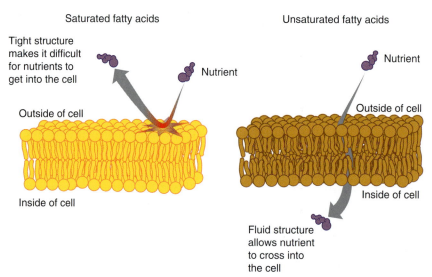

Figure 4.9 Cell membrane.

Omega-6 Fatty Acids

Omega-6 fatty acids are important to epithelial cell function and regulation of gene expression (25). Epithelial cells are "barrier cells" that make up epithelial tissue, which lines most of the surfaces of the body, including the skin, blood vessels, and organs. Linoleic acid is the only essential omega-6 fatty acid; the body cannot make this fatty acid, so it must be consumed in the diet. Insufficient LA can lead to scaly rash and reduced growth. In developed countries, linoleic acid deficiency is rare, and most adults consume several times more linoleic acid than they need (25). LA is a precursor for arachidonic acid, a fatty acid that is a part of membrane structural lipids, serves as a substrate for eicosanoid production, and is necessary for cell-signaling pathways (24, 25). Arachidonic acid, however, can also lead to an inflammatory cascade in the body (82).

Omega-3 Fatty Acids

Three primary omega-3 fatty acids are consumed in the diet: ALA, **eicosapentaenoic acid (EPA)**, and **docosahexaenoic acid (DHA)** (figure 4.10). Each omega-3 fatty acid has a different role in the body and effect on health. **Stearidonic acid (SDA)** is an omega-3 fatty acid found in some seed oils; some fish, including sardines and herring; algae; and GMO (genetically modified organism) soybeans used to create SDA-enriched soybean oil (83, 84). SDA-enriched soybean oil increases red blood cell EPA to a greater extent than ALA, though much less than taking EPA directly (84, 85). Compared with taking EPA directly, conversion of SDA to EPA from SDA-enriched soybean oil is about 17 percent efficient, according to a study in healthy, overweight adults (86). At this rate of conversion, SDA does not improve blood lipids, including triglycerides and HDL cholesterol (85). Consuming

PUTTING IT INTO PERSPECTIVE

HOW FAT AFFECTS CELL MEMBRANES AND CELL FUNCTIONING

Fats are incorporated into cell membranes, and both saturated fat and unsaturated fat are necessary for optimal cell membrane functioning. Saturated fatty acids stack neatly on top of each other in cell membranes. If a membrane were composed of all, or mostly, saturated fatty acids, the tight structure would make it difficult for nutrients to get into cells, compromising cell health and increasing the likelihood of cell injury. Unsaturated fats do not pack neatly on top of each other in cell membranes. They provide a more fluid structure, allowing nutrients to easily cross the cell membrane into the cell and allowing receptors in nerve cells to recognize neurotransmitters (chemical messengers).

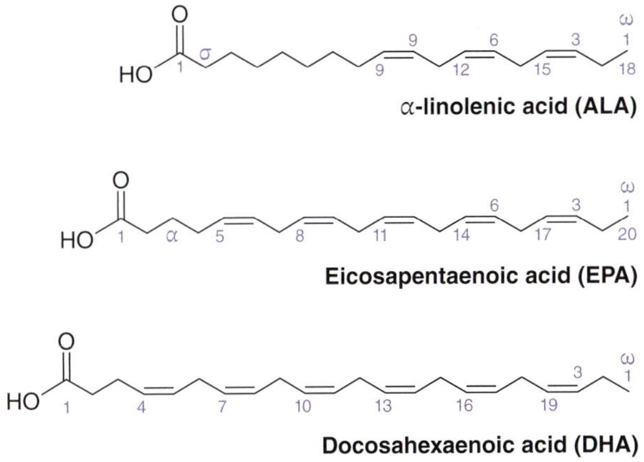

Figure 4.10 Structure of ALA, EPA, and DHA, all polyunsaturated fatty acids. ALA has 18 carbons and three double bonds, EPA has 20 carbons and five double bonds, and DHA has 22 carbons and six double bonds.

SDA does not increase tissue levels of DHA (86, 87). Currently, it is not clear if consuming SDA has an independent effect on cardiovascular disease risk factors or other aspects of health.

Alpha-Linolenic Acid Alpha-linolenic acid is found in soybeans, soybean oil, canola oil, flaxseed oil, black walnuts, flaxseeds, and chia seeds (23). ALA is a precursor to EPA and DHA (24, 88). ALA deficiency, however, can result in scaly dermatitis (25). ALA-rich foods are beneficial for cardiovascular disease risk as a result of the ALA, other compounds found in these foods, or a synergistic effect between the ALA and these compounds (89, 90). Compared with EPA and DHA, much less research-based evidence suggests that ALA is beneficial for cardiovascular disease risk (89). ALA is converted into EPA and DHA in the body. But studies show that only 5 to 21 percent of ALA is converted to EPA and that less than 0.5 to 9 percent of ALA is converted to DHA (91, 92). Diet, health status, genetics, gender, and omega-6 fatty acid competition for elongase and desaturase enzymes (see figure 4.11) influence the conversion rate (26).

Eicosapentaenoic Acid and Docosahexaenoic Acid Sources of EPA and DHA in the diet include fatty

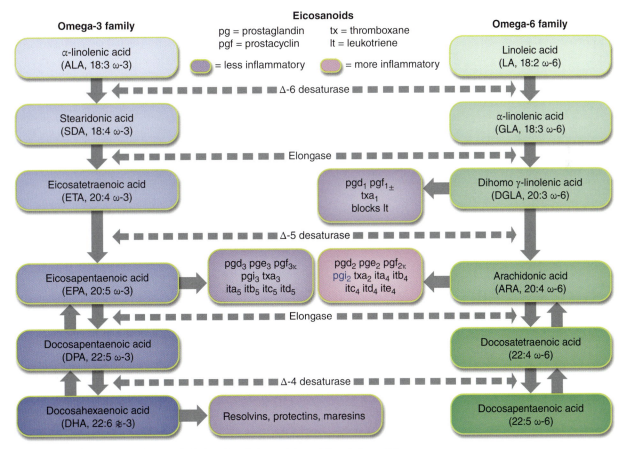

Figure 4.11 Metabolism of alpha-linoleic acid and linoleic acid.

fish such as salmon, mackerel, herring, and halibut. Supplemental sources of EPA and DHA are typically sourced from sardines, anchovies, and some types of algae and krill.

At the top of the food chain increased risk of mercury contamination occurs among certain fish. Shark, king mackerel, swordfish, and tilefish tend to live longer and feed on smaller fish, accumulating substantial methylmercury over their lifetime (figure 4.12). These fish should be avoided, especially by pregnant women, children, the elderly, and those with a compromised immune system (93).

EPA and DHA have distinct roles in the body. EPA is a precursor to eicosanoids, including a group of eicosanoids (series-3 prostaglandins) that may be protective against heart attacks and strokes. EPA helps decrease inflammation by inhibiting the production of proinflammatory compounds. DHA, the major fat found in the brain, is important for brain development and function. DHA is necessary for the production of compounds that help reduce inflammation in the brain from reduced blood flow (strokes for instance). In addition to their distinct roles, together, EPA and DHA decrease triglycerides in a dose-dependent manner (triglycerides decrease in greater amounts with more fish oil consumed) (94), increase HDL cholesterol (94), improve blood vessel functioning in some but not all studies (this may be population and dose dependent) (95, 96), reduce inflammation (97), and lead to a small decrease in blood pressure (98).

Population-based studies and randomized controlled trials examining cardiovascular health and fatty fish or EPA and DHA indicate the following:

> Consuming small amounts of fish is associated with a 27 percent decrease in risk of nonfatal heart attack (99). Consuming at least one serving of fish per week is associated with a reduced risk of sudden death from coronary heart disease (CHD) (100) and a 17 percent decrease in risk of CHD mortality, and each additional serving per week decreases risk an additional 3.9 percent (99).

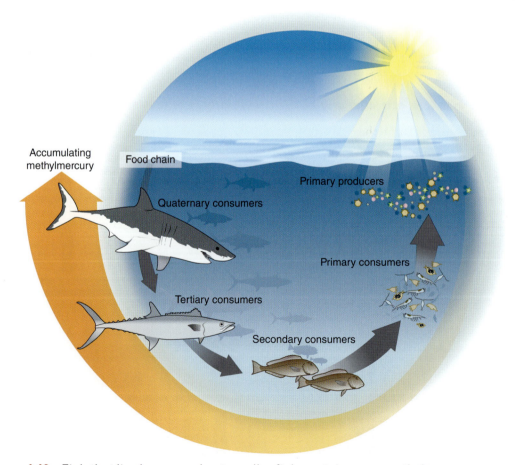

Figure 4.12 Fish that live longer and eat smaller fish contain more methylmercury.

▶ Consuming fish at least once per week is also associated with a decrease in CHD death rate when compared with never eating fish, and consuming fish five or more times per week is associated with a 38 percent decrease in CHD mortality (101).

▶ A pooled analysis of randomized controlled trials found that one to two servings of fatty fish per week or approximately 250 milligrams of EPA plus DHA per day resulted in a 36 percent decrease in CHD death (102).

▶ Modest consumption of fish (one or two servings per week or approximately 250 milligrams of EPA plus DHA per day) reduces risk of CHD by 36 percent and all-cause mortality by 17 percent (103).

▶ Two weekly servings of fatty fish reduced risk of death by ischemic heart disease and reduced all-cause mortality by 29 percent in men with a previous history of heart attack (104).

▶ One capsule containing 850 milligrams of EPA and DHA reduced the risk of all-cause mortality, sudden death, and coronary death in adults with a recent history of heart attack compared with no intervention (105).

▶ Taking 850 to 882 milligrams of EPA and DHA reduced incidence of death and CHD hospitalizations in those with heart failure (106).

Although some studies found that EPA and DHA do not affect cardiovascular disease risk or events, a number of factors might have influenced the results of those studies, including small supplementation amounts; short duration of the study; higher baseline dietary omega-3 intake of the population studied (a higher intake before the start of the study will decrease the potential effect of supplementation); and improvements in cardiovascular disease care and therapies, including use of statin drugs (which lower blood cholesterol), which may mask the effects of EPA and DHA (107-114).

? DO YOU KNOW?

It is currently unclear if there is an ideal ratio of omega-6 to omega-3 fatty acids for health or human performance. In any case, most Americans consume plenty of omega-6 fatty acids, but many need to consume more omega-3 fatty acids.

Omega-3 Fatty Acids and Joint Health, Sport, and Exercise EPA and DHA are incorporated into cell membranes where they make membranes more elastic, more flexible, and less prone to damage. They also influence membrane functioning.

Additionally, EPA reduces COX-2 expression and therefore delays inflammation (several hours after exercise) (115, 116).

Studies show that EPA and DHA can help improve joint functioning, particularly in those with rheumatoid arthritis; decrease the damaging effects caused by concussions (in animal studies); and may help reduce excess soreness after muscle-damaging exercise in untrained people. In addition, studies show that EPA and DHA can improve muscle mass and muscle functioning in older adults.

According to a meta-analysis of 17 randomized, controlled trials, EPA and DHA supplementation, in doses ranging from 1.7 to 9.6 grams per day for 3 to 4 months, reduced patient-reported joint pain intensity, duration of morning stiffness, and number of painful or tender joints in those with inflammatory joint pain from rheumatoid arthritis, inflammatory bowel disease, or painful menstruation (117). Additional research shows that EPA and DHA supplementation decreased both global assessments of pain and disease activity (as assessed by a patient or physician) and the need for nonsteroidal anti-inflammatory drugs in those with rheumatoid arthritis (118).

EPA and DHA may benefit recovery after a concussion (a type of traumatic brain injury) through several mechanisms. DHA makes up 97 percent of the omega-3 fatty acids in the brain and is essential for normal brain functioning (119). EPA and DHA increase fluidity of cell membranes, reduce inflammation, and increase blood flow to the brain. Concussion causes a reduction in blood flow to the brain for up to a month or longer (120). Cell membrane fluidity is important because membranes that are more fluid allow substances to enter cells more easily. Several animal studies show that EPA and DHA supplementation before or after a traumatic brain injury helps limit structural damage and a decline in brain functioning (121-127). In one study, rats starting the study with low brain DHA due to dietary restriction experienced greater cell death, slower recovery of motor function, and greater behavioral anxiety and cognitive deficits after a concussion (128). Although depletion of DHA before a concussion leads to poorer recovery, prophylactic supplementation with EPA and DHA may improve outcomes. A study in mice found that an omega-3-enriched diet consumed for two months before a head injury helped protect against several aspects of short- and long-term behavioral deficits due to a head injury (129).

In a multisite, nonrandomized study with two football teams, supplemental omega-3 fatty acids (2,000 mg DHA, 560 mg EPA, 320 mg DPA) taken for nearly 3 months during the football season led to a reduction in a marker of head trauma, suggesting a neuroprotective effect from omega-3 fatty acids (130).

Although some studies have suggested that omega-3 fatty acids may improve muscle mass and muscle functioning in older adults, the evidence is mixed. The hypertrophic effects (gaining muscle mass) of omega-3s appear to be equivocal when supplementation is combined with a resistance training program. And at this time it remains unclear whether omega-3 supplementation helps muscle functioning in older adults (131).

Few studies have examined omega-3 fatty acid supplementation and exercise-induced muscle damage in resistance-trained people, and at this time the results are inconclusive. Likewise, it is not clear if omega-3 fatty acids are beneficial for decreasing muscle soreness in untrained people (132). Although little research has been done on omega-3 fatty acid supplementation and the prevention of muscle loss during immobilization (if a person is in a cast for instance), one study in young women found that very high-dose omega-3s helped decrease muscle atrophy during immobilization (133).

Trans Fatty Acids

Trans fatty acids are unsaturated fatty acids, although they behave differently from other unsaturated fatty acids (24). Two trans fatty acids—vaccenic aid and elaidic acid—are made by bacteria in the rumen (one of the four chambers of the ruminant stomach) of ruminant animals (such as cows, goats, and sheep) from polyunsaturated fatty acids. These trans fatty acids are found in beef and dairy products. Trans fatty acids make up less than 9 percent of ruminant fat (137, 138). Most trans fatty acids found in the diet are produced from partial hydrogenation of oils. Hydrogenation involves bubbling hydrogen gas through edible oils in the presence of high heat and a catalyst (139). Partial hydrogenation converts some of the unsaturated fatty acids to saturated fatty acids and some of the unsaturated fatty acids from a cis (hydrogen atoms on the same side of the double bond) to a trans configuration (hydrogen atoms are on opposite sides of the double bond) (figure 4.13). Hydrogenated oils are more resistant to spoilage and rancidity (41). Modifying the conditions of hydrogenation alters the amount of trans fatty acids formed, which affects the properties of the end product (solid or semisolid, melting point, mouth feel, etc.) (139). The chemical configuration of trans fatty acids lets them pack neatly on top of each other, forming a semisolid to solid compound.

Industrial Trans Fatty Acids

Clinical trials show that industrially produced (i.e., man-made) trans fatty acids negatively affect several risk factors for coronary heart disease, and observational studies show an association between industrial trans fatty acid consumption and increased risk for coronary heart disease

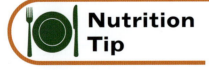

Nutrition Tip

Omega-3 supplements, in doses up to 3 grams per day, are generally recognized as safe (134). Supplemental fish oil does not increase risk for clinically significant bleeding (135). Doses over 3 grams per day, however, should be taken only under the care and guidance of a medical doctor. Although some absorption of EPA and DHA occurs on an empty stomach, for greater absorption EPA and DHA should be taken with a meal. Adverse side effects related to fish oil or ALA supplements are typically minor (such as fish burps and diarrhea) and are resolved by lowering the dose or discontinuing the supplement (136).

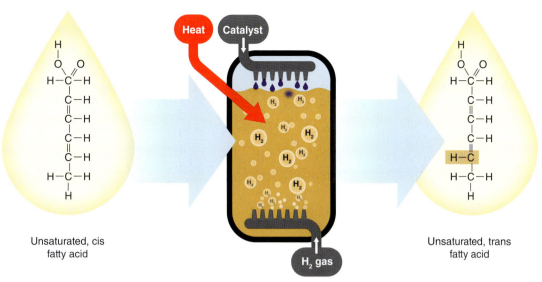

Figure 4.13 Unsaturated fats, which are liquid at room temperature, are made solid by bubbling hydrogen gas through them with a catalyst at a high temperature.

(140). Trans fatty acids from partially hydrogenated oils increase LDL cholesterol, reduce HDL cholesterol, reduce LDL particle size, increase inflammation, and promote blood vessel dysfunction—all risk factors for coronary heart disease (33, 141-145). Some, though not all, studies suggest that trans fatty acids increase triglycerides (141, 146). Trans fatty acids from partially hydrogenated oils also increase inflammation (147) and were found in a randomized trial in overweight postmenopausal women to increase body fat more than other dietary fats (145).

Given the abundance of data indicating that man-made trans fatty acids are harmful for health, in 2015 the FDA removed generally recognized as safe (GRAS) status for partially hydrogenated oils. Partially hydrogenated oils are no longer allowed in the food supply in the United States (148).

> **? DO YOU KNOW?**
> Man-made trans fatty acids are the worst type of dietary fat; even small amounts increase cardiovascular disease risk. No amount of trans fat is considered safe for consumption.

Trans Fatty Acids in Dairy and Meat

Trans fatty acids make up 2 to 5 percent of total fatty acids in dairy products and 3 to 9 percent of total fatty acids in beef and lamb (table 4.2) (137, 138). The amount varies based on feeding practices and geographical and seasonal changes (138, 149).

Table 4.2 Trans Fatty Acid and Conjugated Linoleic Acid Content of Dairy and Meat

Food	TFA content per serving	CLA content per serving
Cheddar cheese, 1 oz	240 mg	36.7 mg
Milk, whole, 1 cup	210 mg	41.6 mg
Yogurt, plain, low-fat, 1 cup	60 mg	37.8 mg
Meat, beef, ground, 20.8% fat, raw, 4 oz	910 mg	103.8 mg

Data from Gebauer et al. (2011).

Total daily intake of vaccenic acid and c9, t11-CLA ranges from 0.4 to 0.8 grams per day and 0.14 to 0.33 grams per day, respectively (150). In the human body, vaccenic acid can be converted to c9, t11-CLA. The conversion rate ranges from 0 to greater than 30 percent, at an average of 19 percent (150-153). Therefore, estimation of dietary intake of c9, t11-CLA alone may not reflect the synthesis of CLA from the vaccenic acid in the body (150).

The effect, if any, of ruminant trans fatty acids, vaccenic acid, and elaidic acid on cardiovascular disease risk factors is unclear. The data are mixed, possibly because of differences in study design. But some studies suggest that lower doses of ruminant trans fatty acids do not affect lipids in lipoprotein, but at higher doses, which are not attainable through diet but instead through supplemental intake, these fatty acids may have effects similar to man-made trans fatty acids, increasing LDL and decreasing HDL (154). In a well-designed, double-blind crossover study in healthy men, four different experimental diets (all contained 2,500 kcal; all food was provided) were given to participants for 4 weeks: (a) high in ruminant trans fats (10.2 g; butter and milk specifically designed for this study to contain high amounts of trans fatty acids), (b) moderate in ruminate trans fats (4.2 g), (c) high in industrial (man-made) trans fats (10.2 g), and (d) low in trans fats from any source (2.2 g). High intake of trans fats, whether from ruminants or industrially produced, increased LDL. Also, HDL cholesterol concentrations were significantly lower after the diet high in ruminant trans fats compared with the diet containing a moderate amount of ruminant trans fats. No significant difference were found in changes in serum cholesterol between the diet containing a moderate amount of ruminant trans fat and the diet containing low trans fats from any source. This study suggests that moderate amounts of trans fats from dairy will not have a substantial effect on blood cholesterol. But trans fats, whether from dairy or industrial production of partially hydrogenated oils, are not heart healthy when consumed in large amounts. Note that the large amount of ruminant trans fats used in this study was beyond the amount of typical human consumption (73).

Supplemental CLA is discussed in more detail in chapter 9.

> **? DO YOU KNOW?**
> According to the World Health Organization, observational studies suggest that ruminant trans fatty acids (those found in dairy and meat) do not increase coronary heart disease risk in typical amounts consumed (139, 155).

Interesterified Fats

Interesterified fats have been used for decades in margarines, cooking oils, and infant formulas (156). Interesterification typically involves blending fats high in saturated fatty acids, which are solid at room temperature, with liquid edible oils (157). Interesterification leads to chemical or enzymatic rearrangement of fatty acids along the glycerol backbone. By altering the chemical structure of a fat and inserting a saturated fatty acid (typically stearic acid), interesterification produces customized fats ranging in melting points and solidity to fit the needs of various food preparations (139).

No trans fatty acids are formed during the production of interesterified fats. Although older studies suggested interesterified fats do not affect blood lipids, any untoward health effects might depend on the type of fatty acid inserted and where it is inserted (158-161). Altering the position of fatty acids along the glycerol backbone may affect lipoprotein metabolism and atherogenesis (162). Additionally, the type of interesterification—chemical or enzymatic—and weight status of the person consuming the fat—obese or nonobese—may determine how interesterified fats affect blood lipids. In a randomized crossover study, obese and nonobese adults consumed 50 grams of carbohydrate from white bread in addition to 1 gram of fat per kilogram body mass of (a) noninteresterified stearic acid-rich fat spread, (b) chemically interesterified stearic acid-rich fat spread, (c) enzymatically interesterified stearic acid-rich fat spread or (d) no fat. Interesterification had no effect on postmeal blood glucose, insulin, free fatty acids, or cholesterol in either group. Obese subjects, however, had an 85 percent increase in triglycerides after consuming the fat that was modified through chemical interesterification compared with noninteresterification. Nonobese subjects' triglycerides were not affected by either fat treatment. Given the extremely large consumption of fat in one sitting, 91 grams for a 200-pound (91 kg) adult, it is unclear whether the results would be different when given lower quantities of the chemically interesterified fat in a meal (163).

A 4-week crossover study examined the effects of different fats on blood lipids and blood glucose when incorporated into a whole-food diet, including a man-made trans-fat-rich partially hydrogenated soybean oil (containing 3.2% trans fat), palm olein (an unmodified fat naturally rich in saturated fat), and an interesterified fat. Both the partially hydrogenated soybean oil and interesterified fat decreased HDL compared with the palm olein and increased fasting blood glucose (almost 20% in the interesterified group). The interesterified fat meal led to a significant rise in postmeal blood glucose (164). Although the results of this study may lead people to believe that all interesterified fats are harmful for blood glucose and insulin, the effect that a modified fat has on glucose and insulin might depend on the position of the fatty acids and the health status of the study subjects. In a crossover trial, healthy men and women aged 20 to 50 years were fed a controlled diet (providing the same percentage of macronutrients and foods) containing (*a*) palm olein, (*b*) interesterified palm oil, or (*c*) high oleic acid sunflower oil for 6 weeks each. The interesterified palm oil did not adversely impair insulin secretion or glucose (165).

> **For heart health, it is best to cook with polyunsaturated fat-rich oil as opposed to ingredients high in saturated fat, such as butter, ghee, or bacon grease.**

It remains unclear at this time if any long-term health effects are associated with consuming interesterified fats (166).

DIETARY RECOMMENDATIONS

No AI, RDA, or UL has been established for dietary fat for anyone above 12 months of age because of a lack of data regarding risk of inadequacy, prevention of chronic disease, or a known dietary fat intake level at which a person will experience adverse health effects (24). If a diet contains adequate calories, carbohydrate can serve as an energy source in place of dietary fat (25). As mentioned in chapter 1, the acceptable macronutrient distribution range (AMDR) for dietary fat is 20 to 35 percent of energy. The lower end of this range helps ensure adequate intake of total energy and essential fatty acids and intake and absorption of fat-soluble vitamins. The lower end of this range also helps prevent low HDL cholesterol and high triglycerides from following a low-fat, high-carbohydrate diet. The upper end of the range supports adequate intake of other nutrients (25) and adequate intake of total energy for those with higher calorie needs (167).

Nutrition experts recommend that people consume less than 10 percent of calories from saturated fat starting at age 2. The National Academies of Sciences, Engineering, and Medicine recommend that dietary cholesterol intake be as low as possible without compromising the nutrition adequacy of the diet (168).

An AI is available for the essential fatty acids (both polyunsaturated fats) linoleic acid and alpha-linolenic acid. The AI for linoleic acid (an omega-6 polyunsaturated fatty acid) ranges from 4.4 grams per day in infants 0 to 6 months of age to 13 grams per day in pregnant and lactating women. The lower end of the range was set based on an amount at which deficiency does not exist in healthy people. The upper end of the range was set based on a lack of evidence of long-term safety and cell studies showing increased lipid peroxidation (breakdown of lipids) and free radicals formed with higher intakes. Lipid peroxidation is considered a potential component in the development of plaque in arteries (25). The AI for alpha-linolenic acid (an omega-3 polyunsaturated fatty acid) ranges from 0.5 grams per day in infants 0 to 12 months of age to 1.6 grams per day in males over the age of 14. The AMDR ranges from 0.6 to 1.2 grams per day for people of all ages. The AMDR is based on maintaining a balance of omega-6 fatty acids, lack of long-term safety data, and cell studies performed in a lab that showed increased free radical production and lipid peroxidation with higher intakes of omega-6 fatty acids (25). The DRIs do not include a recommendation for EPA or DHA. Some organizations list recommendations for EPA plus DHA or fatty fish. For instance, the World Health Organization recommends 250 milligrams per day EPA and DHA for adults (169). The American Heart Association recommends eating one to two seafood meals per week to reduce the risk of congestive heart failure, coronary heart disease, ischemic stroke, and sudden cardiac death, especially when seafood replaces the intake of less healthy foods.

SUMMARY

Dietary fats and oils are sources of energy and aid in the absorption of fat-soluble vitamins A, D, E, and K, as well as certain food components such as carotenoids. But only two types of fatty acids—linoleic acid (LA) and alpha-linolenic acid (ALA)—are considered essential; the human body can make other fatty acids as needed. Small amounts of LA and ALA are necessary for the structural integrity of cell membranes, synthesis of eicosanoids, and cellular communication. Although not considered essential, because the body can make them from ALA (though this process is inefficient), EPA and DHA are beneficial for cardiovascular health. EPA and DHA also help decrease inflammation, and DHA is necessary for optimal brain development and function. Emerging evidence supports a role for EPA and DHA in maintaining joint health, particularly for those with rheumatoid arthritis, decreasing inflammation and restoring muscle function after damaging bouts of resistance exercise in untrained people, and improving strength and muscle mass in the elderly.

Industrially produced trans fats, found in partially hydrogenated oils, are harmful and therefore they are no longer GRAS. Certain saturated fatty acids increase LDL and total cholesterol risk factors for cardiovascular disease. Substituting polyunsaturated fatty acids for saturated fat can help lower total cholesterol and LDL cholesterol, a strategy associated with a reduction in heart attacks and death from heart attacks and improved insulin sensitivity.

FOR REVIEW

1. How does saturated fat affect risk factors for cardiovascular disease?
2. Should dietary saturated fat be replaced with unsaturated fat? If so, what will doing this accomplish?
3. How does high blood cholesterol affect risk for cardiovascular disease?
4. What factors influence how much fat is used during exercise?
5. Why are the essential fatty acids important for health?
6. Describe the cardiovascular benefits associated with fatty fish and fish oil supplements.
7. How does overeating dietary fat compare with overeating carbohydrate?
8. Describe how EPA and DHA can influence muscle.
9. Where is stearidonic acid (SDA) found? Is SDA beneficial for health?

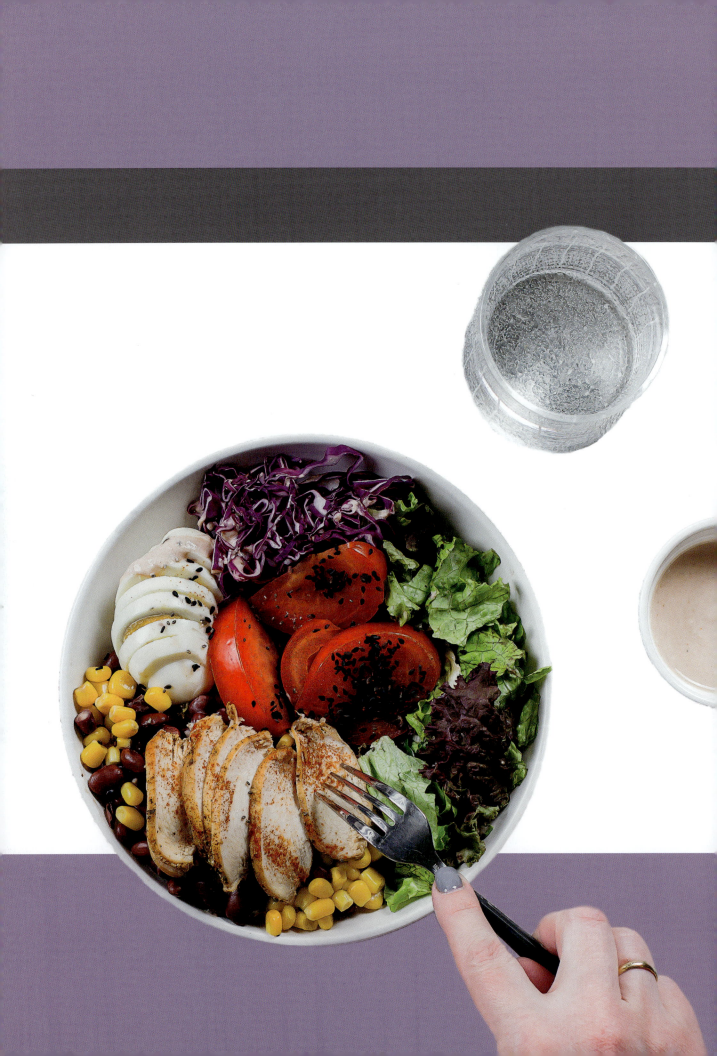

5

Protein

> **CHAPTER OBJECTIVES**
>
> After completing this chapter, you will be able to do the following:
> - Explain the types and basic functions of amino acids.
> - Outline the classification of proteins.
> - Explain the digestion, absorption, and metabolism of proteins.
> - Describe the metabolic fates of proteins.
> - Summarize the concepts and factors affecting protein synthesis.
> - Describe the differences between general protein guidelines and those for athletes.
> - Define vegetarianism and veganism, and explain how these dietary practices affect athletes.

Foods from both animals and plants contain dietary protein. Protein helps build structures in the body and is involved in multiple chemical reactions. The body is efficient at recycling amino acids from proteins broken down through the body. But this process cannot meet all of the human body's needs for amino acid, so dietary protein is necessary to prevent excess breakdown of protein in skeletal muscle to meet the need for amino acids. In this chapter we describe several aspects of protein from amino acid and protein classification to digestion, absorption, and metabolism. We also delve into the unique protein needs of those who are physically active and the way that dietary protein can be manipulated to support health, training adaptations, and competition goals of athletes. Finally, we look at vegetarianism, veganism, and other dietary practices and their implications for athletes.

AMINO ACIDS

Amino acids are the building blocks of protein and make up the sequences of peptide bonds to form protein structures (figure 5.1). In biochemistry, there are multiple ways to classify hundreds of amino acids and simple compounds made of amino acids found in nature. In human nutrition, the primary way to classify amino acids is based on the ability of amino acid to create proteins or serve as precursors to proteins. These amino acids are referred to as **proteinogenic**, and 23 amino acids fit this classification, of which 20 are used by the human body to make a variety of proteins that work to support all structure and function in human physiology. With the exception of the amino acid proline, all amino acids contain carbon and are considered organic compounds. These amino acids are composed of a nitrogen ($-NH_2$) and a carboxylic acid (-COOH) functional group as part of their main structure. Also present is a side chain (R) specific to each individual amino acid. These R chains can vary from a simple hydrogen atom found in glycine to a complex ring of carbon and hydrogen atoms, as in phenylalanine. The R chain gives the amino acid its identity, distinguishing its unique features. Because of these side chains, each amino acid differs in shape, size, composition, electrical charge, and pH.

Within any of the many complex classes of amino acids, considerable differences occur in shape and physical properties, so amino acids are often grouped into their functional subgroups (figure 5.2), of which there are several types. Amino acids with an aromatic group (phenylalanine, tyrosine, tryptophan, and histidine) are often grouped together. The **branched chain amino acids (BCAAs)** consist of leucine, isoleucine, and valine. These amino acids are found in food sources of protein but are most abundant in complete sources of protein that contain all the essential amino acids needed by the body (e.g., most animal sources of protein including beef, poultry, dairy, eggs, fish, and the plant-based protein soy) (1). BCAAs are an important subgroup of amino acids unique in muscle physiology because they are the primary amino acids that are directly taken up by muscle tissue and oxidized for energy. BCAAs also play an important role in supporting muscle adaptation to exercise by triggering the activation of anabolic machinery in the muscle to promote muscle protein synthesis (MPS) and a net positive balance in muscle protein accretion. When studying amino acids in biochemistry, classification can occur in many categories related to their charge, size, and optical activity.

Amino Acid Roles in Metabolism

Amino acids are diverse in their activities in different metabolic pathways and can have fates based on the metabolic needs of the body. As discussed in chapter 2, an amino acid can be oxidized for energy by disposing of its nitrogen group and donating its carbon skeleton to the TCA cycle or can be processed into glucose in

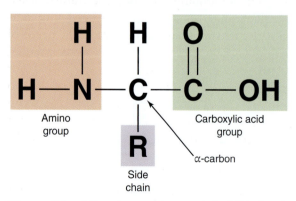

Figure 5.1 All amino acids consist of this basic frame and a unique side chain.

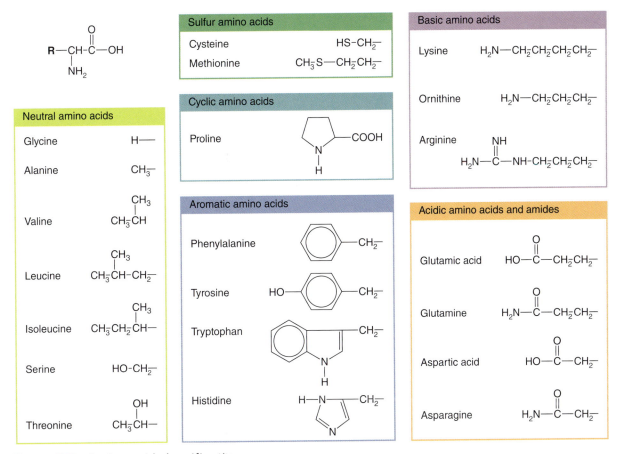

Figure 5.2 Amino acid classification.

the liver. While retaining their nitrogen group, amino acids can be incorporated into proteins in the body or used in the formation of other nitrogen-containing compounds, which includes the synthesis of **nonessential amino acids**. Of the 20 amino acids incorporated into human protein, an important distinction is whether or not the amino acid is essential in the diet or can be made by the body. Nonessential amino acids are also known as *dispensable* because they can be removed from the diet and still be made from other amino acids or from simpler precursors. For several other amino acids, no synthetic pathway exists in the body; these amino acids are termed *essential*, or *indispensable*. Nine essential amino acids are found in our diet, eight of which are clearly indispensable for adults. These eight **essential amino acids** are phenylalanine, valine, threonine, tryptophan, isoleucine, methionine, leucine, and lysine. The ninth, histidine, is essential for infants and believed to be essential for adults in small amounts (2). All other amino acids are considered nonessential—alanine, asparagine, aspartic acid, glutamic acid, and serine; are considered conditionally essential—arginine, cysteine, glutamine, glycine, proline, and tyrosine; or are categorized as simple ammonium (carnitine), nitrogenous (creatine), or gamma (glutathione) compounds. *Conditionally essential* means that particular amino acids are normally synthesized in adequate amounts but become limited when adequate amounts of precursors needed to synthesize them are unavailable to meet the needs of the body. These amino acids can become essential during times of stress, injury, or illness (3). For example, many conditionally essential amino acids are abundant in seafood and meat and can also be synthesized from other amino acids, but the body has trouble meeting synthetic demands, without help from the diet, as a result of trauma, infection, or kidney failure. Glutamine, a normally nonessential amino acid, provides fuel for rapidly dividing cells and is a preferred fuel for intestinal cells. After trauma or periods of critical illness, however, the body has increased need for glutamine, which must be met by the diet. In addition to the essential and nonessential amino acids described that are incorporated into protein, other amino acids appear in the body and have important physiological functions. Hydroxyproline and hydroxylysine are two examples of modifications of amino acids that are produced when proline and lysine are hydroxylated in collagen. **Collagen**, discussed later in the chapter, is the most abundant protein in the human body and provides the scaffolding for the strength and structure needed to hold the body together. Other examples of nonproteinogenic amino acids involve amino acid incorporation into the neurotransmitters GABA and L-Dopa.

Note that other sources discussing amino acids will list 9 essential amino acids but might classify the remaining 11 amino acids under different categories. Such sources might also include other amino acid–like nitrogenous compounds as amino acids. For this reason, some sources cite more than 20 amino acids as important to human physiology. In summary, under normal conditions the adult body has the ability to manufacture the 11 nonessential (includes those classified as conditionally essential) amino acids. Amino acids can be arranged in many combinations; if cells have all 20 amino acids at their disposal, the body can make a bewildering number of combinations to create tens of thousands of different protein chains.

Nine Essential Amino Acids

- Histidine (essential at least for infants and perhaps for adults)
- Isoleucine
- Leucine
- Lysine
- Methionine
- Phenylalanine
- Threonine
- Tryptophan
- Valine

Eleven Nonessential Amino Acids

- Alanine
- Arginine*
- Asparagine
- Aspartic acid
- Cysteine*
- Glutamic acid
- Glutamine*
- Glycine*
- Proline*
- Serine
- Tyrosine*

*Conditionally essential amino acids during stress, illness, or injury

Amino Acids as a Fuel Source

Although the human body prefers to burn carbohydrate and fat to create ATP, protein can also be broken down by the body (catabolized) to be used as an energy source or to make new glucose in the liver (a process known as gluconeogenesis, discussed in chapter 2). Although metabolism is complex and no metabolic pathway, including protein oxidation, is ever shut down, the use of carbohydrate and fat as energy sources allows protein to be used for protein synthesis and the other essential bodily functions. If we do not consume enough energy to sustain vital functions, such as maintaining our blood glucose levels, the body will readily sacrifice its own protein, preferentially from skeletal muscle tissue, to make glucose for use by our nervous system and other vital organs. For protein to be used for energy production, amino acids must be released from their protein structures from a body source or through the process of digestion from the protein foods we eat. Free amino acids from the bloodstream derived from digestion and absorption or from endogenous protein catabolism must then go through a process called deamination to remove their nitrogenous functional unit and free up the carbon skeleton backbone that can enter energy transfer pathways, such as the TCA cycle, within many cells in our body. The roles of amino acids in energy metabolism are further discussed in chapter 2. Figure 5.3 shows several entry points for amino acids into the TCA cycle to help meet the ATP demands of working cells. In the absence of severe metabolic stress and trauma, fortunately, the oxidation of protein as an energy source is

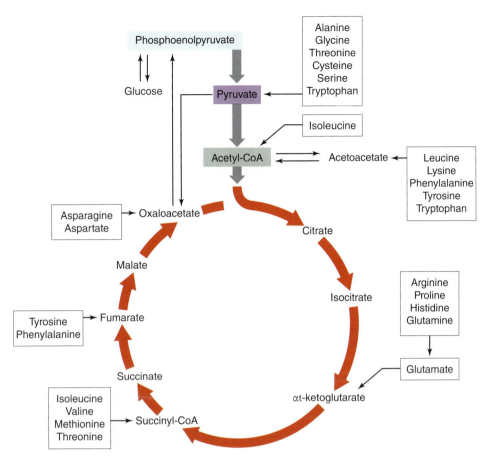

Figure 5.3 Entry points of amino acids.

minimal and takes a back seat to the oxidation of fat and carbohydrate in production of ATP. This process allows protein to be conserved for structural, metabolic, and homeostatic roles within the body.

> **? DO YOU KNOW?**
>
> Diets high in protein have a low risk profile for harming the body and can be quite healthy, especially if you are pursuing an active lifestyle. The healthy body is very efficient at handling waste products associated with protein metabolism. The key to maintaining a healthy high-protein diet is to focus on consuming a variety of foods from all food groups.

CLASSIFICATION AND FUNCTION OF PROTEIN

Amino acids come together to make protein, and protein is second only to water as a component of all plant and animal tissues. Protein plays an integral role in every human cell and is vital to the structure, function, and health of the human body. In many ways, proteins are intricate molecules that can constantly change in response to various stimuli the body encounters daily. Body proteins are constantly broken down, and amino acids from the amino acid pool are used to supply our body with most of the new amino acids required to support constant body protein turnover; thus, more of the amino acids are recycled than are supplied in the diet. The largest portion of protein demands come from body proteins that are broken down by catabolism as part of normal protein turnover to provide building blocks to synthesize body proteins. This is the primary reason we need less protein in our diet when we are not physically active and have minimal physiological stress. That said, dietary protein remains extremely important; when inadequate, increased catabolism of body protein occurs to replenish the amino acid pool, which can lead

PUTTING IT INTO PERSPECTIVE

AMINO ACID POOL

The free amino acids distributed throughout the body in the extracellular fluids and blood make up the amino acid pool (figure 5.4), which is available for protein synthesis at any given time. Amino acids that constantly enter the pool are those that have been catabolized from other tissues, those made in the liver, and those from protein digestion. In addition to protein synthesis, amino acids from the pool can also be broken down to participate in other metabolic pathways. By being broken down, they produce energy and unstable molecules known as amino groups (-NH_2). The -NH_2 is quickly converted into ammonia (NH_3) and expelled by the cells as a toxic by-product taken up for processing by the liver. The liver can detoxify this molecule by combining it with another amino group in the presence of carbon dioxide to generate urea and water. This process is a component of the metabolic pathway known as the **urea cycle**. The nitrogen-rich urea compound is released by the liver and travels to the kidneys, where it is filtered from the blood to form urine, which is then sent to the bladder for excretion. Other nitrogen-containing compounds are also excreted in the urine in small amounts, such as ammonia, uric acid, and creatine. The primary source of nitrogen lost by the body is present in the form of urea, but some nitrogen is also lost through skin and nails, sloughed-off gastrointestinal cells, mucus, and other body fluids. The cycling of amino acids in the amino acid pool is determined based on the metabolic demands of the body. For example, the liver regulates the blood level of amino acids based on tissue needs and breaks down and converts excess amino acids to carbohydrates for energy production.

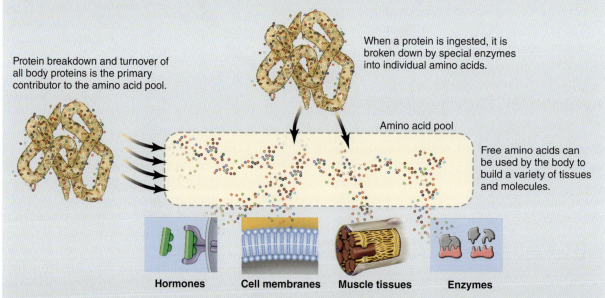

Figure 5.4 The makeup of the amino acid pool is derived primarily from endogenous protein breakdown and supplemented by protein ingestion.

to the breakdown of essential body tissue. This importance is obviously magnified in times of metabolic stress, such as infection, inflammatory disease, and trauma, but is also elevated for athletes who desire to maintain sufficient levels of skeletal muscle, which are crucial to health and performance.

Although the primary sources of protein in the average American diet are beef and poultry (4), all meat, cheese, milk, fish, and eggs are high-quality sources of animal protein. High-quality protein sources contain all the essential amino acids that the body cannot synthesize on its own and are largely found in animal foods. Some plant foods are also a good source (10%–19% of daily needs) or high source (>20% of daily needs) of protein (5). Beans, peas, grains, nuts, seeds, and vegetables all contribute protein to the diet, while also providing vitamins, minerals, and phytonutrients; they typically have the bonus of being low in fat and high in fiber. But not all grains and vegetables are good sources of protein, containing a complete profile of essential amino acids. Table 5.1 presents some common high-protein food sources.

Protein Formation

All protein consumed in our diet, regardless of the source, is digested, absorbed as amino acids, and reassembled in our bodies. Digested animal and plant sources of protein contribute a wide array of amino acids to the protein pool in the body to make new proteins. To support human growth and repair, as well as protein turnover, the proper amount and proportion of amino acids is required. To form protein in the body, amino acids are joined together in long strings by covalent chemical bonds known as **peptide bonds** (figure 5.5). These bonds form when a **carboxyl group** of one amino acid reacts with the amino group of another to form peptide chains that are arranged in a biologically functional way to form

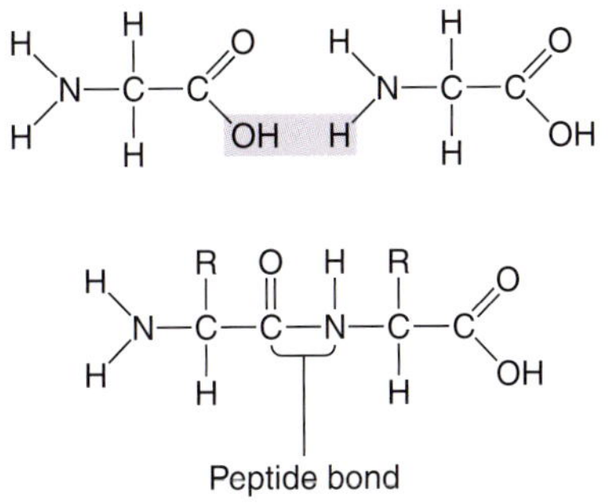

Figure 5.5 A protein peptide bond.

proteins. Their structure and function serve as the centerpiece for the biochemical reactions of life.

When amino acids start linking together by peptide bonds, and eventually form a protein, the complex characteristics work together to determine the specific function of that protein. The number of bonds formed determines the name of the bond. Dipeptides and tripeptides are two and three amino acids joined together by peptide bonds, respectively. A **polypeptide** contains more than 10 amino acids. Strands of proteins (made

Table 5.1 High-Protein Foods

Food	Protein (g)	Calories from protein (%)
3 oz lean beef steak	26	53
3 oz skinless chicken breast (grilled)	16.3	74
3 oz tilapia filet	15	88
3 oz salmon	17	68
3 oz pork loin	24	54
1 cup lentils	9	32
1 cup black beans	15	26
1 cup peas (cooked)	9	27
3 oz tofu	9	40
1 large egg	6.3	32
1 cup milk (1%)	8	31
1 cup soy milk	7	28
1 cup chopped broccoli (raw)	2.6	34
1 cup cooked white rice	4.4	14
1/2 cup quinoa	4	14
2 tbsp peanut butter	7	15
1/4 cup almonds	7	16

Data from U.S. Department of Agriculture and U.S. Department of Health & Human Services (2015).

from polypeptide chains) can be linked together by peptide bonds up to hundreds of amino acids long. The vast number of biological functions that proteins perform in the body depends on their structural arrangement. Proteins can fold into one or more specific spatial conformations through many biochemical interactions. Protein structures can contain tens to several thousand amino acids and can vary greatly in size (6). Additionally, when performing their biological function, these complex protein structures can go through many structural changes, called conformational changes, to modify their function.

Amino acid residues come in several levels of protein structures, referred to as primary, secondary, tertiary, and quaternary structures (figure 5.6). When referring to a protein's primary structure, its sequence of amino acids forms one or more polypeptide chains. The secondary structure of a protein is the coiling or folding of its polypeptide chains and is primarily a result of hydrogen bonding between amino acid chains. The tertiary structure of a protein refers to its three-dimensional shape caused by weak interactions among side groups and interactions between side groups and the fluid environment.

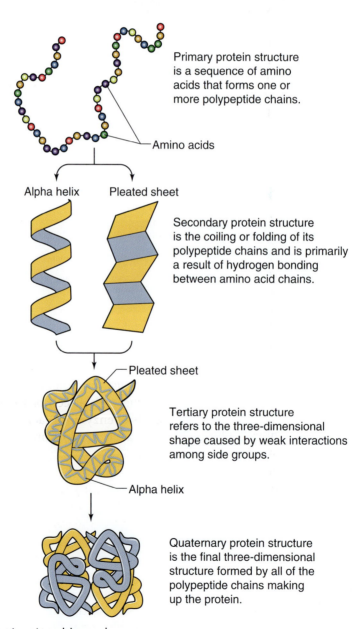

Figure 5.6 Protein structure hierarchy.

Finally, the quaternary structure of a protein is the final three-dimensional structure formed by all the polypeptide chains making up the protein. An example of a quaternary protein structure important in sports nutrition is hemoglobin, an iron-containing protein that is a component of red blood cells. Hemoglobin binds oxygen from the lungs to be delivered throughout the body, including exercising muscles, while picking up carbon dioxide to shuttle back to the lungs for drop-off and exhalation.

Dietary proteins, as well as proteins that make up the body, are long polypeptides; peptide bonds link hundreds of amino acids. Proteins, both small and large, reside in every part of the body, participating in key physiological functions. The largest source of protein in the human body is found in muscle, where a large and diverse family of proteins form contractile fibers and a structural framework that make up muscle tissue. Contractile protein fibers slide alongside each other, shortening and lengthening to contract and relax the muscle tissue.

> **DO YOU KNOW?**
>
> Depending on your hydration status, 1 pound (454 g) of your skeletal muscle tissue consists of approximately 70 percent water, approximately 22 percent proteins, and 7 percent lipid. If you take 22 percent of 454 grams, you get approximately 100 grams of protein in 1 pound of muscle tissue. In comparison, fat tissue contains approximately 50 percent water (7). People with more muscle mass have a higher content of body water.

Protein Functions

Intact body proteins are diverse in human physiology, serving a structural role for muscles, skin, bones, and connective tissue. In fact, the human body contains thousands of different proteins, each with a specific function determined by its shape. For example, **enzymes** work to speed up chemical reactions, whereas **hormones** serve as chemical messengers. **Antibodies** are proteins that make up our immune system and protect us from foreign pathogens. Proteins also serve as regulators by helping pump molecules across cell membranes. They can serve as fluid regulators by attracting water to keep body water in the right place and can influence acid-base balance by releasing or gaining hydrogen ions as needed. Finally, proteins can play a key structural role in serving as transporters of oxygen, vitamins, and minerals for delivery to target cells throughout the body. Key characteristics of the structural and mechanical functions of proteins, enzymes, and hormones and the role of protein in immune function, fluid, and acid-base balance, as well as their role in blood transport, are shown in figure 5.7 and described in detail later in the chapter.

Structure

The most abundant protein in the body of all mammals is collagen. This protein serves as the major constituent of bones and teeth and helps to maintain the structure of every connective tissue within the human body. Collagen relies on its densely packed structure to contribute elastic strength to bones and skin. Keratin is another structural protein that primarily serves to provide the anatomical structure for hair and nails. Motor proteins, such as the contractile fibers described earlier, also provide structure and make up a significant portion of skeletal and smooth muscles. These proteins initiate mechanical movement by harnessing the body's chemical form of energy (ATP) into mechanical work to make muscles contract.

Enzymes

Enzymes are proteins that function to speed up or catalyze chemical reactions in the body to make or change substances that are often referred to as products. Each cell of the body contains thousands of enzymes, each with its own purpose to drive a reaction forward. Enzymes can be thought of as shepherds that steer and regulate a reaction. Enzymes interact with the substrates of a chemical reaction to form new biological products affected by the chemical reaction (figure 5.8). Substrates can bind to the enzyme's active site, causing the active site to change shape, resulting in a better fit for multiple substrates to interact. The enzyme can then maneuver the substrates so that they bind and form the product. The product is then released, and the enzyme can return to its normal shape to interact with other substrates and keep

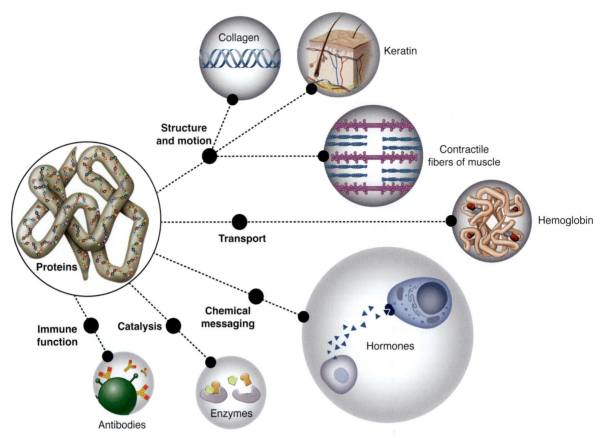

Figure 5.7 Proteins have multiple functions throughout the body.

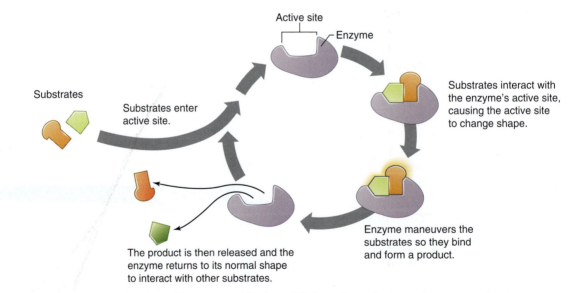

Figure 5.8 Enzyme binding. Enzymes with the addition of a substrate form a product.

the metabolic processes moving. For example, our skeletal muscles contain hundreds of enzymes to catalyze a series of reactions that allow them to break down fuel sources (carbohydrate, protein, and fat) to generate the ATP that facilitates muscle contraction. As discussed in chapter 2, multiple enzymatic reactions work to help decide the fate of pyruvate. Proteins working as enzymes are also prominent every time we digest our food. Multiple enzymes work to target food proteins, carbohydrates, and fats and break them down into smaller particles to prepare them for absorption in the small intestine. Lactase is an excellent example of a digestive enzyme that breaks down the carbohydrate lactose into smaller sugars.

Just as amino acids build proteins that create complex polypeptide bonds that in turn form complicated protein structures, these protein structures are also constantly turning over (i.e., broken down and replaced). A process called protein denaturation is the initial catabolic event responsible for destabilizing a protein's shape. Several forms of stimuli can initiate this cascade of events in the body. Outside the body, many examples of denaturation can be observed by how we prepare the protein foods in our diet for eating. Treating a food with acid, alkalinity, heat, alcohol, oxidation, and agitation can all disrupt a protein's three-dimensional shape, causing it to unfold (**denature**) and lose its shape and function. A good visual example is an egg cooking in a skillet. The heat causes the protein bonds in the egg to break and unfold. The broken proteins then crowd each other tightly to form an opaque egg solid. When lemon juice is added to milk, the milk proteins denature and curdle because of the acid in the juice. In human nutrition, the best example of an acid denaturing dietary protein occurs in the stomach during digestion as hydrochloric acid (HCL) is released by parietal cells found in the stomach lining. This acid denatures dietary proteins, uncoiling them into simpler chains with greater surface area for digestive enzymes to attack their peptide bonds. The process of protein digestion is covered in more detail later in the chapter.

Chemical Messengers

Proteins also play an instrumental role as chemical messengers, called peptide hormones, which interact with cells to signal intracellular events. Insulin (figure 5.9) and growth hormone are two examples of the many peptide hormones made in specific parts of the body that act on cells in other parts of the body. Many of these proteins have important regulatory functions, are relatively

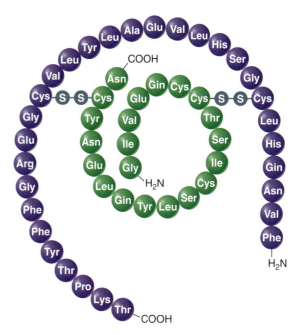

Figure 5.9 Insulin is a polypeptide structure.

fragile, and have a fairly short half-life so that their breakdown can limit the degree of chemical signaling that occurs.

Immunity

Proteins play a key role in bolstering our immune defense against pathogenic invaders such as bacteria and viruses. Antibodies are blood proteins that attack and deactivate these invaders to prevent infection. Antibodies are produced in response to a previous infection so that the body can quickly respond the next time that germ invades. Immune cells can keep a memory of each previous viral invasion to mount a faster response during future invasions.

❓ DO YOU KNOW?

Influenza (flu) vaccines are an example of a public health initiative that provides people with a small amount of a dead or deactivated virus that does not cause an infection but does cue the body to make antibodies to prepare for the potential of a future invasion of the virus. Immune cells retain memory of the protein material provided in the vaccine to mount a fast response if the flu virus invades.

Fluid Maintenance

In addition to serving an important role in immune function, proteins also function in promoting fluid and acid-base balance. In the human body, fluids are found in two basic areas: inside cells (intracellular) or outside cells (extracellular). For the body to function properly, a healthy balance of fluid in each space is partially maintained by specific proteins (figure 5.10). Proteins called globulin and **albumin** are large in size, attract water, and remain inside the blood. They function to attract water within this space to help balance fluid that is lost through the force of the heart pumping blood and pushing the fluid fraction of the blood outside of the blood vessels. Hospitalized patients who experience severe metabolic and catabolic stress resulting from trauma many times become deficient in the blood protein albumin. Albumin deficiency disrupts normal fluid balance and control and results in a form of tissue swelling known as edema. Proteins can also function to stabilize the body's pH by serving as a buffer to pick up extra hydrogen ions when acidity increases (pH decreases). On the other hand, when blood composition becomes slightly basic (rise in pH), proteins can donate hydrogen ions in an effort to neutralize blood pH. The body works hard to keep the pH in tight check, at a neutral measure close to 7.4 on a scale of 0 (acidic) to 14 (basic). Having a blood pH too far outside the range of 7.35 to 7.45 can cause disastrous consequences and has been observed clinically as a result of severe hyperglycemia or trauma. If left unchecked, the unbalance can lead to acidosis and cause death within a matter of hours, primarily by altering the function and activity of many proteins throughout the body.

> **? DO YOU KNOW?**
>
> Your body works hard to maintain an ideal pH balance and tends to succeed. Your body has a complex system of buffers and buffering systems continuously at work to keep pH values somewhere between 7.35 to 7.45. These systems are in place to prevent metabolic and dietary factors from pushing the pH outside of the optimal range. Despite the popular belief that specific diets or high-pH waters can "alkalinize" the body to promote health, the foods and fluids we consume have no significant effect on blood pH.

Cell Transporters

All body cells allow substances to pass into their intracellular space, while also working to excrete various substances. These functions are maintained by protein transporters that act as channels

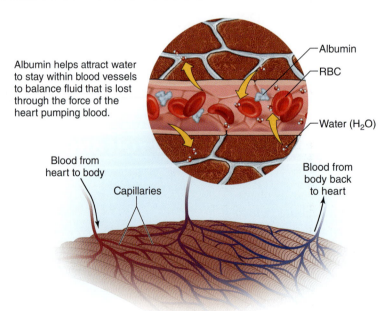

Figure 5.10 Proteins such as albumin assist in the balance of fluid through attraction of water and serve to regulate vascular pressure.

and pumps to regulate intra- and extracellular movement. Protein channels typically work by a process known as diffusion, during which substances freely pass in and out without requiring energy. On the other hand, protein pumps utilize **active transport** that requires energy in the form of ATP to move substances across cellular membranes. Sodium-potassium pumps, often introduced in undergraduate physiology classes, use a significant amount of ATP as a chemical energy source to move sugars and amino acids and to control cell volume and nerve impulses. Proteins also act as carriers to transport important substances to tissues throughout the body. An example of an important protein carrier is a **chylomicron**. This protein carrier is a type of **lipoprotein** that packages lipids from the fats we consume so that these fats can be carried in the blood to peripheral tissues. Have you ever heard the phrase "Oil and water do not mix"? This would be the case with the fat in our water-filled blood without lipoproteins. The chylomicron lipoprotein functions to engulf lipids in the center of its sphere-like core while embedded hydrophilic (water-loving) protein tails toward the outside of this protein molecule to be water soluble and not separate from the blood. Figure 5.11 shows an example of a protein transporter used in amino acid intestinal absorption and a chylomicron.

Protein clearly serves many diverse roles and is of significant importance to human health, function, and athletic performance (table 5.2).

To meet these responsibilities, the diet must provide adequate amounts of amino acids. In addition, the body must have an adequate source of energy (calories) to allow dietary protein to serve optimally in these important roles instead of being used (oxidized) as an energy source. Although a small portion of the protein in the body contributes to ATP synthesis, the proportion of protein used as a fuel source can increase through various stimuli, such as prolonged endurance exercise or

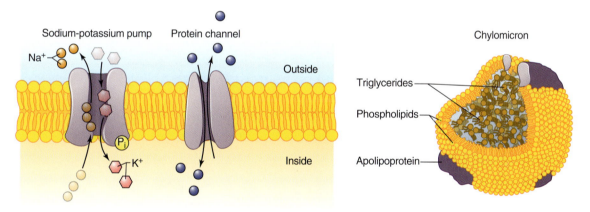

Figure 5.11 The chylomicron is a lipid-containing protein transporter used in the intestinal absorption of fat.

Table 5.2 Protein Functions in the Body

Component	Role
Hormones	Serve as chemical messengers.
Regulators	Help pump molecules across cell membranes to preserve cellular function.
Transporters	Move oxygen, vitamins, and minerals for delivery to target cells throughout the body.
Immune function	Proteins compose antibodies that protect the body from bacteria and viruses.
Fluid and acid-base balance	Attract water and release hydrogen ions; can influence acid-base balance by releasing or gaining hydrogen ions.
Enzymes	Initiate or speed up chemical reactions.
Structure	Cellular integrity; muscle contraction.

> ### REFLECTION TIME
>
> ### PROTEIN IS FOR MUSCLES BUT WHAT ELSE?
>
> We know the importance of skeletal muscle proteins to athletic performance. Now consider several other proteins made in the body that are key to an athlete's success, such as collagen's role in connective tissue and all the protein-containing immune regulators needed to maintain healthy immune function. Without proper formation and function of these proteins, it won't matter if your muscles are bigger and stronger—performance will ultimately suffer. New protein intake guidelines for athletic performance take this into account (9, 10). Although athletes do need more protein than their nonathlete counterparts, they must not overdo protein consumption. Consuming healthy foods from all food groups is important to maintaining diet quality.

starvation. During prolonged endurance exercise (typically greater than 90 minutes), small increases in protein oxidation occur, particularly if limited carbohydrate is consumed (8). The use of protein as an energy source can be problematic in cases of starvation or anorexia nervosa and in chronic situations of inadequate energy intake. In these scenarios, the chronic effect of elevated protein breakdown and oxidation for fuel has deleterious effects on health.

DIGESTION AND ABSORPTION

To appreciate how energy-yielding macronutrients are integrated during metabolism, we must first understand how they are digested and absorbed by the body. The body must first address these important tasks before it can use protein from food to make body protein (figure 5.12). Protein digestion begins in the mouth, where protein in foods is mechanically altered by chewing.

Digestion in the Stomach

In the stomach, proteins are unfolded into long polypeptide chains by the action of hydrochloric acid (HCL). This stomach acid also has a second-

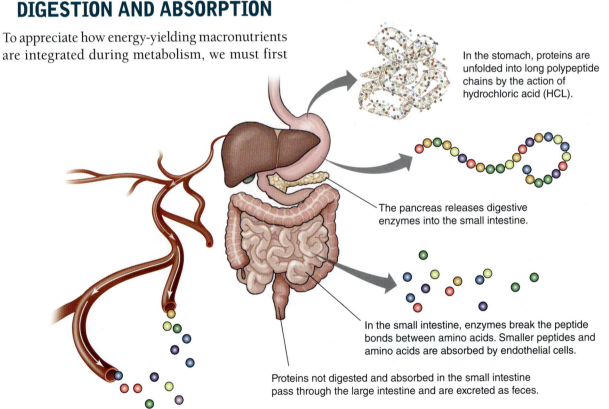

In the stomach, proteins are unfolded into long polypeptide chains by the action of hydrochloric acid (HCL).

The pancreas releases digestive enzymes into the small intestine.

In the small intestine, enzymes break the peptide bonds between amino acids. Smaller peptides and amino acids are absorbed by endothelial cells.

Proteins not digested and absorbed in the small intestine pass through the large intestine and are excreted as feces.

Following intestinal absorption, amino acids are transported via the portal vein to the liver and then released into general circulation.

Figure 5.12 Protein digestion.

ary, but equally important, responsibility. HCL interacts with a **proenzyme** called **pepsinogen** that is released by the cells of the stomach lining. In the stomach cavity, HCL works to unfold and cut off some of the amino acids that make up pepsinogen to change its form and function. This process activates pepsinogen to its active protein digesting form, called **pepsin**. This enzymatic activation step within the gastric cavity and small intestine is common and strategic in the protein digestion process. The activation of these enzymes at the proper time ensures that dietary protein is digested at the right stage of digestion. This process also protects the cells that create the proenzymes, because if each cell created only active forms of these enzymes, the cell would end up digesting itself! In addition to the pathways that activate pepsin, the pepsin generated from this reaction is efficient at clipping peptide bonds of the proteins we consume and will activate more pepsin from additional pepsinogen released into the stomach cavity. When digesting dietary protein, pepsin begins breaking down polypeptides into shorter amino acid chains called peptides. As a result of HCL and pepsin action in the stomach, dietary proteins are digested into smaller polypeptides and approximately 15 percent free amino acids.

Digestion in the Small Intestine

As polypeptides and smaller peptide chains leave the stomach, they enter the small intestine to complete the next phase of digestion and prepare for protein absorption. As partially digested protein enters the small intestine, the **duodenum** detects protein in the partially digested food and signals duodenal cells to release the hormones **secretin** and **cholecystokinin (CCK)** into the bloodstream. These hormones signal the pancreas to release other digestive substances into the small intestine. At the same time, duodenal cells facing the inside of the gastrointestinal (GI) tract release **enterokinases** in the **luminal brush border** to activate additional enzymes to break other peptide bonds. Collectively, these events signal what is called the **protease activation cascade** in the duodenum. Secretin signals the pancreas to release water and bicarbonate in the intestine to neutralize the acidic **chyme**, whereas CCK signals the pancreas to release a family of enzymes that have high specificity for breaking specific amino acid–amino acid peptide bonds. As a result of enzymatic digestion of protein in the stomach (pepsin) combined with the action of pancreatic enzymes (**trypsin**, chymotrypsin, elastase, and carboxypeptidase A and B) and the enterokinases found at the brush border of the small intestine, the protein that was originally consumed now consists of more than 90 percent free amino acids combined with less than 10 percent small peptide chains.

Absorption

All along the small intestine, short peptide chains and single amino acids can be absorbed by intestinal endothelial cells. These cells are aligned back to back on the surface of the intestinal villi. On the brush border membrane of these endothelial cells are at least six different amino acid carriers, also known as channels or transporters, which have overlapping specificity for different amino acids based on their physical and chemical characteristics. Transporters requiring sodium also require ATP to move the amino acid to within the cell. This form of absorption is known as active transport. Other amino acids diffuse across transporters through a process called facilitated diffusion. Most amino acids are transported by more than one transport system (figure 5.13). Normally, proteins in foods supply a healthy mix of several amino acids, so amino acids that share the same transport system are absorbed equally. As amino acids are absorbed in absorptive endothelial cells, other peptidases within the absorptive cells are present to completely break down di- and tripeptides into single amino acids. The individual amino acids are then absorbed into the bloodstream by leaving the endothelial cell. They are absorbed into the capillaries of the larger villi structure and transported to the liver by the **portal vein**. Proteins not digested and absorbed in the small intestine pass through the large intestine and are excreted as feces. In the absence of GI diseases such as celiac disease and cystic fibrosis, generally more than 90 percent of protein is absorbed from the diet in the enterocytes that line the duodenum and jejunum, of which 99 percent enters the blood as individual amino acids. Following absorption, most amino acids and a few absorbed peptides are transported by the portal vein to the liver and then released into general circulation (figure 5.14).

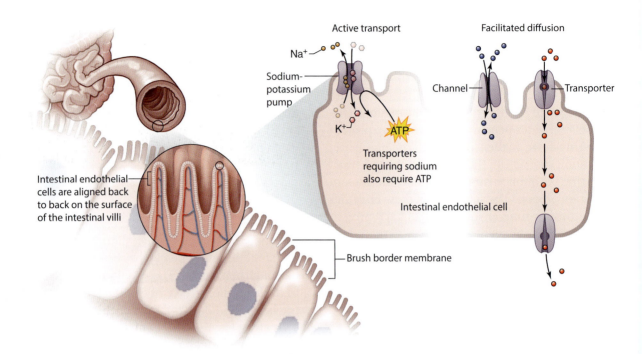

Figure 5.13 The transport of protein can occur through active transport and facilitated diffusion.

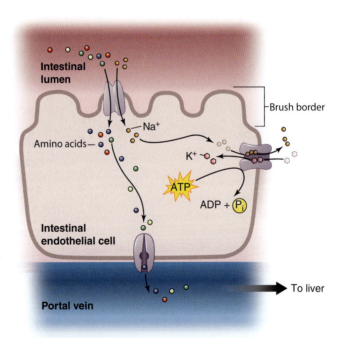

Figure 5.14 Amino acid entry into a portal vein.

METABOLIC FATE OF PROTEIN IN THE BODY

Various metabolic processes use amino acids derived from the liver and the bloodstream following intestinal absorption. As described earlier, these amino acids contribute to what is generically called the liver and blood amino acid pool of the body (see figure 5.4). In the bloodstream, amino acids from this pool are transported throughout the body and are available for synthesizing new proteins. In this section we discuss how the body

PUTTING IT INTO PERSPECTIVE

AMINO ACID COMPETITION FOR ABSORPTION

Consuming a large amount of one particular amino acid can compromise the absorption of other amino acids that share the same transporter. For instance, taking a dietary supplement consisting of a large dose of one amino acid, such as lysine, might interfere with the absorption of other amino acids from the diet. Lysine is classified as a basic amino acid (i.e., nonacidic) and has a specific transporter shared with other basic amino acids, such as arginine. If arginine is consumed in low quantities combined with lysine supplementation, the minimal arginine available will have limited access to absorption transporters saturated with lysine. Although taking single-amino-acid supplements can possibly cause imbalances that might interfere with normal absorption of food-derived amino acids, particularly essential amino acids, not enough research has been done in humans to know at exactly what dosage this can be a problem.

uses this amino acid pool for various synthetic and catabolic processes.

Protein Synthesis

As previously described, cells use peptide bonds to link amino acids and build proteins. The nucleus of every cell provides the blueprint for the synthesis of thousands of proteins that our bodies need to stay healthy and function properly. Our cells store this important genetic information in the form of **deoxyribonucleic acid (DNA)** (11) in the nucleus of each cell. To make new protein, cells signal a specific section with a specific pattern of the DNA, called a gene, to make a special type of **ribonucleic acid (RNA)** called **messenger RNA (mRNA)** (figure 5.15). This mRNA carries the blueprint sequence of amino acids needed in the protein to be synthesized. The mRNA leaves the nucleus and attaches itself to one of the protein-making factories of the cell, called ribosomes,

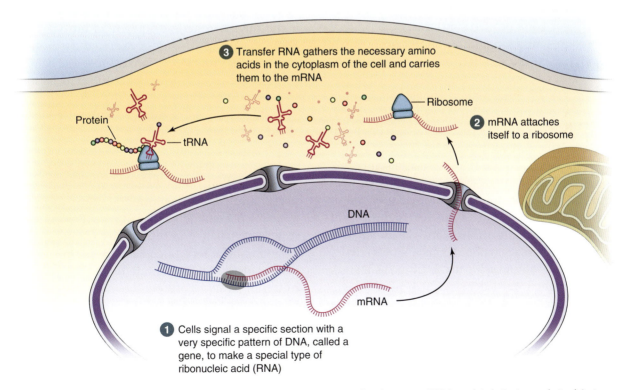

Figure 5.15 Gene expression occurs from DNA transcribed into mRNA, which is translated into a protein.

in the cytoplasm of the cell. During synthesis, the 20 amino acids that are incorporated into human protein are carefully selected from the body's amino acid pool for protein synthesis when coupled to another type of RNA called **transfer RNA (tRNA)** (11). Transfer RNA gathers the necessary amino acids in the cytoplasm of the cell and carries them to the mRNA. To synthesize protein, strands of DNA are transcribed into mRNA, and then tRNA binds to mRNA in three-base groups, where enzymes attach each amino acid to the growing protein chain in the ribosomes of the cell. Different combinations of three consecutive RNA molecules in the mRNA provide a code for the synthesis of different tRNA molecules. The three-base combinations of mRNA, however, are recognized by only 20 different tRNA molecules, and 20 different amino acids are incorporated into protein during protein synthesis. During protein synthesis, thousands of tRNAs each carry their own specific amino acid to the site of protein synthesis, but only one mRNA controls the sequencing of the amino acids for a specific protein. A third type of RNA resides in the ribosome (rRNA) and serves as a ribonucleic acid that is prevalent in the ribosomes that provide a structural framework for protein synthesis and coordinate the many steps involved in protein synthesis.

Protein synthesis requires all the amino acids required to build a specific protein; an insufficient amount of any one might impede or slow formation of a polypeptide chain. If one nonessential amino acid is missing during protein synthesis, the cell can either make that amino acid or obtain it from the pool of amino acids in the liver via the bloodstream. If an essential amino acid is missing, the body may break down some of its own protein to supply the missing amino acid. Without the particular essential amino acid, synthesis of that specific protein will halt, and the incomplete protein that is made will be tagged for breakdown to recycle the amino acids to the amino acid pool. The body then must decide which proteins are most important to make, while sacrificing the structure and synthesis of others. A greater portion of skeletal muscle protein is then catabolized to contribute to the amino acid pool, and some muscle-specific protein-synthetic pathways may be compromised.

Protein Catabolism

On the other side of the protein metabolism equation is protein catabolism, or breakdown. When proteins of a cell are catabolized, the protein's amino acids return back to circulation to contribute to the amino acid pool. The resulting amino acids can also be classified according to the products they produce when metabolized to generate ATP. Amino acids can participate in gluconeogenic (to make glucose) or ketogenic (to make ketones) pathways. There are three metabolic entry points for amino acids following deamination. They include conversion of the amino acid to pyruvate in the cytosol of the cell, conversion to acetyl-CoA in the mitochondria, and conversion to a TCA cycle intermediate. Some of these amino acids may be used again for protein synthesis, whereas others may have their amino groups removed in the liver to produce energy or make molecules such as glucose, DNA, RNA, neurotransmitters, hormones such as thyroxine, histamine, and many other important compounds.

Nitrogen Balance

Traditional attempts to evaluate whether the body is getting enough protein have involved a rudimentary method known as nitrogen balance. Because nitrogen is excreted as proteins are recycled or used, we can estimate the balance of nitrogen in the body. The nitrogen balance equation takes the grams of nitrogen consumed (dietary protein is 16% nitrogen) subtracted by the grams of nitrogen lost (primarily as urea) over the timeframe of 24 hours to determine if someone is in positive or negative nitrogen balance.

Classical nitrogen balance work has been useful for determining minimal protein requirements to prevent deficiency in sedentary humans in energy balance (12). But this technique has also long been recognized as flawed, because of several methodological limitations (13) that minimize its utility in present-day nutrition science. Note that the nitrogen balance technique is only a snapshot of what is occurring with nitrogen at the whole-body level and disregards the fact that protein metabolism and turnover is a complex and dynamic process that is always changing in all the areas of the body. The nitrogen balance technique assumes that all proteins in all body systems and tissues are behaving in the exact same way and relies on a rough estimate of nitrogen excretion that is usually only in the form of a 24-hour urine collection.

Note that determining "need" to prevent deficiency is different from assessing dietary protein amounts that are necessary for proper adaptation to exercise and athletic performance. In the world of physical fitness and sport, athletes do not meet this profile, and achieving nitrogen balance is secondary to an athlete whose primary goal is adaptation to training and performance improvement (13). The nitrogen balance technique cannot provide insight into the kinetics of body proteins, nor does it account for rapidly turning over body tissues. Finally, this technique certainly cannot provide accurate insight on dietary protein intake recommendations for athletes and has created some confusion.

Despite these limitations, the nitrogen balance technique has been used for years to help determine a need or requirement for dietary protein to replaces losses and thus prevent deficiency. Therefore, the technique still has some purpose. A positive nitrogen balance suggests that nitrogen intake exceeds the sum of all sources of nitrogen excretion and has historically been interpreted as achieving adequate protein status to prevent protein malnutrition. A positive balance suggests that the body is adding protein effectively, such as in the case of pregnancy or in supporting child and adolescent growth. Conversely, a negative nitrogen balance implies that nitrogen intake is less than the sum of all sources of nitrogen excretion. Those in a negative balance are thought to be losing protein and may be experiencing starvation, severe illness with fever and infection, extreme weight loss, or recent trauma (13, 14).

General Equation

N intake − (24 h UUN* + 4**) = nitrogen balance

Adding Protein Effectively

14 − 12 = +/− 2.0

Losing Protein

14 − 16 = −2.0

*UUN = urine urea nitrogen; **+ 4 refers to grams of nitrogen from feces, hair, skin, and other body fluids.

DO YOU KNOW?

Nitrogen assessment measures are commonly used to measure protein content in protein powder supplements for food-labeling purposes. To take advantage of this, many manufacturers have added other nitrogen-containing ingredients, such as individual amino acids like glycine and taurine, and portrayed them as grams of protein on the label, even though these proteins are incomplete. How can you avoid amino acid spiking of protein powders? Read the ingredients list to look for added high-nitrogen compounds (glycine, taurine, creatine, glutamine) and make sure that any incomplete proteins sources (e.g., rice) are combined with other protein sources (e.g., pea) to make a complete protein.

PROTEIN IN THE DIET

Many organizations worldwide have recommendations regarding the amount of protein required to contribute to a healthful diet. When we think about the major food groupings that make up our diet, only fruits and fats contain minimal amounts of protein and are not considered protein sources. In the United States and Canada, the recommended dietary allowance (RDA) is the accepted dietary standard for setting protein needs. The RDA for protein was calculated to meet the nutrition needs of most healthy people, but note that the RDA assumes that people are consuming adequate energy and other nutrients to allow their bodies to use the protein they consume for synthesis, rather than for energy. As mentioned earlier, when discussing protein recommendations for athletes, some confusion has surrounded the phrase "protein needs." The RDA, for instance, is meant to prevent protein deficiency and does not take into account additional dietary protein that might be needed to prevent age-related sarcopenia or enhance physiological adaptations to exercise (15, 16).

> ## PUTTING IT INTO PERSPECTIVE
>
> ### CALCULATING PROTEIN NEEDS BASED ON THE RDA
>
> For a college freshman male who weighs 175 pounds (79.5 kg), follow these steps to determine the gram amount of protein intake based on the RDA.
>
> 1. Convert pounds to kilograms: 175 lb / 2.2 kg = 79.5 kg
> 2. Multiply kg body weight × 0.8 g/kg body weight: 79.5 kg × 0.8 g/kg = 63.6 g
>
> This calculation means that a male who weighs 175 pounds (79.5 kg) needs a minimum of 63.6 grams of protein to prevent protein deficiency, assuming he is both healthy and sedentary. Based on current protein intake guidelines for athletic performance, if this college freshman participates in regular exercise or sport, his protein needs rise to at least 1.2 grams per kilogram (9).

Based on studies suggesting increased heart disease risk when diets are low in fat and high in refined carbohydrate (sugar), and increased risk of overweight, obesity, and heart disease when diets are high in fat, the Food and Nutrition Board set the acceptable macronutrient distribution range (AMDR) for protein in adults as 10 to 35 percent of total protein calories consumed (17). Therefore, if a person requires 2,000 kcal per day in their diet to maintain their weight, their protein intake recommendation would range from 50 to 175 grams per day:

$$2{,}000 \text{ kcal} \times (0.10 \text{ or } 0.35) / 4 \text{ kcal per gram of protein}$$

This range of protein intake is typically higher than the RDA.

Protein historically provides about 15 to 16 percent of energy for adults in North America (18). Although the AMDR recommendations for protein are quite wide, and in many cases not very specific, for the first time the AMDR allows flexibility when considering protein needs for active people. This range is broad enough to cover the needs of most active people (19) and is elevated beyond the RDA to match the physical stress that increases the body's need for additional protein. Exactly how much? This question generates conversation and debate among the scientific community and continues to spark scientific inquiry, primarily in exercise science, but also in the aging and clinical nutrition fields of study. Many factors affect the protein needs of physically active people, and these elevated needs are linked to supporting various outcomes that may be important to the athlete. Although training is now widely recognized to increase protein needs, the amount is often less than most people think. It should not be assumed, however, that athletes, particularly female athletes, always consume an adequate amount of protein (13).

How much protein does a person normally consume, and how does this amount compare with the RDA? For a comprehensive assessment of how much protein an individual needs, it is important to understand not only variables, such as physiological stressors or the need of growth and recovery, but also the normal consumption of protein. The most accurate method is to rely on food labels that list the quantity of protein

> ## PUTTING IT INTO PERSPECTIVE
>
> ### DETERMINING PROTEIN NEEDS FOR ATHLETES
>
> The primary method for determining protein needs for athletes is to use the gram per kilogram (g/kg) method. The AMDR is a secondary approach that can be used in conjunction with the g/kg approach, but it should not be used independently. The AMDR provides a wide range of protein intake recommendations for people based on total calorie intake, whereas the g/kg approach gives a more individualized protein intake recommendation.

PUTTING IT INTO PERSPECTIVE

WHEY PROTEIN ISOLATE VERSUS WHEY PROTEIN CONCENTRATE

Protein bioavailability in whey protein concentrate can vary from 25 to 89 percent protein by weight, and many products may contain lactose and fat. Whey protein isolate is a higher-quality protein because over 90 percent, by weight, is protein, and most products are virtually lactose free. Be aware that the two usually taste quite different because of a lack of fat and carbohydrate in whey protein isolate products.

(in grams) in a serving of food. By using food labels, the grams of protein consumed in one day can simply be added together. Clearly, not all foods have food labels, so using other methods to assess the protein quantity of these foods is essential. One method, used for decades, is to rely on food exchange lists. These lists provide serving sizes for most foods and combine this information with a corresponding number of exchanges for carbohydrate, protein, and fat. For example, one protein exchange equals 1 ounce, which corresponds to 7 grams of protein. So a 3-ounce chicken breast equals three exchanges and is estimated to contain 21 grams of protein. Other protein-containing food groups also have exchanges that can be used to estimate protein intake. A vegetable exchange provides 2 grams of protein, whereas a milk exchange provides 8 grams. A starch exchange contributes 3 grams of protein, whereas fat and fruit exchanges contribute zero protein. Those who prefer not to use food exchange lists commonly use other strategies. Food composition tables and "protein calculators" are prevalent online, and computer software programs are available for purchase. The most prudent strategy to ensure accuracy per the RDA is to visit the United States Department of Agriculture's website at www.choosemyplate.gov.

PROTEIN QUALITY

Protein quality measurement is an assessment of the ability of a dietary protein source to fulfill the body's requirement for indispensable (or essential) amino acids. The better the score, the better the food protein meets the body's needs. Generally, protein quality refers to how well or poorly the body uses a given protein. Protein quality can also be defined by how well the essential amino acid (EAA) profile of a protein matches the requirements of the body, the digestibility of the protein, and the bioavailability of the amino acids. Although both animal and plant foods contain protein, the quality of protein in these foods differs. Meat, poultry, fish, eggs, milk, and milk products are all high-quality complete proteins that have at least 20 percent of their calories from protein. Protein isolated from soybeans also provides a complete protein that is equivalent in terms of protein quality to animal protein, with a slightly lower proportion of the amino acids cysteine and leucine. Soy protein may also offer unique health benefits, making it a good choice as a replacement for some of the protein that people consume from animal sources. Table 5.3 describes several methods available to measure the protein quality of food.

Besides ensuring that energy intake is adequate by consuming a wide variety of foods, a strategy to circumvent protein-quality concerns for those who choose to consume a more plant-based diet is to consume complementary proteins. A complementary protein is defined as two or more incomplete food proteins whose assortment of amino acids complement each other's lack of specific EAAs so that the combination provides sufficient amounts of all the EAAs. Grain products tend to be low in the EAA lysine but high in the EAAs methionine and cysteine, whereas legumes such as beans are low in methionine and cysteine but high in lysine. Good examples of complementary proteins found in the diet are beans with rice, peanut butter on bread, pasta with beans, and chickpeas with sesame paste. Each one of these food pairs contain all the EAAs required to make new protein but by themselves (e.g., the peanut butter without the bread) are limited in at least one EAA. Specific pairings of these foods do not need to be consumed together at the same time to

Table 5.3 Protein Quality Methods and Limitations

Protein quality method	Equation	Primary outcome	Limitation of method
Biological value (BV)	BV = N retained / N absorbed or $BV = I - (F - F_0) - (U - U_0) \div I - (F - F_0)$	Represents nitrogen retention as a percentage of nitrogen absorption.	Tedious process that must measure urine and fecal nitrogen loss both on the test diet and the N-free diet.
Net protein utilization (NPU)	Protein ingested ÷ amount protein stored in body	Compares the amount of protein eaten with the amount stored in the body, or how much the body actually used.	Relies on animal nitrogen excretion to determine the nitrogen content retained.
Protein efficiency ratio (PER)	Gain in body mass (g) ÷ protein intake (g)	A score of 1 provides all amino acids needed and is fully digested.	May not correlate well with humans because of reliability on animals for score.
Digestible indispensable amino acid score (DIAAS)	DIAAS % = (amino acid in the protein ÷ amino acid requirement) × amino acid digestibility	Measures protein absorption at the end of the small intestine. Method measures the digestion of individual amino acids to paint a better picture of how protein meets the body's amino acid needs.	Complexity.
Chemical score	AA score = mg AA in 1 g test protein/mg AA in 1 g reference protein × 100	The lowest score for any of the essential AA's designates the limiting AA → chemical score for that protein.	Digestibility and AA availability not taken into account.
Protein digestibility corrected amino acid score (PDCAAS)	Chemical score × % digestibility of a protein	Involves calculating the ratio of amino acids of a food source against the requirements of a 2- to 5-year-old child based on the first limiting dietary EAA within the protein.	Based on young children, so may not serve as best method for determining protein quality for adults.

I = N intake; F = fecal N; U = urinary N; F_0 and U_0 = fecal and urinary N on an N-free diet; AA = amino acid.

make new body protein. Protein complementation is generally only important for people who consume little to no animal proteins. Provided that a variety of low-quality proteins are consumed as part of a healthy diet, the body will have access to all the EAA needed for optimal protein synthesis. Note that even small amounts of animal proteins can also complement the protein in plant foods and further minimize the need for protein complementation.

In addition to assessing the general amino acid composition of foods, people can measure the quality of a protein in many other ways. We know that a high-quality protein provides all the EAAs in the amounts that the body needs, provides enough other amino acids to serve as nitrogen sources for synthesis of nonessential amino acids, and is easy to digest. A protein food that provides all the EAAs but cannot be digested is useless to the body. Each technique to assess protein quality requires information about the amino acid composition and has been traditionally used to help formulate a special diet or to develop new feeding formulas for infants.

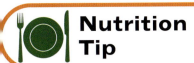

Nutrition Tip

When whole-food protein sources are not convenient, third-party tested supplemental protein powder is an alternative way to meet protein-intake needs. Look for these protein sources:

- Whey—milk protein that is the richest source of BCAAs and has the quickest digestion rate (20), leading to a quick rise in blood amino acids to help muscles adapt to exercise.
- Casein—a milk protein similar to whey but with slower absorption. Casein protein consumption helps stimulate muscle protein synthesis like whey protein but occurs at a slower rate (caused by slow digestion) that might take several hours (21).
- Egg—a high-quality protein; a good option for those who prefer to avoid milk products.
- Vegetable (soy, pea, etc.)—a viable option for vegetarians, vegans, or others. Many soy and hemp products are beneficial because they supply antioxidants, vitamin, minerals, and many essential amino acids. But few plant sources of protein are considered complete because of low levels of certain essential amino acids and lower digestive bioavailability affecting protein quality. Soy is the only complete plant protein when consumed in a typical serving (called a RACC—reference amount commonly consumed). But a single serving of another plant protein may possibly contain all essential amino acids in amounts required to be considered complete if the protein serving size is high enough.

Calculating Chemical Score

Calculating the chemical score (also known as the amino acid score) of a protein is an easy way to determine the protein quality of a food and refers simply to its amino acid profile rated to a standard or reference protein; each amino acid is rated on a scale indicating how much of that amino acid is present compared with the reference protein (table 5.4). The amino acid composition of the reference protein closely reflects the amounts and proportions of amino acids that humans need. Currently, the pattern of amino acids required by preschool children is used as the reference (22). The idea is that if a protein meets the needs of young, growing children, it should meet the needs of all other segments of the population. To calculate the chemical score, the quantity of each of the EAAs in the test food (in milligrams) is divided by the quantity of each of the amino acids found in the reference protein. The resulting numbers for each of the amino acids are then multiplied by 100 to create a percentage score for each amino acid.

The amino acid with the lowest score is the limiting amino acid. This amino acid, by definition, presents in the smallest amount relative to our biological need. The chemical score of the food protein is the same score as its limiting amino acid. The weakness of the chemical score is that

Table 5.4 Protein Chemical Score

	PROTEIN SOURCE					
	Peanut butter		White bread		Brie (cheese)	
Essential amino acid	mg/g	% optimal	mg/g	% optimal	mg/g	% optimal
Lysine	36	**62**	27	**46**	89	154
Threonine	35	102	29	87	36	**106**
Amino acid (chemical) score	62		46		106	

Cheese may be lower in protein in this example but contains higher-quality protein, as indicated by the chemical score.
When comparing amino acids in foods, the amino acid with the lowest percent optimal score (the chemical score) is the limiting amino acid (bold in the table).

it is not used much anymore and is based on an "ideal" reference protein that some suggest is an antiquated concept. Further, the chemical score says nothing about digestion or the way in which the body uses a given protein.

Calculating Biological Value

Biological value (BV), one of the more common methods of measuring protein quality, is simply a measure of how much of the protein absorbed by the digestive tract is retained in the body for growth and maintenance. This concept of nitrogen retention is primarily a function of nitrogen absorption, because technically nitrogen cannot be "retained." Biological value compares protein-in versus protein-out to determine nitrogen absorption as a key element. Based on the calculation used to derive a BV, the highest possible value is 100, meaning that the protein has an amino acid composition most similar to our needs. The protein that entered the bloodstream will be most efficiently retained by the body. The BV is measured through a tedious process that involves feeding subjects a protein-free diet, followed by a measured amount of protein. The amount that is excreted by urine, feces, and skin is estimated, and BV is calculated. The final value represents nitrogen retention as a percentage of nitrogen absorption. For example, the BV of corn protein is 60, meaning that only 60 percent of the absorbed corn protein is retained for use by the body. BV is typically tested at very low protein intakes and can be a source of significant misinterpretation because most adults, especially athletes, consume adequate protein amounts. Further, the number of calories consumed has a significant effect on BV values. Despite these limitations, BV is accurate under conditions of low protein intake, but energy intake (calories) should be meticulously controlled.

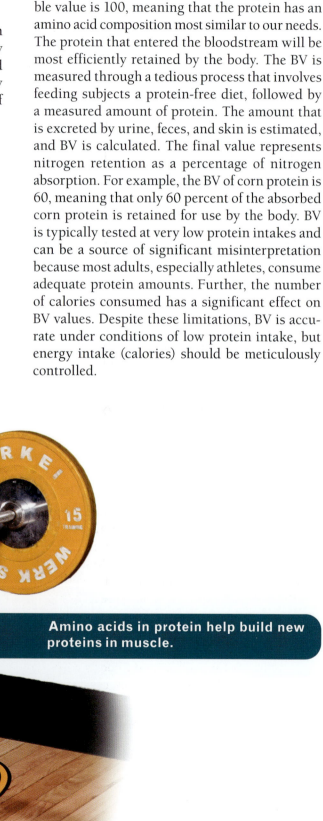

Amino acids in protein help build new proteins in muscle.

Measuring Net Protein Utilization

Net protein utilization (NPU) is similar to BV but simply compares the amount of protein eaten with the amount stored in the body, or how much the body actually uses. BV takes digestion and actual absorption of protein into account, whereas NPU does not. The nitrogen content of the test food is carefully measured and given to laboratory animals as their sole protein source. Animal nitrogen excretion is then measured to determine how much of the food's nitrogen content was retained. How efficiently the animal uses the food protein to make body proteins determines the NPU score.

Measuring the Protein Efficiency Ratio

The protein efficiency ratio (PER) is a measure of the amino acid composition that accounts for digestibility. The amount of weight gain (in grams) of growing animals that are fed a test protein is compared with the weight gain of growing animals that are fed a high-quality reference protein. This method provides information on how well the body can use a test protein by understanding amino acid composition, digestibility, and availability. This PER has been most commonly used to determine the protein quality of infant formulas.

Measuring the Protein Digestibility Corrected Amino Acid Score

The protein digestibility corrected amino acid score (PDCAAS) has been used since the 1990s for scoring protein quality and until recently has been the most common method used. The PDCAAS involves calculating the ratio of amino acids of a food source against the requirements of a 2- to 5-year-old child based on the first limiting dietary EAA within the protein. This method is similar to the chemical score, because it compares the amino acid profile with a reference protein while also considering digestion efficiency by multiplying the chemical score by the percent digestibility of the food protein. Foods with the highest possible PDCAAS of 1.0 are casein, whey, egg whites, and soy proteins. Any score calculated above 1.0 is truncated because any excess protein consumed is thought to be of no added biological value. If a protein has a chemical score of 0.70 and 80 percent of that protein is digestible, then the PDCAAS would be 80 percent of 0.70, or 0.56. The FDA has recognized the PDCAAS as the official method for determining the protein quality of most foods (22), and if the %DV of protein is listed on a food label, it must be based on the PDCAAS of the food. With this requirement, the total grams of protein might be the same per serving for two different foods, but their %DV could be very different because the foods do not contribute equally to the amino acid needs of the body. An example of this is in the comparison of 6 grams of casein protein powder with the same weight of wheat gluten. In this example, casein provides 13%DV whereas wheat gluten provides 3%DV.

Using the Digestible Indispensable Amino Acid Score

Most recently the Food and Agriculture Organization of the United Nations (FAO) has recommended a new method of assessing the quality of dietary protein. The digestible indispensable amino acid score (DIAAS) method builds on previous approaches by accurately measuring the digestion of individual amino acids rather than crude protein digestion. The DIAAS can accurately distinguish between proteins that were previously truncated to a maximum score of 1.0, using the PDCAAS method. Significant improvements in accuracy over the PDCAAS are a result of several advancements. First, measuring protein absorption at the end of the small intestine provides a more accurate assessment of the actual food protein remaining in the GI tract before endogenous proteins are added in the large intestine. This method also measures the digestion of individual amino acids to paint a better picture of how well a protein meets the body's amino acid needs. The DIAAS also does not allow for truncation of scores to 1.0 and recognizes that an excess can make up for any amino acid deficits from consuming incomplete protein foods. Finally, the DIAAS expanded the amino acid reference pattern from the ages of 2 to 5 to account for variation based on age. The DIAAS differentiates between the needs of infants and children with three reference patterns: 0 to 6 months, 6 months to 3 years, and greater than 3 years. With the development of the DIAAS, we are now able to distinguish between protein sources PDCAAS previously classified as the same. The DIAAS can be a useful tool in cases when proteins are consumed in smaller amounts, such as in aging or in clinical applications. When developing new protein formulations by blending protein ingredients, understanding the true value of protein sources is important in formulating the best protein ratio to meet the body's needs.

In summary, many measurements of protein quality are available, including chemical analysis of amino acid content and biological measures of protein digestibility. Ultimately, the most important factors that determine protein quality are the retention of protein in the body to support all amino acid needs and its ability to promote growth.

PROTEIN IN EXERCISE AND SPORT

Many people think that because muscle fibers are made up of protein, building and maintaining muscle must require the consumption of large amounts of protein in the diet. In reality, dietary protein is just one part of the equation to promote an optimal environment for muscles to adapt to physical training. The additional amount of protein required beyond what is already consumed to support optimal muscle adaptation is relatively small. Athletes should note that regular, well-structured training regimens combined with a proper mix of nutrients that meet their energy demands is the cornerstone for achieving their goals. Further, many other factors such as stress, frequent alcohol consumption, and inadequate rest can sabotage even the best diet and exercise plan. This viewpoint is not to say that protein is not important. Research over the last decade has provided much more detail for how dietary protein works to foster muscle hypertrophy (growth) and metabolic adaptations when combined with a proper training program. Dietary protein has four primary roles in an athlete's diet related to sport performance:

1. Maximizing gains in muscle mass and strength
2. Promoting adaptations in metabolic function (e.g., upregulation of oxidative enzymes, an increase in mitochondria size and number, etc.)
3. Preserving lean mass during rapid weight loss
4. Structural benefits to other protein-containing nonmuscle tissues, such as tendons, ligaments, and bones

The science that underpins guidelines for daily protein needs as well as the daily distribution of protein consumed continue to evolve. In this section, we delve into these details and look at how protein metabolism changes during and in response to exercise and how this information melds with other sections of this chapter.

Protein Metabolism and Exercise

Although carbohydrate and fat are the primary macronutrients metabolized for energy in the muscle, protein can also be used during exercise and can be oxidized directly in the muscle. Fortunately, most protein is spared for important synthetic processes, but it is important to remember from chapter 1 that the oxidation of all energy-yielding macronutrient fuel sources is always occurring in the body during exercise. The only thing that changes is the relative proportion of the macronutrients burned. At any one time during exercise, carbohydrate and fat make up more than 85 percent of the energy-yielding macronutrient fuels oxidized, but some protein is always used.

Exercise has a strong effect on protein metabolism. During exercise, the range of protein contribution to meet energy demands (ATP) is generally less than 5 to 10 percent, and in some extreme cases up to 15 percent of total energy expenditure. Many factors affect the percentage of protein oxidized during exercise, including exercise intensity, training level (new versus experienced), and availability of other fuels (e.g., carbohydrate). The type of exercise, or mode of exercise, also has a strong influence. During strenuous resistance training, less than 5 percent of protein is oxidized as an energy source. Conversely, prolonged endurance exercise (>90 min) might result in up to 15 percent of protein to serve as an energy source. A significant increase in protein oxidation, within the 5 to 15 percent range, occurs when muscle glycogen is depleted. As the body's most limited fuel source (carbohydrate) becomes depleted, the body must attempt to keep blood sugar stable to fuel the nervous system. For most people, the process of gluconeogenesis (see chapters 2 and 3) kicks in to help stabilize blood sugar levels by making new glucose from gluconeogenic precursors, including protein. For those following a low-carbohydrate diet, the production of ketones provides more fuel to the nervous system when glucose is limited. Regardless of the amount of carbohydrate in the diet, when muscle glycogen becomes depleted, skeletal muscle BCAA oxidation increases and contributes to the rise in protein use as a fuel source. In such a scenario, exercise intensity decreases. Gluconeogenesis and ketone production cannot keep up with the high ATP demands of high-intensity exercise.

Gluconeogenesis

The most prominent gluconeogenic pathway is the glucose-alanine cycle (figure 5.16). In this metabolic pathway, the gluconeogenic amino acid alanine leaves the muscle to create new glucose in the liver, which contributes to new blood glucose. This process occurs simultaneously with muscle tissue oxidation of BCAAs. As BCAAs are liberated from muscle tissue, their catabolism results in donating their NH_2 group to pyruvate in a process called transamination. The carbon skeletons from the BCAAs can then enter the TCA cycle in the mitochondria of muscle cells as TCA intermediates to contribute to ATP generation. Meanwhile, pyruvate originating from glycolysis can bind with NH_2 that originated from the BCAAs deamination to form the gluconeogenic amino acid alanine. Alanine can freely leave the muscle tissue and travel through the blood to the liver. The liver can then deaminate alanine to reform pyruvate. This liver-generated pyruvate can be further metabolized to form glucose that contributes to blood glucose or liver glycogen. Gluconeogenesis is never really turned off in human metabolism; instead it may occur only at a very low capacity and increase during long bouts of exercise, particularly when carbohydrate stores become limited. A significant limitation of this pathway is that the speed at which it can create new glucose depends on the availability of enzymes needed to drive the reaction. These enzymes must go through the protein synthesis process and are thus not capable of being made fast enough to keep up with the demands of one long endurance exercise bout. As a result, hypoglycemia can eventually occur, which is the primary reason that exercise halts during long events. Although the glucose-alanine cycle is an integral pathway in human metabolism and contributes to exercise metabolism, it is best suited for nonexercise situations during starvation, when key enzymes have time to be upregulated to produce glucose at the expense of muscle protein.

Protein Oxidation

Besides BCAAs, other amino acids from muscle tissue provide substrates for the TCA cycle (glutamine) in working muscle. BCAAs are the only amino acids liberated by the muscle that can be oxidized directly in the muscle. An increased percentage of BCAA oxidation occurs with prolonged aerobic training, with only a marginal carbohydrate-sparing effect that is most appreciable in endurance events lasting longer than 90 minutes. But in these situations there is limited evidence to support BCAA supplementation as a strategy to enhance performance. BCAAs are oxidized at such a low capacity that supplementation has no effect on performance.

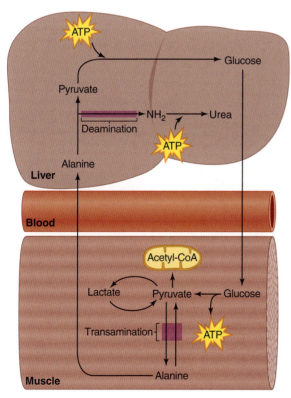

Figure 5.16 Alanine serves as an important gluconeogenic precursor.

Protein needs in athletes are elevated in part to account for increased protein oxidation. This greater need is most pronounced in endurance athletes to support elevated metabolic demand and to allow the muscle to adapt for endurance success by synthesizing more mitochondrial enzymes, producing more and larger mitochondria, and making new capillaries and hemoglobin to transport oxygen to working muscle. Athletes who focus more on strength and power oxidize much less protein during exercise. But because of the nature of their sport and sport-specific training, breakdown of contractile proteins is greater than what is observed with endurance training. Because these protein structures (i.e., the protein fibers that make muscles move) are larger than oxidative enzymes, and at times the breakdown can be significant, protein needs tend to be higher in athletes who participate in strength and power sports. Although these distinctions are clear from a scientific standpoint, from a practical sense, exercising athletes are much more complicated. For instance, many athletes rely on strength, power, and endurance to be successful in their sport and often rely on one aspect more than the others during specific phases of their training. The most prudent strategy to minimize protein oxidation is to have a well-chosen diet that meets both carbohydrate and energy demands of both the endurance athlete (e.g., runners and cyclists) and any athlete involved in a sustained competition in which endurance is a key component (e.g., soccer).

Daily Protein Needs for Athletes

Current guidelines suggest that dietary protein intake necessary to support an athlete's needs (when not in a state of caloric deficit) generally ranges from 1.2 to 2.0 g/kg per day (9). Generally, this daily amount is thought to support metabolic adaptation and repair of muscle and connective tissue by

- repairing and replacing damaged proteins;
- remodeling proteins within muscle, bone, tendon, and ligaments;
- maintaining optimal function of all metabolic pathways that use amino acids;
- supporting accretion of lean mass;
- supporting immune function; and
- supporting the optimal rate of production of plasma proteins.

Note that at any given time, based on training demands, goals, or other physiological stressors, an athlete's protein needs might fluctuate within this range from day to day, week to week, or month to month.

The 2019 International Association of Athletics Federations: Nutrition for Athletics Consensus Statement, recommends approximately 1.5 g/kg of protein per day during intense, heavy training loads and suggests that athletes need approximately 1.6 to 2.4 g/kg per day when weight loss and concurrent retention of muscle mass is desired (10). Although the various recommendations presented can lead to confusion, the best way to decipher this information is to think about the athlete's goals, their training volume, and any changing physical demands required by their sport. If the athlete is planning on maintaining weight while consuming adequate calories to support training and competition, a daily protein intake of 1.3 to 1.7 g/kg per day aligns with recent position papers (9, 10) and will likely be enough to maintain physique and training-related adaptations related to skeletal muscle size, function, and metabolism (23). The higher end of this range (~1.7 g/kg per day) is better suited for well-trained athletes who maintain a high training load. This recommendation is underpinned by data suggesting that increases in skeletal muscle mass and strength as a result of resistance training are maximized with an intake of approximately 1.6 g/kg per day (24).

In some scenarios, short-term intake of protein exceeding 2.0 g/kg might be indicated for athletes during intensified training or when reducing energy intake while pursuing weight loss. Protein needs of athletes are higher when on a lower-calorie diet to minimize the breakdown of skeletal muscle (because more dietary protein will be oxidized as a source of energy) (3). Although some have recommended daily protein intakes up to 3.1 g/kg in specific athlete populations primarily focused on improving physique (25), most competitive athletes are typically concerned with being faster or stronger. Currently, no evidence supports a skeletal muscle adaptive advantage from consuming more than 2.5 g/kg per day (23).

Protein needs for addressing body composition goals are discussed in detail in chapter 13.

Periodization

The aforementioned daily protein intake guidelines provide a general range of daily targets that should be based on adapting to specific sessions of training or competition within a periodized training program. The aim of periodization is to reach the best possible performance in the most important competition of the year and involves progressive cycling of various aspects of a training program during a specific period. These various aspects also include nutrient periodization and certainly involve protein as a nutrient. Changing needs are underpinned by an appreciation of the larger context of athletic goals, nutrient needs, energy considerations, and food choices. Generally, within the recommended daily protein intake range, requirements can fluctuate based on "trained" status (experienced athletes requiring less), training (sessions involving higher frequency and intensity, or a new training stimulus at the higher end of protein range), carbohydrate availability, and most important, energy availability (26, 27). Maintenance of normal bone metabolism and menstrual function are just two of the many body functions that can be negatively affected by low energy availability in athletes. For athletes in heavy training and competition, the consumption of adequate energy, particularly from carbohydrate to help maintain exercise intensity, to match energy expenditure is important so that amino acids are spared for protein synthesis and not oxidized (28). In cases of energy restriction or sudden inactivity as a result of injury, elevated protein intakes as high as 2.0 to 2.4 g/kg per day (9, 10, 29, 30) spread over the day at different mealtimes might be advantageous in minimizing loss of fat-free mass (31) from skeletal muscle (32).

Recommendations for Protein Intake

As shown in table 5.5, the modern view for establishing recommendations for protein intake in athletes clearly extends beyond the DRIs and the AMDR. Focus has shifted to evaluating the benefits of providing enough protein at optimal periodized times to support tissues with rapid turnover and augment metabolic adaptations initiated by a training stimulus. Given the wide range that the AMDR provides for protein intake, its use to determine protein needs in athletes should be limited to double-checking to ensure maximal diet quality (from other energy-yielding macronutrients). The AMDR can also be used after protein needs by body weight (grams per kilogram) are determined to evaluate whether an athlete is consuming a minimal protein amount to meet health needs while not consuming an excessive amount that may displace the intake of carbohydrate and fat. Gram per kilogram recommendations are superior to the AMDR and help fine-tune protein recommendations for athletes depending on their individualized needs during the various training cycles. These recommendations are more specific to the athlete's training demands and goals and are more practical to prescribe. Take, for instance, an athlete who may require 6,000 kcal during heavy training and 3,000 kcal while trying to make competition weight. The daily protein amounts needed based solely on the AMDR would vary greatly for these two calorie requirements combined, with the added variability of having to choose a value to use between 10 and 35 percent. These calculations may either fall significantly short of or exceed current gram per kilogram recommendations. As another example, a competitive athlete might consume as many as 5,000 kcal per day. If that athlete weighed 80 kilograms (176 lb), and if their diet contained only 10 percent of calories as

Table 5.5 Protein Intake Recommendations for Athletes and People With a High Volume of Vigorous Activity

RECOMMENDATIONS BASED ON 1.2 G/KG TO 2.0 G/KG BODY WEIGHT	
Lower end of range	**Higher end of range or exceeding range**
Light- to moderate-intensity physical activity with low to moderate weekly volume	• High-intensity training periods • During reduced energy intake • Recovering from injury or during rehabilitation

protein, they would be getting about 125 grams of protein daily—about 1.6 g/kg body weight. This level of protein is likely adequate to meet the needs of this athlete and would need to be only slightly modified to reach goal intake amounts specific to the current needs described in the literature.

> **? DO YOU KNOW?**
>
> Many athletes and those who are recreationally active tend to "backload" their energy intake, meaning that they tend to consume most of their calories in the evening or at night. Optimal use of protein occurs when smaller, but adequate, amounts of dietary protein are consumed throughout the day. This simple strategy optimizes skeletal muscle protein synthesis in adults as opposed to eating a little here and there throughout the day and one large protein meal at night.

Daily Distribution of Protein in Meals and Snacks

A well-planned distribution of protein containing meals and snacks throughout the waking hours includes eating enough protein after workouts and competitive events to help maximize synthesis of new body proteins every day. This eating schedule also benefits the body's ability to adapt and repair in response to progressive training. Athletes who distribute high-quality protein meals throughout the day at four to six eating occasions, 3 to 4 hours apart, can optimize training adaptations by providing a constant supply of important amino acid building blocks. Target body proteins that benefit from this eating strategy include structural proteins of the skeletal muscle, tendons, ligaments, and vasculature, and smaller "metabolic" proteins to increase mitochondrial size and number, and the essential enzymes involved in carbohydrate and fat metabolism.

Now that you know that the distribution of daily protein intake is important, you likely want to know how much protein is needed per meal or snack. The 2016 Nutrition and Athletic Performance Position Stand recommends a minimum of 0.25 to 0.3 g/kg per meal (9). This translates to approximately 15 to 25 g protein for athletes ranging from 60 to 100 kg (132–220 lb). This recommendation was largely based on acute studies using the isolated dietary proteins whey or soy and are now are thought to represent the minimum per meal protein recommendation (23). The high end of this recommendation (0.3 g/kg) represents a good approximation for people of all body sizes aiming to enhance the repair, remodeling, and synthesis of skeletal muscle tissue after resistance exercise (33).

Although the consensus recommendations seem to fall around 0.3 g/kg per meal, others have recommended higher intakes. The 2017 International Society of Sports Nutrition Position Stand: Nutrient Timing recommends about 0.3 to 0.4 g/kg of protein-rich foods (high in leucine) in athletes with optimal energy intake. This adjustment equates to roughly 20 to 40g protein per meal or snack and has been associated with improved body composition and performance (34). Other athlete circumstances may slightly increase these per meal protein recommendations. Additional research is needed to further elucidate factors that might necessitate greater per meal protein needs such as athlete rehabilitation, joint immobilization after injury, weight loss and meal composition (e.g., choosing a full mixed meal instead of a whey protein supplement), and type of protein (35). For example, Witard and colleagues recommended a target of 0.4 to 0.5g/kg at each meal during periods of weight loss (23).

Factors Affecting Protein Synthesis

Body proteins are constantly turned over through both synthesis and degradation pathways. Although implementing strategies that can augment muscle protein synthesis (MPS) is important, minimizing muscle protein breakdown (MPB) to promote a net increase in muscle protein accretion is also important. Several factors other than protein consumption can affect protein synthesis, including the type, volume, and intensity of exercise. For example, resistance training is the most potent stimulus for muscle building. Progressive resistance training allows athletes to train consistently to complete lifts at higher loads (i.e., weights) and repetitions. The damage to contractile proteins that result from this training is largely what triggers the body to adapt to synthesize more muscle protein to accommodate the increasing loads placed on the dumbbells or barbells. This muscle adaptation associated with exercise occurs with most forms of exercise, albeit to a lesser extent than with progressive resistance training. Exercise is an important variable that can stimulate MPS but is also a moving target, given the wide range of exercises, training volume, intensity, and duration commonly found in any one training program. In addition, the familiarity of the exercise, training program, or sport also is a strong influencer of maximal MPS response. Athletes who complete the same training program and are efficient with the physical movements associated with their sport have a lower MPS response compared with athletes who are new to an intense resistance-training program. The hormonal environment is another factor that works alongside dietary protein and a well-structured exercise program to maximize MPS. Several endogenous hormones, such as insulin-like growth factor-1 (IGF-1), growth hormone, testosterone, and insulin, facilitate the anabolic response. The role of these anabolic hormones is essential to facilitate hypertrophy, but the effect is significant only when maintaining normal hormone levels as a result of youth and exercise. Exercise and nutrition strategies that target these hormones to enhance their ability to promote MPS have been underwhelming; their effect seems to be maximized but not enhanced by proper exercise and nutrition. The negative effect of an unfavorable hormonal environment on MPS is most pronounced as a result of aging, illness, and injury. The major players that initiate significant MPB are malnutrition, inactivity, illness, and injury. These factors promote acute muscle loss from MPB, and minimizing these variables may be as important as optimizing variables associated with MPS.

Although the extremes of these MPB variables are most commonly observed in clinical environments where people are extremely ill from infection or trauma, lesser forms of these variables can significantly contribute to muscle loss in athletes. For example, athletes who chronically train and compete with low energy availability or practice fasting after exercise are at risk of experiencing sustained MPB. Inactivity also serves as the opposite of exercise by removing the exercise stimulus that drives the intracellular MPS machinery to be activated and use proteins from the amino acid pool to make new muscle tissue. Athletic injury (e.g., anterior cruciate ligament (ACL) tear, bone break) and illness promote MPB through two mechanisms. The first is by promoting inactivity or a significant reduction of activity less than required to maximize MPS. Second, acute illness and injury can negatively affect the hormonal environment and promote inflammation that elicits an elevated immune response that may require additional MPB to provide amino acids to support the body's defense of illness or recovery from injury.

Several factors besides total daily protein can affect the body's ability to gain skeletal muscle mass. Other negative factors, including unhealthy lifestyle habits such as smoking and alcohol consumption, can limit MPS, as can high levels of the hormone cortisol, associated with stress and lack of sleep, and inadequate recovery time between workout sessions (37). Diminished blood flow to muscle tissues, such as that observed with peripheral vascular disease, also limits MPS (38). Other positive factors for increasing and maintaining muscle mass include maintaining a positive energy balance (consuming more calories than expended), a consistent meal pattern, pre- and postexercise sports nutrition strategies

PUTTING IT INTO PERSPECTIVE

MUSCLE PROTEIN SYNTHESIS

Muscle protein synthesis (MPS) helps people adapt to exercise by promoting muscle growth, which can further help to increase overall muscle mass and support optimal muscle function. This outcome is accomplished through exercise programs and strategic ingestion of protein after exercise and throughout the day. BCAAs, particularly leucine, are key players in stimulating MPS, and consuming a full complement of essential amino acids (a complete protein) is important to maximize muscle growth over time (36).

to spare muscle protein, and adequate rest to promote recovery between training sessions. The complex nature of MPB mean that simple recommendations such as "eat more protein" can be shortsighted.

Dietary Protein as a Trigger for Muscle Metabolic Adaptation

Dietary protein has been well chronicled to interact with exercise, providing both a trigger and a substrate for the synthesis of skeletal muscle contractile and metabolic proteins (13, 32). Adaptations are thought to occur by (*a*) turning on MPS in response to the amount of leucine consumed in a meal and (*b*) providing an additional outside source of amino acids for incorporation into new skeletal muscle proteins (36). A sample of foods high in leucine is listed in table 5.6.

The role of leucine in initiating MPS is often referred to as the leucine trigger. The leucine trigger hypothesis suggests that a spike in blood leucine occurring in close proximity following exercise is thought to provide a strong anabolic stimulus to trigger and turn on the muscle-building machinery within skeletal muscle to stimulate growth (39). Consuming enough of this amino acid at meals is required to create a rapid rise in blood leucine concentration. Despite heavy interest in leucine, the leucine trigger is thought of as just one part of the story explaining the interaction between dietary protein and exercise in stimulating long-term muscle gains. Although consuming proteins that are naturally rich in leucine and are digested rapidly is important to causing a rapid increase in blood leucine concentrations, athletes also need all EAA to maximize the complete synthetic response to promote muscle growth over time (36). Whey is an example of a dietary protein that is rich in leucine and contains the full complement of EAAs. Because of the convenience of a whey protein dietary supplement, it is highly relevant in postexercise recovery. Although it has been shown that whey protein stimulates a maximal MPS response, note that whole foods high in all EAAs, particularly beef and dairy, have also been shown to cause potent stimulation of MPS following exercise without a rapid rise in blood leucine. So based on the current evidence, what is the take-home message? Protein-containing meals should be evenly distributed and selected not only to provide an adequate protein amount based on grams of protein per kilogram of body weight but also to be of high biological value. Athletes should strive to choose meals containing approximately 10 grams of EAAs and a minimum of 700 to 3,000 mg of leucine (9, 25, 34). When high-quality foods are not convenient or available, the pragmatic use of third-party-tested dietary protein supplements with high-quality ingredients may serve as practical alternative to meet these EAA targets (9). The leucine trigger hypothesis is discussed in greater detail in relation to resistance training in chapter 12.

? DO YOU KNOW?

Getting enough leucine at meals starts with meal planning. Identify and select foods that are rich in leucine to include at each meal.

Table 5.6 Leucine Content of Foods

Food	Approximate amount of leucine (g) per serving*
36 g whey protein isolate	3.2
36 g soy protein isolate	2.4
4 oz (120 g) broiled sirloin steak	2.7
4 oz (120 g) roasted chicken breast	1.4
8 oz (230 g) low-fat yogurt	1.1
8 oz (230 g) fat-free milk	0.8
1 egg	0.5
2 tbsp peanut butter	0.5
1 slice wheat bread	0.1

*Leucine content of food varies slightly based on information source, cut of meat, cooking methods, and processing techniques.

Data from U.S. Department of Agriculture and U.S. Department of Health & Human Services (2015).

Optimal Protein Source for Athletes

High-quality dietary proteins are effective for the maintenance, repair, and synthesis of skeletal muscle proteins (40). Chronic training studies have shown that the consumption of milk-based protein after resistance exercise is effective in increasing muscle strength while also promoting favorable changes in body composition (41-43). Other studies suggest increased MPS and muscle building with whole milk, lean meat, and dietary supplements, some of which provide the isolated proteins including whey, casein, soy, and egg. Dairy proteins are excellent choices, largely because of their leucine content and the digestion and absorptive kinetics of branched-chain amino acids in fluid-based dairy foods (21). Amino acids from whey protein, for example, can appear in the plasma in less than 30 minutes, whereas amino acids from intact animal proteins (beef, fish, etc.) can take 90 minutes or more. Therefore, easily digested, quickly absorbed protein such as whey leads to superior results for acute muscle protein synthesis (as measured within a 3-hour period right after exercise). Acute muscle protein synthesis, however, does not equate to better longer-term results. As an example, although whey is superior to soy for acute muscle protein synthesis within that 3-hour period after lifting weights and consuming protein, a meta-analysis of long-term research (>6 weeks) comparing soy protein with whey and animal protein found no difference between whey and soy or soy and other protein (beef, milk, dairy protein) for promoting a favorable anabolic response immediately after exercise (44).

> **? DO YOU KNOW?**
> Regular protein feedings maximize the number of MPS spikes over a 24-hour period. This schedule is often accomplished with four equally spaced protein-containing meals, with one or more of these coincidentally being close to exercise sessions.

In summary, an athlete's protein needs should be expressed using body weight guidelines (grams per kg body mass) to allow recommendations to be scaled to the large range in body sizes of athletes. Sports nutrition guidelines for protein intake should also consider the importance of the timing and distribution (per meal and snack amounts) of daily protein intake rather than focus only on general daily targets. Note that excess protein may contribute to excess calories, and in some cases may add more weight as fat, not muscle, if an athlete becomes more sedentary and starts to consume more calories than they expend. Although this scenario could degrade an athlete's performance, it does not commonly occur because most athletes are training hard and lifting weights. Additionally, athletes who consume too much fat or carbohydrate are more likely to experience gains of fat mass rather than overconsume protein (45). Finally, most weekend athletes and recreational athletes can easily meet slightly elevated protein needs by simple changes in their diet, and protein supplements are unlikely to help their performance. Competitive athletes should choose adequate calories from a wide variety of foods to help ensure adequate protein intake.

VEGETARIANISM AND VEGANISM

Vegetarians all share the common practice of limiting or completely avoiding meat and meat products; they can, however, differ significantly in their particular dietary choices.

Others may choose a semivegetarian diet, consuming red meat, poultry, or fish no more than once a week. Table 5.7 lists good sources of protein for lacto-ovo-pesco vegetarians, people who eat eggs, milk, and fish but avoid meat, poultry, and products made from meat and poultry. Figure 5.17 lists meatless food options that are high in protein.

Although a vegetarian diet certainly offers many health benefits, certain types of vegetarian choices might pose unique nutrition risks. Vegan diets are the most susceptible to these individual nutrient concerns (e.g., vitamin B_{12}, iron, etc.) because the best sources of these nutrients are from animal foods, and vegan diets contain higher amounts of oxalates and phytates. These compounds are plant-based food constituents that can bind some minerals in the GI tract, making them less available for absorption. Lacto-ovo-pesco vegetarians can easily have a nutritionally complete

Table 5.7 Example Protein Sources for Lacto-Ovo-Pesco Vegetarians

Protein source	Biological value (BV)	Protein (g)	Serving size
Whey isolate	159	16	1 scoop (28.7 g)
Whey concentrate	104	25	1 scoop (28.7 g)
Egg	100	6	1 egg
Milk	90	8	1 cup
Fish	83	22	1 filet (3 oz)
Soybeans	73	9	1 cup
Brown rice	57	5	1 cup
Lentils	50	18	1 cup

Data from U.S. Department of Agriculture and U.S. Department of Health & Human Services (2015).

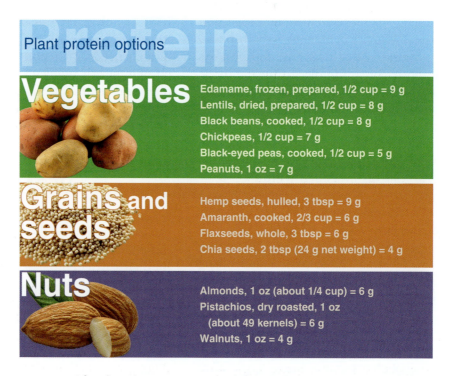

Figure 5.17 Numerous nonmeat food options are sources of protein.

diet providing all protein requirements, but such a diet might also be high in fat and low in iron, particularly if most of the diet is made up of dairy products. Although vegetarian diets can be healthy for most people, followers should be thoughtful of their food choices, taking care to pursue a varied diet and be cautious about any vegetarian diet plan that intentionally excludes multiple food groups. More information on vegetarian diets is found in chapter 14.

Vegetarian athletes committed to frequent training, competition, and success should also be cognizant of the benefits and challenges associated with a vegetarian diet. Vegetarian athletes, particularly vegans, might have an increased risk of lower bone mineral density and stress fractures (46). Additional practical challenges include gaining access to suitable foods during travel, at restaurants, and at training camps and competition venues. Without proper planning, these athletes may underconsume energy and protein, which can significantly affect their training and performance. Vegetarian athletes might benefit from comprehensive dietary assessments, education, and planning. This approach helps ensure that their diets are nutritionally sound enough to support training and competition demands, while also functioning to identify nutrient gaps that can be addressed to support both health and performance.

To meet protein needs, vegetarian athletes and nonathletes alike should focus on protein quality, while striving to consume protein at every meal. Several vegetarian foods have a high PDCAAS score, including eggs, yogurt, and milk, and soy foods, including tofu, edamame, soy milk, and soy yogurt. Consuming multiple small meals and snacks per day also provides the opportunity to add more variety to the diet to include protein-containing foods such as vegetables, legumes, whole grains, and nuts and seeds. Finally, vegans who avoid all animal products should supplement their diets with a reliable source of vitamin B_{12}, such as fortified soy milk, other fortified foods, or a dietary supplement. A more detailed discussion of vegetarian diets is provided in chapter 14.

PROTEIN DEFICIENCY AND EXCESS PROTEIN

Given the important role of protein to virtually all body systems and processes, it is no surprise that protein deficiency can create several problems affecting normal human physiology. As a reminder, a lack of essential amino acids will stop the synthesis of body proteins, leading to increased rates of body protein catabolism to fulfill the body's amino acid demands. Protein intake may also be inadequate to support training adaptations in training and competition when protein needs are elevated. During growth and development, childhood and adolescent dietary protein deficiency can lead to inadequate growth (stunting). Risk of protein deficiency can also become elevated because of physiological stress presenting in the form of an injury, trauma, pregnancy, or other medical conditions. These stressors increase the rate of body protein catabolism. Protein consumption that was adequate before the onset of these physiologic stressors might not be adequate when stressors are present. The ability to meet elevated protein synthesis needs alongside elevated catabolism will be compromised without the consumption of additional dietary protein.

Although protein deficiency is widespread in poverty-stricken communities in underdeveloped countries, in North America it is most common in clinical settings where patients experience severe metabolic stress and do not have the ability to meet their elevated protein needs through their diet. In industrialized countries, most people face the opposite problem of protein excess, which in many cases is a product of consuming more calories than needed. But dietary protein excess is more difficult to define in terms of specific daily intake of protein and cut points above the RDA. Also, the Food and Nutrition Board has not provided an upper intake level for protein because of insufficient evidence to support the link to chronic health problems (47). Despite the lack of a clear definition of "excess protein intake," we know that the average American consumes above the RDA for protein. As described earlier, in many cases this concern is justified. When examining specific protein intakes in relation to body weight, anecdotal reports of dehydration and kidney stress have been associated with protein intakes greater than 2.0 g/kg per day, but a consensus is developing in the scientific literature that protein intakes at and slightly above this level are safe (48, 49). Although the kidney must excrete the products of protein breakdown, high protein intake may only strain kidney function in people with uncontrolled diabetes and specific types of kidney disease. Furthermore, in healthy people, there is no indication that high-protein diets contribute to dehydration. Despite the established beneficial role of higher-protein diets on satiety and weight control, the most common concern regarding chronic high protein intake is that the protein foods chosen to reach this level of protein intake might be displacing a variety of other nutrient-dense foods (e.g., fruits, vegetables, grains, etc.) that have a strong connection to chronic disease prevention and longevity. Foods that have potential for being displaced may also be higher in fiber, contain fewer calories and fat, and provide some protective benefits against obesity and cancer. Table 5.8 outlines how choosing a wide variety of protein-containing foods can help maintain high diet quality.

Table 5.8 Nutrients Found in Different Categories of Protein Foods

Protein-containing food categories	Insufficient source of nutrients	Good source of nutrients providing 10%–19% of daily value
Common animal proteins: beef, chicken, egg, fish	Fiber, calcium, folate, vitamin C, thiamin, vitamin K, beta-carotene	Vitamin B_6, iron, zinc, vitamin B_{12}, niacin, phosphorous, pantothenic acid
Dairy proteins: milk, cheese, yogurt	Beta-carotene, vitamin C, iron, vitamin E	Calcium, riboflavin, phosphorous, vitamin B_{12}
Plant proteins: whole grains and legumes	Vitamin B_{12}, DHA, heme iron	Fiber, most B vitamins, iron, zinc, magnesium, vitamin E, vitamin K
Plant proteins: nuts and seeds	Vitamins A, C, B_{12}, K	Most B vitamins, fiber, vitamin E, magnesium, ALA

Based on the FDA's Guidelines for Reference Amounts Customarily Consumed (RACC) and USDA Nutrient Database; Data from Institute of Medicine (US) Committee on Examination of Front-of-Package Nutrition Rating Systems and Symbols; Wartella et al. (2010); and U.S. Department of Agriculture, Agricultural Research Service (2020); USDA Food and Nutrient Database for Dietary Studies (2017-2018).

SUMMARY

Amino acids are the building blocks of both body and dietary protein. Protein is the key structural component that makes up not only muscle but also all other connective and organ tissues. Protein also has an essential role in making up hormones, enzymes, and antibodies and can be used as an energy source to make ATP. High-quality dietary proteins are effective for repair, synthesis, and maintenance of all body proteins. Consuming protein at appropriate amounts and at the right times helps skeletal muscle recover and adapt to exercise. Dietary protein can be obtained through animal and vegetable sources, as well as in supplement form, and must be digested and absorbed before being utilized. Vegetarians can meet their protein needs by planning a well-chosen diet. Most people can easily meet their protein needs by consuming a source of dietary protein with every meal and snack. For athletes, special attention should be given to the total amount of protein consumed per day, the type of protein, and the timing of intake. Careful planning of protein feedings for the athlete allows optimal skeletal muscle utilization of these food-derived amino acids.

FOR REVIEW

1. Describe the various functions and roles of protein.
2. What is an enzyme? How does it function?
3. Can essential amino acids be made by the body? What amino acid group is important for promoting MPS?
4. Describe the primary, secondary, tertiary, and quaternary structure of proteins (if necessary, review figure 5.6).
5. Describe protein digestion.
6. How would you begin to recommend protein intake for a sedentary, active, and extremely active person? Explain the steps you would take.
7. What are potential concerns for athletes trying to meet their protein needs with a vegetarian diet?
8. What is gluconeogenesis? List the gluconeogenic precursors.

PART III

ROLE OF MICRONUTRIENTS, WATER, AND NUTRITIONAL SUPPLEMENTS

This section of the book covers vitamins (chapter 6), minerals (chapter 7), water and electrolytes (chapter 8), and nutrition supplements (chapter 9). Vitamins and minerals do not provide energy, but they facilitate chemical reactions in the body that help generate energy. In addition, vitamins are important for growth and development, organ functioning, and building and maintaining structures in the body, including protecting the body from damage. Minerals help build structural components of the body and are necessary for a variety of functions that support health and athletic performance. Deficiencies in certain vitamins and minerals can impair health and in some cases also athletic performance.

Because minerals are electrolytes, they conduct electricity in the body and affect fluid balance and muscle pH and function. Electrolytes and water go hand in hand because overconsumption or underconsumption of fluid can alter electrolyte balance. Water is also a medium for transportation in the body. Dietary supplements may include macronutrients, micronutrients, or a variety of compounds intended to support good health, aid athletic performance, or fill in dietary gaps.

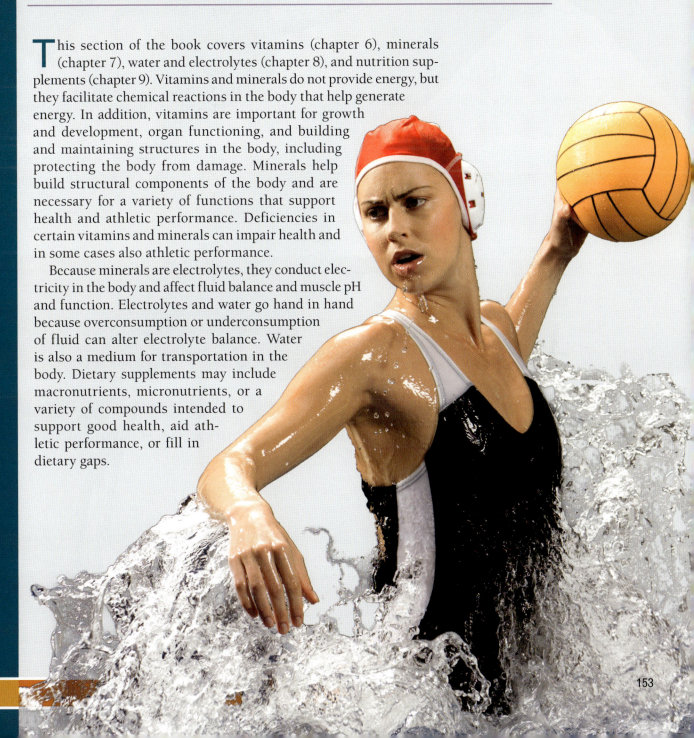

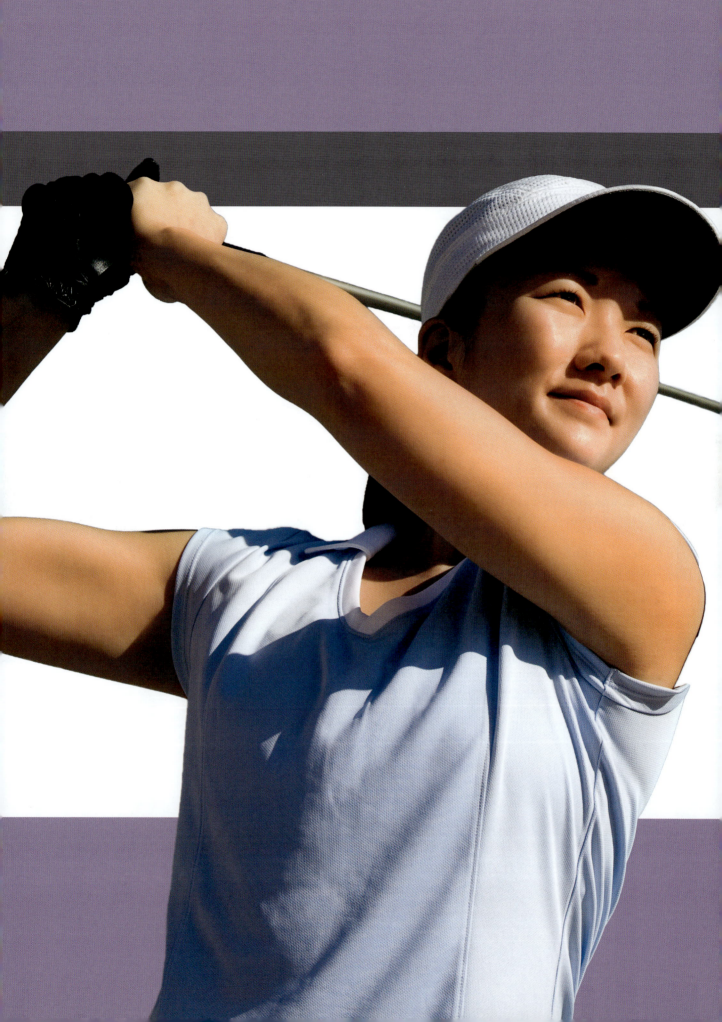

6

Vitamins

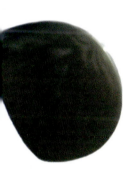

> **CHAPTER OBJECTIVES**
>
> After completing this chapter, you will be able to do the following:
> - Discuss why vitamins are important for overall health and training.
> - Describe how training and exercise affect vitamin needs.
> - List the vitamins that most people are not getting enough of through their diet.
> - List the vitamins that are toxic when consumed in excess.
> - List a few good food sources for each major vitamin.
> - Explain factors that may increase a person's need for a specific vitamin.

Vitamins are necessary for metabolism, proper growth and development, vision, and organ and immune functioning. They also aid human performance by facilitating energy production; supporting muscle contraction and relaxation, as well as oxygen transport; building and maintaining bone and cartilage; building and repairing muscle tissue; and protecting the body's cells from damage. The human body can make vitamin D, and gut bacteria can make vitamin K; all other vitamins must be consumed in the diet to meet dietary requirements. Although deficiencies or insufficiencies in certain nutrients can impair training adaptations and performance, no current data indicate that excess nutrient intake, beyond the requirements for general health, will improve athletic performance (1). In some cases, excess consumption of specific vitamins may interfere with performance, training adaptations, and recovery. Figure 6.1 illustrates the importance of many vitamins discussed in this chapter.

FAT-SOLUBLE VITAMINS

Vitamins A, D, E, and K are **fat-soluble** vitamins. They are stored in the body's fat tissues and more easily absorbed when consumed with dietary fat.

Vitamin A

Vitamin A helps form healthy teeth, bones, soft tissue, skeletal tissue, mucous membranes, and skin. Vitamin A also promotes good vision, particularly night vision, and is necessary for growth, development, tissue repair, cellular communication, and immune system functioning, as well as the formation and maintenance of several organs, including the heart, lungs, and kidneys (2). Vitamin A refers to a group of fat-soluble retinoids including retinol, retinal, and retinyl esters. Two types of vitamin A are found in food:

❯ **Preformed vitamin A** (retinol and retinyl ester) is found in some animal foods. Retinol is a type of preformed vitamin A found in animal liver, whole milk, and some fortified foods. Preformed vitamin A must be metabolized to retinal and retinoic acid, the active forms of vitamin A in the body that are used to support biological functions (3). In Western countries like the United States, on average more than 70 percent of vitamin A intake comes from preformed vitamin A in animal products. In developing countries, less than 30 percent of vitamin A intake comes from preformed vitamin A (4).

❯ **Provitamin A carotenoids**, including beta-carotene, alpha-carotene, and beta-cryptoxanthin, are the dark-colored pigments found in red palm oil and in several fruits and vegetables, notably carrots, mango, cantaloupe, squash, sweet red bell peppers, seaweed, and spinach. These carotenoids are converted to the active form of vitamin A in the body, a process that depends on several factors, including the food matrix, food processing, and dietary fat intake, as well as genetic differences (4, 5). Therefore, the conversion of carotenoids to vitamin A in the body can vary tremendously. Beta-carotene is the most important carotenoid because more if it is converted to vitamin A compared with other carotenoids. Approximately 45 percent of the Western population are considered "low converters" of beta-carotene to the active form of vitamin A in the body, a factor that can affect vitamin A levels over time if a large portion of vitamin A intake comes from carotenoids (5). See figure 6.2 for sources of provitamin A carotenoids.

> **❓ DO YOU KNOW?**
>
> Consuming carotenoid-rich foods with a source of fat improves carotenoid bioavailability (7). Chop up mango and have it alongside a full-fat yogurt or with some nuts and seeds; eat carrots with peanut butter and salad with dressing that contains some fat (preferably low in saturated fat for heart health), avocado, or nuts and seeds to ensure optimum carotenoid bioavailability.

More than 600 types of carotenoids are found in nature; many, though not all, have provitamin A activity. Nutrition data exist for alpha-carotene, beta-carotene, and beta-cryptoxanthin, all of which are pro-vitamin A carotenoids and act as **antioxidants**. Certain antioxidants protect plants from pests and disease (8, 9) and protect cells in the human body from **free radical** damage (10). Figure 6.3 shows the interaction between free radicals and antioxidants.

Free radicals are reactive oxygen and nitrogen species generated in the body through metabolism

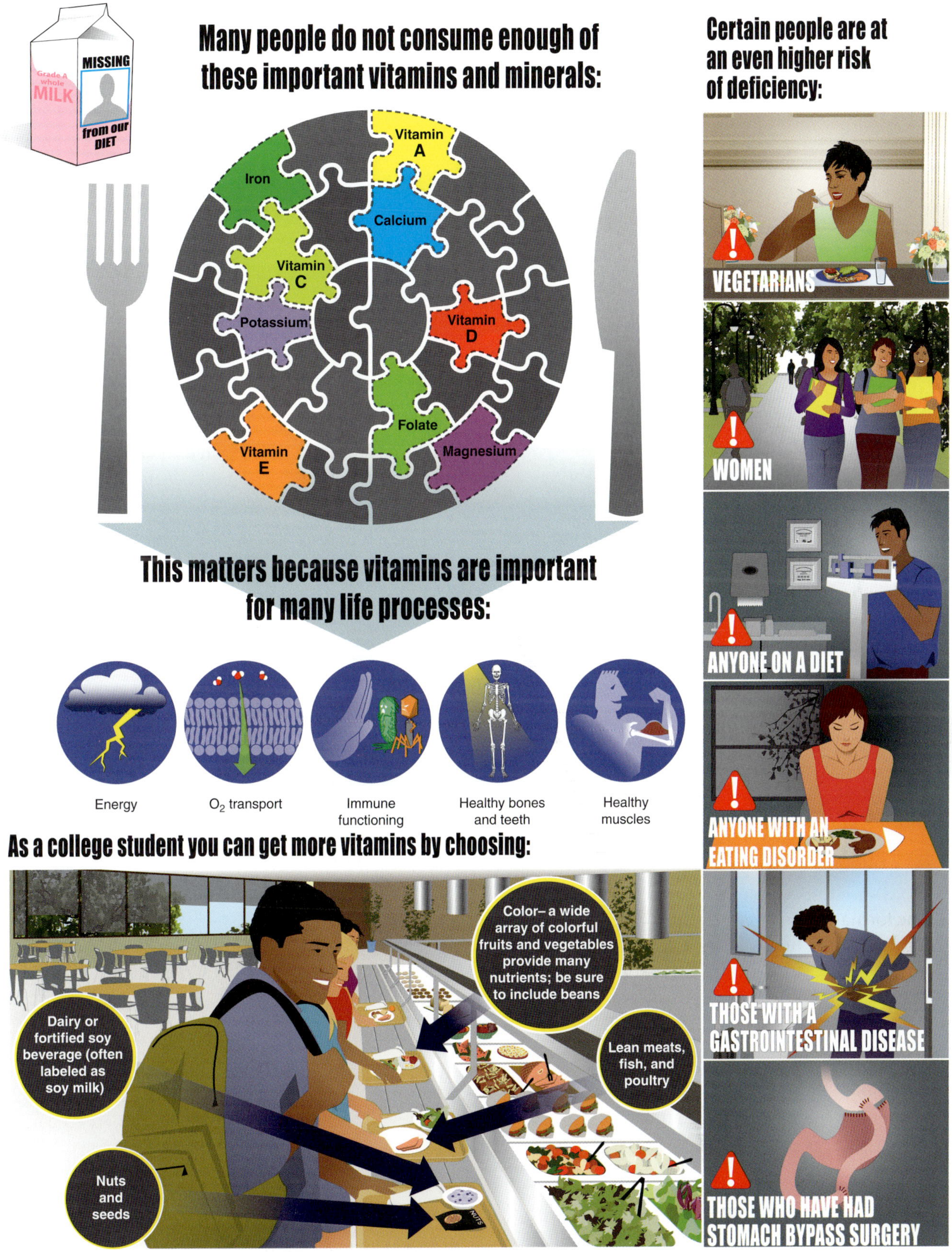

Vitamins 157

Many people do not consume enough of these important vitamins and minerals:

- Vitamin A
- Iron
- Calcium
- Vitamin C
- Potassium
- Vitamin D
- Vitamin E
- Folate
- Magnesium

This matters because vitamins are important for many life processes:

- Energy
- O₂ transport
- Immune functioning
- Healthy bones and teeth
- Healthy muscles

As a college student you can get more vitamins by choosing:

- Dairy or fortified soy beverage (often labeled as soy milk)
- Nuts and seeds
- Color—a wide array of colorful fruits and vegetables provide many nutrients; be sure to include beans
- Lean meats, fish, and poultry

Certain people are at an even higher risk of deficiency:

- VEGETARIANS
- WOMEN
- ANYONE ON A DIET
- ANYONE WITH AN EATING DISORDER
- THOSE WITH A GASTROINTESTINAL DISEASE
- THOSE WHO HAVE HAD STOMACH BYPASS SURGERY

MISSING from our DIET

Figure 6.1 What you need to know about vitamins.

158　Nutrition for Sport, Exercise, and Health

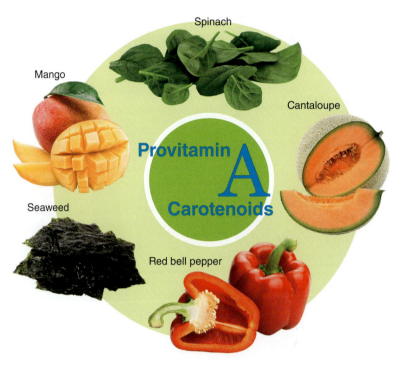

Figure 6.2 Provitamin A carotenoids include beta-carotene, alpha-carotene, and beta-cryptoxanthin. Beta-carotene is considered the most important source of provitamin A (6).

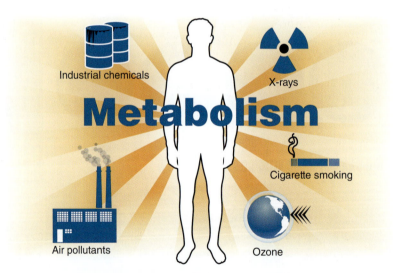

Our bodies create free radicals, and we are exposed to free radicals through our environment.

Figure 6.3 Free radicals are naturally produced in the body and made upon exposure to various environmental insults and diseases. Some antioxidants can help attenuate oxidative damage resulting from free radicals running amok.

Data from U.S. Department of Agriculture (2013).

and exposure to various physiological conditions or disease states. Free radicals are essential for health, but they can be harmful when they go into overdrive. For normal physiological functioning, the body must maintain a balance between free radicals and antioxidants (not getting too much or too little of either; supplemental antioxidant intake may actually increase oxidative damage to cells or impair adaptations to resistance training). Overproduction of free radicals, when combined with an inability to regulate them, leads to **oxidative stress** and subsequent damage to cellular lipids, proteins, and DNA in addition to initiating a number of diseases (11).

Sources of Vitamin A and the RDA

The RDA for vitamin A is given in micrograms (mcg) of retinal activity equivalents (RAE) to account for sources of vitamin A. Although 1 mcg of retinol is equal to 1 mcg RAE, it takes 12 mcg beta-carotene or 24 mcg alpha-carotene or beta-cryptoxanthin to equal 1 mcg RAE. Making matters more confusing, vitamin A is listed on dietary foods and supplements in international units (IUs). The conversion between IU and RAE depends on the source of vitamin A (table 6.1).

Vitamin A Deficiency and Toxicity

Vitamin A deficiency is rare in North America yet common in developing countries (12, 13), where it is a leading cause of preventable blindness in children (14-16). Xerophthalmia—dry eyes caused by inadequate tear production—which can lead to night blindness, is an early sign of vitamin A deficiency. Vitamin A deficiency can also suppress immune system functioning and increase risk of infection (17). In the United States and other developed countries, groups at risk of deficiency include premature infants and people with cystic fibrosis (18, 19).

Preformed vitamin A is stored in the body, particularly the liver, and can be toxic when taken in one single massive dose or in large doses over time. Acute overdose can lead to very dry skin, inflammation and cracking of the lips at the corners of the mouth (**cheilosis**), gingivitis, muscle and joint pain, fatigue, depression, and abnormal liver tests. Signs and symptoms of chronic consumption of extremely high intakes of vitamin A might include increased cerebrospinal fluid pressure, dizziness, blurred vision, vomiting, nausea, bone and muscle pain, headaches, and poor muscular coordination (20). Vitamin A toxicity can also lead to liver damage (that is not always reversible), coma, and death (2, 21). Excess dietary intake (from food) or supplements could potentially lead to toxicity, but most cases of vitamin A toxicity are from therapeutic retinoids

Table 6.1 Excellent or Good Sources of Vitamin A

Food	Serving size	RAE per serving (mcg)	IU per serving	%DV
Beef, variety of meats and by-products, raw liver	4 oz (113 g)	32,000	106,670	2,133
Sweet potato, baked or boiled (no skin)	1 cup mashed (145 g)	2,581	51,627	1,033
Pumpkin, canned	1 cup (245 g)	1,906	38,129	762
Goose liver (raw)	1 liver (94 g)	8,750	29,138	582
Carrots (frozen, cooked, boiled, drained)	1 cup sliced (146 g)	1,235	24,715	494
Carrots (raw)	1 cup chopped (128 g)	1,069	21,384	428
Turkey liver (raw)	1 liver (78 g)	6,285	21,131	422
Collards (frozen, chopped, cooked, boiled, drained)	1 cup chopped (170 g)	978	19,538	391
Kale (frozen, cooked, boiled, drained)	1 cup chopped (130 g)	956	19,115	382
Spinach (cooked, boiled, drained)	1 cup (180 g)	943	18,866	377
Swiss chard (cooked, boiled, drained)	1 cup chopped (175 g)	536	10,717	214

Data from U.S. Department of Agriculture (2013).

(medicines prescribed in high doses for the treatment of acne, psoriasis, and other conditions). A considerable amount of time must pass for tissue stores of vitamin A to decline after discontinuing intake (2).

Provitamin A carotenoids are considered nontoxic, although over a long period, excess beta-carotene from dietary supplementation can lead to yellow-orange skin. Skin will return to its natural shade after beta-carotene intake is discontinued (2). Although beta-carotene does not build up in the body, studies show that very high doses (33,000-50,000 IU supplemental beta-carotene) taken over the course of 5 to 8 years increased risk of lung cancer and cardiovascular disease in current and former smokers (22-24). In a controlled supplementation trial in male smokers spanning 6 years, high-dose beta-carotene (66,600 IU beta-carotene/day) increased risk of hemorrhagic stroke (caused by rupture of a weak blood vessel), and alpha-carotene (50,000 mcg/day) increased risk of hemorrhagic stroke and death from hemorrhagic stroke, yet lowered risk of ischemic stroke (caused by a blockage in the blood vessel) (25).

Vitamin A and Exercise

Because of the body's ability to store vitamin A and a lack of data on vitamin A status in athletes, there is no evidence or plausible reason to suggest that athletes or recreational gym-goers are more likely to be deficient in this vitamin (1). Further, data on vitamin A supplementation in athletes are insufficient to suggest that supplementation is beneficial for performance or recovery, especially beyond the RDA and in the absence of deficiency.

Vitamin D

Vitamin D comes from food and dietary supplements and is made in the body when skin is exposed to UVB rays from the sun (figure 6.4). Vitamin D synthesis in the body upon sunlight exposure is considered one of the main sources of vitamin D given that dietary sources are limited (26). All of these forms are inert and must be converted to the active form, calcitriol (1,25-dihydroxyvitamin D). **Calcitriol** is a steroid hormone that promotes calcium absorption, helps maintain blood calcium and phosphorus levels for normal bone mineralization, reduces inflammation, and has important physiological effects on cell growth, muscle, and immune system functioning (27-31).

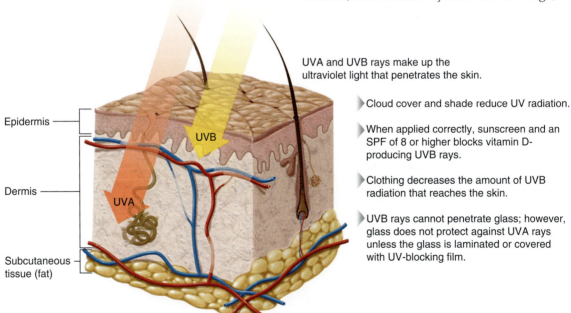

Figure 6.4 UVA rays penetrate the middle layer of skin (dermis). UVB rays are shorter in wavelength and extend only to the outer layer of skin (epidermis). UVB rays, as well as combined UVB and UVA rays, increase the body's production of vitamin D (32, 33).

PUTTING IT INTO PERSPECTIVE

TANNING BEDS AND VITAMIN D

Tanning beds damage skin and might be worse for your vitamin D levels than no light at all. Tanning beds emit either UVA radiation only or a combination of UVA and UVB radiation (34). UVB radiation helps the body produce vitamin D. UVA plus UVB radiation (sunlight contains both) also increases vitamin D production in the body. But some research shows that UVA1 radiation (UVA rays include UVA1 and UVA2 rays) alone leads to a significant reduction in blood vitamin D (calcidiol) (32, 33). Both UVA and UVB rays damage skin. A tan is an injury to the skin resulting from UV radiation. Tanning bed use (both newer and older models) is associated with a significant increase and risk of melanoma (a form of skin cancer that can be deadly). Therefore, tanning beds are not a safe way to get vitamin D and are not FDA approved as a way to increase vitamin D levels (35-37).

Vitamin D controls hundreds of genes and might have a beneficial role in outcomes related to cancer, autoimmune disease, cardiovascular disease, and diabetes, although the research results on vitamin D in relation to those diseases are not entirely clear at this time (38-40).

Sources of Vitamin D

The two types of vitamin D are vitamin D_2 (ergocalciferol) and vitamin D_3 (cholecalciferol). Vitamin D_2 is made from UV light irradiation of fungus, such as mushrooms and yeast (41). This form of vitamin D is found in vegan supplements and vegan-fortified foods, including soy milk, almond milk, and other nondairy beverages. Vitamin D_2 is also sometimes given in prescription doses (50,000 IU per week or every 2 or 4 weeks). Vitamin D_3 is naturally found in cod liver oil and oily fish, including halibut, mackerel, salmon, and trout, and in much smaller amounts in egg yolks, cheese, and beef liver. Vitamin D_3 is in fortified foods, notably milk, and made from lanolin in sheep's wool for dietary supplements (42). In addition to natural and fortified food sources of vitamin D_3, this vitamin is produced in the body when skin is exposed to UVB rays (see figure 6.4). See figure 6.5 for more information on sources of vitamin D.

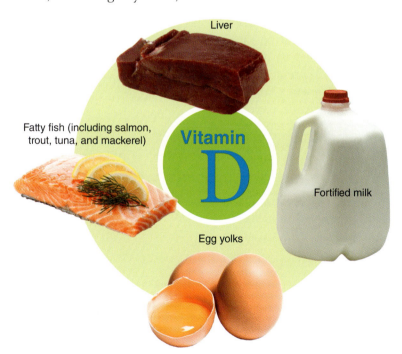

Figure 6.5 Sources of Vitamin D. In addition to food sources of vitamin D_3, mushrooms exposed to UV radiation are a source of vitamin D_2.

> **PUTTING IT INTO PERSPECTIVE**
>
> ### FOOD FORTIFICATION AND ENRICHMENT
>
> Although many people use the terms *fortification* and *enrichment* interchangeably, they have distinct meanings. Food **fortification** refers to the addition of nutrients to food to improve the nutrition content. Fortification started with the mineral iodine in 1924 as a systematic approach to correcting nutrient deficiencies and nutrient deficiency diseases. Food manufacturers follow a "standard of identity"—an established type and level of fortification for a staple food. Enrichment refers to the addition of vitamins and minerals that are lost during food processing. For instance, white flour is enriched with iron, thiamin, riboflavin, niacin, and folic acid in levels that occur naturally in flour before nutrient losses that occur during processing (43, 44).

Several studies suggest that vitamin D_3 is superior to vitamin D_2 for maintaining serum 25(OH)D concentrations (45, 46). Serum 25(OH)D, or 25-hydroxyvitamin D, is used to assess vitamin D status in the body.

For optimal absorption, vitamin D supplements should be taken with a meal that contains fat, rather than with a fat-free meal or on an empty stomach. Absorption of a single 50,000 IU vitamin D_3 supplement was 32 percent greater when taken with a meal containing fat compared with a fat-free meal (47).

Vitamin D Deficiency and Insufficiency

Serum-circulating calcidiol—also referred to as 25-hydroxyvitamin D or 25(OH)D—is used to assess vitamin D levels. But comparing rates of deficiency or health effects based on deficiency is not always easy because different values for vitamin D deficiency, insufficiency, and sufficiency have been used in scientific papers and corresponding data briefs, media reports, and other consumer-related communications (48). In addition, blood levels of vitamin D (25[OH]D) are largely composed of vitamin D bound to vitamin D binding protein (85%–90%) followed by 10 to 15 percent bound to albumin and only 1 percent free circulating vitamin D. Some research suggests free circulating vitamin D might be a better predictor of bone mineral density (BMD) in an ethnically diverse population compared with looking at blood levels of vitamin D. But even this measure alone may be insufficient without also examining genetic differences in binding proteins and the vitamin D receptor (49). Moreover, the enzymes involved in vitamin D metabolism are dependent on magnesium. Therefore, optimal levels of magnesium may be necessary for adequate levels of vitamin D (50).

In 2011, the Endocrine Society issued vitamin D guidelines based on the role of vitamin D in bone and muscle health. These definitions, along with the Institute of Medicine's guidelines, are provided in table 6.2 and will be used for this chapter (51).

Table 6.2 Vitamin D Definitions

	Endocrine Society (51)	Food and Nutrition Board, Institute of Medicine (52)
Deficiency (ng/ml)	<20 ng/ml (50 nmol/L)	0–11 ng/ml (<30 nmol/L)
Insufficiency (ng/ml)	21–29 ng/ml (52.5–72.5 nmol/L)	12–20 ng/ml (30–50 nmol/L)
Sufficient levels (ng/ml)	>30 ng/ml (75 nmol/L)	>20 ng/ml (>50 nmol/L)
Toxicity (ng/ml)	It is not clear what the safe upper limit is for serum-circulating 25(OH)D to avoid hypercalcemia. According to the Endocrine Society, studies in both adults and children show blood levels may need to be above 150 ng/ml (375 nmol/L) before risk of harm.	>150

Based on serum-circulating calcidiol.

Data from Holick (2011); U.S. Institute of Medicine (1998).

National Health and Nutrition Examination Survey (NHANES) data from 2011 to 2014 found that 5 percent of the population studied was deficient in vitamin D (<12 ng/ml) and 18.3 percent of the population had insufficient levels of vitamin D (12–20 ng/ml). Rates of deficiency were highest in those aged 20 to 39. Also, rates of deficiency and insufficiency were highest among Blacks at 17.5% and 35.8%, respectively (53). Other sets of population-based survey data have shown much higher rates of deficiency and insufficiency. For instance NHANES data from 2011 to 2012 found that 39.9 percent of the population was deficient (they defined deficiency as <20 ng/ml) (54).

In non-vitamin D-supplemented athletes, variations were found in serum vitamin D levels. This result is likely explained by when they tested (summer versus winter), practice time and clothing or equipment needs (limiting sunlight exposure), and differences in dietary intake (55). But studies show that vitamin D deficiency and insufficiency is widespread in athletes (56). Black athletes and indoor athletes with little exposure to sunshine are more likely to be deficient (57). Two separate studies found that 38 percent and 11 percent of healthy endurance athletes were deficient, and 91 percent of Middle Eastern sportsmen were deficient. Two studies in NFL players found that 26.3 percent and 30.3 percent of players, respectively, were deficient in vitamin D (57-61). NBA combine data from 2009 to 2013 found that 32.3 percent were deficient and 47 percent had insufficient levels (62). Other research has found that 36 percent of Liverpool's pro soccer players were deficient or insufficient (63). In addition to high deficiency rates, a high percentage of athletes also have insufficient levels of vitamin D to support optimal muscle and, potentially, bone health (57, 58, 61). The body's production of vitamin D through exposure to sunlight (UVB rays) is a significant source of vitamin D, so athletes who test normal in the summer might be deficient in the winter months (64).

Groups with a higher risk of vitamin D deficiency or insufficiency include the following (65-68):

- The elderly, because aging alters vitamin D synthesis in the body after sunlight exposure.
- Obese people.
- People who have had gastric bypass surgery.
- Those who avoid the sun (homebound people), those who wear attire or sporting equipment that covers their body and head, and those who regularly use sunscreen with an SPF of 8 or higher. Sunscreen with an SPF of 8 will not fully protect skin from the damaging effects of UV rays, but it will decrease (by 95 percent or more) the body's ability to synthesize vitamin D.
- Infants exclusively or partially breastfed.
- People who have medical conditions leading to fat malabsorption, including cystic fibrosis, celiac disease, and Crohn's disease.
- People with dark skin—the pigment melanin provides natural protection from the sun yet decreases the body's ability to produce vitamin D upon exposure to sunlight.

Additionally, athletes who live in northern latitudes and those who train primarily indoors throughout the year are at risk for poor vitamin D status. Poor dietary intake also contributes to low levels of vitamin D in athletes. In several studies, most athletes surveyed do not meet the RDA for vitamin D through food alone; one study found that less than 5 percent of athletes surveyed obtained the RDA for vitamin D through dietary intake (64, 69-72). This result is in line with research in the population at large, which shows that more than 90 percent of Americans do not consume an adequate amount of vitamin D from food alone (73).

Vitamin D deficiency decreases calcium and phosphorus absorption 10 to 15 percent and 50 to 60 percent, respectively (79). In children, vitamin D deficiency can lead to rickets, a disease characterized by soft bones and skeletal deformities resulting from impaired bone mineralization (80). In adults, deficiency can lead to osteomalacia, resulting in weak bones, bone pain, and muscle weakness (65, 81). Chronic vitamin D deficiency can also lead to secondary hyperparathyroidism. This combination of hyperparathyroidism and vitamin D deficiency can result in excessive mobilization of calcium out of bones to help maintain blood calcium. Over time, however, this can decrease BMD (82). Vitamin D deficiency is also associated with chronic low-back pain, which

> ### PUTTING IT INTO PERSPECTIVE
> #### WILL THE RDA HELP US MEET OUR VITAMIN D NEEDS?
>
> The RDA for vitamin D was established primarily based on bone health (65) and obtaining adequate serum blood levels of 25-hydroxyvitamin D for skeletal health (>20 ng/ml). But several questions have been raised about both the RDA and the range set for sufficient vitamin D status in blood. Bone researchers suggest that the lowest acceptable cutoff level for optimal skeletal health should be 30 ng/ml (74), based on evidence from a large randomized controlled study showing 33 percent lower rates of osteoporotic fractures when serum vitamin D was increased from 21 to 29 ng/ml (75), as well as research in older adults suggesting that risk of fractures is lower in those with vitamin D levels above 30 ng/ml and above 40 ng/ml for certain fractures (76, 77). In addition, if dietary intake is the sole source of vitamin D (e.g., when a person avoids the sun), the RDA is not enough to keep serum vitamin D level at 10 ng/ml—an amount far below adequacy (74).
>
> Some scientists question whether the RDA for vitamin D is adequate for the general population. High rates of vitamin D deficiency and insufficiency in a wide range of climates—from sunny California to colder areas—support the case for increasing the RDA. In most cases, the RDA is set to meet the needs of 97.5 percent of healthy people, which means that if the RDA were adequate, 2.5 percent, or less, of the healthy population would be vitamin D deficient—yet rates are much higher than that. Two separate groups of scientists reviewed the studies and estimates used to determine the RDA. They found that an estimated daily intake of 7,000 to 8,895 IU of vitamin D from all sources, including 3,875 IU vitamin D per day from food, might be necessary to achieve adequate blood levels of vitamin D in 97.5 percent of the population (78).

improves after vitamin D supplementation (83-85). Maintaining vitamin D levels at or above 20 ng/mL is associated with a decreased risk of fractures, cardiovascular disease, colorectal cancer, diabetes, depressed mood, cognitive decline, and death, though the association with fractures and cardiovascular disease has not been seen in Black people (86).

Note that in consistency with the Endocrine Society's guidelines, before vitamin D treatment, current vitamin D status should be measured through a blood test.

Identifying and Treating Vitamin D Deficiency

When determining if people should get their vitamin D levels tested, the following factors should be considered:

- Risk factors for and symptoms of vitamin D deficiency
- Health history, including injuries, particularly stress fractures and bone and joint injuries
- Muscle pain or weakness
- Frequent illness
- Use of medications or herbal supplements that interfere with vitamin D metabolism, such as anticonvulsants, kava kava, and St. John's wort (87, 88)

Anyone with excess body fat or darker skin and those taking medications affecting vitamin D metabolism might need to consume more vitamin D to raise their blood levels (51). High-dose prescriptions of vitamin D are sometimes used to raise blood levels quickly. These prescription doses, however, should be taken only under medical supervision.

One study found that prescription weekly doses of 35,000 IU or 70,000 IU of vitamin D led to a drop in the active form of vitamin D in the body (1,25[OH]2D3) even though it raised blood levels of vitamin D (the nonactive form of vitamin D that is tested for it because it has a longer half-life). These study data imply that high supplemental doses of vitamin D_3 lead to a negative feedback loop that decreases the active form of vitamin D in the body. It is not clear that this condition negatively affects bone (89). Because of seasonal changes in vitamin D status, some experts recommend that those with vitamin D deficiency be tested at least twice a year—in the winter and summer. (51). Treatment guidelines are listed in table 6.3.

Table 6.3 Prevention and Treatment of Vitamin D Deficiency (74)

Age group (yr) or health condition	Treatment for deficiency (<20 ng/ml)	Maintenance plan after achieving 30 ng/ml
1-18	• 2,000 IU vitamin D_2 or D_3 for at least 6 weeks or • 50,000 IU vitamin D_2 once per week for at least 6 weeks	600-1,000 IU/day
18	• 50,000 IU vitamin D_2 or vitamin D_3 once a week for 8 weeks or • 6,000 IU of vitamin D_2 or vitamin D_3 daily	1,500-2,000 IU/day
Obese, malabsorption syndromes, those on medications that affect vitamin D metabolism	At least 6,000-10,000 IU/day of vitamin D	3,000-6,000 IU/day
Hyperparathyroidism	Treatment as needed; monitor blood calcium levels	Treatment as needed; monitor blood calcium levels

Data from Heaney (2011).

Although treatment guidelines exist for vitamin D supplementation to correct deficiency or insufficiency, changes in blood vitamin D levels in response to supplementation vary among individuals based on body size, baseline vitamin D status, and genetics (90, 91). There is no consensus on vitamin D supplementation guidelines in athletes (92). Also, to date, there is no evidence of **ergogenic** effects when athletes with sufficient vitamin D supplement with vitamin D.

Excess Intake and Vitamin D Toxicity

As a fat-soluble vitamin, vitamin D can accumulate in tissues and become toxic when levels are very high. Toxicity can occur over time with supplemental or prescription doses. The human body cannot produce toxic levels of vitamin D from exposure to UV light (either through sunlight or tanning beds), and consumption of toxic levels through food is highly unlikely (93, 94). Patients with chronic granuloma-forming disorders, including sarcoidosis and tuberculosis; chronic fungal infections; or lymphoma might overproduce vitamin D, which can lead to high blood calcium or high levels of calcium in the urine. These patients should have their vitamin D and calcium levels monitored regularly (51). Data from animal studies suggest that vitamin D_2 may be less toxic in high doses as compared with vitamin D_3 (65).

Vitamin D toxicity has a wide range of effects, including anorexia, weight loss, large volume of dilute urine, heart arrhythmias, and high blood calcium levels that can result in calcification of tissues leading to damage to the heart, blood vessels, and kidneys (65). The upper intake level (UL) for vitamin D is 4,000 IU per day for adults (65). Both low and high serum levels of vitamin D (in the form of calcidiol) are related to higher risk of certain diseases (28, 95, 96). Table 6.4 lists signs of vitamin D toxicity and includes information on many vitamins throughout the chapter.

Vitamin D and Exercise

Vitamin D influences muscle functioning by regulating calcium transport and uptake of inorganic phosphate, which is used to produce ATP (97-99). In particular, vitamin D affects type II fast-twitch fibers—the kind used for short, rapid-fire bursts of activity such as jumping and sprinting. Vitamin D deficiency leads to weak type II fibers, impaired muscle contraction and relaxation, decreased strength, and a potential decline in athletic performance (99, 100). Vitamin D deficiency and insufficiency are also associated with an increased risk of bone injuries, including fractures; impaired immune system functioning; and increased incidence of upper-respiratory infections (99, 100).

Higher serum vitamin D status, compared with deficiency, is associated with greater muscle strength, power, and force; jumping performance;

Table 6.4 Vitamin Sources and Symptoms of Excess and Deficiency

Vitamin	Excellent sources (>20% DV) based on standard serving size	Good sources (>10% DV) based on standard serving size
Vitamin A (as preformed vitamin A, beta-carotene, alpha-carotene, beta-cryptoxanthin, or a combination of these compounds)	Beef liver, goose liver, turkey liver, sweet potato, pumpkin, cantaloupe, sweet red bell peppers, mangoes, broccoli, apricots.	Herring, tomato juice, ricotta cheese.
Biotin	Data on the amount of biotin in food are not available, although it is found in a wide range of foods, including turkey breast, beef, whey protein, soybeans, and chickpeas.	
Folic acid or folate	Beef liver, spinach, black-eyed peas, cooked rice, asparagus, enriched spaghetti.	Cooked broccoli, raw spinach, avocado, white bread, kidney beans, green peas, boiled mustard greens.
Niacin	Turkey (all parts or breast alone), peanuts, tuna fish, pork loin, brown or white rice, anchovies, beef, chicken, mackerel, salmon, potatoes.	Greek yogurt, gluten-free pasta made with corn and rice flour, flaxseeds, chestnuts, blue cheese.
Pantothenic acid	Turkey breast, sunflower seeds, shiitake mushrooms, beef liver, lamb liver, avocado, sockeye salmon, brown or white rice, canned mushroom gravy.	Sweet potato, orange juice, egg, blackberries, peanuts, burrito with beans, cream of potato soup, wild Atlantic salmon.
Vitamin B_1 (thiamin)	Enriched breakfast cereals, long-grain white rice, egg noodles, pork chops, trout, black beans, mussels.	Whole-wheat macaroni, acorn squash, bluefin tuna.
Vitamin B_2 (riboflavin)	Some fortified breakfast cereals, instant oats, yogurt, milk, beef, clams.	Almonds, Swiss cheese, egg, chicken, salmon, plain bagels, portabella mushrooms.
Vitamin B_6 (pyridoxine)	Chickpeas, beef liver, tuna, sockeye salmon, potatoes, banana, marinara sauce.	Winter squash, cottage cheese, bulgur, ready-to-eat waffles, ground beef.
Vitamin B_{12}	Clams, trout, sockeye salmon, beef liver, haddock, some fortified breakfast cereals, sirloin.	Milk, Swiss cheese, beef taco, ham, egg.
Vitamin C	Sweet red or green pepper, orange juice, orange, grapefruit juice, kiwifruit, broccoli, Brussels sprouts, grapefruit, tomato juice, cantaloupe, cabbage, cauliflower, potato, tomato.	Spinach, frozen green peas, pumpkin, prune juice, teriyaki rice bowl with chicken, peaches, hash brown potatoes, summer squash, yellow corn, edamame, okra, butternut squash.
Vitamin D (D_3 or cholecalciferol)	Cod liver oil, swordfish, sockeye salmon, tuna fish, orange juice fortified with vitamin D (check label), yogurt fortified with 20% DV vitamin D, milk.	Egg (in the yolk), sardines.
Vitamin E	Wheat-germ oil, sunflower seeds, almonds, sunflower oil, safflower oil, hazelnuts.	Peanuts, corn oil, spinach, peanut butter.
Vitamin K	Natto, collards, turnip greens, spinach, kale, broccoli, soybeans, soybean oil, edamame, pumpkin, pomegranate juice.	Pine nuts, blueberries, iceberg lettuce, grapes, chicken breast, canola oil, cashews, carrots, olive oil, vegetable juice cocktail.

Based on Allen et al. (2006); U.S. Institute of Medicine (1998); U.S. Institute of Medicine (2001); U.S. Institute of Medicine (2011).

Common forms in food and dietary supplements	Deficiency signs and symptoms	Excess intake and toxicity signs and symptoms
Beta-carotene.	Deficiency is rare in developed countries but prevalent in undeveloped countries. Signs and symptoms include xerophthalmia (abnormal dryness and inflammation in the eyes) and night blindness.	• Increased intracranial pressure, dizziness, nausea, headaches, skin irritation, joint and bone pain, coma, and death. • Above 33,000–50,000 IU beta-carotene may increase risk of lung cancer in smokers.
Biotin.	Rare unless a person is frequently eating raw egg whites.	Excess is excreted.
Found in supplements as folic acid; in food, it is found as folate.	Although deficiency is rare, women of childbearing age have an increased need for folate or folic acid. Folic acid can reduce the risk of birth defects of the brain and spine in newborn babies.	Excess folic acid can mask a vitamin B_{12} deficiency and might interfere with certain medications.
Niacin	Rare; niacin is found in protein-rich foods.	Flushed skin, rashes, and liver damage.
Pantothenic acid.	Deficiency is rare in developed countries. Signs and symptoms include numbness and burning of the hands and feet, headache, extreme tiredness, irritability, restlessness, sleeping problems, stomach pain, heartburn, diarrhea, nausea, vomiting, and loss of appetite.	Excess is excreted through diarrhea, and water retention may result.
Thiamin.	Rare.	Excess is excreted.
Riboflavin.	Rare except in those who are severely malnourished.	Excess is excreted.
Pyridoxine.	Rare.	Large doses over time can cause nerve damage.
Cobalamin.	Vegetarians, vegans, and the elderly are at risk.	Low toxicity, no UL established.
Ascorbic acid.	Rare.	Excess is excreted, though very large amounts (over 1,000 mg/day) may cause diarrhea and upset stomach.
D_3 or cholecalciferol.	Low intake levels are more common in people who are not exposed to sunlight, as well as the elderly.	Excess is stored in the body and can be toxic. Quantities above 10,000 IU/day can cause hypercalcemia, hypercalciuria, kidney stones, and soft tissue calcifications.
Natural vitamin E (d-alpha tocopherol) is more active than the synthetic form of vitamin E (dl-alpha tocopherol); approximately 50% more of the synthetic form is needed to compare with the natural form.	Very rare unless fat malabsorption is present.	• Few side effects have been noted, even in doses as high as 3,200 mg. • In vitro data suggest that high doses inhibit platelet aggregation. The tolerable upper limit (UL) was set because of the potential for hemorrhagic effects.
Phylloquinone, phytonadione, menadione.	Rare.	Few side effects noted.

$\dot{V}O_2$max; and speed (101, 102). Additionally, higher serum vitamin D is associated with greater strength recovery after intense exercise (103). And supplementation with vitamin D in those with "sufficient" baseline vitamin D status (30.5 ng/ml) led to faster recovery of muscle force compared with a placebo (104). Increasing vitamin D levels may have the greatest effect on muscle strength in those with severe deficiency (<12 ng/ml) and the elderly (105, 106). Higher vitamin D levels are also correlated with greater $\dot{V}O_2$max, and the strongest correlation is found in those with low levels of physical activity (107).

Professional male athletes deficient in vitamin D improved 10-meter sprint time and vertical jump (both recruit mainly type II fibers) after taking 5,000 IU vitamin D_3 per day for 8 weeks (raising mean levels from 11.6 ng/ml to 41 ± 10 ng/ml) compared with no change in athletes with deficient or insufficient levels who were given a placebo (55, 108, 109). In one study with almost 70 percent of the athletes deficient (<20 ng/ml) at the start of the trial, 5,000 IU vitamin D taken daily for more than 8 weeks led to a statistically significant improvement in vertical jump height compared with taking a placebo (55). Adult male judoka athletes who took a bolus dose of vitamin D to improve their levels from 13 to 17 ng/ml improved muscle strength by 13 percent in 8 days (110). In contrast, a meta-analysis of five randomized controlled trials found no difference in strength after vitamin D supplementation. The trials in which athletes started below 20 ng/ml, however, did observe strength gains. This outcome suggests that improvements in athlete strength following vitamin D supplementation may occur only in athletes who start with vitamin D deficiency (111).

Vitamin D and Illness

Vitamin D deficiency is associated with increased risk of illness, whereas maintaining sufficient levels of vitamin D may reduce risk of infectious illness (64). In one study, 27 percent of athletes with vitamin D levels above 48 ng/ml experienced one or more upper-respiratory tract infections over a 4-month period, compared with 67 percent of those with levels below 12 ng/ml. Athletes with vitamin D below 12 ng/ml also experienced more total symptomatic days compared with athletes with vitamin D levels above 12 ng/ml (58). These results are in line with studies in nonathletes; adults with vitamin D levels below 10 ng/ml had a significantly higher risk of respiratory infections when compared with adults with vitamin D levels greater than 30 ng/ml (109). A study in British adults found respiratory infections peak in the winter and decrease as the weather gets warmer, and also found a 7 percent decrease in risk of respiratory infections with each 4 ng/ml increase in blood vitamin D up to the average study participant high of 28.8 ng/ml in September (116). Another study found that blood serum concentrations of vitamin D equal to or greater than 38 ng/ml were associated with a significant reduction in risk of acute respiratory tract infections and percentage of days ill (108).

PUTTING IT INTO PERSPECTIVE

CAN YOU MEET YOUR VITAMIN NEEDS THROUGH FOOD?

Whether dining in the cafeteria or cooking in your own apartment, it is possible, though not always easy, to meet the RDA for all nutrients through a nutrient-dense diet (but note that some scientists question whether the RDA for vitamin D is adequate, as discussed earlier in the chapter). Research shows, however, that many Americans are falling short on several vitamins, including vitamins A, C, D, E, and folate (folic acid) (73, 112). Research in athletes shows that those who restrict their calorie intake, follow diets that cut out food groups or energy-yielding macronutrients (ketogenic diets, for example, are very high-fat, moderate-protein diets containing less than 5% carbohydrate), eat a nutritionally poor diet, or follow a vegetarian or vegan diet are more likely to fall short on several vitamins (113-115). What does this mean for you? If you are following a restrictive diet or cutting calories, chances are you are falling short on several nutrients, including vitamin D. Check out table 6.4 for excellent and good sources of each vitamin.

Vitamin D and Injuries

An association is evident between vitamin D insufficiency and deficiency and injuries, including stress fractures, as well as chronic musculoskeletal pain. In one study of Marine recruits, those deficient in vitamin D (<20 ng/ml) had a 60 percent higher incidence of stress fractures than recruits with higher levels of vitamin D (117). Likewise, a study in NFL players found lower vitamin D in those who suffered at least one bone fracture (57). Also, a study in over 800 NCAA Division I athletes found that the rate of stress fracture was 12 percent higher for athletes with vitamin D levels less than 40 ng/ml compared with those who maintained or improved their vitamin D levels through supplementation to 40 ng/ml or greater (118). Although maintaining higher levels of vitamin D to decrease risk of stress fractures seems sensible, there is no scientific consensus on the role of vitamin D in fracture healing (63).

A study examining NFL players found that those with at least one muscle injury (muscle strain, tear, or pull) resulting in at least one missed practice or game during the season had significantly lower vitamin D levels compared with players with no reported muscle injuries during the same period (19.9 ng/ml and 24.7ng/ml, respectively) (61). Another NFL study found that 59 percent of players had inadequate vitamin D levels, and players with a history of lower-extremity muscle strain or core muscle injury were more likely to have inadequate vitamin D levels compared with uninjured athletes (119). Moreover, athletes with inadequate vitamin D levels had 1.86 higher odds for lower-extremity strain or core muscle injury and 3.61 higher odds of hamstring injury. In another study, conducted with players from the Pittsburgh Steelers, significantly lower vitamin D levels were found in players with at least one bone fracture compared with those with no bone fractures (after correcting for total number of NFL seasons played because years played influences risk). Also, significantly lower vitamin D levels were observed in players released during the preseason (because of injury or poor performance) when compared with levels in those who played the entire regular season. Athletes with serum vitamin D above 41 ng/ml played more seasons than those with serum vitamin D levels below 21 ng/ml (57). In addition to the association between vitamin D and risk of injury, vitamin D might also improve surgical recovery. Patients with levels below 30 ng/ml (75 nmol/L) had delayed strength recovery after anterior cruciate ligament surgery (120).

> **? DO YOU KNOW?**
>
> At this time experts have not come to a consensus on the optimal vitamin D status (25(OH)D levels) for athletes for bone health or reducing fracture risk (121). The IOM states that levels greater than or equal to 20 ng/ml are sufficient for most of the population, but some studies suggest that levels of 30 ng/ml or more are sufficient for bone health. Other studies suggest that levels of 40 ng/ml are required for both bone and muscle health.

Vitamin E

Vitamin E is incorporated in the body's cellular and subcellular membranes, where it helps to prevent oxidative damage to the fats in cell membranes. This oxidative damage can disrupt cell membrane structure and function as well as function of the cell overall (122-124). Vitamin E is also

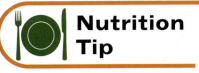

Nutrition Tip Some companies list total antioxidant capacity (TAC) scores of a food, beverage, or supplement on the label based on antioxidant testing methods such as ORAC (oxygen radical absorbance capacity). TAC scores provide a measure of the capacity of a food to scavenge free radicals. Although these scores are useful for research purposes, they do not tell us anything about human health because TAC scores do not take into account how the body absorbs and uses antioxidants. So these scores should not be used as a way to compare foods, beverages, or supplements or to suggest that one food is healthier than another (125).

involved in immune functioning, cell signaling, metabolic processes, blood vessel dilation, and inhibiting platelets from clumping together (122).

Sources of Vitamin E

The eight naturally occurring forms of vitamin E are alpha-, beta-, gamma-, and delta-tocopherol and alpha-, beta-, gamma-, and delta-tocotrienol.

Although gamma-tocopherol is the most prevalent form found in the diet, only alpha-tocopherol is maintained in human blood in significant amounts. It is therefore the form considered most biologically important and the one used to estimate vitamin E requirements. See figure 6.6 for excellent sources of vitamin E.

Vitamin E Deficiency and Toxicity

Vitamin E deficiency is rare, seen only in people with fat malabsorption disorders and those with rare inherited disorders that prevent maintenance of normal blood concentrations of vitamin E. Symptoms of deficiency may include peripheral neuropathy, loss of control of body movements (ataxia), skeletal muscle weakness, and retina damage. Vitamin E deficiency can also lead to hemolytic anemia, the type of anemia characterized by ruptured red blood cells.

> **? DO YOU KNOW?**
>
> National survey data suggest that Americans do not consume adequate amounts of vitamin E through food, although total vitamin E intake might have been underestimated if oil used during cooking was not accounted for in surveys assessing dietary intake (126).

No health effects have been observed from vitamin E intake through dietary sources. Lab studies suggest, however, that large supplemental doses of vitamin E can inhibit platelet clumping and thereby increase risk of bleeding. Such supplementation may be particularly dangerous when large doses of vitamin E are taken with anticoagulants, especially in conjunction with low vitamin K intake. Additionally, the Selenium and Vitamin E Cancer Prevention Trial found that men who supplemented with 400 IU vitamin E each day for an average of 5.5 years had a 17 percent increased risk of prostate cancer (127). The tolerable upper limit for vitamin E in adults 19 years of age and older is 1,000 mg (1,500 IU).

Vitamin E and Exercise

Free radicals, produced in muscle, have important roles in supporting normal skeletal muscle adaptations to exercise. These functions include cell signaling, production of muscle force, muscle growth, and recovery. A healthy balance is important, because excess free radicals can damage plasma membranes, impairing muscle contraction and contributing to muscle fatigue and delayed-onset muscle soreness (128, 129). The stress of exercise, particularly exercise with high oxygen demand (high oxygen demand means that more free radicals are produced) or muscle-damaging exercise, damages cell membranes—the barrier that protects cells. Vitamin E protects cells from the damaging effects of free radicals and is essential for cell membrane repair, so it might support training adaptations and recovery (128). Vitamin E–deprived muscle cell membranes do not heal properly.

Although vitamin E is critical for muscle cell health, studies examining the role of vitamin E in athletics have yet to find that supplemental vitamin E above the amount provided in the average diet improves athletic performance or decreases

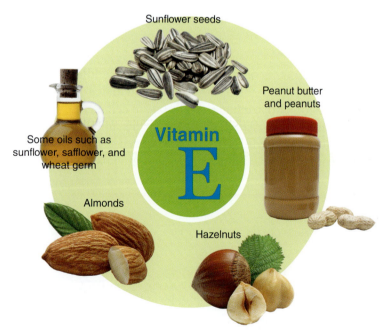

Figure 6.6 Excellent sources of Vitamin E, containing more than 20% DV per serving (6).

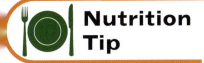

Nutrition Tip: Several factors affect the body's ability to absorb plant compounds, including antioxidants from food, form of the food (liquid or solid), foods consumed at the same time, composition of gut bacteria, overall health, and age. Chewing foods into smaller pieces before swallowing can increase antioxidant absorption, and the presence of fat in the gut can enhance absorption of fat-soluble antioxidants such as carotenoids and vitamin E.

muscle damage (130-133). In fact, in high doses, vitamin E may interfere with training adaptations as noted later in this chapter.

Vitamin K

Vitamin K is a fat-soluble vitamin composed of vitamin K_1 and several forms of vitamin K_2. In the body, vitamin K is a coenzyme involved in the synthesis of proteins necessary for blood clotting and bone metabolism. Additionally, scientists are working to determine how vitamin K_2, as part of a vitamin K–dependent protein, might reduce calcification in arteries (arterial calcification contributes to arterial plaque and blockage within arteries, which increases risk of chronic kidney disease and cardiovascular disease) (138, 139). Vitamin K is also found in the brain, liver, heart, and pancreas (2).

Vitamin E interferes with clotting activity of vitamin K, although interindividual differences seem to occur in response to vitamin E intake that influences its effect on clotting as well as bleeding (140).

Sources of Vitamin K

There are two types of vitamin K:

> Vitamin K_1 (phylloquinone, phytomenadione, or phytonadione) is made in plants and can be converted to vitamin K_2 by bacteria in the human body. Vitamin K_1 is found in high concentrations in green leafy vegetables, soybeans, soybean oil, and canola oil. Vitamin K_1 is less bioavailable from greens than from oil or supplements. Consuming dietary fat at the same time as vegetables improves vitamin K_1 absorption from vegetables.

> Vitamin K_2 comes in several forms (menaquinones) and is found in animal livers, some Chinese dishes, and some fermented foods, such as natto. In addition, most menaquinones are produced by bacteria in the human gut (2, 6). See figure 6.7 for good and excellent sources of vitamins K_1 and K_2.

Vitamin K Deficiency and Toxicity

Vitamin K status, as measured by the time it takes for blood to clot (prothrombin time), is not typically tested unless a person is taking anticoagulants (medicines that help prevent blood clots, which antagonize the action of vitamin K; warfarin is an example) or has a bleeding disorder. Vitamin K deficiency can cause bleeding

---

PUTTING IT INTO PERSPECTIVE

IMPROVING JOINT PAIN

If you exercise regularly or participate in sport, you might experience joint pain. In particular, some athletes feel pain or stiffness in their knees, especially if they sit for a long time with knees bent (in a lengthy class lecture, movie theater, or on an airplane, for instance) because of worn-down cartilage. Some athletes may have osteoarthritis, a degenerative joint disease characterized by pain, stiffness, and swelling in joints. Osteoarthritis is a disease that primarily affects cartilage, the tissues that provide cushioning between joints, allowing them to move over one another smoothly. Studies suggest that higher dietary intake of vitamin C, beta-carotene, and vitamin E can support joint health by attenuating the development of osteoarthritis (134-137).

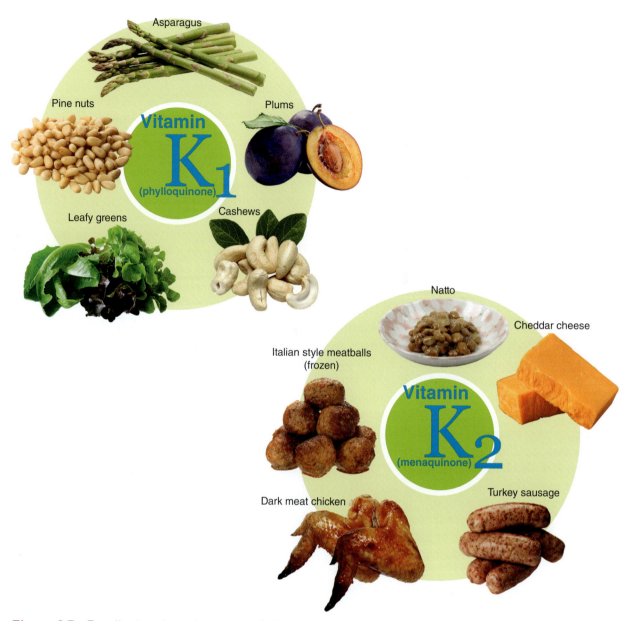

Figure 6.7 Excellent and good sources of vitamin K₁ and vitamin K₂. Note that chicken and meat products contain vitamin K₂ only if the animals' feed contained a synthetic form of vitamin K. (The animals produce vitamin K₂ from the vitamin K in their feed.)

and hemorrhage and might also decrease bone mineralization, thus possibly contributing to osteoporosis. Infants not treated with vitamin K at birth and those with malabsorption syndromes and GI diseases (including celiac disease, cystic fibrosis, and ulcerative colitis) are at risk for vitamin K deficiency. (Vitamin K interacts with certain medications, notably anticoagulants, a type of blood thinner.) Such people require close monitoring and consistent intake of vitamin K–containing foods and supplements (as directed by a physician). Note, too, that changes in vitamin K intake can increase or decrease the effectiveness of some anticoagulants (2). No evidence suggests that vitamin K interferes with a different category of blood thinners that prevent platelets from sticking together to form clots; aspirin and clopidogrel are examples. To be on the safe side, patients on blood thinners, regardless of which type, should always check with a medical professional about vitamin K from dietary supplements and food.

DO YOU KNOW?

No known association exists between vitamin K and athletic performance or recovery.

WATER-SOLUBLE VITAMINS

Unlike fat-soluble vitamins, most water-soluble vitamins are not stored in the body, and any excess is excreted in the urine. Therefore, these vitamins must be consumed regularly.

B Vitamins

B vitamins work together and are catalysts necessary for the metabolism of carbohydrate, fat, and protein, as well as for energy production (52). As such, B vitamins are critical for health and human performance. Each B vitamin also has other functions in the body. Few studies have examined consistently low intake of B vitamins and the effect on athletic performance, although one study found that dietary restriction of thiamin,

PUTTING IT INTO PERSPECTIVE

CAN I USE THE NUTRITION FACTS PANEL TO MAKE SURE I AM MEETING MY VITAMIN NEEDS?

The Nutrition Facts label (figure 6.8) can be used to compare foods that include nutrients that many Americans are not getting in adequate amounts, including vitamin D, calcium, potassium, and iron. Getting enough of these nutrients helps to reduce the risk of some diseases or disease risk factors, while improving health. The FDA requires that food labels list the total content of these micronutrients on the Nutrition Facts label. The daily value (DV) was developed to help consumers see the nutrient levels in a standard serving size of food compared with their approximate requirement for that nutrient. The %DV is based on a 2,000 kcal diet and thus provides a reference you can use to compare foods, even if you consume more or less calories each day (141). A food is "high," "rich in," or an "excellent source of" a nutrient if it contains 20 percent or more of the DV for a standard serving size. It is considered a "good source," "contains," or "provides" if it contains 10 to 19 percent of the DV for a standard serving size (142). In addition to specifying the amounts of these four micronutrients—vitamin D, calcium, potassium, and iron—some companies voluntarily list the amount of other vitamins and minerals.

Nutrition Facts

8 servings per container
Serving size 2/3 cup (55g)

Amount per 2/3 cup
Calories 230

	% Daily Value*
Total Fat 8g	10%
Saturated Fat 1g	5%
Trans Fat 0g	
Cholesterol 0mg	0%
Sodium 160mg	7%
Total Carbohydrate 37g	13%
Dietary Fiber 4g	14%
Total Sugars 12g	
Added Sugars 10g	20%
Protein 3g	
Vitamin D 2mcg	10%
Calcium 260mg	20%
Iron 8mg	45%
Potassium 235mg	6%

*The % Daily Value (DV) tells you how much a nutrient in a serving of food contributes to a daily diet. 2,000 calories a day is used for general nutrition advice.

Figure 6.8 Companies must list the DV for vitamin D, calcium, potassium, and iron on the Nutrition Facts label.

riboflavin, and vitamin B_6 resulted in decreased peak aerobic capacity and peak power in trained male cyclists (143). No evidence suggests that a greater intake of B vitamins, beyond what the body needs, improves athletic performance.

According to national survey data, few people consume below the estimated average requirements (EAR) for thiamin, riboflavin, niacin, or vitamin B_6. There are no nationally representative estimates of pantothenic acid intake, but this vitamin is widely distributed in food. Low calorie intake may increase an athlete's risk for low thiamin, riboflavin, and vitamin B_6 (144, 145). Despite low intake, B vitamin deficiencies are uncommon, although certain groups have a higher risk of developing a vitamin B_{12} deficiency. For instance, adults over the age of 50 might benefit from supplemental vitamin B_{12} or higher amounts of vitamin B_{12} from fortified foods because of a potential decrease in absorption of vitamin B_{12} (52).

Biotin

Biotin is found in a wide range of foods, including turkey breast, beef, whey protein, soybeans, and chickpeas (6). Biotin deficiency can occur during pregnancy or with long-term tube feeding, rapid weight loss, or consumption of raw egg whites over a long period. Raw egg whites contain a protein called avidin, which binds biotin so it cannot be absorbed in the body (146). Biotin deficiency can lead to dermatitis (red, scaly skin rash), conjunctivitis, hair loss, central nervous system abnormalities, and seizures. In infants, biotin deficiency can lead to lethargy, developmental delay, withdrawn behavior, and hypotonia (floppy baby syndrome). Biotin toxicity has not been observed in humans (52). Research to assess the effect of biotin supplementation on athletic performance has been insufficient.

> **? DO YOU KNOW?**
>
> Many skin, hair, and nail supplements contain biotin because a biotin deficiency can cause skin rashes and hair loss (52).

Choline

Americans get most of their choline in the diet from milk, meat, poultry, fish, eggs and egg-based dishes, bread, and grain-based dishes such as pasta (147). Eggs, turkey, beef, soybeans, chickpeas, and lima beans are excellent sources of choline (6).

Choline is a methyl donor necessary for lipid metabolism and transport, cell functioning, brain development and functioning, and creatine formation. Choline is the precursor for the neurotransmitter acetylcholine, phospholipids, and betaine (52, 148). National survey data suggest that many people are falling short of their choline needs; mean choline intakes for children and for all age ranges of men and women are below the AI (147).

Choline deficiency leads to fat infiltration in the liver and to liver and muscle damage (149). High supplemental doses of choline (10 g/day) might slightly reduce blood pressure. High dietary intake of choline, especially choline magnesium trisalicylate, is associated with potential side effects that include ringing in the ears and mild liver toxicity.

Although humans placed on a choline-deficient diet for 3 weeks experienced a decline in muscle functioning (150), there is no evidence of choline deficiency caused by exercise, and choline supplementation does not benefit either brief, high-intensity anaerobic exercise or prolonged aerobic exercise (151).

Dietary Folate and Folic Acid

Dietary folate is found naturally in food. Excellent dietary sources of folate include beef liver, dark green leafy vegetables, beans and peas, rice, fortified cereals, and wheat germ (6). Folic acid is the term used for the synthetic form of folate found in dietary supplements and fortified foods. For our purposes, both folate and folic acid will be called "folate" unless otherwise specified. Folate is necessary for normal metabolism and healthy red blood cells (52).

Folate status can be assessed by measuring red blood cell (erythrocyte) folate levels. Deficiency can lead to megaloblastic or macrocytic anemia, a type of **anemia** characterized by large, immature (not completely developed) red blood cells (figure 6.9). Anemia is a condition in which blood fails to carry enough oxygen throughout the body. Signs and symptoms of megaloblastic anemia include fatigue, shortness of breath, weakness, pale skin, and sore mouth and tongue. Babies born to pregnant women deficient in folate have an increased risk of neural tube or spinal defects. In addition to consistently low intake of dietary folate or folic acid, malabsorptive diseases, chronic heavy alcohol intake, smoking, and genetic variations in folate metabolism can contribute to the risk of folate deficiency. Many women and adolescent females capable of becoming pregnant do not meet their folate needs (152). Several medicines may interfere with folate metabolism, including long-term therapeutic doses of nonsteroidal anti-inflammatory drugs (NSAIDs), such as ibuprofen (52). The Institute of Medicine encourages every woman who could become pregnant to get 400 mcg of folic acid every day from fortified foods, supplements, or a combination of both to decrease the risk of birth defects.

No adverse effects are associated with folate consumption through food. Excess folic acid intake can mask a vitamin B_{12} deficiency, thereby correcting megaloblastic anemia without addressing the side effects caused by a B_{12} deficiency.

Although folate status in athletes appears to mirror that of the general population, with women more likely to be deficient than men (52, 153-156), folic acid supplementation in athletes deficient in folate, yet not anemic, does not improve athletic performance (155).

Niacin

Niacin is important for metabolism, digestive system function, and skin and nerve function. Niacin is found in a wide variety of foods, including beef, milk, eggs, legumes (including peanuts), poultry, fish, and rice (6). Niacin deficiency leads to the disease pellagra. Symptoms of pellagra include inflamed skin, mental impairment, and digestive issues. Niacin toxicity is associated with nausea, vomiting, and liver toxicity (52).

> **❓ DO YOU KNOW?**
>
> Consuming high amounts of niacin can lead to flushing or a warm, itchy, or tingly feeling of the face, neck, arms, and upper body, as well as to GI effects and vision changes.

No evidence suggests that niacin supplementation is necessary for athletic performance. In fact, niacin supplementation might block the release of fatty acids from fat tissue, increasing the body's reliance on carbohydrate, which could potentially lead to faster depletion of muscle glycogen and impaired endurance performance (157-159).

Pantothenic Acid (Vitamin B_5)

Pantothenic acid is an important part of a coenzyme involved in fatty acid metabolism. Deficiency is uncommon under normal circumstances and has been observed only in experimental conditions in those fed a diet void of pantothenic acid. There is no evidence of toxicity from pantothenic acid. Major sources of pantothenic acid include chicken, beef, potatoes, tomato products, whole grains, and egg yolks (52). We have no reason to believe that pantothenic acid, beyond that obtained from dietary intake, is necessary for athletic performance (160).

Riboflavin (Vitamin B_2)

Riboflavin (figure 6.10) is a component of two coenzymes necessary for metabolism, energy production, cellular function, growth, and development.

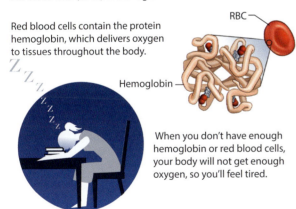

Figure 6.9 Deficiencies in several nutrients can result in anemia.

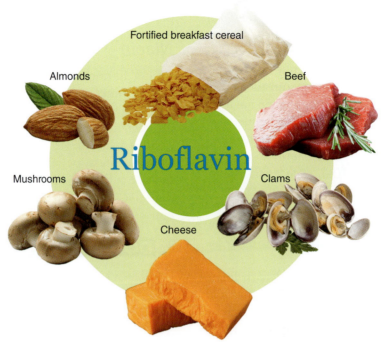

Figure 6.10 Good or excellent sources of riboflavin (6, 52).

Most Americans consume enough riboflavin through their diet, so riboflavin deficiency is rare in the United States (73), although endocrine abnormalities can lead to deficiency. Signs and symptoms of deficiency include skin issues, edema in the mouth and throat, cracks at the corners of the mouth (called angular stomatitis or angular cheilosis), hair loss, sore throat, itchy red eyes, liver and nervous system abnormalities, and reproductive problems (52, 161).

Exercise might increase riboflavin needs, which can be met through increased calorie intake of nutrient-dense foods. Athletes who are dieting may fall short of their riboflavin intake (153, 162-164). Little research has looked at the effect of riboflavin supplementation on performance, although one study found correcting low riboflavin status improved endurance performance in adolescents aged 12 to 14 (165).

Thiamin (Vitamin B$_1$)

Thiamin (figure 6.11) is essential for the activity of enzymes involved in carbohydrate, lipid, and amino acid metabolism. In the United States and many other countries, grain products, including breads and cereals, are fortified with thiamin. Cooking food decreases thiamin content to about 50 to 60 percent of precooked levels. The greatest thiamin losses are from boiling, followed by baking, poaching, and frying. High temperature, high pH, and high chlorine content in water all accelerate thiamin losses (166).

Thiamin Deficiency and Toxicity Most people in the United States consume enough thiamin. Thiamin deficiency, often caused by chronic alcoholism, leads to the neurological disorder Wernicke-Korsakoff syndrome (167). Thiamin deficiency can also lead to beriberi, a disease that is now extremely rare in the United States because of thiamin fortification in grains. Older adults have a higher risk of thiamin deficiency, which may be caused by low dietary intake, chronic diseases, nutrient-drug interactions, or a decrease in thiamin absorption (168, 169). People with HIV or AIDS, diabetes, or with a history of bariatric surgery have a greater risk of developing thiamin deficiency (170-173). Signs of thiamin deficiency include weight changes, mental changes, apathy, impaired short-term memory, confusion, irritability, muscle weakness, and enlarged heart (52).

Thiamin and Exercise Studies in athletes on calorie-restricted diets indicate they might be con-

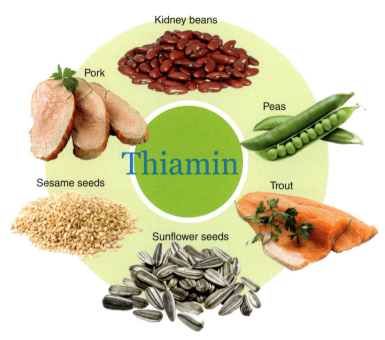

Figure 6.11 Excellent sources of thiamin (6).

suming less than the RDA for thiamin (113-115). Therefore, anyone on a reduced-calorie diet should include foods that are a good or excellent source of thiamin. Several studies show no benefit for muscle strength or endurance performance from thiamin supplementation (160, 164, 174, 175).

Pyridoxine (Vitamin B₆)

Pyridoxine is necessary for metabolism and immune functioning (52). Excellent sources of pyridoxine include chickpeas, tuna, salmon, chicken breasts, and fortified cereals (6). Most people in the United States consume adequate amounts of pyridoxine. Pyridoxine deficiency is rare by itself but instead typically occurs alongside other B vitamin deficiencies. Deficiency leads to microcytic anemia, characterized by small, pale red blood cells; abnormalities in the electrical activity of the brain; dermatitis; cheilosis; swollen tongue (glossitis); depression; confusion; and suppressed immune functioning. Kidney diseases, malabsorption diseases, autoimmune diseases, alcoholism, and some genetic diseases can cause a pyridoxine deficiency. No toxic effects of vitamin B₆ from food sources are known, but chronic high-dose supplemental intake can lead to neuropathy, loss of control of body movements, painful dermatological lesions, sensitivity to sunlight, and GI symptoms (52, 176-178).

Exercise increases pyridoxine losses, so athletes on reduced-calorie diets might fail to meet the RDA for pyridoxine (163, 164, 179-181). It remains unclear if supplemental pyridoxine intake will enhance performance, because few studies have assessed this matter.

Vitamin B₁₂ (Cobalamin)

Vitamin B₁₂ is necessary for the formation of red blood cells, neurological functioning, and DNA synthesis (52). Vitamin B₁₂ is naturally found in many animal foods. Excellent sources include clams, beef, beef liver, salmon, haddock, trout, and tuna fish, as well as fortified breakfast cereals and some types of nutritional yeast (6, 52).

Vegetarians, particularly vegans (those who eat no animal foods) who do not take a multivitamin containing vitamin B₁₂ or a separate vitamin B₁₂ supplement, and who do not regularly consume foods fortified with vitamin B₁₂, have an increased risk of developing marginal vitamin B₁₂ status or deficiency (182), which can lead to megaloblastic anemia. People with pernicious anemia, caused by an autoimmune disease that affects the stomach lining, infections, surgery, medicine, or diet, cannot absorb vitamin B_{12} (52, 183) and require vitamin B_{12} shots. Without shots, they will develop megaloblastic anemia and neurological disorders (52, 184). People with reduced stomach acid or intestinal disorders might have problems absorbing vitamin B_{12} from food, putting them at risk for deficiency (185). Elderly women are more likely than men and younger women to have malabsorption, putting them at greater risk of developing a B_{12} deficiency or marginal B_{12} status (186, 187).

Signs and symptoms of pernicious and megaloblastic anemia include pica (the desire to eat nonfood items such as ice or clay), diarrhea or constipation, nausea, poor appetite, loss of appetite, pale skin, pale nail beds and gums, difficulty concentrating, lightheadedness, dizziness, shortness of breath during exercise, swollen red tongue, and bleeding gums. Chronic vitamin B_{12} deficiency can lead to nerve damage and related symptoms, including tingling and numbness in the hands and feet, difficulty walking, irritability, memory loss, dementia, depression, and mental illness (188). No evidence suggests vitamin B_{12} supplementation, beyond correction for deficiency, improves athletic performance (189). But data on vitamin B_{12} and athletic performance are limited.

? DO YOU KNOW?

Vitamin B_{12} is the only water-soluble vitamin stored in the body. Rather than being excreted in the urine, it can be stored in the liver for several years.

Vitamin C (Ascorbic Acid)

Vitamin C is an antioxidant that

- protects cells in the body from free radical damage,
- helps regenerate other antioxidants, including vitamin E (190),
- affects immune system functioning,
- helps produce collagen,

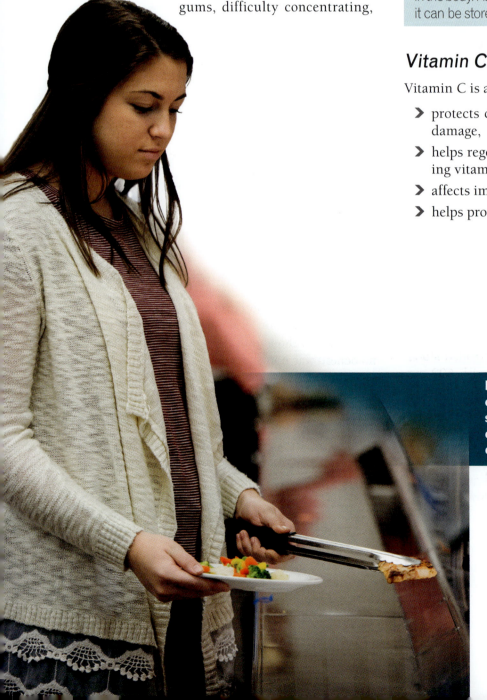

Look for nutrient-packed options including a variety of steamed vegetables, grilled chicken, and potatoes in college dining halls.

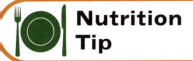

Nutrition Tip: Water, light, and heat decrease the vitamin C content in foods. Instead of boiling vegetables (and throwing out a good amount of vitamin C in the water they are boiled in), consider microwaving or steaming vegetables or eating them raw. Try cutting fruits and vegetables soon before you eat them instead of buying precut produce or leaving cut produce out of the refrigerator for long periods before eating. The more surface area (smaller pieces of produce) exposed to heat and light, the greater the amount of vitamin C lost. If you are in a dorm room, consider vegetables you can microwave or eat raw.

- helps repair and maintain cartilage and bone (122),
- keeps capillary and blood vessel walls firm, which helps prevent bruising,
- keeps skin and gum tissue healthy, and
- helps the body absorb plant sources of iron (non-heme iron; this form is not absorbed by the body as well as heme iron, the kind found in animal foods).

Excellent sources of vitamin C include oranges, grapefruit, tomatoes, bell peppers, peaches, kiwi, strawberries, and broccoli (6).

Does Vitamin C Prevent Illness?

Although vitamin C is necessary for immune system functioning (122), several studies show that vitamin C supplementation may not benefit such functioning (191-193). In athletes, however, the research is mixed and the effectiveness of supplementation might depend on regular dietary intake of vitamin C, supplemental vitamin C dose and duration, and the level of exercise stress. A double-blind, placebo-controlled study found that daily supplementation with 600 mg of vitamin C for 21 days before a 90-kilometer (56 mi) race reduced self-reported symptoms of upper-respiratory tract infections during the 2-week period after the race, compared with placebo. Nonrunning controls also benefited from vitamin C supplementation (194). Another randomized, double-blind, placebo-controlled study showed no differences in immune markers between runners who took 1,500 mg of vitamin C daily for 7 days before an 80-kilometer (50 mi) race, compared with those who took a placebo (193). Additionally, a randomized, double-blind study found that 500 mg of vitamin C consumed three times a day for several days before a 120-minute bout of indoor cycling at a moderate pace in a hot and humid environment did not affect incidence of upper-respiratory tract infections or immune system functioning, as measured by salivary immunoglobulin A (195). A meta-analysis of research studies found that supplemental vitamin C taken daily before getting a cold was beneficial for marathon runners, skiers, soldiers, and people participating in subarctic exercises. An 8 percent reduction in common cold duration was observed for adults with intakes of 200 mg or more daily, and an 18 percent reduction in common cold duration was seen in children taking 1 to 2 grams daily. Taking vitamin C after the onset of cold symptoms yielded no benefit. Although vitamin C supplementation before getting a cold was beneficial for those undergoing extreme exercise, no benefit was noted for the general public (196).

Vitamin C and Exercise

Regular exercise can increase vitamin C needs, and low vitamin C status negatively affects performance (197). Correcting a vitamin C deficiency or suboptimal intake can increase work capacity and aerobic power (143, 198).

PUTTING IT INTO PERSPECTIVE

CAN ANTIOXIDANTS IMPROVE RECOVERY AND DECREASE MUSCLE SORENESS?

Muscles produce tissue-damaging free radicals (reactive oxygen and nitrogen species) and serve as signaling molecules to help promote muscle adaptation to exercise (199). Free radicals play important roles in the production of muscle force, muscle growth, and recovery. A healthy balance of free radicals is necessary because high levels can damage cells, impair muscle contraction, and contribute to muscle weakness, fatigue, and dysfunction (200, 201). Dietary intake of antioxidants, including vitamins C and E, as well as carotenoids, might protect against excess muscle cell damage caused by free radicals (128). Therefore, consuming a diet rich in antioxidants may protect muscles from the damaging effects of excess free radicals. But no evidence supports supplemental doses for this purpose; in fact, taking high doses of antioxidant supplements can potentially shortcut the essential actions of free radicals. Most of the studies that examined supplemental doses of vitamins C and E found no positive effects on muscle strength or hypertrophy; instead, the studies found that these antioxidants can interfere with training gains by decreasing expected training adaptations that are triggered by the presence of free radicals. Free radicals are important for strength, power, and muscle repair after strength training (133, 199-204). Daily supplements of 1,000 mg vitamin C plus 235 mg (261 IU) vitamin E (as dl-alpha tocopherol acetate) interfere with cell signaling after resistance training, impair increases in muscle strength in response to strength training, and interfere with cellular adaptation to endurance training (205, 206). Supplemental doses of greater than 1,000 mg vitamin C alone impaired sport performance in at least four studies (207).

SUMMARY

Exercise stresses many vitamin-dependent pathways. Vitamins are important for health and have several important roles related to exercise and athletic performance, including energy production, oxygen transport, immune functioning, building and maintaining bone density, and synthesizing and repairing muscle tissue. The body can make vitamins D and K, although vitamin D production depends on exposure to UVB rays and the ability to convert vitamin D to its active form in the body. Many Americans are not making adequate amounts of vitamin D in their bodies or getting enough from food. Other vitamins commonly underconsumed include vitamins A, C, D, E, and folate. Athletes who are dieting or cutting out food groups or who generally consume a nutritionally poor diet have an increased risk of deficiency in one or more vitamins. Water-soluble vitamins, with the exception of vitamin B_{12}, need to be replenished daily, because excess is excreted in urine. Several vitamins, including folate and vitamins B_6 and B_{12}, are important for oxygen transport throughout the body, including to muscle tissues. In addition to monitoring overall dietary intake, people should consider the effect of cooking methods on water-soluble vitamin content. Supplemental intake must also be considered to get a good overall picture of a person's vitamin intake. Although vitamin deficiencies can negatively affect performance, excess intake has not been shown to enhance performance and in some cases might be detrimental.

FOR REVIEW

1. Discuss the vitamins affected by cooking methods and cooking methods that contribute to vitamin losses.
2. List some of the signs and symptoms associated with vitamin C deficiency.
3. Discuss methods to help the body absorb antioxidants from food.
4. How does vitamin D deficiency or insufficiency affect athletes? Discuss how excess intake of antioxidants might affect muscle.
5. List a day's worth of vitamin-rich meals.

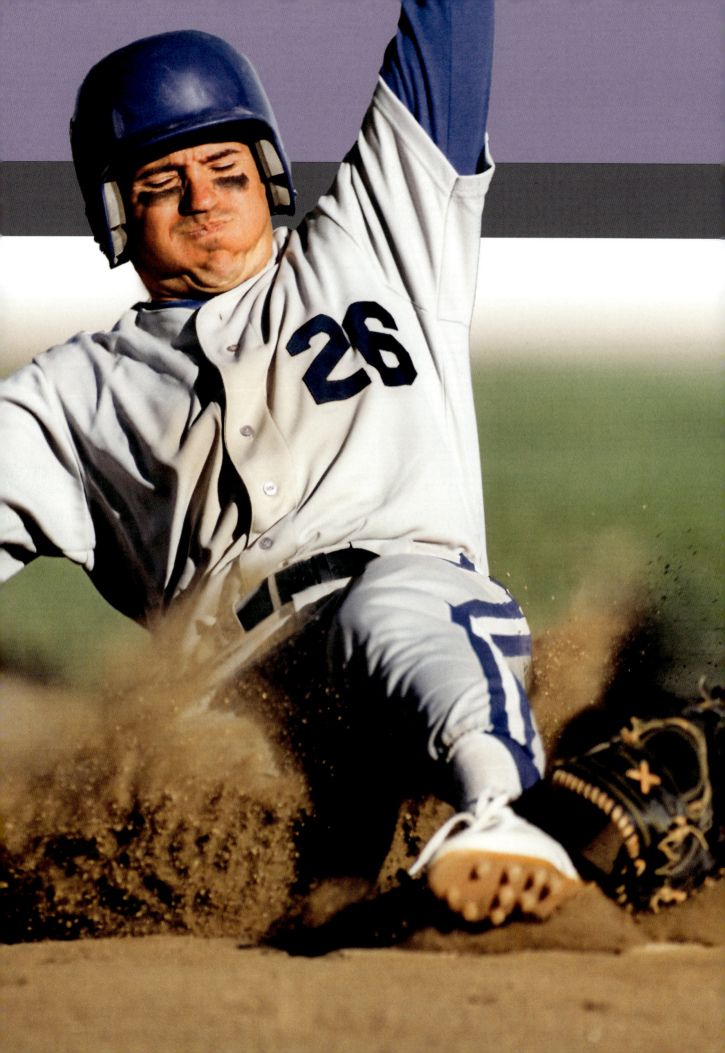

7

Minerals

> **CHAPTER OBJECTIVES**
>
> After completing this chapter, you will be able to do the following:
> - Discuss why minerals are important for training and overall health.
> - Explain how training and exercise affect mineral needs.
> - List the minerals that athletes are most likely not getting enough of through their diet.
> - Discuss potential hazards of excess mineral intake.
> - List a few good food sources for each major mineral.

Minerals help regulate fluid balance, muscle contraction (including heartbeat), nerve impulses, oxygen transport, immune functioning, and muscle (and connective tissue) building and repair. Minerals are structural components of many body tissues, including bones, nails, and teeth. Additionally, they are part of enzymes that facilitate several metabolic functions (1). Sodium, chloride, potassium, calcium, magnesium, and phosphorus are **electrolytes**—they conduct electricity in the body. Electrolytes affect fluid balance, muscle pH, and muscle functioning (2).

Minerals are essential for health and athletic performance; deficiencies can lead to health consequences and performance decrements (1). Mineral needs depend on gender and life stage (pregnancy, lactation, etc.). Table 7.1 includes the dietary reference intakes (DRIs) for adults aged 19 to 30. Although minerals are vital, no evidence suggests that increased intake of minerals, beyond the DRIs, will improve training adaptations or measures of performance (3).

MACROMINERALS

Minerals needed by the body in larger amounts are called macrominerals. These include calcium, phosphorus, magnesium, sodium, potassium, chloride, and sulfate. Each mineral, with the exception of sulfate, has a DRI. Sulfur-containing amino acids provide the body with enough sulfate to meet dietary requirements, so sulfate has no EAR, RDA, or AI. In addition, data are insufficient to establish an UL (4).

Calcium

Ninety-nine percent of calcium is stored in bones and teeth in the form of **hydroxyapatite**, where it supports the structure and function of these tissues. Less than 1 percent of total body calcium is found in blood (serum), muscle, extracellular fluid, and other tissues. All cells, however, require calcium. Calcium is required for hormone secretion and nerve transmission, constricting and dilating blood vessels, and muscle contraction.

Table 7.1 Dietary Reference Intakes for Minerals for Adults 19 to 30 Years Old

Mineral	Males	Females	Pregnancy	Lactation
Calcium	**1,000 mg	**1,000 mg	**1,000 mg	**1,000 mg
Chloride	*2.3 g	*2.3 g	*2.3 g	*2.3 g
Chromium	*35 mcg	*25 mcg	*30 mcg	*45 mcg
Copper	**900 mcg	**900 mcg	**1,000 mcg	**1,300 mcg
Fluoride	*4 mg	*4 mg	*3 mg	*3 mg
Iodine	**150 mcg	**150 mcg	**220 mcg	**290 mcg
Iron	**8 mg	**18 mg	**27 mg	**9 mg
Magnesium	**400 mg	**310 mg	**350 mg	**310 mg
Manganese	*2.3 mg	*1.8 mg	*2.0 mg	*2.6 mg
Molybdenum	**45 mcg	**45 mcg	**50 mcg	**50 mcg
Phosphorus	**700 mg	**700 mg	**700 mg	**700 mg
Potassium	*3,400 mg	*2,600 mg	*2,900 mg	*2,800 mg
Selenium	**55 mcg	**55 mcg	**60 mcg	**70 mcg
Sodium	*1,500 mg	*1,500 mg	*1,500 mg	*1,500 mg
Zinc	**11 mg	**8 mg	**11 mg	**12 mg

All values are estimated average requirements (EAR) unless otherwise indicated.
*Specifies adequate intake (AI). An AI is set if data are insufficient to set an RDA.
**Specifies recommended dietary allowances (RDA). An RDA is the average daily intake level sufficient to meet the nutrient needs of nearly all (97%–98%) healthy people in a group.
Data from U.S. Institute of Medicine (1997); U.S. Institute of Medicine (2001); U.S. Institute of Medicine (2011).

The endocrine system keeps calcium levels in the blood within a tight range (typically ranging from 8.5 to 10.2 mg/dl, though some labs use a slightly different range) (5, 6). All organs, particularly nerves and muscles, depend on an adequate supply of calcium in blood and cells (7). When serum calcium drops, the body readily pulls this mineral from bone to maintain a normal concentration of calcium in serum, muscle, and intracellular fluids that supports critical metabolic processes (8, 9). Therefore, high or low levels of calcium in the serum are primarily due to certain health conditions affecting calcium regulation instead of changes in dietary calcium intake (8).

Sources of Calcium

Excellent sources (foods containing 20% or more of the DV per standard serving) of calcium include dairy foods such as milk, cheese, and many brands of yogurt. The DV for calcium and other minerals is shown in table 7.2. Dairy foods are the top sources of calcium in the diets of Americans over the age of 2 years (10). Calcium-fortified orange juice, soy beverages, almond drinks, and tofu prepared with calcium sulfate are excellent or good sources of calcium (11). Some leafy green vegetables contain calcium. For instance, one cup of raw kale contains 53 mg of calcium, and one cup of raw spinach contains 30 mg of calcium—a small fraction of the RDA for men and women aged 19 to 30 years, which is 1,000 mg calcium per day (8, 11). See figure 7.1 for the calcium content in common foods. Approximately 30 percent of

Table 7.2 Daily Values for Minerals

Food component	DV (13)
Sodium	2,300 mg
Potassium	4,700 mg
Calcium	1,300 mg
Iron	18 mg
Iodine	150 mcg
Magnesium	420 mg
Zinc	11 mg
Selenium	55 mcg
Copper	0.9 mg
Manganese	2.3 mg
Chromium	35 mcg
Molybdenum	45 mcg
Chloride	2,300 mg

Keep in mind DV is an indicator of how much of one serving of a food item contributes to a person's nutrition needs, based on a 2,000 kcal diet.

Data from U.S. Food and Drug Administration (2016).

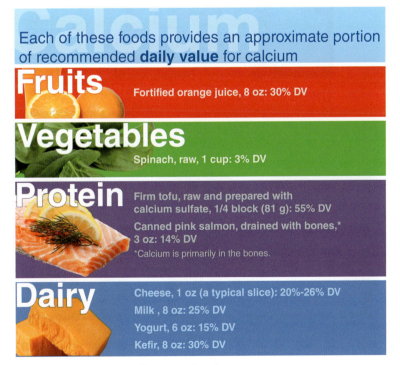

Figure 7.1 Calcium content of commonly eaten foods.

Text based on U.S. Department of Agriculture (2013).

calcium from food is absorbed, though the exact amount varies by the type of food consumed (8). Several factors affect calcium absorption, as noted in figure 7.2. For instance, the bioavailability of calcium from spinach is poor because of its high oxalate content, a compound that reduces the absorption of minerals from food (12). Phytic acid in plant-based foods might also decrease calcium absorption (4). The DRI, however, takes into account potential factors that decrease mineral absorption.

> **? DO YOU KNOW?**
>
> If raw spinach were the only source of calcium in your diet, you would need to eat 33 cups a day to meet the DV for calcium.

Both vitamin D and inulin, a prebiotic dietary fiber, increase calcium absorption (14, 15). Additionally, calcium absorption varies based on other compounds found in food (16). For instance, naturally occurring compounds found in plants including oxalic acid and phytic acid can bind calcium and other minerals, making them unavailable for absorption (17, 18). Because of the high oxalic acid content in spinach, the absorption of calcium from spinach is only 5 percent, whereas 28 percent of calcium is absorbed from milk (19). Other foods high in oxalic acid include collard greens, sweet potatoes, rhubarb, and beans.

Also, when using supplements, calcium and zinc intake must be balanced for optimal calcium absorption. For instance, when calcium intake is low (230 mg/day), a higher level (140

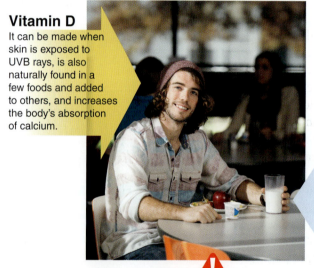

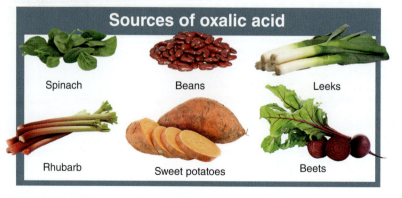

Figure 7.2 Factors that affect calcium absorption.
Based on U.S. Institute of Medicine (1997).

mg) of supplemental zinc interferes with calcium absorption, but 100 mg zinc per day does not. At higher calcium intakes (800 mg/day), a higher level of supplemental zinc (140 mg) has no effect on calcium absorption (20).

Calcium absorption decreases as the amount of calcium consumed in a serving increases. For maximum absorption, up to 500 mg of calcium should be taken at once (8). In addition, absorption of calcium from food increases with lower total calcium intakes compared with higher intakes. As an example, calcium absorption from food is about 45 percent when total calcium is 200 mg/day, whereas consuming calcium intakes higher than 2,000 mg/day decreases calcium absorption to about 15 percent (21). Calcium absorption is highest in infants and young children who need a good amount of calcium to build bone. Calcium absorption decreases with age, reaching about 25 percent in adulthood (4).

In addition to compounds that affect calcium absorption, other factors can increase calcium excretion. Caffeine has a minor effect on calcium excretion; studies show that one cup of coffee resulted in a 2 to 3 mg calcium loss (22, 23). Phosphorus intake has a minor impact on calcium excretion (24). Foods high in phosphorus include yogurt, milk, salmon, mozzarella cheese, lentils, cashew nuts, and beef. A high-protein diet increases calcium loss in urine, but it also increases calcium absorption and influences hormones in such a way to set the stage for using calcium to build bones (25-28). For instance, in one study, consuming 2.1 grams of protein/kg increased calcium absorption and excretion compared with 1.0 gram of protein/kg (26). Additionally, protein is also a major structural component of bone, making up half of bone volume and one-third of bone mass (25, 29). Most population-based studies show either no adverse effect of a high-protein diet on bone health or a positive effect of long-term high-protein intake that increases bone mineral density (30, 31). Given the fact that most studies show no adverse effect of a high-protein diet on bone health, the wise approach is to follow the recommended protein intake based on the guidelines in chapters 5 and 12.

> **? DO YOU KNOW?**
>
> Calcium carbonate and calcium citrate are two of the more common forms found in fortified foods and supplements. For optimal absorption, take calcium carbonate with food. You can take calcium citrate at any time of the day, with or without food (32).

Calcium Deficiency and Inadequacy

If calcium intake is insufficient to meet physiological needs, the body will withdraw calcium from bone to keep serum calcium constant and prevent hypocalcemia, or low blood calcium (also referred to as calcium deficiency) (33). Chronic low calcium intake affects bone health, because too many withdrawals weaken bone (figure 7.3) (7).

The skeleton is an organ that provides support, mobility, and protection for the body and stores the essential minerals calcium and phosphorus. The brittle bone disease osteoporosis

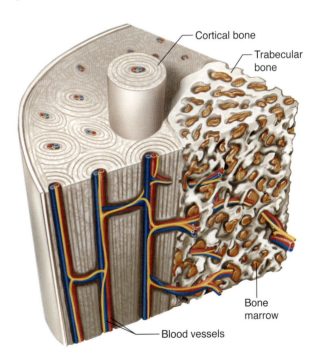

Figure 7.3 The two types of bone are cortical and trabecular. Trabecular bone, sometimes called spongy bone, has a honeycomb-like structure that makes up the inside of bone. Cortical bone is hard and forms the outer layer of bone.

is characterized by low bone mass, which can lead to structural abnormalities, including bent posture (7).

Bone is a dynamic, metabolically active tissue that responds to genetics, exercise, and diet. Lifestyle choices have a profound effect on bone, influencing 20 to 40 percent of peak bone mass (34). During childhood and adolescence, bone is sculpted by modeling; new bone is formed at one site within bone, and old bone is removed at another site on the outside of bone. During this process, bones shift and grow longer, denser, and stronger. During puberty, bones become thicker as formation occurs both inside and on the outer surface of bone (7). Up to 90 percent of peak bone mass, maximum bone strength and density, is attained during late adolescence (1), but 100 percent peak bone mass is generally not reached until the early 20s to about age 30 (7, 35). In children, consistent inadequate dietary calcium intake or poor calcium absorption can lead to rickets, a disease characterized by weak bones that do not grow properly. Remodeling, removal of old bone and replacement with new bone at the same site, occurs throughout life; the adult skeleton is replaced approximately every 10 years (7). Remodeling repairs small cracks or deformities in bone and prevents buildup of older bone, which can become brittle (7). In older adults, bone breakdown (resorption) exceeds bone formation, leading to a net loss in bone mass and increased risk of developing brittle bones, termed osteoporosis (8). To prevent or delay the onset of osteoporosis, it is critical to build peak bone mass during the early years and slow bone loss after peak bone mass is reached. Figure 7.4 provides information on food that helps to build peak bone mass.

Despite the detrimental effects associated with low calcium intake, national survey data show that over 40 percent of Americans do not meet the EAR for calcium (figure 7.5) (10, 36). Females,

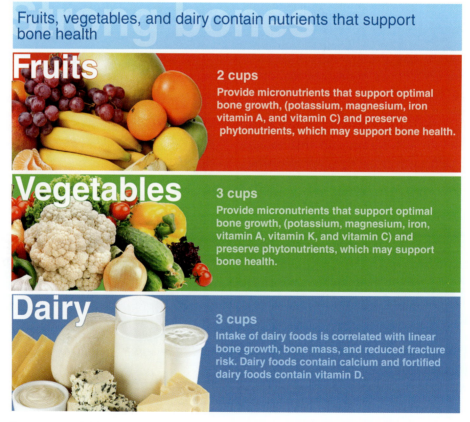

Figure 7.4 Recommended servings of dairy, fruits, and vegetables for peak bone mass for adults aged 19 to 30.

Based on Weaver et al. (2016).

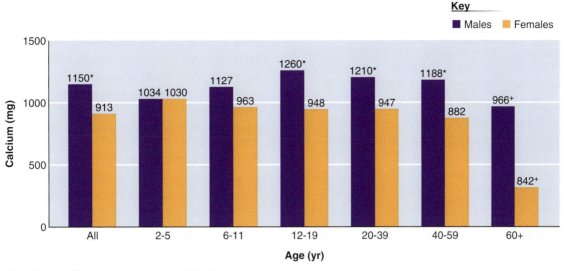

*Significantly different from females (p<0.001)
+Within gender, significantly different than other age groups combined (p<0.001)

Figure 7.5 Calcium intake of the U.S. population.
Reprinted from Hoy and Goldman (2009).

particularly preteens and teenagers, are most likely to consume inadequate amounts of calcium (9). Although females have higher calcium density than males—more calcium per the amount of calories they consume—they consume fewer overall calories and therefore less total calcium (10). Older adults also consume less calcium than other age groups, in part because of lower calorie intake (10). Average calcium intake is lower for African Americans than for whites or Hispanics. Those from lower-income households also consume less than people from higher-income households (10).

Excess Calcium Intake

High calcium intake can cause constipation and interfere with iron and zinc absorption. Also, some studies suggest supplemental calcium intake is related to risk of kidney stones (8).

Although typically associated with primary hyperparathyroidism, very high intakes of calcium can cause high blood calcium, **hypercalce-** mia (8, 37), which can lead to vascular and soft tissue calcification, excessive calcium in the urine, kidney stones, and renal insufficiency (8).

Calcium and Exercise

Because of its role in bone health, calcium is extremely important for fitness enthusiasts and athletes. Among other variables, including training, biomechanics, and overall nutrition intake, chronically low calcium intake can lead to low bone mineral density, resulting in increased risk of stress fracture (38). For females, chronically low energy availability (not consuming enough total calories to meet the body's needs) combined with delayed menarche (first menstrual cycle), a history of oligomenorrhea (light or infrequent menstrual cycles or cycles more than 35 days apart), or amenorrhea (absence of three or more menstrual cycles in a row) all increase risk for low bone mineral density and subsequent fracture risk (39).

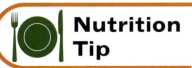

Use it or lose it. Whether you are in a cast, on prolonged bed rest, in a wheelchair, or on a flight in space, immobilization leads to rapid bone loss (7). The best way to ensure that your bones will allow you to be active in your 70s, 80s, and 90s is to use them throughout life.

Phosphorus

Phosphorus is essential for the formation of bones and teeth, helps the body use carbohydrates and fats, and is important for growth, maintenance, and repair of cells and tissues, as well as for maintaining normal pH. Phosphorus plays an essential role in nerve signaling, blood vessel functioning, regular heartbeat, and muscle contractions (as part of ATP and PCr). All cells throughout the body contain phosphorus and rely on this mineral for functioning (7). Bones and teeth contain most of the body's phosphorus stores (40). When phosphorus is in short supply, the body takes it from bone to meet physiological demands (7).

Think of bone like a bank account—calcium and phosphorus are deposited in bone and removed by hormones when levels are insufficient to meet vital functions in the body. Removal decreases the amount of calcium and phosphorus stored for later use unless you deposit (consume) more. Over time, constant withdrawals with no, or minimal, deposits leads to weaker bones (figure 7.6) (7).

Sources of Phosphorus

Phosphorus is found in a wide variety of foods, including poultry, seeds, nuts, beans, dairy, meat, poultry, and fish. The standard American diet, the typical dietary pattern of most Americans, contains roughly two to four times more phosphorus than calcium, and national survey data indicate that many Americans get more than enough phosphorus in their diet, suggesting that sources of phosphorus are both popular among and readily available to U.S. consumers. That said, not all groups have an adequate intake of phosphorus.

Inadequate or Excess Phosphorus Intake

People who eat a lot of dairy foods or drink several servings of soft drinks per day tend to have a high phosphorus intake. Soft drinks higher in phosphorus include Coca-Cola, Cherry Coke, Vanilla Coke, and Dr. Pepper, although a 12-ounce (360 ml) serving of each contains only about 4 percent of the RDA for those 9 to 18 years of age. By comparison, 12 ounces (360 ml) of Revive fruit punch vitamin water contains 31 percent of the RDA for those ages 9 to 18 (this product is several times higher than other vitamin water flavors). Root beer, ginger ale, and Sprite have a negligible amount of phosphorus (41). Females 12 to 19 years of age are the only group with an average phosphorus intake below the RDA (42, 43).

Hypophosphatemia, low blood phosphate, is not common, though it can develop from starvation, anorexia nervosa, starting enteral or parental nutrition (2 to 5 days after due to the change from a catabolic to an anabolic state), excessive alcohol intake, and chewing or swallowing issues. Hypophosphatemia can lead to anemia, muscle weakness, bone pain, rickets, osteomalacia, general physical weakness, increased risk of infection, paresthesia (a tingling or pricking feeling), ataxia (loss of body movements), confusion, anorexia, and possible death (40).

Excess phosphorus intake can lead to **hyperphosphatemia**, abnormally high phosphorus levels in blood. Risk of hyperphosphatemia is greatest in those with end-stage renal disease or vitamin D intoxication. Hyperphosphatemia can lead to decreased calcium absorption and calcification of nonskeletal tissues, such as the kidneys (8).

Phosphorus and Exercise

Given the many roles that phosphorus performs in the body, including in muscle, a deficiency of

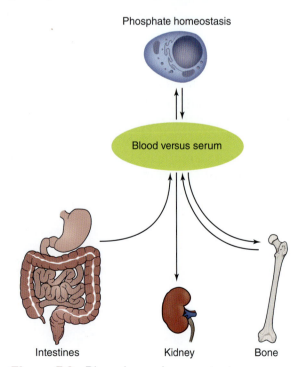

Figure 7.6 Phosphorus homeostasis.

> **PUTTING IT INTO PERSPECTIVE**
>
> **HOW DO I KNOW IF I'M MEETING MY MINERAL NEEDS?**
>
> To determine if you are meeting your needs for each mineral, regularly monitor the foods you are eating. Keep a food diary for at least 3 days without changing your normal eating habits. Are you eating foods that are good or excellent sources of each mineral?

this mineral could, theoretically, impair athletic performance. Because phosphorus deficiency is rare, however, implications of low phosphorus intake or deficiency and potential effect on athletic performance have not been studied.

Magnesium

Magnesium is a cofactor in over 300 biochemical reactions in the body that regulate a wide array of functions, including protein synthesis, nerve and muscle function, glucose control, and blood pressure regulation. Magnesium is essential for maintenance of intracellular calcium and potassium levels, metabolism, and energy production. Magnesium is a structural component of bone and is necessary to synthesize RNA, DNA, and glutathione, an antioxidant that helps to suppresses muscle fatigue resulting from prolonged exercise (40, 44). Approximately half of the body's magnesium stores is found in bone. The remaining amount is in soft tissues, and less than 1 percent of the body's magnesium stores is found in blood. The amount of magnesium in blood is tightly regulated and has little correlation to the amount of magnesium found within specific tissues (40). When more magnesium is consumed, the body absorbs less. Likewise, lower magnesium intake leads to an increase in intestinal absorption (4).

Low magnesium intake is associated with insulin resistance, endothelial dysfunction, and hypertension (high blood pressure) (45). A meta-analysis examining the effect of magnesium supplementation on blood pressure summarized 22 trials with 3 to 24 weeks of follow-up and a supplemented elemental magnesium range of 120 to 973 mg (mean dose 410 mg). Combined, the trials found a small, yet clinically significant mean decrease in systolic blood pressure, 3 to 4 mmHg, and diastolic pressure, 2 to 3 mmHg. Results were greater in crossover trials with a supplemental intake of greater than 370 mg per day (46). Another meta-analysis of 34 trials found that a median magnesium dose of 368 mg per day for a median duration of 3 months significantly reduced systolic blood pressure by 2 mmHg and diastolic blood pressure by 1.78 mmHg (47).

Higher magnesium intake is associated with lower fasting insulin concentrations (lower concentrations of the hormone insulin are measured during fasting) in both adults and obese children. Lower fasting insulin concentrations may correspond with greater insulin sensitivity (greater insulin sensitivity means muscle, fat, and liver cells respond better to insulin; insulin signals cells to absorb glucose from the bloodstream) (48-51). Additionally, approximately 25 to 38 percent of people with type 2 diabetes have low magnesium concentration (52). Despite the associations between dietary magnesium intake, fasting insulin concentrations, and type 2 diabetes, clinical trials examining how magnesium supplements affect fasting blood glucose and insulin sensitivity in type 2 diabetics have led to mixed results (53-58). A meta-analysis of 40 prospective cohort studies, however, found that increasing dietary magnesium was associated with a reduced risk of stroke, heart failure, type 2 diabetes, and all-cause mortality, but not CHD or total CVD (59).

Sources of Magnesium

Magnesium is found in nuts, seeds, legumes, leafy green vegetables, and whole grains (figure 7.7). Excellent dietary sources of magnesium (those containing 20% or more of the DV) include pumpkin seeds, almonds, boiled spinach, soybeans, cowpeas, Brazil nuts, and cashews. Good sources of magnesium include kidney beans, peanuts, brown rice, wild rice, and walnuts (11, 60).

When examining a magnesium supplement, the total amount of actual magnesium (referred to as "elemental magnesium"), as well as the body's ability to absorb the specific source of

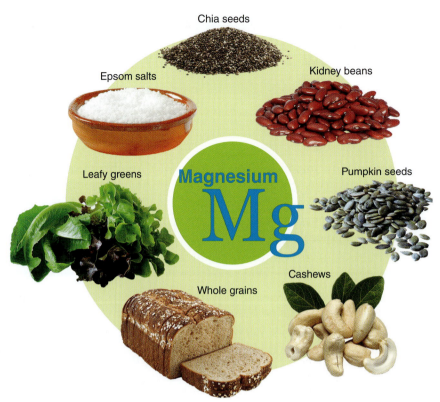

Figure 7.7 Sources of magnesium, including Epsom salts, which is absorbed through the skin during a bath and should not be eaten.

magnesium, should be considered. Dietary supplements contain varying amounts of magnesium. Manufacturers are required to list the amount of elemental magnesium on the supplement label, which is a fraction of the magnesium-containing compound. The absorption of supplemental forms of magnesium also varies. Magnesium aspartate, citrate, lactate, and chloride are better absorbed and more bioavailable than magnesium oxide and magnesium sulfate (61-65). Magnesium is a large mineral, so single-pill multivitamin mineral supplements do not contain anywhere near 100 percent of the DV for magnesium.

Inadequate Magnesium Intake

Poor magnesium intake is prevalent among several groups in the United States (66-71). According to national survey data, mean magnesium intake in U.S. adults is 82 to 85 percent of the current RDA (72). A large percentage of American teenagers, along with men and women 71 years of age or older, are consuming below EAR for magnesium (73). Those who consume dietary supplements are more likely to meet their magnesium needs, yet many women who use supplements still fall short of the RDA (66, 74).

Symptomatic magnesium deficiency in otherwise healthy people is rare. Gastrointestinal diseases, type 2 diabetes, alcoholism, and regular use of specific medications can lead to magnesium deficiency (75-77). Those with cardiovascular disease, neuromuscular disease, malabsorption syndromes, renal disease, and osteoporosis may have an increased risk for depleted magnesium levels (4). In addition, older adults have an increased risk of deficiency caused by decreased magnesium absorption and increased excretion. Older adults are also more likely to have chronic diseases or take medications that affect magnesium status (78, 79). Symptoms of magnesium deficiency include decreased appetite, nausea, vomiting, fatigue, weakness, numbness, tingling, muscle contractions and cramps, twitches or spasms, seizures, personality changes, abnormal heart rhythms, hypocalcemia (low serum calcium), hypokalemia (low serum potassium), and coronary spasms (80, 81). Magnesium deficiency can disrupt muscle cell functioning; impair carbohydrate uptake by muscle cells; lead to impaired cardiovascular functioning, muscular fatigue, and muscle cramping; and impair athletic performance (82-85). Low magnesium levels are also associated with chronic inflammation (86, 87). Based on animal research, magnesium deficiency may lead to structural and functional damage to proteins and DNA, as well as decreased antioxidant capacity (88, 89). Different methods are used to test magnesium status (see figure 7.8).

Excess Magnesium Intake

Healthy people typically excrete excess magnesium. No adverse effects have been noted from magnesium intake through food (4). Excess magnesium intake from medications, supplements, and magnesium-containing antacids or through intake of multiple servings of magnesium-rich sports drinks or greens drinks can lead to nausea, stomach cramping, and diarrhea (4). Magnesium toxicity is associated with nausea, vomiting, facial flushing, fatigue, muscle weakness, breathing difficulty, extreme hypotension (low blood pressure), irregular heartbeat, and cardiac arrest (78). Poor kidney functioning increases risk of magnesium toxicity caused by a decline in the body's ability to remove excess magnesium (78).

Magnesium and Exercise

Given the many roles of magnesium in the body that affect athletic performance, including ATP synthesis, carbohydrate and fat metabolism, bone strength, and muscle functioning, this mineral is clearly important for athletic performance and recovery (40, 88, 89). That said, relatively few studies have examined the effects of magnesium supplementation on sport performance (90).

Observational data accessing dietary recalls from adolescent athletes, ultraendurance athletes, rhythmic gymnasts, young adult male athletes (aged 19 to 25 years old), male collegiate soccer (football) players, male collegiate rugby players, and elite female athletes from a wide variety of sports suggest that many athletes are not meeting their magnesium requirements (91-98).

Even marginal magnesium deficiency can impair exercise (99). A study in elite male basketball, handball, and volleyball players found that magnesium intake, as assessed by a 7-day diet record, was directly associated with maximal

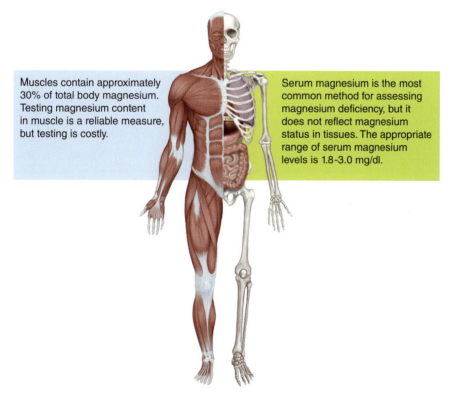

Figure 7.8 Red blood cell magnesium might be the best method for testing magnesium status, but it does not correlate well with total body magnesium status.
Based on Elin et al. (1994).

isometric trunk flexion, rotation, handgrip, jumping performance tests, and all isokinetic strength variables, independent of calorie intake (84). Despite the associations between magnesium and factors that affect performance, only a few studies suggest that magnesium supplementation, particularly in the absence of low magnesium status as identified through testing, can improve athletic performance (90).

In a double-blind, 7-week strength-training study, untrained males aged 18 to 30 were given a magnesium oxide supplement, a poorly absorbed form of magnesium (to bring total intake to 8 mg/kg body weight per day based on dietary intake as assessed by a 3-day diet record) or placebo. In a double-blind study, both the researchers and participants are unaware of the intervention. In this study, the researchers and participants did not know if they were taking the supplement or placebo. At the end of the 7-week period, quadriceps torque was measured. Both groups gained strength, but the supplemented group had a greater gain in absolute torque, relative torque adjusted for body weight, and relative torque adjusted for lean body mass, compared with the placebo group (100).

Twenty-five professional male volleyball players were given either 350 mg magnesium or 500 mg maltodextrin each day for 4 weeks. The group supplemented with magnesium experienced a significant decrease in lactate production and up to 3-centimeter increases in countermovement jump and countermovement jump with arm swing (the athlete stands upright, flexes knees, moves arms back while squatting, and then swiftly extends knees and hips to jump vertically), whereas no change occurred in the placebo group, suggesting improvement in immediate energy anaerobic metabolism (101).

Magnesium supplementation may also help reduce muscle soreness in those with low dietary magnesium intake as indicated by a study in resistance-trained college-aged males and females. At baseline, only 2 of the 22 study subjects met or exceeded the RDA for magnesium, and 50 percent of subjects consumed less than 50 percent of the RDA as determined by analysis of a 7-day food diary. Subjects performed the bench press on day 1 to induce muscle soreness. They also took either 350 mg of magnesium glycinate or a placebo for 10 days. Two days later they came back to the lab for a performance baseline test on the bench press (three sets of bench press to failure at 65%, 75%, and 85% of estimated 1RM with a 3-minute recovery between sets). On day 8 they repeated the eccentric soreness test from day 1, and on day 10 they repeated the performance trial. Those taking magnesium experienced significantly less muscle soreness 24, 36, and 48 hours after their bench press on day 10 compared with those taking a placebo. Compared with baseline, perceived recovery status improved after magnesium intake but not for those taking the placebo (102).

Magnesium supplementation may also benefit fitness in older people. A study in postmenopausal women found that low magnesium intake led to lowered magnesium stores in muscle and red blood cells; the women required more oxygen during exercise and were more likely to fatigue quickly during submaximal work (85). A randomized, controlled trial in elderly women attending a fitness program found that supplementing with 300 mg magnesium oxide daily led to improvements in performance, particularly in women consuming lower than the RDA for magnesium (103).

Although magnesium is critical for exercise performance and recovery and many athletes are underconsuming this mineral, relatively few studies have examined the effect of magnesium supplementation in athletes. Given the relative lack of research and fact that magnesium status is

BE WARY OF DETOX CLEANSES

Many detox diets and cleanses rely on a combination of ingredients, foods, or beverages that often include laxatives and diuretics. Magnesium is a common ingredient in some laxative products (104). If your detox diet or cleanse contains magnesium carbonate, chloride, gluconate, or oxide, you are more likely to experience diarrhea (61). Also, very large doses of magnesium can lead to magnesium toxicity, particularly in those with impaired kidney functioning (40).

rarely tested for, a good starting place for athletes is to examine the amount of magnesium in their diet and improve intake of magnesium-rich foods if warranted.

Potassium

Potassium helps maintain fluid volume inside and outside cells, making this mineral important for proper cell structure and function, smooth and skeletal muscle (including muscle contraction) functioning, acid-base balance, and nerve transmission. A diet rich in potassium can help decrease the adverse effects that sodium can have on blood pressure, reduce the risk of recurrent kidney stones, and potentially decrease bone loss (105). Potassium levels must be maintained within normal limits, because either high or low potassium levels can lead to serious health effects (105).

DO YOU KNOW?

Despite the safety data reported in some studies, potassium supplements should be taken only under the guidance of a physician or registered dietitian because high blood potassium can lead to cardiac arrhythmia (abnormal heart rate or rhythm) and is associated with increased risk of death (112). For more information on potential risks to high blood potassium, see the section Excess Potassium Intake.

Potassium intake and stroke risk are inversely associated; higher levels of potassium intake are associated with lower risk of total, hemorrhagic, and ischemic stroke (113-115). This relationship between potassium and stroke risk remains even after adjusting for the effect that potassium has on lowering blood pressure. In a systematic review, researchers found that the highest dietary intake of potassium was associated with a 13 percent reduced risk of stroke compared with the lowest dietary intake. A potassium intake of 3,500 mg was associated with the lowest risk of stroke (113).

Sources of Potassium

The average American over age 2 consumes 2,640 mg of potassium per day. Women over 20 years of age consume an average of 2,408 mg of potassium, and men over age 20 consume an average of 3,172 mg of potassium (116). As with many other nutrients, potassium intake is related to calorie intake. Those who consume more calories each day generally consume more potassium as well. Average total daily potassium intake is greater in men than women because of higher total daily calorie intake (116). National dietary survey data suggest that less than 1 percent of women consume at least 4,700 mg of potassium per day, which is the DV for potassium. Non-Hispanic Black females consumed the least amount

PUTTING IT INTO PERSPECTIVE

A POTASSIUM-RICH DIET MIGHT HELP LOWER BLOOD PRESSURE

Population-based research shows that higher potassium intake is associated with lower blood pressure (106). Additional evidence supporting the role of potassium in healthy blood pressure comes from randomized clinical trials showing that increasing dietary potassium intake leads to a small, though statistically significant, decrease in blood pressure in those with normal blood pressure or hypertension (107), particularly when dietary sodium intake is high (108). Randomized placebo-controlled trials suggest that potassium supplementation in doses of 235 to 7,820 mg taken for several weeks is safe in the population studied with no adverse effects and has a modest yet statistically significant effect on blood pressure (109). There is a dose-response relationship between potassium and reduced systolic and diastolic blood pressure (109). Potassium supplementation has the greatest effect on lowering blood pressure in those who are high sodium consumers, subjects not on medications to lower blood pressure, and those with the lowest potassium intake before supplementation (110).

Potassium decreases blood pressure by relaxing smooth muscle, which opens up blood vessels to allow greater blood flow and a subsequent drop in blood pressure (111). In addition, supplemental potassium intake increases the excretion of sodium chloride in urine (111). The next time you drink a cup of potassium-packed, 100 percent orange juice or add slices of tomatoes to your sandwich, you will be supporting healthy blood pressure levels.

of potassium, followed by Hispanic women and non-Hispanic white females (116).

Vegetables, beans, and fruits are among the highest dietary sources of potassium. All beans (soybeans, lima beans, mung beans, white, black, kidney, pinto, etc.) are excellent sources of potassium, containing more than 25 percent of the AI per half-cup serving. Potatoes, apricots, tomatoes, orange juice, prunes, and beet greens are also some of the best dietary sources of this nutrient (11). In the average American diet, the highest contributors of potassium include fruits and vegetables (20%), milk and milk drinks (11%), meat and poultry (10%), and grain-based mixed dishes (10%) (116).

Inadequate Potassium Intake

Moderate potassium deficiency can lead to increased blood pressure, salt sensitivity, increased risk of kidney stones, and a potential increase in cardiovascular disease, especially stroke. Severe potassium deficiency, called hypokalemia, can lead to muscle weakness, glucose intolerance, and abnormal heart rhythm. Excess intake of diuretics or laxatives, prolonged vomiting or diarrhea, as well as kidney and adrenal disorders, contribute to potassium deficiency (105, 117, 118). Sodium intake, as tested up to 3.2 grams per day, does not increase potassium excretion (119). At levels above 6.9 grams per day, however, there is a net loss of potassium (at least over the short term—it isn't clear whether the body adjusts to consistently higher sodium intake) (120).

Excess Potassium Intake

A UL for potassium consumption has not been established because the kidneys excrete excess intake through urine, helping prevent high blood potassium (105). But potassium can build up in the blood, a condition called hyperkalemia, in those with poor kidney functioning and impaired ability to excrete excess potassium. Potassium-sparing diuretics, hemolytic anemia (premature destruction and removal of red blood cells), severe bleeding in the stomach or intestines, tumors, excess potassium intake from salt

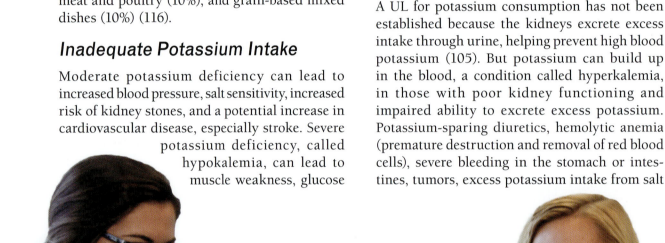

Reach for healthy snacks like fruits, vegetables, and hummus to keep up your energy for long study sessions.

substitutes or dietary supplements, and certain heart medicines (ACE inhibitors, angiotensin receptor blockers) can also lead to hyperkalemia. Nonsteroidal anti-inflammatory drugs (NSAIDs) such as ibuprofen, aspirin, and naproxen may also increase risk of hyperkalemia, particularly in those with poor kidney functioning. Hyperkalemia can lead to nausea, slow or irregular heartbeat, sudden collapse, and cardiac arrest (121). Those who have impaired ability to excrete excess potassium should keep their total daily intake below 4.7 grams (105, 117).

Potassium and Exercise

Relatively small changes in extracellular potassium levels can affect nervous system function, muscle contraction, and blood vessel function (105). The role of potassium in athletic performance is discussed in chapter 8.

Sodium

Sodium regulates the amount of fluid in blood, and extracellular fluid balance (blood volume) is necessary for nerve and muscle functioning, helps transport molecules across cell membranes, and is involved in the electrical potential across cell membranes. Combined with sodium, chloride helps maintain fluid and electrolyte balance and makes up sodium chloride, otherwise known as table salt (4). The AI for sodium is 1.5 grams per day (3.8 g/day sodium chloride, or table salt) for young adults, 1.3 grams per day for those 50 to 70 years of age, and 1.2 grams per day for anyone 71 years of age or older. This level ensures that the diet provides enough sodium to cover normal sweat losses in those not acclimated to the heat yet exposed to high temperatures, while also ensuring adequate intake of other nutrients. The AI is not applicable for those who may need to consume more sodium, such as competitive athletes, workers exposed to extreme heat stress, or anyone else who loses large volumes of sodium through sweat (4).

The body regulates fluid balance by monitoring blood volume and sodium level. When blood volume or sodium is too high, the kidneys increase sodium excretion. Additionally, the pituitary gland releases antidiuretic hormone in response to low blood volume. Antidiuretic hormone triggers the kidneys to conserve fluid. If blood volume drops too low, the kidneys secrete the hormone aldosterone to retain sodium and excrete potassium. Increased sodium retention leads to a decrease in urine production and subsequent rise in blood volume.

As people age, fluid balance is not well regulated. Older adults are more likely than younger adults to have an altered thirst mechanism and thus are less inclined to drink enough fluids. Kidney function changes with age, excreting more fluid in urine. Older adults have less total body water, so a slight drop in body water can lead to more serious health consequences than would occur in younger adults. Also, older adults are more likely to take multiple medications, which can increase fluid excretion, and to have diseases or conditions (impaired walking, swallowing difficulty, dementia) that alter their ability or desire to drink a sufficient amount of fluid.

Sources of Sodium

Most sodium consumed in the United States comes from salt, and the greatest source by far is processed foods, contributing to approximately 77 percent of salt intake. Only 6 percent of the average person's salt intake comes from the salt shaker, and only 12 percent is from the sodium chloride naturally found in food (4).

Inadequate Sodium Intake

The human body has a remarkable ability to adapt to low intake of sodium by conserving sodium in the body (4). Low serum sodium and chloride levels are rare in healthy people. Severe vomiting may lead to excess sodium losses, low chloride levels, and metabolic alkalosis (blood that is too alkaline). Prolonged or intense exercise, particularly in the heat without proper sodium intake, can lead to dangerously low blood sodium levels, a condition called hyponatremia (4), which is discussed in chapter 8.

Excess Sodium Intake

Healthy people excrete excess sodium intake. Continuous high sodium chloride (table salt) intake over time, however, is associated with an increase in blood pressure, a risk factor for stroke, heart disease, and kidney disease (4). This increase in blood pressure appears to be greatest in older adults, African Americans, and those with chronic kidney disease (4). Higher dietary potassium intake increases sodium excretion, reducing the rise in blood pressure associated with sodium intake (4). Higher potassium intake has the greatest effect on blood pressure when sodium intake is high (4).

Changes in blood pressure in response to changes in sodium intake can vary tremendously among people (122). Salt sensitivity refers to the change in blood pressure after a reduction or increase in salt intake (105). Older adults, African Americans, and those who are obese or have metabolic syndrome are more likely to be salt sensitive; their blood pressure increases in response to an increase in sodium intake and decreases in response to a lower-sodium diet (123-125). Both genetic and environmental factors appear to influence salt sensitivity (126). Twenty-five to 50 percent of those with normal blood pressure are salt sensitive; in this group, salt sensitivity seems to predict future high blood pressure (122, 127). Forty to 75 percent of those with high blood pressure are salt sensitive (127). Those who are salt sensitive and have high blood pressure are more likely to experience changes in blood pressure in response to salt intake (122).

According to *2020-2025 Dietary Guidelines for Americans*, almost all men and about 80 percent of women consume too much sodium (128). The AI for sodium in adults is 2,300 mg. The Institute of Medicine reviewed the research on sodium intake and health outcomes and found a positive relationship between higher sodium intake and risk of cardiovascular disease (CVD). But they found no benefit associated with a sodium intake below 2,300 mg per day in the general population. The institute also found no evidence for benefit, but perhaps for a greater risk of harm, with sodium intakes between 1,500 and 2,300 mg per day in those with diabetes, kidney disease, or CVD (129). In addition, a study examining over 100,000 people found that a sodium intake between 3 and 6 grams per day was associated with lower risk of death and CVD events compared with higher- or lower-sodium diets (130). Average daily sodium intake in the United States is approximately 4,274 mg per day for males and 3,142 mg per day for females (128). Most adults consume far above the AI for sodium; see figure 7.9.

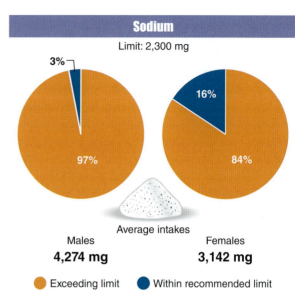

Figure 7.9 Although *Dietary Guidelines for Americans* recommends that Americans limit their sodium intake to 2,300 mg per day, most Americans consume much greater amounts of sodium. The average intake for men and women is 4,274 mg and 3,142 mg per day, respectively.

Reprinted from U.S. Department of Agriculture and U.S. Department of Health and Human Services (2020).

Independent of its effect on blood pressure—that is, whether it raises blood pressure or has no effect—a high-sodium diet (although there is no universal definition for high sodium) might have other adverse effects in the body. In those with normal blood pressure, 4,600 mg of sodium per day decreased nitric oxide activity—the molecule that opens blood vessels for greater blood flow (131). Nitric oxide is an important molecule for healthy blood pressure and one that is a target of active people—arginine and beetroot juice support nitric oxide activity to help increase blood flow to working muscles. Adults with normal blood pressure experienced a temporary decrease in blood vessel dilation after a single high-salt meal (1,500 mg sodium) (132), and overweight or obese adults with normal blood pressure saw improvements in blood flow while on a low-sodium diet (1,150 mg sodium), compared with when they were on a high-sodium (3,450 mg) diet (133). High sodium intake seems to damage the inner lining of blood vessels (endothelial lining), which is involved in blood clotting, nitric oxide release, immune function, and other important processes (122), while also increasing artery stiffness (stiff arteries do not expand as well as normal arteries to accommodate increases in blood pressure) (134). Also, a link exists between high dietary salt intake, increased inflammation among immune system cells, and impaired immune regulation (127).

Sodium and Exercise

Sodium chloride has two main functions during exercise—it helps the body retain fluid consumed (135) and helps restore electrolytes for proper muscle functioning. Sodium is the top electrolyte lost through sweat, followed by chloride. Sodium chloride losses vary tremendously among athletes, so sodium chloride recommendations should be individualized as much as possible (2, 136, 137), a topic revisited in chapter 8.

Chloride

Chloride is essential for maintaining extracellular fluid volume and plasma osmolarity. Most dietary chloride comes with sodium in the form of salt (sodium chloride). As a part of hydrochloric acid, chloride is also a component of gastric fluid. Approximately 98 percent of sodium chloride is absorbed. In healthy people with little sweat loss, most sodium chloride leaves the body through urine, and the amount excreted is almost equal to the amount consumed (4). Because chloride is bound to sodium, the AI for chloride is based on the AI for sodium (i.e., the AI equals the amount of chloride in the quantity of salt containing the AI for sodium). Much more sodium chloride is derived from processed foods than from salt added to food from the saltshaker. Chloride deficiency is rare, caused mainly by a loss of hydrochloric acid. Diuretics can increase water, sodium, and chloride. Those with cystic fibrosis have an unusually high sodium and chloride content in sweat and thus require more sodium and chloride. Excess intake is related to high blood pressure in those who are salt sensitive (4).

Sulfur

Many metabolic intermediates, including the antioxidant glutathione, contain sulfur. Sulfur is found in the diet through sulfur-containing amino acids and water. Sulfur is also created in the body from the amino acids methionine and cysteine. Deficiency is rare in those with adequate protein intake. There is no UL for sulfur because of an absence of sufficient data. Excess sulfur intake, from water high in inorganic sulfate, can lead to osmotic diarrhea (4).

TRACE MINERALS

Trace minerals are those that the body needs in small amounts. They include iron, manganese, iodine, zinc, chromium, copper, selenium, and fluoride. Table 7.3 summarizes sources and signs of deficiency and excess intake of some minerals.

Iron

Iron is necessary for growth, development, cell functioning, immune functioning, and the synthesis and functioning of some hormones. Iron is also essential for energy production and oxygen transport by the proteins hemoglobin and myoglobin. Hemoglobin transfers oxygen throughout the body; myoglobin transports oxygen to muscles (149-153).

IF I EAT TOO MUCH SALT NOW, WILL I GET HIGH BLOOD PRESSURE LATER IN LIFE?

Many factors contribute to high blood pressure, including genetics and obesity. There is no evidence that a high-sodium diet causes high blood pressure in healthy people with normal blood pressure. According to the Institute of Medicine, however, most Americans consume too much salt—and not enough potassium—for health and reducing risk of some chronic diseases (105). Recall that potassium can help diminish the possible deleterious effects of a high-sodium diet on high blood pressure.

Table 7.3 Excellent and Good Sources for Select Minerals

Mineral	Excellent sources (>20% DV) based on standard serving size (4, 8, 11, 40, 138-141)	Good sources (>10% DV) based on standard serving size (4, 8, 11, 40, 138-141)	Deficiency signs and symptoms (4, 8, 40, 138-141)	Excess intake and toxicity signs and symptoms (4, 8, 40, 138-141)
Calcium	Some types of yogurt, some brands of calcium-fortified orange juice (11, 142).	Milk, some calcium-fortified plant beverages (soy milk for instance), some brands of tofu made with calcium sulfate, canned salmon with bones (142).	Inadequate calcium intake produces no symptoms in the short term because blood calcium levels are tightly regulated.	Impaired kidney function and decreased absorption of other minerals.
Chromium*	Chromium is in a wide array of foods, typically in small amounts, including meats, whole grains, some fruits, vegetables, spices, grape juice, and potatoes (143). But there are no reliable methods to determine the chromium content of grains, fruits, and vegetables accurately because agricultural and manufacturing processes have a significant influence on chromium content (143).		There are no reports of chromium deficiency in healthy people.	• Isolated case reports suggest that chromium supplements may cause some adverse effects including anemia, liver dysfunction, dermatitis, renal failure, and hypoglycemia. • Chromium can interact with certain medications including medicines for diabetes and thyroid disease (143).
Copper	Lamb liver, veal liver, beef liver pork, lobster, oysters, cocoa powder, cashew nuts, pecans, sunflower seeds, Brazil nuts, hazelnuts, walnuts, mashed potatoes, blackberries.	Peas, peanuts, figs, sesame seeds, pink or red lentils, chestnuts, dried seaweed, peanut butter, kidney beans, potatoes, spinach.	Deficiency is not common although symptoms may include anemia, hypopigmentation, hypercholesterolemia, connective tissue disorders, osteoporosis, bone defects, abnormal lipid metabolism, ataxia, and increased risk of infection.	Copper is fairly nontoxic, but chronic exposure can lead to organ damage and gastrointestinal symptoms including cramps, nausea, diarrhea, and vomiting. Chronic exposure can come from consuming water containing high levels of copper from stagnant water sitting in copper-containing pipes and plumbing. Wilson's disease also increases risk of copper toxicity (144).
Iron	Oysters, white beans, dark chocolate, iron-enriched hot cereals such as cream of wheat or cream of rice, cereal fortified with 100% of the DV.	Sardines, kidney beans, ground beef, tofu, spinach, lentils, chickpeas.	General weakness, fatigue, irritability, poor concentration, headache, decreased athletic performance, hair loss, pale skin, cracks at the sides of the mouth, cold hands and feet, shortness of breath, dry mouth (145-147).	Risk of excess iron intake from dietary sources is low. High-dose iron supplements can cause constipation, nausea, vomiting, or diarrhea. Acute iron toxicity can lead to alterations in functioning of the cardiovascular system, central nervous system, kidney, and liver.

Mineral	Excellent sources (>20% DV) based on standard serving size (4, 8, 11, 40, 138-141)	Good sources (>10% DV) based on standard serving size (4, 8, 11, 40, 138-141)	Deficiency signs and symptoms (4, 8, 40, 138-141)	Excess intake and toxicity signs and symptoms (4, 8, 40, 138-141)
Magnesium	Pumpkin seeds, chia seeds, watermelon seeds, Brazil nuts (11, 60).	Peanuts, almonds, spinach, cashews, soymilk, black beans, edamame (11, 60).	Decreased appetite, nausea, vomiting, fatigue, and weakness; as magnesium deficiency worsens, numbness, tingling, muscle contractions and cramps, seizures, personality changes, abnormal heart rhythms, and coronary spasms can occur.	Doses over 350 mg per day can cause loose stools and diarrhea (40).
Phosphorus	Soy protein powder, sesame seeds, pumpkin seeds, mixed seeds, sunflower seeds, some bran cereals.	Plain yogurt, milk, salmon, scallops, mozzarella cheese, chicken, cashew nuts, 90% lean ground beef, cod, wheat germ, turkey, Brazil nuts, white beans, Swiss cheese, sirloin steak, ground beef.	Anorexia, anemia, bone pain, rickets, osteomalacia, general debility, increased risk of infection, paresthesia, ataxia, confusion, possible death.	Decreased calcium absorption and calcification of nonskeletal tissues, especially the kidneys.
Potassium		Yams, lentils, acorn squash, bananas, chili with beans, white beans, kidney beans.	Constipation, skipped heartbeats, palpitations (heart racing or pounding), abnormal heart rhythm (which may lead to feeling faint or lightheaded), fatigue, muscle damage, muscle weakness or spasms, tingling or numbness. If potassium levels are very low, the heart can stop.	Muscle fatigue; weakness; paralysis; slow, weak, irregular pulse; arrhythmias (abnormal heart rhythms); sudden collapse due to slow heartbeat or no heartbeat; nausea (148). Dietary supplements typically contain tiny amounts of potassium because high potassium can be extremely dangerous.
Zinc	Oysters, red meat, crab, lobster, pork chop, baked beans, some fortified breakfast cereals.	Pumpkin seeds, low fat yogurt, cashews, dark meat chicken, chickpeas, Swiss cheese.	Impaired immune functioning, loss of appetite, and growth retardation. In more severe cases, hair loss, diarrhea, impotence, eye and skin lesions, taste abnormalities, delayed wound healing, weight loss, mental fatigue.	Nausea, vomiting, loss of appetite, diarrhea, headaches, abdominal cramps.

*No DV.

Based on Allen et al. (2006); Otten, Hellwig, and Meyers (2006); U.S. Department of Agriculture (2013); U.S. Food and Drug Administration (2016); U.S. Institute of Medicine (1997); U.S. Institute of Medicine (1998); U.S. Institute of Medicine (2001); U.S. Institute of Medicine (2011).

Sources of Iron

Two types of iron are found in food: heme iron and non-heme iron (figure 7.10). Heme iron, derived from hemoglobin, is found in foods that contain hemoglobin—animal foods such as red meat, fish, and poultry. Approximately 15 to 35 percent of heme iron is absorbed (154). Dietary factors do not affect heme iron absorption (4). Vegetables, grains, iron-fortified breakfast cereal, and other non-meat-based foods contain non-heme iron; 2 to 20 percent of non-heme iron is absorbed (155). Phytic acid (the storage form of phosphorus in plants), polyphenols, phytates (legumes, whole grains), vegetable proteins, and calcium decrease non-heme iron absorption (4, 156-159), whereas vitamin C enhances non-heme iron absorption (4). Animal protein appears to increase non-heme iron absorption (4).

Inadequate Iron Intake

Iron deficiency is the most prevalent nutrient deficiency in the world, largely because of iron-poor diets in developing countries (160). In the United States, higher rates of iron deficiency and iron-deficiency anemia are seen in infants and toddlers, women of childbearing age, teenage girls, women aged 20 to 49, pregnant women, and female endurance athletes, partially because of poor dietary iron intake (161, 162). Approximately 15 to 35 percent of female athletes are iron deficient, whereas 5 to 10 percent of male athletes are iron deficient (163).

The following people have a higher risk of developing iron-deficiency anemia:

- women because of blood loss during menstruation;
- endurance athletes because of exercise-related gastrointestinal tract bleeding, subclinical exercise-induced inflammation, and foot strike hemolysis (see the sidebar Do You Know?);
- and vegetarians because of inadequate dietary intake (161, 162, 164).

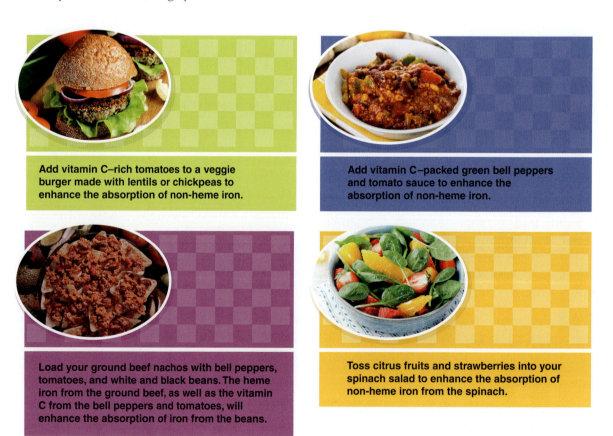

Figure 7.10 Are you getting enough iron each day? Here are some easy ways to incorporate more iron in your diet and enhance the absorption of non-heme iron.

Additionally, people with excessive intake of antacids, anyone who has had bariatric surgery (weight-loss surgery involving the stomach or intestines), and those with digestive diseases, such as celiac disease, have an increased risk of developing iron-deficiency anemia (140, 165). Blood donation can also affect iron status (147).

> **? DO YOU KNOW?**
>
> Foot strike hemolysis is the destruction of red blood cells in the bottom of the foot caused by activities involving running or jumping. Foot strike hemolysis might explain the association between greater exercise duration and intensity and lower hemoglobin, hematocrit, and ferritin (the storage form of iron in the body) in trained athletes (166).

Iron deficiency occurs in three progressive stages: iron depletion, marginal deficiency (also referred to as iron-deficient erythropoiesis), and iron-deficiency anemia (167, 168). General symptoms of compromised iron status may include fatigue, feeling cold, lightheadedness, pale skin, elevated heart rate and respiratory rate, and dyspnea (difficult or labored breathing) (169). Marginal deficiency and iron-deficiency anemia can cause irritability, poor concentration, headache, decreased athletic performance, hair loss, and dry mouth (145-147, 170).

Iron deficiency alters immune system functioning and the immune system's response to inflammation and infection. Iron-deficiency anemia is also associated with an increased risk of infection (171). Given the role of iron in the formation of hemoglobin and myoglobin, low levels of iron commonly lead to fatigue and reduced aerobic endurance performance (figure 7.11). Untreated iron-deficiency anemia can potentially lead to depression, heart problems, and cognitive development delays in children.

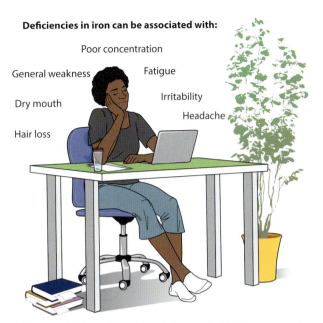

Deficiencies in iron can be associated with:
- Poor concentration
- General weakness
- Fatigue
- Dry mouth
- Irritability
- Headache
- Hair loss

Figure 7.11 Marginal iron deficiency and iron-deficiency anemia might make studying more difficult.

Excess Iron Intake

Risk of excess iron intake from dietary sources is low. High-dose iron supplements can cause constipation, nausea, vomiting, or diarrhea. Acute iron toxicity can lead to alterations in functioning of the cardiovascular system, central nervous system, kidney, and liver. Though there is some question about excess iron intake (through food or supplements) and coronary heart disease and cancer, the association, if any, remains unclear (4). People at greater risk for developing high iron levels include those with hereditary hemochromatosis, chronic alcoholics, those with cirrhosis caused by alcoholism, and those with blood disorders (thalassemias) (4).

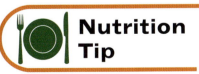 **Nutrition Tip**

Ibuprofen, aspirin, and other nonsteroidal anti-inflammatory drugs (NSAIDs) are commonly used to prevent and treat pain, inflammation, fever, arthritis, and other conditions. Long-term use of these drugs can damage the lining of the small intestine, causing inflammation, upset stomach, and bleeding, which can lead to iron-deficiency anemia (172, 173). If you experience adverse side effects or have concerns, talk to your physician. Iron supplements can also cause upset stomach; do not take iron supplements with an NSAID unless directed to do so by your physician.

> ### REFLECTION TIME
> ### I'M TIRED—SHOULD I TAKE AN IRON SUPPLEMENT?
>
> If you feel tired and grouchy, have difficulty concentrating, or notice that exercise is tougher than usual, you could have marginal iron deficiency or iron-deficiency anemia. Review the best sources of iron in table 7.3. On average, are you are getting enough iron in your diet each day? If you are not meeting your iron needs, increase your intake of iron-rich foods and consider taking a multivitamin that has 100 percent (or less) of the DV for iron. Consider seeing your physician for a diagnosis. Never take high doses of iron without consulting a qualified health care provider first. In addition to the side effects associated with iron supplements, acute iron toxicity is extremely harmful to the body.

Iron and Exercise

Marginal iron deficiency and iron-deficiency anemia can impair endurance performance and reduce exercise capacity (146, 147, 152, 174). Without adequate iron, oxygen transport to working muscle is impaired. Improving iron status through supplementation may or may not improve endurance performance (3, 175). According to a systematic review, when supplementing iron-deficient nonanemic athletes, the greatest likelihood of a performance benefit may be seen in those with ferritin stores of less than 20 micrograms/L. Iron deficiency might also affect cognitive functioning. A study of 127 females aged 18 to 35 found that those with better iron status had better reaction time and faster planning time (176).

Manganese

Manganese is important for bone formation and enzyme activity involved in amino acid, carbohydrate, and cholesterol metabolism. Manganese has no AI because data are insufficient to set an EAR. Grain products and vegetables make up large amounts of the manganese in the American diet (4). Beef, nuts, and beans are among the highest dietary sources of manganese (11). Clinical symptoms associated with low intakes are generally not observed, even among those with poor dietary intake of manganese (4, 177). Symptoms of manganese deficiency include dermatitis, decreased levels of clotting proteins, and low blood cholesterol. Miners exposed to manganese-laden dust have developed symptoms of toxicity, including neurological symptoms classified as manganese-induced Parkinsonism (note that Parkinsonism is different from Parkinson's disease), involving tremors, involuntary muscle contractions, impaired postural reflexes, and slow movements (177, 178).

Iodine

As a component of thyroid hormones, iodine is important for proper thyroid function. Thyroid hormones regulate a number of processes in the body, including metabolism and protein synthesis. Thyroid hormones affect several organs, including the brain, muscles, heart, pituitary gland, and kidneys. Seafood contains high amounts of iodine. Dairy products, fruits, and vegetables contain lower levels. The amount of iodine in fruits and vegetables can depend on iodine content in soil, fertilizer used, and irrigation. The addition of iodine to salt is mandatory in Canada and optional in the United States, where approximately 50 percent of salt is iodized. Iodized salt is one of the main sources of iodine in the U.S. and Canadian diet. Seafood might contain more iodine than many other foods because of the iodine content of seawater. Processed foods might also contain higher amounts of iodine because of the addition of iodized salt or other additives that contain iodine.

Excess iodine intake through food and dietary supplements is highly unlikely. Although rare, overt symptoms of iodine deficiency can lead to impaired cognitive development in children and hypothyroidism and goiter (enlarged thyroid) in adults. Iodine deficiency is particularly damaging to the developing brain, because it can lead to neurological damage. Excess intake of iodine can alter thyroid function (hypothyroidism or hyperthyroidism) and cause inflammation of the thyroid gland (4).

PUTTING IT INTO PERSPECTIVE

ARE PROCESSED FOODS UNHEALTHY?

Processed foods are not necessarily unhealthy. Although countless magazine articles and blogs are devoted to warning consumers about processed foods, many of the authors do not understand the true (FDA) definition of processed food. For example, frozen broccoli, frozen chicken breasts, dried beans, and dried pumpkin seeds are all examples of processed foods.

A processed food is

> any food other than a raw agricultural commodity (food that is in its raw or natural state, including all fruits that are washed, colored, or otherwise treated in their unpeeled natural form prior to marketing) and includes any raw agricultural commodity that has been subject to processing, such as canning, cooking, freezing, dehydration, or milling. (179)

If you have a busy day ahead studying for exams, you might want to spend less time chopping, prepping, and cooking and more time studying. Enjoy a nutrition-packed, easy-to-prepare, healthy dinner that includes such processed foods as steamed frozen vegetables, a chicken breast that has been thawed from frozen and then grilled, and 5-minute whole-grain couscous with a glass of milk. Do not believe everything you hear about processed foods. They can provide diet versatility, good nutrition, and convenience, often at a good price.

Zinc

Zinc is essential for immune system functioning. This mineral promotes wound healing and helps maintain skin integrity, one of the first lines of defense against pathogens. Zinc is essential for the metabolism of carbohydrates, proteins, and fats, gene expression, red blood cell functioning, protein synthesis, glucose use, hormone metabolism, normal taste and smell, and growth and development. Zinc is not stored in the body and thus must be consumed daily (180).

Sources of Zinc

Many foods are good or excellent sources of zinc. Oysters are among the highest sources, containing nearly 500 percent of the DV for zinc in just 3 ounces. Red meat is another excellent source, and poultry, fish, baked beans, and cashews are good sources. Diets high in protein provide substantial amounts of zinc (11).

Inadequate and Excess Zinc Intake

National survey data suggest that few people consume below the EAR for zinc (36), but several studies in athletes show low dietary intake or low zinc status. This research shows that various athletes are not consuming enough zinc through their diet, including a small group of competitive male swimmers in Brazil, male and female adventure race athletes, male and female U.S. national figure skaters, trained female cyclists, and female high school gymnasts (91, 116, 190-192). Vegetarians, athletes consuming very high-carbohydrate, low-fat diets, and those who don't meet their daily calorie needs are more likely to fall short of rec-

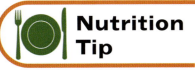

Some, though not all, studies show that zinc gluconate lozenges taken within 24 hours of the onset of cold symptoms may be helpful for decreasing the duration and severity of the symptoms (181-185). Other studies have used different forms of zinc, so it remains unclear what dose, formulation, and duration of zinc consumption is best (185, 186). When using a zinc lozenge or other zinc supplement, consume the zinc according to package directions for a few days at the early onset of symptoms. Do not take a zinc supplement long term, because this can lead to adverse side effects, including suppressed immune system functioning (140, 187). Excess zinc may decrease magnesium balance and copper absorption, so monitor the number of zinc lozenges you take, especially when combined with a multivitamin mineral supplement with over 100%DV for zinc (188, 189).

ommended intake levels for zinc (186, 191, 193). Because of lower overall energy intake, female athletes are less likely than male athletes to meet their zinc needs (194, 195). See figure 7.12 for sample dietary patterns (vegetarian and nonvegetarian) that meet most micronutrient needs including those for zinc.

Although zinc deficiency is considered rare (4), inadequate zinc intake can impair energy production and measures of athletic performance (196, 197). The primary symptom of zinc deficiency is growth retardation. Additional symptoms include hair loss, diarrhea, eye and skin lesions, poor appetite, and delayed sexual maturation (4). Zinc deficiency can also delay wound healing, suppress immune system functioning, and cause weight loss (187, 195). Excess supplemental zinc intake over a long period can suppress immune system functioning, lower HDL, and inhibit copper absorption, potentially leading to copper deficiency (140).

> **? DO YOU KNOW?**
>
> **Chelated** means attached to another compound. Chelated minerals are often attached to an amino acid. In some, though not necessarily all, instances, chelation improves absorption.

Zinc and Exercise

Zinc is part of the red blood cell enzyme carbonic anhydrase, which picks up carbon dioxide for the lungs to exhale, an important step for chemical balance in muscle cells. Zinc deficiency leads to a decline in carbonic anhydrase activity, a reduction in peak oxygen uptake and peak carbon dioxide output, and a decrease in respiratory exchange ratio, suggesting that the body had insufficient oxygen to use carbohydrates efficiently (197).

Low zinc levels lead to a decline in muscle strength and power output. Marginal zinc deficiency is associated with low levels of testosterone, thyroid hormones, and IGF-1, a hormone that promotes muscle growth and metabolism (196, 198). Correction of zinc deficiency with zinc or iron and zinc improves red blood cell functioning in those with anemia (199, 200). Although zinc has an important role in athletic performance, at this time there is little quality evidence that zinc can improve athletic performance (201).

Chromium

Chromium is important for the functioning of insulin, a hormone involved in the metabolism and storage of fat, protein, and carbohydrate. Chromium is found in small amounts throughout the food supply, although food processing can decrease the chromium content of whole grains and other foods (140). Chromium deficiency is rare and has been observed only in hospitalized patients fed intravenously (before chromium was added to intravenous solutions). Deficiency can impair glucose tolerance, leading to weight loss and neuropathy (202).

Although chromium deficiency can impair the action of insulin and glucose tolerance, the safety and efficacy of chromium supplementation as a treatment for insulin resistance and type 2 diabetes has not been backed by science (140). In a review of 15 trials, all but 1 showed that chromium supplementation had no effect on glucose or insulin concentrations in people with and without diabetes (203).

Copper

Copper is necessary for the functioning of several enzymes, including the enzyme that turns on collagen synthesis, helps the body make hemoglobin, and assists with energy production. The highest sources of copper are lamb, beef, shellfish, whole grains, beans, and nuts. Copper deficiency is rare, although it has been observed in premature malnourished infants; deficiency can lead to brittle bones, the blood disorder neutropenia, and anemia. As zinc intake increases, copper decreases in the body (204). High copper intake through dietary sources has not been observed in humans. But drinking water with high levels of copper due to stagnant water sitting in copper plumbing has resulted in cramps, nausea, abdominal pain, diarrhea, and vomiting (4).

Selenium

Selenium-rich proteins are important for thyroid functioning and defend the body against **oxidative stress**, an imbalance between the production of

IDEAL MENU—18-YEAR-OLD ACTIVE FEMALE, 2,400 KCAL

This dietary pattern meets or exceeds the DRIs for all vitamins and minerals except chromium, fluoride (which can be obtained from drinking water and toothpaste), molybdenum, choline, and iodine (which can be obtained from iodized salt). The DRIs are the average recommended intake over time. Therefore, you do not need to meet the DRIs every single day. In this example, the college student can consume more molybdenum, choline, and iodine from food and beverages on other days.

Breakfast
- 4 oz (120 g) nonfat plain Greek yogurt
- 2 tbsp hemp seeds
- 1/2 cup (75 g) strawberries
- 1 slice whole-wheat bread and one-half avocado
- 1 cup (240 ml) fortified orange juice

A.M. Snack
- 1 medium apple
- 2 tbsp peanut butter
- 1 cup (240 ml) fortified nonfat milk

Lunch: Burrito Bowl
- 1 cup (200 g) brown rice
- 1-1/2 cup salad mix
- 3 oz (90 g) chicken
- 1/2 cup black beans
- 1/2 cup tomato, 1/2 cup bell pepper, 1/4 cup onion

P.M. Snack
- 1/4 cup unsalted almonds
- 1/4 cup grapes
- 1/4 cup hummus and 2 oz (60 g) wheat crackers

Dinner
- 5 oz (150 g) sockeye salmon
- 1 cup asparagus
- 1 cup sweet potatoes cooked with 1 tbsp olive oil and 1/4 tsp salt

IDEAL MENU—18-YEAR-OLD ACTIVE VEGETARIAN MALE, 3,200 KCAL

This dietary pattern meets or exceeds the DRIs for all vitamins and minerals except chromium, fluoride (which can be obtained from drinking water and toothpaste), molybdenum, and iodine (which can be obtained from iodized salt). The DRIs are the average recommended intake over time. Therefore, you do not need to meet the DRIs every single day. In this example, the college student can consume more molybdenum and iodine from food and beverages on other days.

Breakfast
- Scramble: 2 eggs, 1 cup spinach, 1/2 cup bell pepper
- Cooked in 2 tsp olive oil
- 2 slices whole-wheat bread
- 1 cup (240 ml) fortified nonfat milk

A.M. Snack
- 6 oz (180 g) vanilla Greek yogurt
- 1/4 cup slivered almonds
- 1/2 cup blueberries

Lunch: Stir Fry
- 8 oz (230 g) tofu, 2 cups brown rice, 1/2 cup broccoli, 1/2 cup carrots, 1/4 cup mushrooms, 2 tbsp teriyaki sauce
- Cooked in 2 tsp olive oil

P.M. Snack
- 1 cup oatmeal, 2 tbsp peanut butter
- 1 medium apple
- 1 cup (240 ml) fortified nonfat milk

Dinner: Burrito
- Large whole-wheat tortilla
- 1 cup black beans
- 1 cup brown rice
- 1/2 cup lettuce
- 1/4 cup tomatoes
- 1/4 cup corn
- One-half avocado
- 2 tbsp shredded cheese
- 1 tbsp salsa

Figure 7.12 Dietary patterns that meet most micronutrient needs.

> ### PUTTING IT INTO PERSPECTIVE
>
> #### SHOULD YOU TAKE A MULTIVITAMIN SUPPLEMENT?
>
> According to *2020–2025 Dietary Guidelines for Americans*, "because foods provide an array of nutrients and other components that have benefits for health, nutritional needs should be met primarily from food." *Guidelines* continues, "In some cases, fortified foods and dietary supplements are useful when it is not possible to otherwise meet needs for one or more nutrients" (128). This point is important because foods also contain fiber and plant-based compounds necessary for good health. In some instances, a beneficial synergistic effect between the compounds is found in various foods that cannot be replicated in a supplement. Multivitamins cannot take the place of consuming healthy foods (206).
>
> If you want to ensure you're meeting your mineral needs, eat a wide variety of nutrient-dense foods. Greater variety means you are more likely to get a wide array of compounds found in food that are necessary for good health. But even with a healthy diet, getting enough of certain minerals can be tough, especially if you do not consume at least 2,000 kcal per day (more food means more opportunities to consume nutrients). Even if you meet energy needs, research shows that many athletes, active adults, and nonathletes are not meeting their nutrient needs (207). Women, people who avoid certain food groups, and those who are dieting are particularly likely to fall short of their micronutrient needs. Women consume far less than the dietary reference intakes set for calcium, iron, magnesium, and potassium. Also, some people have higher needs for specific minerals because of medications, previous surgery (such as gastric bypass), or health conditions. Fortified foods or a multivitamin mineral supplement can help fill in dietary gaps (208, 209).
>
> According to the National Institutes of Health, groups likely to benefit from taking certain nutrients found within multivitamin mineral supplements include the following:
>
> - Pregnant women have higher iron needs, so their physicians might recommend a prenatal multivitamin mineral with iron or a separate iron supplement.
> - Postmenopausal women might need more calcium to increase bone strength and reduce fracture risk.

free radicals and the body's antioxidant defenses (205). Selenium is in a wide variety of foods, including seafood, cereals, fruits, vegetables, grains, dairy, and meat. Selenium content of foods can vary tremendously based on the selenium content of soil. Selenium deficiency is rare, although it is possible in those with vegetarian diets consisting of food grown in low-selenium soil. Symptoms of deficiency include alteration in cardiac functioning and diseased cartilage. Selenium toxicity is also rare, although it can lead to GI disturbances, brittle hair, and nails (4).

Fluoride

Fluoride is essential for bone and teeth. This mineral helps protect against dental cavities and stimulates the formation of new bone. The primary source of fluoride in the U.S. diet is through fluoridated water. Other sources include beverages such as tea (fluoride builds up in tea leaves) and some marine fish (particularly if the bones are eaten). Inadequate fluoride intake can increase risk of developing cavities. Infants and children living in areas where water is not fluoridated will have difficulty meeting the AI for fluoride. Excess fluoride intake can lead to discolored or pitted teeth. Teeth might have opaque white spots or brown stains. Young children who swallow too much toothpaste or mouth rinse might get too much fluoride (4).

SUMMARY

Minerals have many essential functions throughout the body. For fitness and athletic performance, minerals are essential components of bone and help regulate fluid balance, metabolism, pH balance, oxygen transport, nerve impulses, and muscle contractions. Minerals are also important for supporting muscle building and repair. Low intake of calcium can increase risk of developing a stress fracture. Low intake of other minerals and overt mineral deficiencies, particularly in the case of iron, can affect health and human performance and, in some instances, lead to athletic performance decrements. Despite the importance of minerals, with the exception of iron, measuring mineral status can be challenging because serum markers do not always reflect tissue stores. Although inadequate intake of minerals can affect health and performance, no evidence to date suggests that consuming more than the RDI will improve health or athletic performance. Also, excess intake of certain minerals, such as zinc, can be detrimental to health and affect the balance of other minerals in the body.

You can find several forms of minerals in dietary supplements. Many might interact with other supplements or medications, so anyone considering taking a supplement should talk to their pharmacist or RDN first.

FOR REVIEW

1. Name the minerals that many Americans do not consume in adequate quantities and discuss why.
2. How does iron deficiency affect fitness and athletic performance?
3. What are the stages of iron deficiency?
4. Which minerals are important for bone health?
5. List common sources of magnesium.
6. How does zinc deficiency affect physical performance?
7. Discuss the roles of sodium and potassium for blood pressure regulation.

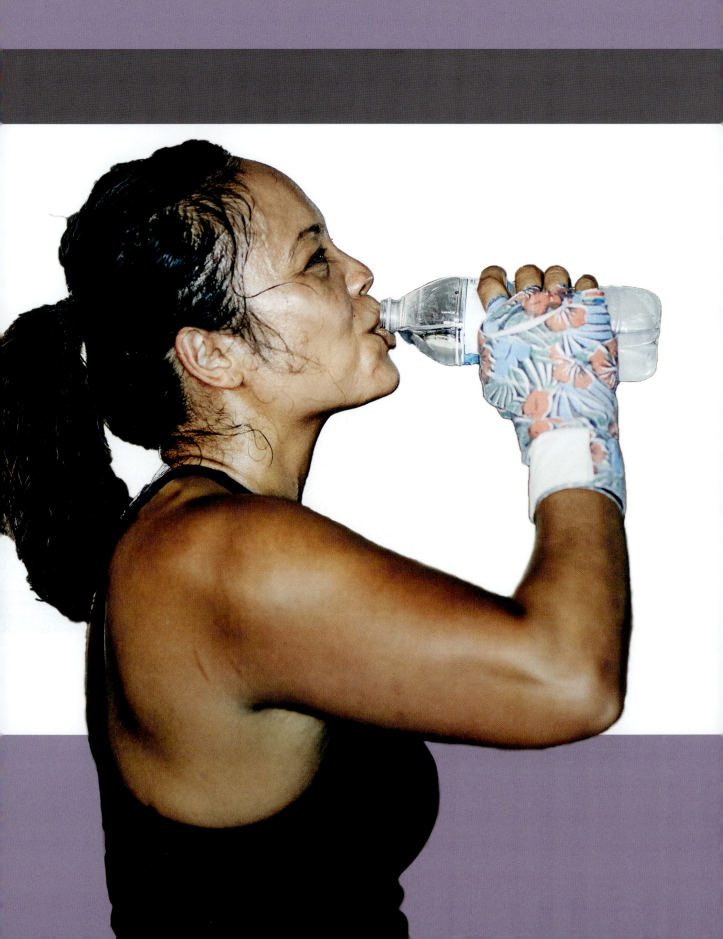

8

Water and Electrolytes

> **CHAPTER OBJECTIVES**
>
> After completing this chapter, you will be able to do the following:
> - Discuss the role that water plays in health and performance.
> - Discuss factors that affect a person's fluid and electrolyte needs.
> - Describe the major electrolytes lost through sweat and their health and physical performance implications.
> - Calculate sweat rate.
> - Describe tools that measure hydration status, including their ease of use and efficacy.
> - Describe signs and symptoms of hyponatremia.
> - Discuss risk of developing hyponatremia.

Water and electrolytes are essential for optimal health and athletic performance. Water lost through sweat cools the body, but if it is not replaced, health and athletic performance can be compromised. When fluid losses that are not replaced reach significant levels, risk of heat illness increases. Electrolytes conduct electricity. They are essential for muscle and nerve functioning and thus critical for the heart and skeletal muscles. Several factors affect fluid and electrolyte losses, making measurements in different environments essential for developing an individualized hydration plan for each athlete.

WATER

Water is critical for **homeostasis** (a state of balance or equilibrium). Water is a solvent for biochemical reactions, helps maintain blood volume, and serves as a means to transport nutrients and remove waste products (1). Water helps regulate body temperature by absorbing heat from metabolic processes and dissipating heat through **insensible perspiration** (fluid that evaporates through pores in the skin by sweat glands before the body recognizes it as moisture on the skin) and sweating. As sweat evaporates, skin is cooled. See figure 8.1 for the functions of water in the body. Low water intake is associated with some diseases, although evidence is insufficient to establish water intake recommendations for specific populations as a means to reduce risk of chronic disease (1).

For optimal functioning and health, total body water must be kept within a narrow range. Fluid intake, through food and beverages, increases total body water. Total body water loss stems from respiratory loss, insensible perspiration, urinary loss, gastrointestinal tract water loss (during metabolism), and fecal loss. See figure 8.2 for further information on daily fluid gains and losses. Excessive body water losses from fever,

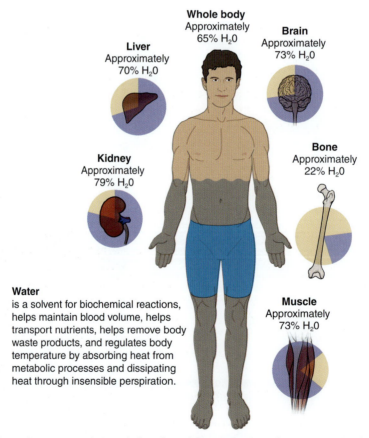

Figure 8.1 The body gains water through food and beverages, whereas typical water losses stem from respiration, insensible perspiration, metabolism, urine, and feces.

Data from U.S. Institute of Medicine (2005).

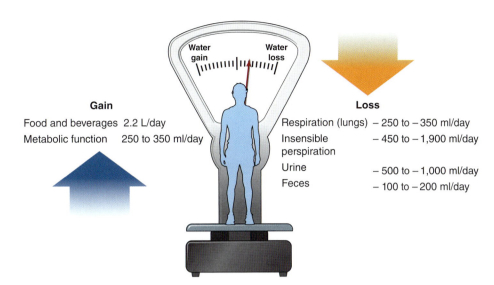

Figure 8.2 How we gain and lose fluid.

Data from Riebl and Davy (2013); U.S. Institute of Medicine (2005).

burns, diarrhea, vomiting, trauma, heat exposure, or exercise can impair health (1). **Hyperhydration** from excessive intake of low- or no-sodium fluids can increase body water and dilute blood sodium levels, potentially leading to **hyponatremia**—dangerously low blood sodium (1).

As the largest part of the human body, total body water makes up 45 to 75 percent of body weight in healthy people. Sixty-five percent of total body water is found in intracellular fluid; the remaining 35 percent is found in extracellular fluid (1, 2). Differences in body water among individuals of the same body weight are typically due to variations in body composition. Muscles contain approximately 70 to 75 percent water, whereas fat tissue contains 10 to 40 percent water (1). Athletes typically have high total body water compared with their sedentary counterparts because of higher levels of muscle mass and muscle glycogen (1).

Fluid Needs

Many factors affect fluid requirements, including age, body size, physical activity, environmental heat, altitude, health status, medications used, and use of particular dietary supplements. People who exercise or reside in hot climates might need more water.

Additionally, fluid needs vary from day to day (3). The AI for total water intake each day from foods and beverages for healthy, sedentary adults in temperate climates is 2.7 liters (91.3 fl oz, or 11.4 cups) for women and 3.7 liters (125.1 fl oz, or 15.6 cups) for men. The AI for pregnant and lactating women is 3.0 liters (101.4 fl oz, or 12.7 cups) and 3.8 liters (128.5 fl oz, or 16.1 cups) per day, respectively. All sources of fluid contribute to meeting the AI. Most of a person's water intake, approximately 81 percent, comes from water and beverages. The remaining amount, about 19 percent, comes from food (1). Table 8.1 shows the amount of water in select foods. Regardless of its source (food, water, other beverages), fluid is absorbed and treated the same in the body (1).

❓ DO YOU KNOW?

The advice to "drink eight 8-ounce glasses of water each day" isn't backed by science.

To determine how well various fluids keep a person hydrated, study authors assessed how a variety of drinks affected short-term hydration over a 4-hour period after intake. In this study in recreationally active healthy men at rest, full-fat milk, skim milk, and an oral rehydration beverage drink were the best at keeping the men hydrated (as measured by less urine output) over a 4-hour period after consumption. In this study they tested 13 beverages including still water, sparkling water, cola, diet cola, sports drink, an oral rehy-

Table 8.1 Water Content of Selected Foods and Beverages

Food or beverage	Ounces of water	% water based on weight
Water, 8 oz	8	100
100% vegetable juice, 8 oz (243 g)	7.7	94
Watermelon, 1 cup diced (152 g)	4.7	92
Milk, 1% fat, 8 oz (236 g)	7.2	90
Soup, garden vegetable, 1 cup (246 g)	7.2	87
Yogurt, plain, Greek, nonfat, approximately 1 cup (200 g)	5.7	85
Grapes, American, 1/2 cup (46 g)	1.2	81
Egg, scrambled, 1 whole, large, scrambled (61 g)	1.6	76
Chicken breast, sliced, 3 oz (85 g)	2.1	74
Banana, medium (118 g)	2.6	64
Fish, salmon, Atlantic, cooked in dry heat, 3 oz (85 g)	1.7	60
Bread, wheat, 1 slice (29 g)	0.3	34
Peanuts, raw, 1/4 cup (36.5 g)	0.1	7

Percentage water calculated based on the amount of water in the food (in gram weight) as compared with the total weight of the food.
Based on U.S. Department of Agriculture (2013).

dration beverage (80 kcal/L, 1,265 mg sodium/L), orange juice, lager, coffee, tea, cold tea, full-fat milk, and skim milk. They found that the drinks with the highest macronutrient and electrolyte contents were most effective at maintaining fluid balance. Macronutrients slow the movement of fluids through the stomach, keeping you hydrated for a longer period. Therefore, both the volume of fluid consumed and the composition of the drink influence hydration. The presence of other factors can influence fluid retention, including electrolytes such as sodium and potassium, diuretic agents such as alcohol, total calories, and the emptying speed of carbohydrate, fat, protein, and alcohol from the stomach. Consuming fluids that keep you more hydrated for hours after intake may be especially beneficial when taking breaks to urinate is inconvenient or when access to fluids is limited (4). Body weight and gender do not influence the short-term hydration potential of beverages consumed (5). For easy to implement tips on staying hydrated, see figure 8.3.

Body Fluid Regulation

Water and electrolytes are tightly regulated through coordination of neural pathways in the brain, kidneys, heart, sweat glands, and salivary glands. When the body is dehydrated, sensors in the brain, kidneys, and heart detect increases in plasma **osmolarity** (the concentration of solutes, particularly sodium, in the blood), as well as decreases in fluid volume, and set off a cascade of actions to preserve fluid volume (figure 8.4).

> **? DO YOU KNOW?**
> The kidneys are responsible for filtering blood and urine. On average, 1.5 liters of urine is produced each day. Urine contains water, electrolytes, and waste products (1). The kidneys function best when water is abundant (15).

Dehydration, the process of losing body water, causes a drop in blood volume (1, 16). When blood volume is low, the kidneys set off a cascade of events to maintain healthy blood pressure. Blood vessels are constricted, increasing blood pressure; sodium and water are reabsorbed from the water filtered by the kidneys so that less urine is produced; blood volume starts to rebound, leading to an increase in blood pressure; and a message is sent to the brain to stimulate thirst. But during dehydration, thirst sensation can lag behind fluid

- ✓ Drink from a 24- or 32-ounce (720 or 950 ml) water bottle each day. Do not refill the bottle until it is completely empty.
- ✓ Set goals for the number of bottles to drink each day. Schedule timeframes when you will consume them. For instance, you may take two 16-ounce (480 ml) drinks with you to class and consume them from 8 a.m. to 1 p.m. When studying at home from 2 p.m. to 4 p.m., drink one more 16-ounce bottle.
- ✓ Drink 16 ounces (480 ml) with every meal.
- ✓ Set a reminder on your phone for a time to take a few sips or drink 4 to 6 ounces (120 to 180 ml) of fluid.
- ✓ Drink something that tastes good. Sparking water, 100% juice, milk, kombucha, or other beverages you enjoy will help you drink more fluid.
- ✓ Try a smoothie for breakfast or a snack.
- ✓ Try 100% juice popsicles or make your own popsicles in the hot months with any combination of fruit, 100% fruit juice, and yogurt
- ✓ Add a hot or cold vegetable-based soup or whole fruits (not dried) or vegetables to every meal.

Figure 8.3 Practical solutions to increase fluid intake.

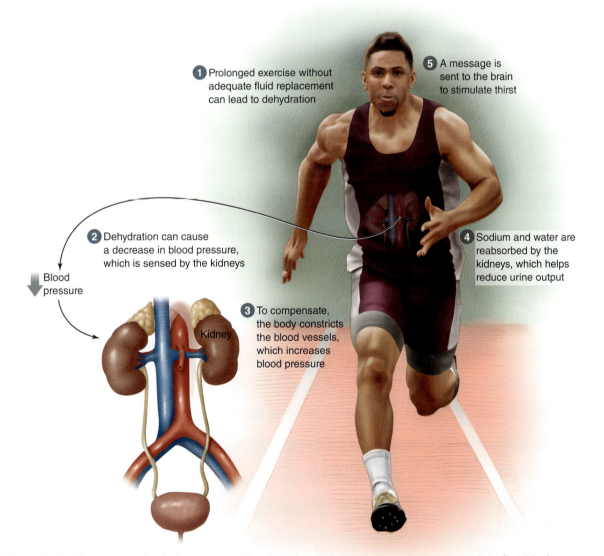

Figure 8.4 The human body has several feedback mechanisms in place to regulate fluid balance.
Based on Popkin et al. (2010); U.S. Institute of Medicine (2005).

> **PUTTING IT INTO PERSPECTIVE**
>
> ### DO CAFFEINE-CONTAINING BEVERAGES CAUSE DEHYDRATION?
>
> Caffeine is the most widely used legal central nervous system stimulant in the world. Caffeine temporarily increases alertness and memory, decreases fatigue, and improves mental functioning (6). Although caffeine has a mild diuretic effect, caffeine consumption in doses of less than 400 mg in a sitting (amounts higher than this have not been studied) does not lead to excessive fluid loss at rest (7). Additional research has found that 6 mg caffeine per kg body mass consumed during exercise in the heat did not influence fluid balance (8). Caffeine is considered safe and should not have a negative effect on fluid balance (9). That said, individual responses to caffeine vary tremendously because of genetics, so until you know your limits, be mindful of your caffeine intake. Caffeine can cause anxiety or jitteriness, especially in large doses (10, 11). Caffeine is completely absorbed within 45 minutes, although its effects peak anywhere between 15 and 120 minutes. The half-life of caffeine—that is, the amount of time it takes for caffeine concentration to decrease by half—is between 1.5 and 9.5 hours, a wide range that can be affected by several factors, including oral contraceptives, obesity, smoking, altitude, genetics, and intake of other stimulants (12). Although some research suggests that caffeine improves reaction time, attention, and vigilance after sleep deprivation, other research suggests that caffeine has limited potential to reduce errors that result from sleep loss (13, 14). Therefore, caffeine might help you study, but it may also do more harm than good if it interferes with sleep.

loss. Also during dehydration, stretch receptors in the aorta and carotid arteries detect a decrease in blood pressure and signal antidiuretic hormone (ADH) release to increase the amount of water absorbed by the kidneys, which helps maintain blood volume and, in turn, sufficient blood pressure for adequate blood delivery to tissue (1).

> **? DO YOU KNOW?**
>
> Dehydration might reach a 2 to 3 percent decrease in body weight before you feel thirsty. At this point, especially in the heat, athletic performance might already be compromised.

When blood volume is higher than normal, stretch receptors in the heart send a signal inhibiting ADH release. The thirst mechanism is inhibited, and the kidneys excrete more water.

Dehydration and Hypohydration

Whereas dehydration refers to the process of losing body water, **hypohydration** is the uncompensated loss of body water (18). Depending on the amount of body fluid lost, hypohydration can be mild, moderate, or severe. Symptoms of mild to moderate hypohydration include thirst, dry mouth, low urine production, dry and cool skin, headache, muscle cramps, and dark urine (not to be confused with bright yellow or orange urine from B vitamins, carotene, or certain medications). Signs and symptoms of severe hypohydration include the following:

- Increased core body temperature
- Decreased blood pressure (hypotension)
- Decreased sweat rate
- Rapid breathing
- Fast heartbeat
- Dizziness or lightheadedness
- Irritability
- Confusion
- Lack of urination
- Sunken eyes
- Shock
- Unconsciousness
- Delirium
- Dry, wrinkled skin that doesn't bounce back quickly when pinched
- Reduced stroke volume and cardiac output
- Reduced blood flow to muscles
- Exacerbated symptomatic exertional **rhabdomyolysis** (serious muscle injury)
- Increased risk of heat stroke and death (1, 19-22)

> **PUTTING IT INTO PERSPECTIVE**
>
> ### CAN I USE DIURETICS, DETOXES, OR CLEANSES TO LOSE WEIGHT QUICKLY?
>
> Diuretics increase urine production, so you lose water weight, temporarily. As soon as you rehydrate, you gain the weight back. Many detoxes and cleanses claim to remove toxins from your body, causing you to lose weight. Typical approaches include one or more of the following:
>
> › Consuming juice only or a liquid diet for several days
> › Laxatives, enemas, or colonics
> › Various dietary supplements that increase urine production
>
> No concrete evidence suggests that typical detoxes and cleanses remove toxins or improve health. If the detox or cleanse diet or program is lower in calories, compared with what you typically consume, you might lose weight. According to the FDA and the Federal Trade Commission, some detox or cleansing products or programs can be harmful. Both agencies have taken action against several companies for selling illegal and potentially harmful ingredients, making false claims suggesting that their products could treat serious diseases, or promoting unapproved uses of medical devices for colon cleanses. Other issues identified include the following:
>
> › Unpasteurized juices might contain harmful bacteria (pasteurization kills bacteria) that could make people sick, particularly those with weakened immune systems, the elderly, and children.
> › Because of high levels of oxalate, high intake of juice could be harmful for those with kidney disease.
> › Laxatives can lead to diarrhea, dehydration, electrolyte imbalances, and dependence.
> › Anyone with diabetes could experience serious side effects resulting from an imbalance between prescribed medication and diet, causing low blood sugar.
> › Fasting and very low-calorie diets could lead to headaches, fainting, weakness, dehydration, and other issues (17).
>
> In chapter 13 we look at safe and effective strategies for losing weight.

During exercise, hypohydration occurs when fluid intake doesn't match water lost through sweat (25). Risk for hypohydration is greater in hot, humid environments and at altitude (26-28). Clothing, equipment, heat acclimatization, exercise intensity, exercise duration, body size, and individual variations in sweat rates all affect risk of hypohydration (25). With repeated exposures to hot environments, the body adapts to heat stress by normalizing cardiac output and stroke volume and conserving sodium. These adaptations help reduce the risk for heat-related illness.

Because of larger body size, equipment, and exercising outdoors in the heat, American football players, particularly linemen, have an increased risk of dehydration (19). A study in NFL players found that smaller players lost significantly less fluid through sweat during practice than larger players.

Sickle cell trait, cystic fibrosis, diabetes medications, diuretics, and laxatives increase risk of dehydration. Children and the elderly also have an increased risk of dehydration (29, 30).

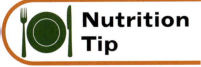

Nutrition Tip

Your hydration level might affect your ability to study and do well on tests. A body water loss of just 1 to 2 percent (1.5–3 lb for a 150 lb person [0.7–1.4 kg for a 68 kg person]) can impair concentration and short-term memory, while increasing reaction time, moodiness, and anxiety (23, 24).

> **REFLECTION TIME**
>
> **WILL SUPPLEMENTS MAKE ME DEHYDRATED?**
>
> Certain ingredients commonly found in detox products, cleanses, and weight-loss supplements will increase water lost through urine. Some of these products include uva ursi, dandelion (*Taraxacum officinale*), burdock root, horsetail, and hawthorn. Although many people believe creatine increases dehydration, no research supports this view (31, 32).

Several studies suggest that children are at greater risk than adults for dehydration and heat illness. Children have more body surface area relative to their body weight, leading to greater heat gain from the environment. They have a lower sweat rate and thus a decreased ability to dissipate heat through sweat (though this conserves body water) and higher skin temperature. Children also take longer to acclimatize to heat (25, 33-35). Some studies suggest that children rehydrate as well as, if not better than, adults (36-39), whereas other studies show that children, like adults, do not drink enough to replace fluid losses adequately in warm temperatures, even when they have sufficient access to fluids (38, 40, 41). Sweat sodium concentration is lower in children than in adults, however, a factor that may help children retain fluid (42). Signs and symptoms of heat illness are presented in figure 8.5.

Older adults do not have a sensitive thirst mechanism, so they generally drink less fluid than younger adults. In addition, the kidneys do not conserve water as well with age. Older people on certain medications might have increased fluid requirements or increased fluid losses. Some elderly people have limited access to food and fluids because of impaired motor skills, injuries, diseases, or surgeries that limit mobility. All these factors put the elderly at greater risk for heat stress, dehydration, and hypohydration.

Hyperhydration

Hyperhydration, sometimes referred to as overhydration or water intoxication, is an excess of total body water resulting from excessive intake of low- or no-sodium fluids, such as water (1). Hyperhydration is rare in healthy individuals. Those with heart, kidney, or liver disease, as well as people who have damage to the thirst mechanism, have an increased risk of hyperhydration because of the kidneys' reduced ability to excrete excess water. Athletes, particularly those competing in prolonged endurance events and consuming only water or low-sodium beverages, might also be at risk for hyperhydration (47).

Signs and symptoms of hyperhydration (48, 49)

Confusion
Inattentiveness
Blurred vision
Muscle cramps or twitching
Poor coordination
Nausea or vomiting
Rapid breathing
Acute weight gain
Weakness
Paralysis

Hyperhydration can result in cellular edema and hyponatremia, which is a dangerously low blood sodium level, defined by plasma sodium below 135 mmol/L (1). When blood sodium levels fall below 125 mmol/L, a person might experience intracellular swelling, headaches, nausea, vomiting, muscle cramps, swollen hands and feet, restlessness, and disorientation. When blood sodium drops below 120 mmol/L, risk of developing cerebral edema, seizures, coma, brainstem herniation, respiratory arrest, and death increases (21, 50-52). Hyponatremia can occur during an event or up to 24 hours afterward. In athletes, hyponatremia might result from high water intake during prolonged endurance or ultraendurance events, particularly for athletes with slower race times (52). Because slower athletes take a longer time to complete a race, they have more time to overconsume water or low- or no-sodium sports drinks, which will increase their risk of developing hyponatremia.

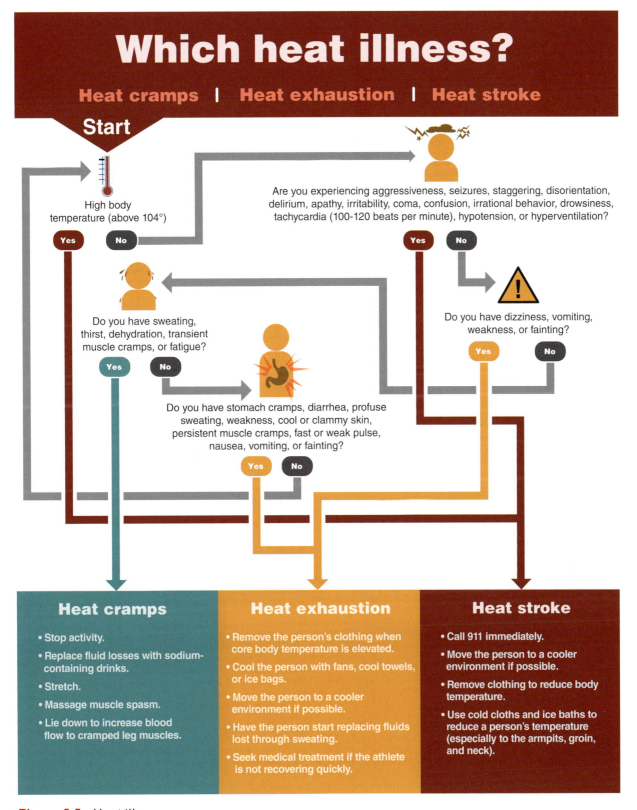

Figure 8.5 Heat illness.
Based on Binkley (2002).

Signs and symptoms of hyponatremia
Core body temperature less than 40 degrees Celsius (104 degrees Fahrenheit) during or following exercise
Nausea
Vomiting
Swelling of the hands and feet
Low blood sodium level
Progressive headache
Confusion
Lethargy
Altered state of consciousness
Apathy

PUTTING IT INTO PERSPECTIVE

WHY DOES ALCOHOL GIVE YOU A HANGOVER?

We all know that drinking too much alcohol can lead to a hangover. But why? And how can we prevent it? Hangover symptoms include fatigue, headache, poor sleep, thirst, nausea or vomiting, dizziness, and sensitivity to light, among others. Unfortunately, the mechanisms that lead to a hangover are not entirely clear. Although alcohol causes hangovers, there appears to be no way to prevent them other than the obvious—not drinking or drinking less. But among the factors that can reduce the severity of a hangover, two are in our control: getting enough sleep and not smoking (44).

In addition to causing hangovers, an acute bout of heavy alcohol consumption can harm the body in other ways. Alcohol decreases the amount of ADH produced, leading to a larger volume of urine and increased dehydration (45). Alcohol shrinks and disrupts brain tissue, throwing neurotransmitters off course, so you feel sleepy and function in slow motion—both physically and verbally. A single night of heavy drinking can also compromise your immune system, decreasing the ability of white blood cells to handle pathogens (46).

To prevent or reduce some of the negative side effects of overdrinking, try these strategies for drinking less. Know how much alcohol is in your drink (figure 8.6) and alter your pace accordingly. Drink a glass of water after each alcoholic drink. Eat something—eating slows the absorption of alcohol so that you have more time to metabolize what you are drinking. Also, for academic performance, don't drink, or at least limit drinking, the night before tests, exams, or days of intense studying.

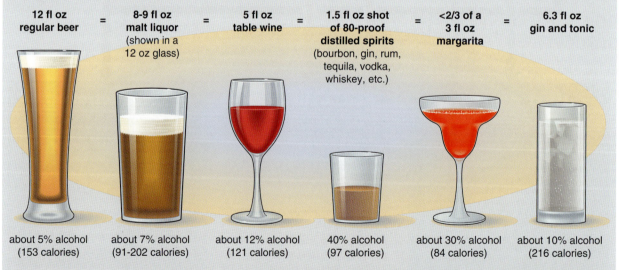

Figure 8.6 Percent alcohol by volume in alcoholic beverages. To find out the amount of alcohol in a drink, multiply the percent alcohol by the volume of the drink. Each one of the drinks pictured contains 0.6 ounce (18 ml) of alcohol. Interactive calculators to help you determine both the caloric content and amount of alcohol in various drinks are available online.

Adapted from National Institute on Alcohol Abuse and Alcoholism (2010).

Pulmonary edema

Cerebral edema

Seizures

Rhabdomyolysis (skeletal muscle injury)

Coma

Based on Coris (2004); Sawka et al. (2007); U.S. Institute of Medicine (2005).

ELECTROLYTES

Electrolytes are essential for muscle contraction and nerve conduction, so an electrolyte imbalance could certainly impair athletic performance (19, 21). **Electrolytes** lost in sweat include sodium, chloride, potassium, calcium, and magnesium (figure 8.7) (21).

Because of the high amount lost through sweat, sodium losses are the greatest concern, ranging from 230 to greater than 2,277 mg/L (10 to 99 mEq/L), followed by chloride, which is lost along with sodium (1, 19, 21). Sodium influences fluid regulation by helping the body retain more of the fluid consumed (less fluid consumed is lost through urine) (53). With greater sodium losses, risk of muscle cramping increases (54, 55). Athletes who exercise intensely or for several hours and hydrate excessively with only water or a no- or low-sodium beverage can dilute their blood sodium levels, increasing risk of cramping and possibly developing hyponatremia (21, 50, 51). To avoid hyponatremia, fluid intake shouldn't exceed sweat losses, and athletes should consume sodium in food or sports drinks (21, 56).

Hypernatremia, elevated blood sodium, is defined as a blood sodium concentration greater than 145 mmol/L. Hypernatremia is typically associated with dehydration and can be extremely dangerous, even causing death (57, 58).

Some sports drinks provide very small amounts of potassium, but others provide no potassium. In a healthy person, blood potassium is well regulated. High doses of supplemental potassium can be extremely dangerous, possibly fatal (1).

Calcium is lost in sweat in very small quantities. When blood calcium levels drop, the body can pull calcium from bone tissue to maintain blood calcium within a tight range. Although magnesium is lost in sweat and urine during exercise, it is redistributed in the body to accommodate metabolic needs (59). In addition, the average amount of magnesium lost through sweat, approximately 10 mg/L, is a tiny fraction of a person's magnesium needs each day (240–420 mg/day for those 9 years old and up, depending on life stage) (21, 60).

❓ DO YOU KNOW?

Sodium is the primary electrolyte lost through sweat. Increased sodium losses can increase an athlete's risk of cramping, particularly when combined with substantial fluid losses.

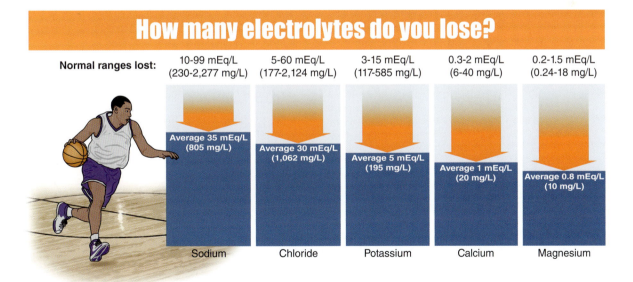

Figure 8.7 Average amounts of electrolytes lost through sweat.
Data from Coris (2004); American College of Sports (2007); Institute of Medicine (2005).

WATER, ELECTROLYTES, AND EXERCISE PERFORMANCE

During exercise, muscular contractions produce heat, which must be dissipated through sweat to help cool skin and body temperature. When fluids are consumed to maintain normal body water (euhydration), sweating remains an effective compensation for increased core temperatures. But as discussed earlier, thirst lags behind fluid needs. A 2 to 3 percent loss in body mass from fluid may have to occur before thirst kicks in (40). Thus, thirst might not be a sufficient stimulus to prevent significant dehydration during exercise, particularly in hot, humid conditions (figure 8.8) (25). If sweat losses are not replaced with fluid, hypohydration will lead to a decrease in sweat rate and evaporative heat loss, an increase in core body temperature, a drop in blood volume, a decrease in blood pressure, and cardiovascular strain, as well as altered metabolic and central nervous system functioning (18, 61). Factors increasing dehydration risk include wearing multiple layers of clothing or protective equipment (pads, helmets); heat; humidity; participating in multiple practices per day; intentional dehydration; and other unsafe weight-loss practices, including diuretics, using the sauna, manipulating water and sodium balance to "make weight," excessive spitting, self-induced vomiting, laxative abuse, and inappropriate use of thermogenic aids (compounds that purportedly increase calorie burning) (20, 62-67).

Hypohydration of less than 1 percent of pretraining body weight is not likely to have a negative effect on performance, unless the athlete begins training with a significant fluid deficit (68). Sweat losses reaching 1 to 3 percent body weight loss can increase core body temperature and sweat losses of 2 percent or more, especially in the heat, can negatively affect athletic performance by increasing fatigue; decreasing motivation; impairing attention, psychomotor, and immediate memory skills; decreasing sprint performance; increasing rate of perceived exertion; and impairing neuromuscular control, accuracy, power, strength, and muscular endurance (26, 69-77). Significant fluid deficits may result from poor hydration practices such as inadequate rehydration following exercise or alcohol consumption the night before an early morning practice.

In endurance-trained cyclists, dehydration of 4 percent of body weight in the heat decreased blood flow to muscles (20). Cardiac output, sweat production, and blood flow to skin and muscle decrease when sweat fluid losses rise to 6 to 10 percent of body weight, while risk for heat illness increases (18, 19, 21, 78).

Many athletes and recreational exercisers start training in a hypohydrated state, making it

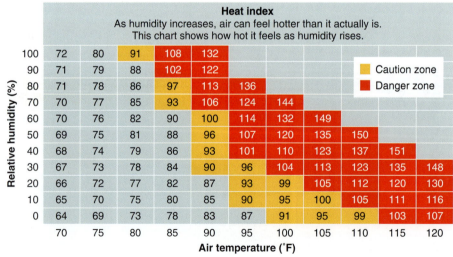

Figure 8.8 The heat index is a measure of how hot it really feels outside when humidity is taken into account along with temperature.

Reprinted by permission from C.B. Corbin, G.C. Le Masurier, and K.E. McConnell, *Fitness for Life*, 6th ed. (Champaign, IL: Human Kinetics, 2014), 76.

difficult to achieve euhydration during training (56, 67, 68, 79-81). A study in NCAA Division I athletes found that 66 percent started practice in a hypohydrated state and 13 percent in a significantly hypohydrated state as measured by urine specific gravity (USG). USG is a tool used to assess hydration status by measuring the concentration of particles in urine (82). Additional research studies found that many teenage male and female tennis players, female Canadian junior elite soccer athletes, and more than 50 percent of the athletes on Canada's junior men's hockey team began practice in a hypohydrated state (65, 68, 83). Pro indoor and outdoor athletes follow similar patterns as younger athletes—many start in a hypohydrated state (56).

Starting in a hypohydrated state can be especially detrimental in athletes who undergo large fluid losses during exercise. Yet many athletes start in a hypohydrated state. For instance, a study examining 29 NBA players during indoor summer league competition found that 52 percent started the game in a hypohydrated state and 5 players lost more than 2 percent body mass (measured before the game) during the game. When starting in a hypohydrated state, athletes cannot compensate for pregame hypohydration during the game (56). Figure 8.9 illustrates how basketball performance suffered as dehydration increased.

Available data show that fluid losses during exercise typically range from 0.3 to over 4.6 L/h in athletes (21, 56). Losing over 3 liters per hour is not common and is typically associated with extreme circumstances such as hot and humid environments, high exercise intensity, or large body mass (84). But sweat rate varies between sports not only because of the nature of the sport but also because of athlete body size, equipment, environmental conditions, and so on. The highest sweat fluid losses are reported for American football players followed by endurance athletes, basketball players, soccer players, and baseball players (85). Significant hypohydration (>2% loss of body weight), however, has been most reported in soccer players, whereas sports with high sweat rates generally report mild fluid disturbances (participants may sweat a lot but they make up for sweat losses by drinking). These findings suggest that many sports offer sufficient drinking opportunities to help offset sweat losses but this is not the case for soccer (85).

Even though a mere 2 percent loss of body mass due to uncompensated sweat losses led to skill decline in basketball players, higher levels of hypohydration, a 3 to 4 percent loss of body mass, which is not routinely observed, is more likely to impair cognition, technical skill, and physical performance in team sport athletes, particularly in the heat. Team sports are defined as those characterized by intermittent bursts of high-intensity exercise over 1 to 2 hours. Performance is also more likely to decline when dehydration is due to heat stress from the environment or high-intensity exercise. Across studies, higher levels of perceived

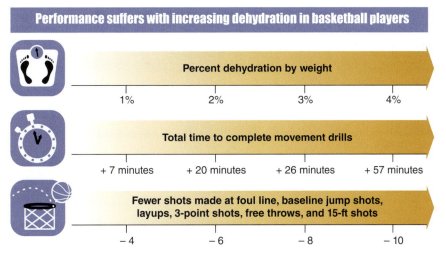

Figure 8.9 Skill decreases in basketball with progressive dehydration.
Data from Baker (2007).

exertion (exercise feels harder than it really is) and higher subjective ratings of fatigue accompany hypohydration in team sports and therefore may, in part, explain performance impairments due to hypohydration. In endurance athletes the threshold is lower; hypohydration of greater than 2 percent can impair performance (85).

Substantial sweat sodium losses can increase an athlete's risk of muscle cramping (55), poor performance, and, when combined with overhydration, hyponatremia (21, 50-52). A study in NCAA Division I football players found that sweat sodium losses were two times higher in those with a history of heat cramps compared with age-, weight-, race-, and position-matched players who had never cramped (54). Sweat sodium losses are generally expressed in g/L; the range reported in the literature is from 230 to greater than 2,277 mg/L (10 to 99 mEq/L), followed by chloride, which is lost along with sodium (1, 19, 21). This can mean that substantial sweat sodium losses can occur in athletes. For instance, a study in hockey players found that those in the American Hockey League lost 1.68 ± 0.74 grams of sodium per hour (86). See figure 8.10 for sweat sodium losses in NFL players and figure 8.11 for a sample hydration plan based on estimated hydration needs and measured sweat losses. For reference, *Dietary Guidelines* recommends that people limit their sodium intake to 2.3 grams per day.

In addition to the importance of hydrating before and during exercise, rehydrating after

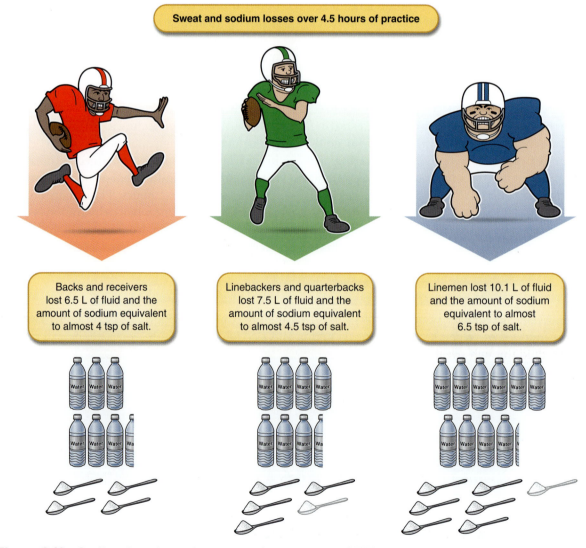

Figure 8.10 Sodium lost through sweat in three groups of NFL players over 4.5 hours of practice in the heat.

AI for sedentary men in moderate climates: 125 ounces (3.7 L)/day.

81% of this is typically from fluid (the rest is from food): 101 ounces (3.0 L) from fluid.

Incorporate this amount of fluid during the day and add additional fluid for practice and postpractice weight loss. Measure USG the next day and adjust this plan accordingly.

Prepractice weight: 301.8 lb

Postpractice weight: 294.4 lb

Weight lost during a 50-minute practice: 7.4 lb

% dehydration (7.4/301.8 × 100): 2.5%

Water consumed during practice: 36 ounces (1.1 L)

Sweat loss [(7.4 × 16) + 36]: 134 ounces (4.0 L)

Sweat rate: 4.8 L/h (161 oz/h)

Sweat sodium loss: 1,187 mg/L; 5,653 mg/h

Breakfast (7 a.m.)
- 8 oz (240 ml) of 100% orange juice
- 8 oz (240ml) of water

Meetings and lifting weights
- 16 oz (480 ml) of a sports drink
- Postlift shake containing 10 oz (300 ml) of milk

Lunch (11 a.m.)
- 8 oz (240 ml) of water
- 8 oz (240 ml) of a sports drink

Practice (1–2:30 p.m.)
Drink 1.5 liter per hour to start and gradually move up to 2 liters per hour (if tolerated) and then 2.5 liters per hour (if the athlete can handle this amount; be sure to include electrolytes).

Note: Because of his extreme fluid losses, this athlete will not be able to make up for much more than 2.5 liters per hour (if he can even get to this amount because it depends on his tolerance and the number of fluid breaks that players are given during practice) without getting an upset stomach.

Postpractice
Drink 20 to 24 oz (600 to 720 ml) of fluid in the form of a sports drink, water, and carbohydrate- and protein-rich shake for every pound (0.5 kg) loss. This amount may not be entirely feasible at first given his extreme fluid losses. When he dials in his hydration and electrolyte plan during practice, he will not lose as much fluid through sweat.

Postpractice meetings
Drink 32 oz (950 ml) of fluid.

Dinner
Drink 20 oz (600 ml) of fluid before, during, or after dinner.

Evening
Drink a 10 oz (300 ml) shake before bed and 6 oz (180 ml) of water.

Note: If the calculated ideal amount of fluid is too much for an athlete to drink, make sure they do not force drink fluid because this method may have the unintentional effect of decreasing the amount of food they eat and may potentially lead to stomach upset during practice.

Figure 8.11 NFL player hydration plan in season.

exercise takes time. In one small study, subjects had their food and fluid intake restricted and exercised in moderate heat to achieve hypohydration by 0 percent, 3 percent, 5 percent, and 7 percent of their body weight on 4 separate trials (each subject experienced each level of dehydration). For a period of 1 hour afterward, they were allowed to drink as much as they wanted. All subjects didn't consume enough fluid during this time to rehydrate back to baseline body weight, suggesting that adequate rehydration after hypohydration takes time, even when subjects have access to plenty of fluid (87).

Athletes should drink enough fluid to prevent water weight losses exceeding 2 percent of body weight, while also restoring electrolytes lost through sweat to prevent adverse effects on health and athletic performance. In addition, restoring fluid intake after exercise and before the next training session is important (21). Given the wide range of fluid and electrolyte losses through sweat, all athletes should have their own individualized hydration plan. The first step to developing an individualized hydration plan is an assessment of daily hydration status, as well as fluid and electrolyte losses during exercise.

HYDRATION ASSESSMENT

Hydration status can be measured in several ways, varying in cost, ease of use, and ability to detect small changes in hydration (16). No measurement method is perfect for all situations, although plasma osmolality is generally considered the most effective overall (1, 89). Plasma osmolality measures the concentration of solutes in the blood. When an athlete sweats, plasma volume and extracellular water decrease with fluid losses, while plasma osmolality increases (more fluid is lost than solutes). Plasma osmolality alters with acute changes in hydration status (1). In sport settings, commonly used measures of hydration status include urine osmolality (UOsmol), USG, changes in body weight, sweat patches, and bioelectrical impedance analysis (89). Urine markers, including UOsmol and USG, and serum osmolality measure the concentration of particles in urine and serum, respectively. Both are sensitive (effective) indicators of hydration status (1). As discussed earlier, USG measures the concentration of particles in urine and provides an assessment of hydration status and kidney function (82). Although serum osmolality is considered the gold standard for measuring hydration status in healthy people, it is not practical to use outside a clinical setting (88). USG is easy to use, inexpensive, and practical. USG and UOsmol should be measured first thing in the morning; values may be misleading during acute periods of dehydration (as can happen when athletes sweat profusely during exercise) or if urine is assessed after rehydration (16, 21). Both devices show delayed dehydration-related changes (16). If dehydrated athletes consume a large volume of hypotonic fluid, they will produce a large volume of urine before becoming adequately rehydrated (euhydration). During this period of rehydration, USG and UOsmol are misleading. Both values will indicate that athletes have achieved euhydration when in fact they are still dehydrated (21, 90). UOsmol is misleading and a poor indicator of hydration for at least 6 hours after exercise (91). USG values increase with increasing water deficit, although this varies considerably among individuals. USG values cannot predict the extent of water deficit (1). See table 8.2 for more information on meas-

PUTTING IT INTO PERSPECTIVE

DO RECREATIONAL ATHLETES NEED MORE SALT DURING TRAINING AND COMPETITION?

Hyponatremia occurs more often in recreational athletes than in competitive athletes, which suggests that recreational athletes need to be more cognizant of their fluid and sodium intake. Staying well hydrated, yet not overhydrated, and replacing electrolytes will help you perform your best and make the most of your workout. All athletes, no matter their level of competition, should know the basics of dehydration, hyponatremia, and sodium replenishment.

Table 8.2 Measuring Hydration With USG

USG value	Status	% body weight change from pretraining weight*
1.001–1.012	May indicate overhydration	Weighing more posttraining as compared with pretraining indicates overhydration.
<1.020	Euhydration	0%-2%
1.020–1.030	Hypohydration	>2% of body mass
>1.030	Severe hypohydration	>5% body mass

*Note that USG does not correspond to or predict body weight changes.
Some studies consider 1.010 to 1.020 as minimal dehydration and less than 1.010 as euhydration. Others consider 1.001 to 1.010 as indicative of possible overhydration.
Both USG and percent body weight change (from a state of euhydration) can be used to assess hydration status, although USG values do not correspond to or predict percent changes in body weight (for example, a USG of 1.020 does not correspond to a 3%–5% change in weight).
Data from Armstrong (1994); Popowski (2001).

uring hydration with USG. Note that assessing urine at one point in time during the day does not necessarily reflect 24-hour hydration status (92).

A wide range of values is normal for urine UOsmol—50 to 1,200 mOsmol/L (94). Given this range, increasing urine UOsmol can be used to determine increasing levels of dehydration, although it is not considered a good indicator of hydration status (1, 95, 96).

> **? DO YOU KNOW?**
> USG testing is often part of routine testing of urine samples. The next time you provide a urine sample at your physician's office, check the report for your USG value. USG is also measured during drug testing to determine if athletes have attempted to manipulate the test by overhydrating in an attempt to dilute their urine.

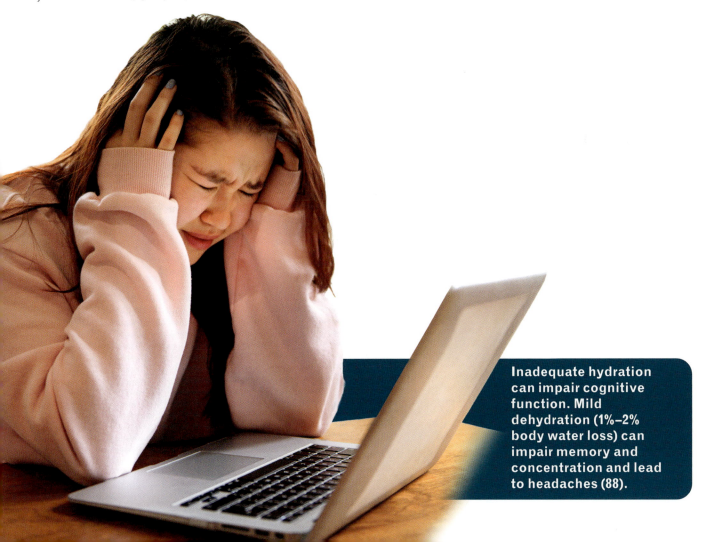

Inadequate hydration can impair cognitive function. Mild dehydration (1%–2% body water loss) can impair memory and concentration and lead to headaches (88).

Many athletes underestimate their sweat losses by 50 percent or more. Heavier sweaters are more likely to underestimate sweat fluid losses and underestimate them to a greater extent (97). Measuring changes in weight can help identify athletes who are dehydrated. Acute changes in body weight often reflect fluid fluctuations in athletes who are in a state of caloric balance—that is, consuming enough calories each day to maintain their weight. Athletes can estimate day-to-day hydration changes by weighing in the nude or in minimal clothing each morning after using the bathroom and before eating or drinking. See figure 8.12 for accurately estimating sweat losses through changes in body weight. Athletes can estimate sweat-related fluid losses, and therefore sweat rate, by weighing pre- and postworkout (21, 98). Although body weight changes can be used to estimate acute changes in hydration status, over a longer period, food intake, bowel movements, and alterations in body composition will confound the use of weight as an indicator of changes in hydration status (98).

Athletes are sometimes advised to check their urine color (figure 8.13) to assess their hydration status; darker urine is more concentrated with solutes and a sign of dehydration or hypohydration, whereas pale yellow urine is less concentrated and considered a sign of euhydration. Urine color charts are an effective tool that athletes can use to assess their hydration status. But urine color should be assessed after a urine sample is collected in a clear container and then evaluated in adequate light. Urine should not be assessed in

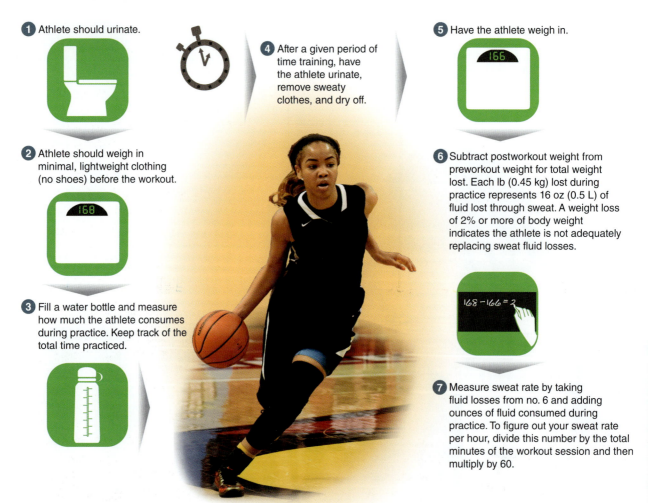

Figure 8.12 Estimating sweat losses through weight changes.

Urine color chart

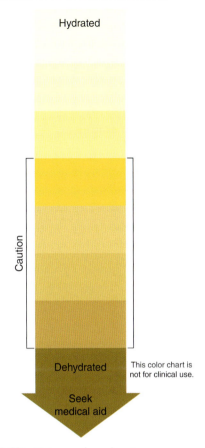

Figure 8.13 Urine color chart.

a toilet bowl because the urine sample is diluted with water and therefore it cannot be compared with a urine color chart (93).

Anyone using a urine color chart should understand that assessing urine color is subjective; it can be imprecise and open to interpretation (1, 21). Several food ingredients, nutrients, and medications can influence the color of urine (82, 99, 100), as can phase of the menstrual cycle, acute changes in body weight, environmental conditions, and time of day when urine is collected (88). Also, urine color is not an accurate measure for at least 6 hours postexercise (91).

Urine will be pale in color during the immediate rehydration period after dehydration, even though the athlete is still dehydrated (21). See table 8.3 for more information on factors influencing urine color.

Sweat patches are placed on an athlete's forearm or another part of the body to collect fluid and electrolyte losses. These patches are easy to use and provide valuable information for developing an individualized hydration and electrolyte (sodium chloride) plan. Bioelectrical impedance analysis (BIA) is an easy, quick method of assessing hydration status. BIA uses a frequency passed through the skin. There is greater resistance to the current when water and electrolyte content in tis-

Table 8.3 Common Causes of Changes in Urine Color

Color or appearance	Medical reasons	Potential food and drug causes
Pale yellow or clear	• Hyperhydration • Diabetes insipidus	Diuretics Alcohol consumption Mannitol
Cloudy	• UTI (urine might also smell bad) • Phosphaturia (excess phosphorus in urine) • Chyluria (presence of a milky white lymphatic fluid) • Renal disease • Hyperoxaluria (recurrent kidney and bladder stones)	Diet high in purine-rich foods such as anchovies, asparagus, liver, mushrooms, herring, gravy, sweetbreads, game meats, dried beans and peas, brains, beef kidneys, mackerel, muscles, sardines, or scallops

Milky	• Bacteria (UTI)
	• Substances in urine:
	  • Crystals
	  • Lipids
	  • White or red blood cells
	  • Mucus
	• Chyluria (a tropical disease more common in poverty-stricken populations)
		No known food or drug causes

>continued

Table 8.3 >continued

Color or appearance	Medical reasons	Potential food and drug causes
Brown	• Bile pigments • Myoglobin (a protein that carries oxygen in heart and skeletal muscles)	• Fava beans • Antimalarial drugs • Antibiotics (Flagyl) • Medications to treat Parkinson's disease or UTIs
Dark brown	• Excess bilirubin in the urine leading to liver disorder such as acute viral hepatitis or cirrhosis • Muscle injury causing myoglobin (a protein found muscle) in urine; among the many types of muscle injury is rhabdomyolysis (rapid breakdown of muscle tissue leading to leakage of muscle contents into blood)	• Cascara (a plant used as a laxative) • Senna (a laxative) • Medications to treat Parkinson's disease or high blood pressure (methyldopa) • Medicine used to treat bacterial infections (metronidazole therapy)
Brownish black	• Bile pigments • Melanin • Methemoglobin	• Cascara • Certain drugs for Parkinson's disease • Certain antihypertensive medications • Senna
Green or blue	• Bilirubin • Medications to treat depression, ulcers, allergies (Phenergan) • Diuretics (triamterene) • UTI	• Food coloring (indigo carmine) • Methylene blue (used to treat UTI) • Diuretics (triamterene) • Antidepressants (amitriptyline) • Anti-inflammatory drugs (indomethacin)
Purple	Malabsorption and bacterial overgrowth syndromes	• No known food or drug causes • Purple tubing and bags in hospitals that can discolor urine in long-term catheterized patients
Orange or dark yellow	• Hypohydration (especially if dark, scanty urine is produced) • Bile pigments • Laxatives • Medications such as phenazopyridine, rifampin, warfarin, pyridium, phenothiazines	• Antibiotics used to treat bacterial infections (rifampicin) • Carrots • Cascara
Pink, red, or light brown	• Hemolytic anemia • Injury to the kidneys • Porphyria • Injury to the urinary tract or urinary tract disorders that lead to bleeding • Blood in urine • Medications such as phenolphthalein, rifampin (Rifadin)	• Beets, blackberries, rhubarb • Some food colorings • Senna, anthraquinone, and phenolphthalein-containing laxatives, doxorubicin, rifampin, and phenothiazine
Bright yellow	No known medical reasons	• Carrots • B vitamins

UTI = urinary tract infection

Based on Gerber and Brendler (2011); Raymond and Yarger (1988); Sharma and Hemal (2009); Simerville, Maxted, and Pahira (2005); U.S. Department of Agriculture (2013).

sues is higher (101). In euhydrated and chronically hyperhydrated or hypohydrated subjects, BIA provides a good estimate of total body water and hydration status (98, 102). But fluid shifts between intracellular and extracellular water during exercise, increased blood flow to working muscles and skin, and sweating can confound BIA measures in athletes. BIA is also independently influenced by water and electrolyte content, as well as by changes in electrolyte content in intracellular fluid and extracellular fluid. So, for instance, when plasma (extracellular fluid) sodium concentration increases, resistance decreases, which can also confound its use for estimating hydration status (98). For these reasons, BIA is not an accurate method for assessing hydration status in athletes because their hydration status changes frequently (1, 98). Table 8.4 presents methods for measuring hydration status.

Table 8.4 Measuring Hydration Status

Measure	Practicality	Advantages	Measures acute or chronic hydration status or both	Normal values	Higher than normal values may suggest	Lower than normal values may suggest
Total body water (based on dilution—a lab method)	Low	Accurate, reliable	Both	<2%	• Overhydration • Disease state	• Dehydration • Disease state
Plasma osmolality	Medium	Accurate, reliable	Both	290 mOsml/kg	• Dehydration • Diabetes • High blood sugar level • High level of nitrogen waste products in the blood • Hypernatremia • Stroke or head trauma resulting in decreased ADH secretion	• Hypothyroidism • Hyponatremia • Overhydration • Adrenal gland not working properly • ADH oversecretion • Conditions related to lung cancer
Urine-specific gravity	High	Easy to use	Chronic	<1.020	• Glycosuria • Alterations in ADH • Dehydration	• Overhydration • Diuretic use, diabetes, adrenal insufficiency, aldosteronism, impaired renal function
Urine osmolality	High	Variable—can be used to measure level of dehydration yet not a good measure of hydration status	Chronic	<700 mOsmol/L	• Heart failure • Dehydration • Renal artery stenosis • Shock • Sugar in the urine • Poor ADH secretion	• Overhydration • Damage to the kidneys • Kidney failure • Kidney infection
Body weight	High	Easy, quick	Both*	<1%–2%	Overhydration	Hypohydration

*Chronic changes (over a few days) can be estimated in an athlete in a state of caloric balance.

Based on Kavouras (2002); Sawka et al. (2007); Tilkian, Boudreau, and Tilkian (1995).

HYDRATION RECOMMENDATIONS FOR EXERCISE

Given the wide variety of conditions that affect sweat fluid losses—including climate, training or athletic event, clothing, equipment, acclimation, and individual differences in sweat rates and electrolyte losses—it is impossible to develop general fluid guidelines sufficient for all people in all situations. But the following research-based recommendations can be adjusted based on a thorough assessment of an individual's fluid and electrolyte losses in different environmental conditions.

Before Exercise

Many athletes and active people start training or exercise in a hypohydrated state, making it difficult to achieve euhydration during training (56, 67, 68, 80, 81). Thus, the preexercise goal is to achieve euhydration by prehydrating, when necessary, several hours before exercise to allow time for fluid absorption and urine production. If using USG, the measurement should read below 1.020 for the first morning void (21).

Four hours before exercise, athletes should slowly drink enough fluid to urinate approximately 5 to 10 ml/kg body weight (2–4 ml/lb) to allow sufficient time to void excess fluid (21, 103). The addition of sodium, through a sports drink or table salt, to a preworkout meal or snack will help the athlete retain more of the fluid consumed (104).

> **❓ DO YOU KNOW?**
> Athletes should start training or competition in a hydrated state, avoid losing more than 2 percent of body weight (through sweat loss) during exercise, and rehydrate completely after exercise before the next training session.

During Exercise

The average person loses approximately 0.3 liters per hour through insensible perspiration and sweating when sedentary (1). Sweat fluid losses during training range from 0.3 to over 4.6 liters per hour, and sodium losses range from 230 to 2,277 mg or more per liter of sweat. Given this variation, the best approach is to use an individualized hydration plan that helps limit fluid losses of greater than 2 percent, replenishes electrolyte losses, and avoids overhydration (21, 56). Most athletes can maintain adequate hydration by consuming 0.4 to 0.8 liters per hour (13–27 oz/h) of fluid. Athletes with high sweat rates (>1.2 L/h) or salty sweat or those exercising for more than 2 hours are more likely to have considerable sodium losses and should choose a beverage that contains sodium during exercise. A carbohydrate concentration of 6 to 8 percent might be ideal, because sports drinks containing more than 8 percent carbohydrate delay gastric emptying (i.e., how quickly the drink is emptied from the stomach), which could result in an upset stomach (21, 105). Cool, but not cold, beverages are recommended: 10 to 15 degrees Celsius (50–59 degrees Fahrenheit) (80).

> **❓ DO YOU KNOW?**
> When sports drinks are ingested at high rates during intense or prolonged exercise, athletes might consume more carbohydrate than their stomach can process quickly, which could result in an upset stomach.

A drink containing multiple types of carbohydrate, such as glucose and fructose or maltodextrin combined with fructose, can increase the speed of gastric emptying and thus decrease the risk of upset stomach (106). During prolonged periods of training, athletes can consume 30 to 60 grams of carbohydrate per hour to help sustain energy. Research, mainly conducted during long bouts of cycling, suggests that aerobic endurance athletes could increase total carbohydrate intake to 90 grams per hour if their sports drink contains multiple types of carbohydrate (107).

Children and Adolescents

A sports drink with flavor and sodium may increase drinking at one's pleasure. Children should be offered a choice of fluids so that they can decide which one they prefer (25).

The American Academy of Pediatrics suggests enforcing periodic drinking in children to ensure adequate fluid intake during exercise. Drinks should contain a sodium chloride concentration of 15 to 20 mmol/L (1 g per 2 pints), which has been shown to increase voluntary hydration by 90 percent when compared with unflavored water (41, 108, 109). According to the academy's guidelines

> children weighing 40 kg (88 lb) should drink 5 ounces (150 ml) of cold water or a flavored salted beverage every 20 minutes during practice, and

> adolescents weighing 60 kg (132 lb) should drink 9 ounces (270 ml) every 20 minutes, even if they do not feel thirsty.

Adults

Athletes should follow an individualized hydration plan. In general, a sports drinks should contain 20 to 30 mEq of sodium (460–690 mg, with chloride as the anion) per liter, 2 to 5 mEq of potassium (78–195 mg) per liter, and 5 to 10 percent of carbohydrate (110). Given the available literature on tennis players, recommendations specific to their sport suggest aiming for approximately 200 to 400 ml (approximately 7–14 oz) fluid per changeover, with some of their fluid coming from a carbohydrate and electrolyte sports drink (111).

All guidelines for children, adolescents, and adults might need to be adjusted to fit the needs of individual athletes.

After Exercise

Many athletes, whether competitive or recreational, finish exercising with a fluid deficit. They might continue sweating afterward and lose additional fluid through urine. For those reasons,

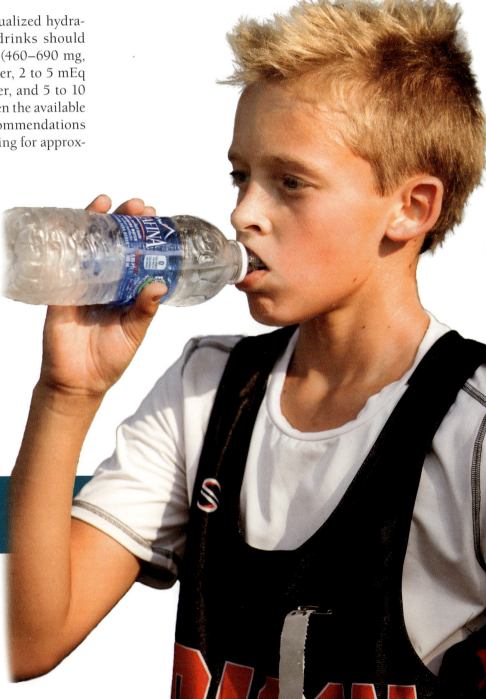

A child participating in any sport should have plenty of breaks to ensure proper hydration.

PUTTING IT INTO PERSPECTIVE

FACTORS THAT CONTRIBUTE TO GREATER FLUID CONSUMED

Given the importance of hydration and the potential adverse health effects that can result from dehydration, hypohydration, and heat illness, coaches and parents should create an environment that encourages fluid consumption. They can do this by providing access to fluids (both water and flavored sports drinks), scheduling breaks during training, and educating athletes and parents about the importance of hydration, while also providing instructions for maintaining optimal hydration (114).

the athlete needs more fluid than lost through sweat to replace total fluid losses and restore fluid balance. They should aim to consume 125 to 150 percent of the fluid deficit (20–24 oz per lb body weight lost or approximately 1.5 L fluid for each kg body weight lost). Plain water is not effective at restoring fluid balance during recovery (112). If sodium is not consumed with the beverage (or through food intake after exercise), much of the fluid consumed postexercise will lead to increased urine output (90). Sodium content of a postworkout drink should contain more sodium than the sodium content in sweat to restore fluid balance (this is often more than what is in a typical sport drink; 460–575 mg/L) (112). Therefore, sodium should be consumed in postworkout drinks, meals, or snacks both to replace sodium and to enhance rehydration. Additional salt can be added to foods when sodium losses are substantial (1, 21, 90). This strategy helps make up for increased urine production following consumption of a large volume of fluid (21, 113). In addition, adding carbohydrate (likely through food or fluid) enhances fluid retention (112).

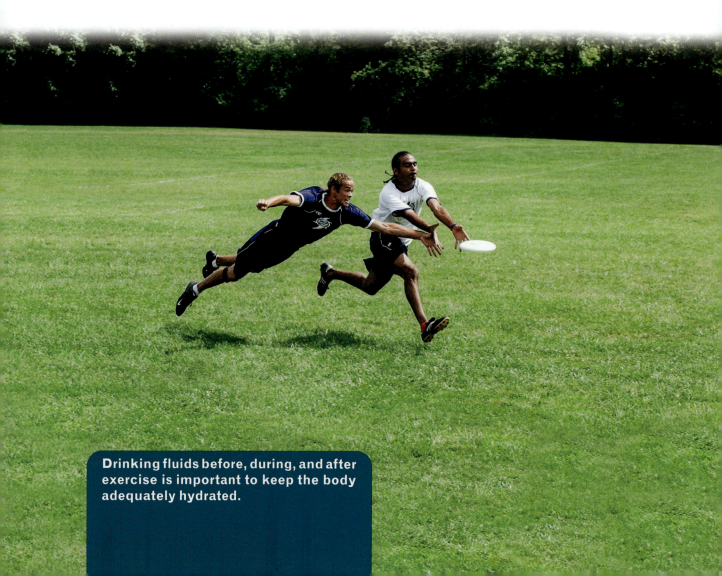

Drinking fluids before, during, and after exercise is important to keep the body adequately hydrated.

SUMMARY

Water and electrolytes are essential to health and athletic performance, but many factors affect hydration needs, so no one recommendation fits everyone. The AI can be used as guidance and adjusted accordingly based on individual needs. Daily hydration status, as well as hydration and electrolyte losses from activity, can be measured and used to develop individual hydration strategies to ensure adequate daily hydration and prevention of excessive loss of body fluid and sodium during exercise. In instances when hydration status is not measured (possible reasons include lack of measuring devices and sensitivity about body weight), the athlete's coach (or parent) must pay close attention to the athlete and educate them on frequency and quantity of urination, as well as symptoms of hypohydration. Despite access to fluids, many athletes and recreational exercisers start training in a hypohydrated state, lose significant quantities of sweat while training, and cannot quickly replace body fluid losses because of continued sweating and urinary losses postexercise.

FOR REVIEW

1. Why is body water important for athletic performance, exercise, and fitness?
2. Discuss the factors that affect a person's fluid needs.
3. Discuss the role of sodium in the body and its importance for athletic and exercise performance.
4. List the methods used to calculate sweat rate. Which methods are more accurate than others?
5. Discuss the symptoms associated with hyponatremia.
6. Which people are most at risk of developing hyponatremia? Why is their risk increased?

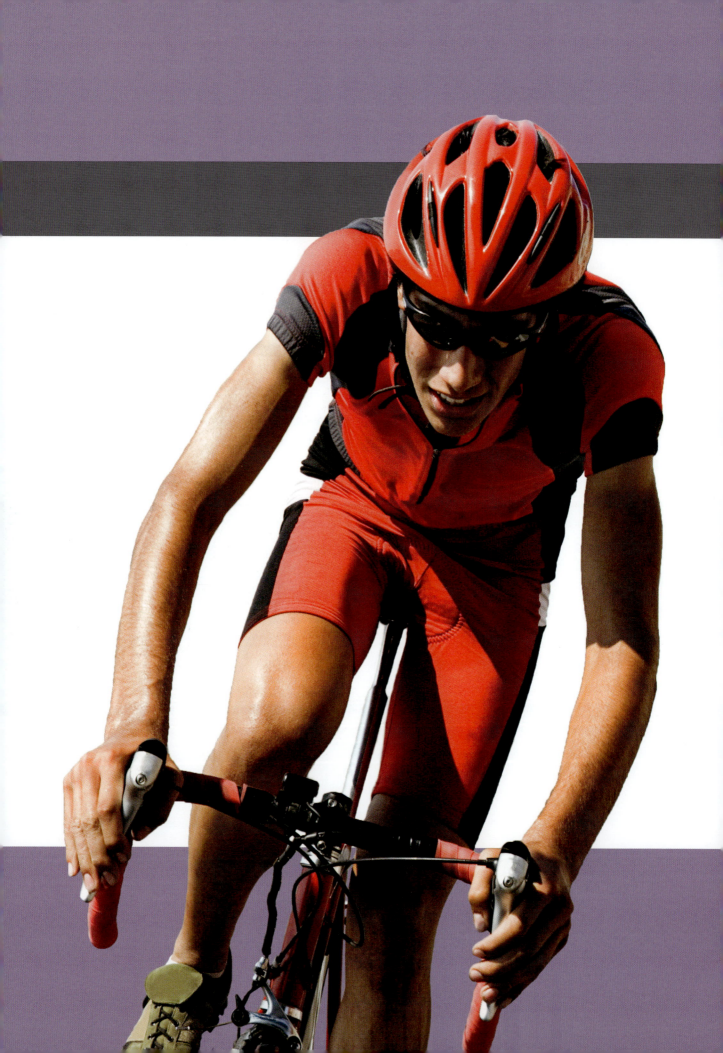

9

Nutritional Supplements and Other Substances Commonly Used in Sport

> **CHAPTER OBJECTIVES**
>
> After completing this chapter, you will be able to do the following:
>
> › Explain how dietary supplements are regulated by the FDA.
> › Describe the categories of claims used with dietary supplements.
> › Discuss the process for evaluating the safety and efficacy of dietary supplements.
> › Identify common supplements used in different sports and discuss their efficacy and safety.
> › Describe illegal and other drugs commonly used in sport and their consequences.
> › Discuss the effects of alcohol on sport performance.

People choose to take supplements for many reasons including but not limited to the following: to maintain or improve health, to boost energy levels, to meet macronutrient needs that accompany increased training demands, to enhance athletic performance, to improve recovery from training, to change body composition, and to compensate for nutrients not consumed in adequate amounts through intake of food and beverages (1-3). When used correctly, many dietary supplements can indeed support health, training, and athletic performance. But some dietary supplements are not beneficial, and some are harmful in certain circumstances (depending on a person's health, what else they are taking, and several other factors) (4-7). For athletes, poor manufacturing practices or intentional spiking of a supplement with a prescription drug or illegal substance could result in a positive drug test. In any case, both competitive athletes and others must ensure the safety of any dietary supplement they choose to take.

POPULARITY OF SUPPLEMENT USE IN SPORT

The prevalence of dietary supplement use among athletes is difficult to quantify because of insufficient studies, inconsistent methodology, poor research design, and a lack of homogeneity among published studies. An estimate of supplement use internationally ranges from 37 to 89 percent. The greatest use is seen among elite and older athletes, in which the specific age is defined by the sport (3). A review and meta-analysis reported the prevalence of dietary supplement use among athletes using data from 159 previously published studies (8). These data suggest that supplement use is higher among elite athletes compared with their nonelite counterparts; use is similar for men and women, with a few exceptions (men use more vitamin E, protein, and creatine, whereas women use more iron); prevalence of dietary supplements use has been relatively high over time; and a larger percentage of athletes use supplements compared with the general U.S. adult population.

The most commonly used supplements cited from this study include vitamins and minerals, amino acids and protein, creatine, herbal supplements, omega-3 fatty acids, caffeine, and energy drinks. Many more products are on the market, and new ones are being introduced on a regular basis. Note that many supplements are safe and some are effective in providing people—athletes and nonathletes alike—with the benefits they seek that are not gained through their regular eating habits or nutrition programs.

REGULATION OF DIETARY SUPPLEMENTS

Dietary supplements are regulated by the U.S. Food and Drug Administration (FDA) (13), whereas the **Federal Trade Commission (FTC)** (14) protects consumers by regulating potentially unfair, deceptive, or fraudulent practices in the marketplace. The Dietary Supplement Health and Education Act (DSHEA) of 1994 legally defined a dietary supplement as

> a product taken by mouth that contains a "dietary ingredient" intended to supplement the diet. The "dietary ingredients" in these products may include vitamins, minerals, herbs or other botanicals, amino acids, and substances such as enzymes, organ tissues,

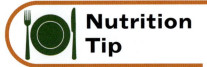

Nutrition Tip

Many supplements marketed for energy contain caffeine, but companies are not required to list the caffeine content on the label of dietary supplements (9). According to a study conducted by the United States Department of Agriculture, the caffeine content of dietary supplements ranged from 1 mg to more than 800 mg for a daily dose—800 mg is equivalent to approximately eight cups of coffee (8 oz of home brewed) (10, 11). Caffeine affects people in different ways, so consumers should use caution when taking a caffeine-containing supplement, especially if consuming other caffeinated foods or beverages (12). When taking supplements with caffeine, start slow, monitor your body's reaction, and proceed accordingly.

glandulars, and metabolites. Dietary supplements can also be extracts or concentrates, and may be found in many forms such as tablets, capsules, soft gels, gel caps, liquids, or powders. (13, 15)

If any of these compounds are in other forms, such as a nutrition bar, the information provided on the product label cannot represent the product as a conventional food and cannot imply that it can replace a meal or substitute for a diet composed of foods. Under this act, dietary supplements are regulated separately and under a set of regulations different from food and drugs (13).

A working group within the International Olympic Committee (IOC) who wrote a consensus statement on dietary supplements and the high-performance athlete, believe that the definition of a dietary supplement set forth by the FDA is not adequate because it does not factor in the quality of the diet. These authors defined a dietary supplement as "a food, food component, nutrient, or non-food compound that is purposefully ingested in addition to the habitually consumed diet with the aim of achieving a specific health and/or performance benefit." The IOC authors acknowledge that dietary supplements come in many forms such as enriched, fortified, and functional foods; single nutrients; food and products specifically created for athletes or those providing a convenient source of energy and nutrients; and multi-ingredient products (2).

The FDA does not approve dietary supplements for safety or effectiveness before these products reach the store shelves for purchase by the consumer. The manufacturer is responsible for ensuring that the Supplement Facts label and ingredient list are accurate, the dietary ingredients are safe for use as intended, and the amounts of each active ingredient matches the amount declared on the label. After a product is marketed and sold, the FDA is responsible for demonstrating that a dietary supplement is harmful or unsafe before taking action to restrict the use of the product or remove it from public purchase. Manufacturers and distributors of dietary supplements must record and investigate any reported adverse reactions from their product and forward any reports to the FDA. The FDA is able to review reported adverse reactions from manufacturer reports, or information reported by health care providers or consumers, to identify the potential presence of safety risks to the public. A safety alert or consumer advisory has been issued on some common products, including pure powdered caffeine, caffeinated energy drinks, red yeast rice, and botanicals added to conventional foods (11, 13, 16). The FDA website provides a complete list and updates (16).

Marketing Supplements

Supplement manufacturers are required to notify the FDA of their intention to sell a product if it contains a "new dietary ingredient." This term refers to an ingredient that meets the established DSHEA definition of a dietary ingredient and was not sold in the United States in a dietary supplement before October 15, 1994. If a manufacturer and distributor of the supplement intends to use a new ingredient, they are responsible for determining whether the ingredient meets this definition and demonstrating to the FDA that their proposed ingredient has a reasonable expectation of safety for use in their product, unless it has been recognized as a food substance and is present in the food supply. Any supplements that do not contain new ingredients do not need approval from the FDA before they are marketed and sold to the consumer (13).

Manufacturers can voluntarily provide information to the FDA or consumers about the safety and efficacy of their product, if they choose to do so (13). Each manufacturer can establish its own policy regarding this disclosure to either the FDA or its customers.

In June 2007 the FDA published comprehensive regulations for **current good manufacturing practices (GMPs)** for those who manufacture, package, or distribute dietary supplement products. These regulations focus on practices that ensure the identity, purity, quality, strength, and composition of dietary supplements. The existence of GMPs may help ensure that the ingredients on the label are present in listed quantities and that products are free from contaminants and impurities. These published GMPs do not govern marketing or claims made about the product, so the consumer must contact the manufacturer of a product if they want more information (13).

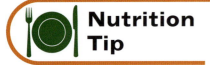

Nutrition Tip: The FDA and the National Institutes of Health's Office of Dietary Supplements provide research-based information about dietary supplements. If you are considering taking a supplement, visit the websites of these government organizations for basic information and useful tips (13, 15).

Supplement Facts Labels

Regulations control the information that must appear on the labels of dietary supplements. All supplement labels must include "a descriptive name of the product stating that it is a 'supplement'; the name and place of business of the manufacturer, packer, or distributor; a complete list of ingredients; and the net contents of the product." The FDA further requires that most dietary supplements have a Supplement Facts label on the product (figure 9.1). This label must list each dietary ingredient contained in the product; those ingredients not included in the label must be listed in the "other ingredients" statement printed beneath the label. Other ingredients may include the source of dietary ingredients, other food ingredients (e.g., water and sugar), additives, colors, preservatives, flavors, or other processing aids. FDA regulations do not limit a serving size or the amount of a nutrient or ingredient in a dietary supplement. The recommended serving size on the product label is determined by the manufacturer and does not require FDA approval (13, 17).

Dietary Supplement Claims

Manufacturers generally employ three types of claims with their dietary supplements (9, 17):

1. Nutrient content claims
2. Authorized health claims that meet the significant scientific agreement (SSA) standard
3. Structure or function claims

Nutrient Content Claims

Nutrient content claims describe the quantity of a nutrient in a product and can be used for both foods and dietary supplements. Common examples refer to calories, fat, sugar, and sodium. Other terms, such as "light" or "healthy," are also defined. Examples include "low-fat," "sugar-free," "low-calorie," "good source," and "high potency." Some of these terms compare the level of the nutrient in a product to the daily value (DV) for that nutrient (e.g., "excellent source"), whereas others may compare one product with another similar product (e.g., "reduced" or "more"). Detailed descriptions of FDA-approved nutrient content claims can be found on the FDA website (9, 13, 17). Any changes to existing terms or the addition of new terms appears on this website.

Authorized Health Claims That Meet the Significant Scientific Agreement (SSA) Standard

The second category of claims that the FDA oversees and issues regulations regarding the use of, in both foods and dietary supplements, is authorized health claims that meet the significant scientific agreement (SSA) standard (9, 13, 17). These claims

Figure 9.1 Supplement Facts label.

Supplement Facts
Serving Size: 1 capsule
Servings Per Container: 30

	Amount Per Serving	%DV
Ester C	50mg	83%
Vitamin E (dl-alpha tocopherol)	20IU	67%
Vitamin B6 (pyridoxine hci)	25mg	1250%
Vitamin B12 (cyanocobalamin)	25mcg	416%
Vitamin B1 (thiamine)	1.5mg	100%
Vitamin B2 (riboflavin)	1.5mg	88%
Aloe Vera Powder	50mg	-
Alpha Lipoic Acid	50mg	-
BioPerine Standardized Extract	1.5mg	-
Collagen Type II (from chicken)	250mg	-
CoQ10	10mg	-
Curcumin C3 Complex	25mg	-
Hyaluronic Acid	10mg	-

*Daily Value (DV) not established.

Other Ingredients: Vegetable Capsule (Hydroxypropyl Cellulose)

describe a relation between a nutrient or ingredient (component of food or dietary supplement) and reduced risk of a health-related condition or disease. Both components in this relationship must be present to be a health claim. To be an FDA authorized health claim, there must be SSA among leading, qualified experts in the field agreeing that the claim being made is supported by the available scientific evidence for the relationship being claimed. For example, the FDA-approved health claim regarding calcium and osteoporosis lists both components in its model claim: "Adequate calcium throughout life, as part of a well-balanced diet, may reduce the risk of osteoporosis." On the other hand, dietary guidance statements do not fulfill this requirement (e.g., regular fruit and vegetable consumption is good for health). For the FDA to approve a health claim for use on a food or supplement product, significant scientific agreement must support the proposed claim. A limited number of health claims have been approved for use. The complete list can be found on the FDA website (9, 13, 17). The site lists any new health claims that have been approved. Dietary supplement manufacturers cannot legally use any health claim not approved by the FDA. For example, manufacturers cannot promote or print on a label that the product is a treatment, prevention, or cure for a specific disease or condition.

Structure/Function Claims

The third category of claims related to foods and dietary supplements is called **structure/function claims**. Two claims are under the regulatory requirements of the DSHEA:

1. Claims of general well-being
2. Claims related to a nutrient deficiency disease

Structure/function claims may state how the product, nutrient, or ingredient intends to affect the normal structure or function within the body (e.g., calcium helps build strong bones) or how it acts to maintain a particular structure or function (e.g., fiber helps keep you regular; antioxidant nutrients help maintain cell integrity). Structure/function claims cannot explicitly or implicitly link or associate the claimed effect of the nutrient, component, or dietary ingredient to a specific disease or state of health leading to a disease.

The FDA does not preapprove these claims, but the manufacturer must submit notification of the claim to the FDA no later than 30 days after marketing the dietary supplement. The manufacturer must have scientific evidence to substantiate their claim and verify that their claim is truthful and not misleading. If the structure/function claim is used with the product, the product must include a disclaimer stating that the claim has not been evaluated by the FDA. The disclaimer must also state that the dietary supplement product is not intended to "diagnose, treat, cure or prevent any disease" because the product is a dietary supplement, and only drugs can legally make such claims about a disease (17).

EVALUATION OF DIETARY SUPPLEMENTS

A wide array of dietary supplements are available for sale, and more are arriving on the market regularly. With many products to choose from and many similar products competing with each other, it is easy to be confused. When considering a dietary supplement, the guidelines that follow are helpful. Of course, this information is not meant to replace advice given by a medical provider.

ADVERSE SUPPLEMENT REACTIONS CAN BE REPORTED TO THE FDA

You or your health care provider can anonymously report an adverse reaction or illness suspected to be caused by a dietary supplement or problems with packaging, contamination, or other quality defects to the FDA. The FDA website has a safety-reporting portal that you should use if you experience an adverse reaction (13).

Product Labels

The first step in evaluating a dietary supplement is to view the product label. The brand, product name, claims, and name and quantity of key ingredients should be listed. This information, however, says nothing about the quality or efficacy of the product. The limited, and sometimes confusing, regulations associated with the DSHEA can make the process of product evaluation difficult for consumers. Health professionals must go above and beyond any advertising or simple label reading to determine the safety and effectiveness of a product.

Peer-Reviewed Scientific Evidence

Many printed sources of information are available about dietary supplements. Laypersons might commonly turn to search engines, social media, or magazine articles because these media tend to cover current, popular topics. Articles published in these sources may or may not be from experts in the field qualified to write about the topic, and you may not know authors' qualifications or potential conflicts of interest (are they receiving money from a company to write a good review?). Registered dietitian nutritionists and other allied health professionals possessing knowledge of dietary supplements should keep up with both the lay information being presented to the public and the scientific evidence presented in peer-reviewed journals. Peer-reviewed journal articles, also called refereed or scholarly journal articles, are written by experts in the field who have conducted the research study being published or by those who are reviewing the current available literature. Peer review refers to a blinded review of journal articles by fellow experts. Not all journals go through the process of peer review before publishing their articles.

Resources Regarding Quality and Banned Substances

Well-established resources are available for health professionals and consumers to use to minimize chances of purchasing a supplement that is adulterated or contaminated.

Because dietary supplements do not require FDA approval before being sold, athletes may want to consider using supplements that are third-party tested for banned substances. Although no third-party testing program can guarantee that a supplement is 100 percent safe, these programs add a layer of assurance for athletes. Third party means that the certifying company is independent from the supplement manufacturer, has no financial interest or other conflicts of interest, and has no official governmental regulation authority. A third-party certifying company must be accredited by the International Standard Organization (ISO) 17065—Conformity Assessment—Requirements for Bodies Certifying Products (18). This accreditation standard means that the program

REFLECTION TIME: WHAT JOURNALS ARE PEER REVIEWED?

To investigate whether or not a journal is peer reviewed, visit the homepage of the journal on the Internet. Many journals describe their peer-review process and also include a list of people on their editorial board (the editorial board is in charge of finding experts to review the articles). If still in doubt, a reference librarian at a university library can likely help you.

Peer-reviewed journals in the fields of nutrition and exercise sciences include the following:

- *Journal of Nutrition*
- *Journal of the Academy of Nutrition and Dietetics*
- *International Journal of Sports Nutrition and Exercise Metabolism*
- *Medicine and Science in Sports and Exercise*
- *Journal of Athletic Training*
- *Journal of Strength and Conditioning Research*

has strict standards for testing, record keeping, manufacturing practices, ongoing monitoring, and strict standards established for a mark or seal used on the dietary supplement label. If a product meets the set standards set by the third party of choice, the product is considered certified and a particular seal (a stamp of approval) can be used on the label. Although the supplement testing and certification industry has evolved over the last decade, each third-party certification program differs. Therefore, nutrition educators and supplement users need to understand the various dietary supplement certification programs (19).

Banned Substances Control Group (BSCG) (20), Informed Choice (5), ConsumerLab (21), **NSF International** (22), and the U.S. Pharmacopeia Convention (USP) (23) are among the organizations that have assessment programs (24). An assessment should not be confused with a recommendation for use. Manufacturers who use third-party testing do so voluntarily because testing is not required to sell products. No testing company tests for all the substances banned by the NCAA, MLB, NFL, or **WADA (World Anti-Doping Agency)** (25). In addition, any list of banned substances is subject to change as new substances become available.

BSCG (20) tests for banned substances through antidoping and sports drug testing and also provides a variety of certification, testing and good manufacturing practice (GMP) compliance services to manufacturers of dietary supplements. BSCG offers analytical testing to product manufacturers, ingredient suppliers, athletic organizations, or individual athletes or consumers who want to verify that the products purchased are not contaminated with drugs or other agents that can lead to health concerns or positive drug tests. BSCG offers several certification programs:

- BSCG Certified Drug Free provides protection against over 491 substances on the WADA Prohibited List as well as prescription, over-the-counter (OTC), and illegal drugs not banned in sport.
- BSCG Certified Quality verifies ingredient identity and label claims specifications as well as analyzes for heavy metals, microbiological agents, pesticides, and solvents.
- BSCG Certified GMP provides onsite audits to verify that manufacturers compliant with current good manufacturing practice (cGMP).
- BSCG Certified CBD analyzes THC (tetrahydrocannabinol) limit for drug-testing protection, screens for WADA-prohibited substances, verifies THC and CBD (cannabidiol) content, tests for contaminants, screens for synthetic cannabinoids, and evaluates claims and cGMP compliance.

NSF International (22) provides third-party certification, meaning that this independent organization has reviewed the manufacturing process of a dietary supplement product and has independently determined that the final product complies with specific standards for safety, quality, and performance. NSF certification and the NSF mark on the nutritional supplement label indicates the product complies with all NSF standard requirements. NSF conducts periodic facility audits and product testing to verify that the product continues to comply with their standards. These certifications do not indicate that the product has been tested for banned substances.

The NSF Certified for Sport (22) mark indicates that the product is free from or below testing limits of banned substances tested for (remember that no testing company tests for all possible banned substances) and therefore can help athletes minimize their risk of testing positive for banned substances.

Informed Choice (5) is a quality-assurance testing and certification program specifically designed for sports nutrition products and their manufacturers and suppliers. This program ensures products are not inadvertently contaminated with substances prohibited in sport by WADA, but they do not test for everything on the prohibited list (25).

Informed Choice has banned substances testing services that include the Informed Choice mark with their language "We test—you trust." Supplements that carry the Informed Choice logo complete a full manufacturing audit. There is assurance that the supplement manufacturing facility is equipped with proper critical control procedures, that the raw materials used in manufacturing are not prohibited or contain naturally occurring banned substances, and that product is regularly tested for a wide variety of WADA-banned substances. A second label mark specific to sports supplements is Informed Sport. In addition to the manufacturing audits procedures mentioned earlier, this mark ensures that these certified products are presumed safe for athletes, and every single batch of product is tested for banned substances before they hit the market for sale. The Informed Choice website offers numerous educational resources that health professionals can use with their patients and clients to provide reputable information on understanding the manufacturing auditing process, the process of testing for banned substances, and the risk with using supplements in sport.

The U.S. Pharmacopeial Convention (USP) (23) is a scientific, worldwide, nonprofit organization with a 200-year history that sets standards for the identity, strength, quality, and purity of medicines, food ingredients, and dietary supplements manufactured and distributed for sale. The USP is proactive in working with manufacturers to ensure they have the appropriate quality assurance protocols in place to produce a quality product before it reaches the public for sale. USP staff meet the company proprietors, inspect their manufacturing facilities, review files to determine how ingredients for products are sourced, examine how the supplements are made, and examine the methods used to test both ingredient quality and the final products. USP determines whether the testing methods used are appropriate for the product being made and are sensitive enough to identify harmful contaminants including heavy metals, pesticides, and microbes. In addition to testing products made by other manufacturers, USP conducts their own facility audit by pulling product off store shelves and testing them to ensure they continue to meet high-quality standards.

USP offers third-party, voluntary, independent verification of dietary supplements in an attempt to limit the presence of adulterants and contaminants in supplement ingredients and final products sold to consumers. A supplement successfully meeting the rigorous standards and testing criteria may display the USP Verified Mark. This mark means that the supplement

1. contains the ingredients listed on the label in the specified strength and amounts,
2. does not contain harmful levels of specified contaminants or impurities,
3. is made according to FDA and USP good manufacturing practices,
4. uses sanitation principles, and
5. will break down and dissolve within a specified amount of time so that the active ingredients can be released and absorbed by the body.

> **? DO YOU KNOW?**
>
> Although third-party certification programs are available for supplement manufacturers, they are voluntary. The manufacturer of the product may choose whether to participate in this process.

The FDA provides valuable resources to consumers to help them reduce the risk of encountering a product marketed as a dietary supplement but containing hidden ingredients. The FDA's Medication Health Fraud website (26) lists some of the potentially hazardous products that contain hidden ingredients marketed and sold to consumers. Products more likely to be contaminated are

REFLECTION TIME: ARE SEALS ON SUPPLEMENT LABELS A GUARANTEE?

Although many of the verification, certification, and label seal (mark) programs can be useful when making a supplement selection, they do not guarantee purity (the supplement is free from contamination) or safety. Independent, third-party auditing programs can test dietary supplements for substances that are banned or restricted by sport organizations. These testing facilities use a standard (ISO 17025 accreditation standard) that provides a better assurance that a tested supplement is free of banned substances tested for and thus can help decrease the likelihood that an athlete has a doping violation or loss of eligibility (18, 19).

those promoted for weight loss, sexual enhancement, and bodybuilding (7, 27, 28).

The FDA advises caution when considering products with these potential warning signs (7, 27, 28):

- They claim to be alternatives to FDA-approved drugs or to have effects similar to prescription drugs.
- They claim to be a legal alternative to or one step away from anabolic steroids.
- They are marketed primarily in a foreign language.
- They are marketed through mass emails.
- They are marketed as sexual-enhancement products promising rapid or long-lasting effects.
- They include small print about the possibility of testing positive on a drug test.

Dietary Supplement and Drug Testing Specific to Competitive Athletes

Some athletes in competitive sports are tested for banned substances such as steroids. Therefore, they must be careful when choosing supplements because they may contain prohibited substances not declared on the label. Contamination of a supplement can occur because of poor manufacturing practices, intentional doping from the manufacturer, or through deliberate intent on the part of the athlete. Whether a supplement was contaminated at the outset or through a conscious choice of the athlete can be difficult to discern. Athletes who test positive for a banned substance often blame the positive test on a supplement, when in reality they were taking the substance intentionally. Most sport organizations with banned substances policies have strict liability. This provision means that even when athletes innocently ingest the substance and then test positive, they are not allowed to compete.

Drug Free Sport International (29) is a worldwide provider of drug-free prevention services for professional athletic organizations and is a leader in sport drug-testing programs. Some of the professional organizations served include the NFL, the NCAA, Major League Baseball's Minor League program, the PGA and LPGA Tours, NASCAR, the NBA and WNBA, and hundreds of educational institutions such as universities, colleges, and high schools.

Drug Free Sport International works exclusively with sport organizations and their athletes. In addition to testing athletes for banned substances, they offer antidoping education services for sports teams, athletic organizations, and educational institutions. These programs include educational subscription services, customized webinars, blogs, and a speakers' bureau.

The **U.S. Anti-Doping Agency (USADA)** (30) is a national antidoping organization in the United States for Olympic, Paralympic, Pan American, and Parapan American sport. USADA manages the antidoping program that includes both in and out of competition testing, manages the results of testing, provides drug reference resources, and provides sports education focused on awareness and prevention of doping for all sport national governing bodies recognized by the United States Olympic and Paralympic Committee (USOPC), their athletes, and their events. In addition, the USADA oversees the UFC Anti-Doping Program and contributes to the promotion and advancement of clean sport through scientific research and education. The Supplement 411 section of USADA's website (30) educates athletes on how to recognize supplement red flags that indicate an increased risk of testing positive from the supplement, how to reduce the risk of testing positive, and how to avoid developing adverse side effects. Frequently asked questions are included, and an area is available where users can submit a question to the expert panel. Before competing, all athletes would benefit from knowing the rules regarding banned or prohibited substances in their particular sport.

Considerations for Choosing a Supplement

People can take three steps to assess a supplement for potential safety or efficacy concerns. First, they can examine the brand to determine if the product is made by a widely recognized national company or a small obscure brand. Many national brands have good manufacturing practices in place and want to maintain a sound reputation.

This assertion does not mean that smaller companies make poor products, but brand reputation is one factor to consider. Also, consumers should be wary of manufacturers whose products target weight loss, bodybuilding, or sexual enhancement because research indicates that products in these three categories have the highest level of tainted supplements (27). Second, consumers should be beware of complicated products with long lists of ingredients, unfamiliar ingredients, or **proprietary blends**. These blends are used in supplement labeling and marketing and are combination of ingredients used solely by the supplement manufacturer selling the product. Other companies do not make the same combination of ingredients. With proprietary blends, knowing the quantities of individual ingredients and comparing them to information in the scientific literature is impossible, because the literature specifies the quantity of an ingredient or ingredients. If the proprietary blend has different amounts of ingredients than those used in the research studies, a product might not have an efficacious dose of the active ingredient or ingredients. Manufacturers sometimes add useless ingredients to make a product appear more robust and appealing. Third, consumers should be concerned if a product claims to have the same effect as a prescription drug. Many such claims are false. Finally, users should not be fooled by the term "natural." This term is not defined by the FDA and is not an indication of safety (31). Many herbal products are natural yet contain compounds that have pharmaceutical activity or that can interfere with the action of over-the-counter or prescription drugs (13, 15). For example, kava kava should not be used with alcohol or with many antidepressant drugs prescribed by psychiatrists, and black cohosh might interfere with commonly prescribed statin drugs (32).

WHAT SHOULD I CONSIDER BEFORE TAKING A SUPPLEMENT?

You should think about many factors when deciding whether to take a supplement or which one to take.

Here are some questions to consider:

- Do you have a diagnosed nutrient deficiency? If so, you should be under the care of a qualified health care practitioner. A supplement may or may not be the answer. Sometimes a nutrient deficiency can be corrected through medical nutrition therapy.
- Do a product's claims sound too good to be true? Do they sound exaggerated or unrealistic? If so, research the product thoroughly or ask an RDN who is versed in supplements before purchasing and taking the product.
- Are a product's claims only from testimonials? If so, use reason before believing these claims.

The Australian Institute of Sport (AIS) created and published some guiding principles used in their Sports Supplements Framework (33). The AIS emphasizes the importance of asking the following questions before considering using a sports supplement:

- Is it safe? Lack of scientific evidence of harm does not mean that the product is safe. It might mean only that no research is available.
- Is it permitted in sport? Banned substances can result in loss of eligibility to compete.
- Is there evidence that it works? You should review the scientific evidence instead of just believing the claims.

You need to understand the answers to these questions before deciding to use a supplement. The resources mentioned previously can be searched to determine if a product or substance is permissible for use. Besides being knowledgeable about the position papers referenced, the fitness professional must be able to complete a through peer-reviewed literature search and understand the scientific evidence available regarding safety and efficacy.

COMMON PRODUCTS AND SUPPLEMENTS USED FOR PERFORMANCE ENHANCEMENT

The Australian Institute of Sport (AIS) created an ABCD classification system ranking sports foods and supplement ingredients into four groups. The scientific evidence is carefully evaluated and reviewed and then sports foods and supplements are categorized by efficacy, safety, and other practical considerations for use of the product. Group A supplements are supported for use when using evidence-based protocols in specified situations. Group B products could be considered for use under a research protocol or monitored, evidence-based protocol but warrant further research. Group C products have little proof of a beneficial effect. Group D products are banned or at high risk of contamination and should not be used (33).

The International Olympic Committee published a consensus statement regarding dietary supplements and performance in athletes (2). In this review, they categorized sports supplements into the following areas:

- Sports foods and functional foods used to provide a practical form of energy and nutrients
- Supplements taken to prevent or cure specific nutrient insufficiencies or deficiencies
- Supplements with strong evidence of efficacy of performance improvements for specific activities
- Supplements claiming to improve training capacity, recovery, muscle soreness, and rehabilitation from injury
- Supplements claiming to enhance immune health
- Supplements claiming to alter body composition by increasing lean mass and reducing fat mass

Although the overall research publication pool is getting larger each year, there is a huge disparity in the quantity and quality of research conducted and published about the various kinds of products. For example, carbohydrate- and electrolyte-containing sports drinks, caffeine, and creatine have a large amount of research available, whereas other products have far less published data available to evaluate their efficacy in improving health or performance. This chapter provides more information on the products with the most research and less on those supplements that have prompted fewer research studies and publications. Because the scientific literature concerning dietary supplements and sports supplements is expanding, consulting the literature is the way to keep current on the latest updates.

Portable and Convenient Sports Products

Although nutrient guidelines are well established for athletes in different sports and a "food first" approach can often meet nutrient needs, turning to sports foods and products often serves a purpose. Athletes may face difficulties with food preparation, food storage, time-consuming training schedules, and digestive distress. Alternatives to traditional foods can provide convenient and palatable options to meet nutrient intake goals. The most common products that fit into this category are sports drinks, gels, and gummies containing carbohydrate and electrolytes, sports bars containing a variety of energy-nutrient combinations, protein drinks or powders, electrolyte replacements, and energy drinks usually containing carbohydrate and caffeine and sometimes additional vitamins and compounds (2). Details of the ideal use of these products are addressed in chapters 5, 8, and 11 in this book.

Supplements to Prevent or Cure Specific Micronutrient Insufficiencies or Deficiencies

Athletes and nonathletes alike are subject to nutrient deficiencies if dietary needs are not met. Details about micronutrient needs of athletes and active people are discussed in chapters 6 and 7 in this book. The micronutrients most often of concern are vitamin D, iron, calcium, and antioxidants (3). The first step is to attempt to meet all nutrient needs through the diet. If this is not possible because of increased physiological demand coupled with food intake challenges, or the person has a deficiency or insufficient intake, a physician or RDN may recommend supplementation. Keep in mind that more is not always better for health or performance.

Supplements With Evidence of Efficacy of Performance Improvements

Some supplements have enough scientific evidence to support their use in specific sport situations using evidence-based protocols. Using these products outside the established parameters may not enhance performance and may lead to unwanted side effects.

Caffeine and Energy Drinks

Caffeine can be found naturally in food and beverages, added to food and beverage products, or purchased as a dietary supplement. Some of the common herbal sources of caffeine often used in weight-loss products include guarana, kola nut, and yerba maté.

Caffeine is the most widely consumed legal psychoactive agent (i.e., a substance that affects brain functioning) in the world. It occurs naturally in the leaves, nuts, and seeds of over 60 plants, yet it can also be made synthetically for use in over-the-counter medications and dietary supplements. Caffeine is consumed by billions worldwide. The major dietary sources are coffee, tea, and soft drinks, which typically contain 30 to 200 mg of caffeine per serving. Chocolate is another common source, but the caffeine content is significantly lower (usually less than 15 mg/oz) (10). Over-the-counter medications such as pain-relieving headache medications may contain 100 to 200 mg of caffeine per tablet. In over-the-counter medications, the amount of caffeine is listed on the label. Caffeine can be toxic in high doses, such as 15 mg/kg body weight, and these toxic effects can be exacerbated when caffeine is combined with other stimulants (34, 35). Caffeine content is not required on food labels, so exact quantities in some products, such as coffee, are difficult to determine and can be quite variable depending on the source and brewing method (10). If caffeine is added to a food or beverage, it must be included in the list of ingredients on the label, but there is no requirement to disclose the quantity of caffeine (36).

Caffeine has been studied and used for decades to improve physical performance. The original rationale for its use was related to the physiological finding of enhanced free fatty acid (FFA) release. The assumption at that time was that these FFAs would be a preferential fuel source for working skeletal muscle during exercise and thus glycogen would be spared. Some research has demonstrated that although FFAs are released into the bloodstream with caffeine ingestion, FFA oxidation (use) does not increase in the skeletal muscle, nor is glycogen spared. In other words, the fatty acids go through circulation and then travel back to the adipose cells again to be stored and skeletal muscle (2, 37-39). Newer studies report that moderate doses of caffeine (3 mg/kg) increased fat oxidation (use) in cyclists (40). But more research is needed on this purported mechanism of action and factors such as fasting versus fed states, trained versus untrained people, and intensity of training need. Figure 9.2 illustrates the potential for caffeine ingestion to increase fat oxidation, but this may only occur during lower-intensity exercise. The translation to altering fuel usage (e.g., sparing carbohydrate) is not clear, and more research is needed.

It appears that another **ergogenic**, or performance-enhancing, benefit of caffeine is most likely related to its role as a central nervous system stimulant. Adenosine, a compound found in all cells in the body, plays an important role in energy metabolism. Adenosine prepares the body for sleep by blunting communication between nerve cells while widening blood vessels to increase oxygen flow. Caffeine and adenosine compete for the same receptors in the brain. When levels of adenosine are reduced because of higher levels of caffeine competing for binding, the result is an increased feeling of alertness. In exercise performance, the main benefit is a heightened sense of awareness and decreased perception of effort (2, 37-39).

Caffeine is generally recognized as safe by the FDA and has been consumed for centuries as part of coffee and tea. Considerable research supports the use of caffeine as an ergogenic aid, and studies have most commonly examined doses ranging from 3 to 6 mg/kg body weight. This dosage range is the amount typically used to stimulate central nervous system functioning. Some organizations ban the use of caffeine in higher doses or have limits to urinary caffeine levels. Higher doses are considered to be in the range of 10 to 13 mg/kg. For a 70 kg (154 lb) athlete, this

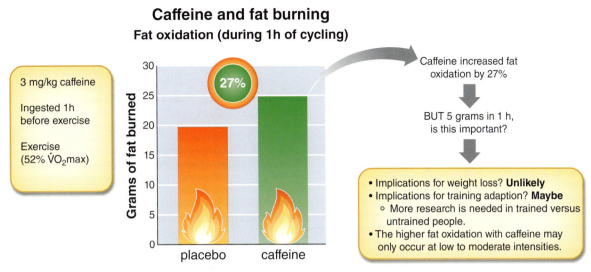

Figure 9.2 Caffeine and fat burning.

Adapted from A. Jeukendrup, "Study Shows That Caffeine Increases Fat Burning, but Does It Matter?" Mysportscience Ltd, accessed March 30, 2023, www.mysportscience.com/post/caffeine-increases-fat-burning.

is equivalent to 700 to 900 mg of caffeine, or in 7 to 9 cups of coffee. This amount is far greater than what the average athlete consumes. Doses in this range may come with significant side effects, including elevated heart rate and elevated levels of catecholamine, lactate, FFAs, and glycerol. Furthermore, undesirable feelings of gastrointestinal distress, jitteriness, mental confusion, anxiety, problems concentrating or focusing, and sleep disturbances may accompany such doses. Symptoms might be more pronounced in people who usually use no or low doses of caffeine and then suddenly increase the dose for an event (2, 37-39).

Although moderate doses of caffeine (3–6 mg/kg body weight) have often been used in research studies and demonstrate an ergogenic effect on endurance performance without undesirable side effects, other research has found that lower doses (2–3 mg/kg) can also be ergogenic. It appears that doses greater than or equal to 9 mg/kg body weight do not offer an enhanced performance benefit and, more important, are likely to induce the negative side effects of nausea, anxiety, restlessness, and insomnia. In addition to quantity, timing is an important consideration. Caffeine is rapidly absorbed in the body, appearing in the blood stream 5 to 15 minutes after ingestion and reaching peak concentrations after 40 to 80 minutes (2, 37-39).

DO YOU KNOW?

Dehydration itself results in reduced urine output, but less is known about the effects of caffeine ingestion in people who are already dehydrated (41). Any possible minor diuretic effect caused by caffeine appears to be insignificant and does not lead to impaired performance. In fact, caffeine, when used properly, can be a safe ergogenic aid. Research also suggests that coffee, when consumed in moderation by caffeine-habituated males, provides similar hydrating qualities to water (42).

A final consideration is whether the ergogenic effects of caffeine use are more pronounced with acute use or chronic use and whether an ergogenic difference occurs among athletes who metabolize caffeine at different rates (43). This question has not been fully resolved in the literature and therefore must be included in trial periods. Chronic users may need a higher dose during competition to see a benefit. But caution should be used by those who are not habitual caffeine users. There are genetic differences in caffeine metabolism, and a person not accustomed to caffeine could be sensitive to it (39). Limited research identified a CYP1A2 gene that affects caffeine metabolism, and different genotypes have been recognized.

> **? DO YOU KNOW?**
>
> People often avoid coffee because they believe that its consumption causes dehydration and that it cannot be a beverage used to maintain fluid balance. Fortunately for coffee lovers, we have data suggesting that moderate coffee consumption in habitual users provides hydrating qualities similar to water (42).

People with one genotype had improved performance with 2 to 4 mg/kg caffeine, whereas the same dose resulted in no change or diminished performance in people with other genotypes (43). As with any change in diet, athletes who want to test their response to caffeine should experiment during the preseason or early in the training season, not during competition or precompetition.

The guidelines for the consumption of energy drinks are different from those for caffeine because energy drinks contain a variety of other ingredients, such as sugar, carbonation, herbs, amino acids, vitamins, minerals, and other stimulants (4).

> **? DO YOU KNOW?**
>
> The caffeine content in beverages like coffee and tea are generally too variable to determine a specific dose. Factors such as brew time, origin and type of plant, and preparation methods can all affect caffeine content.

Sodium Bicarbonate

Sports involving heavy use of anaerobic glycolysis as the predominant energy system result in the metabolic fatigue associated with progressive increased intracellular acidity. Athletes may consume sodium bicarbonate in an attempt to neutralize the hydrogen ions and thus extend the time of high-intensity activities before fatigue sets in. Athletes participating in sporting events of high intensity lasting approximately 60 seconds, such as high-intensity sprints, might benefit the most from bicarbonate. But participants in other sports lasting much longer in duration (e.g., 30–60 minutes) that include surges of increased intensity, or in sports with intermittent periods of high intensity, might also benefit, but the research data are less clear. The recommend protocols for use are (a) a single, acute dose of 0.2 to 0.4 g/kg body weight taken 60 to 150 minutes preexercise, (b) several smaller doses of the same total quantity taken over 30 to 180 minutes, or (c) three or four smaller doses per day for 2 to 4 consecutive days before an important training day or competitive event (2, 3, 44, 45).

Sodium bicarbonate is inexpensive and readily available in all grocery stores as baking soda, but it might not be palatable. Commercial products available in capsules or tablets might be more desirable. Potential side effects reported with use of sodium bicarbonate include nausea, vomiting, stomach pain, and diarrhea, which clearly result in performance impairment, not improvement. To minimize gastrointestinal distress, athletes may consider using sodium citrate instead of sodium bicarbonate, split it into smaller doses, and take it in conjunction with a carbohydrate-dense meal containing approximately 1.5 g/kg body weight of carbohydrate. Athletes should try different protocols for tolerance before an important day of training or competition (2, 3, 44, 45).

Beta-Alanine

Carnosine is a dipeptide composed of beta-alanine and histidine and thought to serve as a buffer for skeletal muscle during high-intensity activities. Beta-alanine is a beta-amino acid, differing from most alpha-amino acids found in the human diet. Synthesis of muscle carnosine is limited by the availability of beta-alanine, the rate-limiting substrate. Supplementation with beta-alanine might enhance natural carnosine production and subsequent skeletal muscle carnosine content and provide an ergogenic, buffering effect during exercise lasting 30 seconds to 10 minutes (2, 3, 46, 47).

Several research studies examining beta-alanine supplementation have reported increased skeletal muscle carnosine content and an ergogenic effect of reducing perceived exertion (i.e., exercise feels like less effort) and biochemical markers of muscle fatigue. Common supplementation protocols include daily consumption of approximately 65 mg/kg body weight ingested in a split dose regimen of 0.8 to 1.6 grams every 3 to 4 hours over a 10- to 12-week period before competition. More research is needed to examine the potential benefits for sport-specific activities, especially those of longer durations. This supplement might benefit endurance athletes who have intermittent, high-intensity requirements, sprinters, those engaged in repeated sprint activity (such as in soccer or American football), or those who focus on strength training. Note that there may be large interindividual variations in skeletal muscle carnosine synthesis and that content and benefits of supplementation may be less in well-trained individuals. Paresthesia, tingling in the skin, and skin rashes are potential side effects (3, 45-47).

Nitric Oxide Boosters

There are three main types of nitric oxide (NO) boosters. Beets and other nitrate-rich vegetables work through the nitrate-nitrite-NO pathway, one that functions when oxygen is not as readily available (during high-intensity exercise such as sprinting up and down a soccer field). L-arginine works through a far different pathway, one that requires the presence of enzymes and oxygen and thus is not effective during high-intensity exercise. Finally, certain polyphenols, including those found in Concord grape juice, acai juice, cranberry juice, carrot juice, and pomegranate juice, turn on proteins that signal the endothelial cells to make more endothelial nitric oxide synthase (eNOS, one of the enzymes responsible for the majority of nitric oxide produced; eNOS helps produce nitric oxide from arginine), boosting levels of eNOS for up to a full day. The endothelial cells treated with Concord grape juice increased nitric oxide levels by 50 percent (48, 49).

Inorganic nitrate helps open blood vessels to increase blood flow, supporting cardiovascular health and athletic performance. It is naturally found in beetroot juice, green leafy vegetables such as spinach and arugula, celery, commercial vegetable juices, carrot juice, and pomegranate juice (3, 50). But the amount of dietary nitrate varies in beets and other vegetables based on growing conditions, including the nitrate content of the fertilizer used, the level of nitrate in the water supply, soil conditions, time of year, and the way in which the vegetables are stored (51).

Once consumed, inorganic nitrate (NO_3^-) is metabolized to bioactive nitrite (NO_2^-), which is converted to nitric oxide (NO). The initial conversion of inorganic nitrate to nitrite begins in the mouth with the help of salivary bacteria; the conversion rate is approximately 20 percent (50, 52). Antibacterial mouthwash and antibiotics kill bacteria in the mouth, which significantly reduces this initial conversion (50). Once swallowed, the conversion to nitric oxide occurs in many phases in the stomach, gut, and other organs. Although research is limited, the bioavailability (the amount that reaches the circulation) of nitrite has been reported to be 95 to 100 percent (50, 52).

Nitric oxide exerts its action by signaling the lining of blood vessels (the endothelium) to relax, subsequently enhancing blood flow. This enhanced blood flow is thought to improve exercise performance and recovery. Nitrate intake might result in enhanced exercise tolerance and improved performance. Most of the research on nitrate has reported improved time to exhaustion in activities lasting less than 40 minutes and enhanced type II skeletal muscle fiber function in activities of high-intensity, intermittent, or team sport activity ranging from 12 to 40 minutes long. Research has shown that both acute (2-3 hours) and chronic (3-15 days) supplementation of nitrate improve activities for men and women of all ages, including both trained and untrained people (50). Further reports, however, suggest that the positive effect is more pronounced in untrained and recreationally active people compared with elite competitors (3, 53). The recommended protocol for chronic ingestion includes acute intake of 310 to 560 mg (5-9 mmol) for 3 or more days. Consuming more than 1,041 mg (16.8 mmol) compared with the recommended range does not appear to benefit performance further. This recommended quantity is equivalent to approximately 2 cups (480 ml) of pure (nothing added) beetroot juice. For athletes choosing to stick with foods rather than traditional dietary

? DO YOU KNOW?

Inorganic nitrate found in beets and other vegetables are not the same as nitrite salts (sold over the Internet), which can be harmful, and even deadly in low doses. Organic nitrates and nitrites are also very different from inorganic nitrate. Organic nitrates and nitrites are potent vasodilators (substances that open blood vessels) found in the drugs nitroglycerine and amyl nitrite, used to treat angina (chest pain), and should be prescribed and used only under the care of a medical doctor.

supplements, consumption of beetroot juice and other green leafy vegetables, such as arugula and spinach, may provide some benefits. Ingestion of nitrate in typical amounts from foods does not cause adverse health consequences in healthy people. Less is known about the safety of supplementation with high doses in the supplemental form, although there are no known safety issues with supplementation at recommended doses in healthy people (2, 50, 52).

> **? DO YOU KNOW?**
>
> Beets and beetroot juice might turn your urine red. This outcome is harmless. For more information on substances that change the color of your urine, see chapter 8.

Arginine is a conditionally essential amino acid that plays a role in boosting NO synthesis. The body usually makes plenty of arginine, but it becomes essential (and must therefore be consumed through food) during times of illness and metabolic stress. Some athletes attempt to boost their intake of arginine through foods or supplements in hopes of observing a performance benefit. The form found in food and supplements is commonly referred to as L-arginine. L-arginine is found in fish, meat, eggs, and dairy foods and plant sources including beans, brown rice, oats, and nuts. The ergogenic effect of L-arginine supplementation is not well established, and when taken alone this amino acid may have a limited effect on NO production. When combined with other compounds, it may reduce perceived exertion in sedentary people or moderately trained, but not highly trained, athletes. Another amino acid, L-citrulline, may promote a higher level of extracellular L-arginine and enhanced NO production. Some research reported that L-citrulline and L-citrulline combined with malate improved skeletal muscle efficiency and improved high-intensity aerobic exercise performance. Further research is needed before absolute recommendations can be made regarding a performance benefit (2).

Creatine

Approximately 95 percent of the body's creatine stores are in skeletal muscle, and about 60 percent of total creatine content is in the form of phosphocreatine (PCr). Creatine is used in the ATP-PC energy system, where PCr can rapidly **rephosphorylate** adenosine diphosphate (ADP) to adenosine triphosphate (ATP). ATP is then used as the energy source for the contracting muscle. This process generally occurs in high-intensity activities lasting only seconds. Creatine can be produced by the body, primarily in the kidney and liver, though ingestion of 1 gram per day from the diet helps maintain creatine homeostasis (3, 39, 45, 55).

Primary dietary sources include meat and fish, but many athletes choose to take creatine in the supplemental form to maximize skeletal muscle size and improve performance. The recommended supplementation protocol consists of a 20-gram-per-day loading phase for 5 to 7 days, followed by a maintenance phase of 3 to 5 grams per day

---

PUTTING IT INTO PERSPECTIVE

BAD RAP FOR NITRATE?

Nitrate is a naturally occurring chemical compound found in plants, soil, and within the human body. Sodium nitrate is also naturally occurring and is used as a preservative in processed meats. When this compound interacts with the bacteria naturally found in meat, it is converted to sodium nitrite. Sodium nitrite can also be added directly to meats for the purpose of preservation. Nitrites have received much attention because, when heated, they can create nitrosamines, which are reported to be carcinogenic in animals. Nitrate and nitrite are still abundant in the human diet. Vegetables are a larger source of nitrates than processed meat is, and plant foods are generally considered healthy; greater intake is linked to a reduced risk of cancer and CVD. Since the initial scare, newer scientific evidence has become available suggesting that these compounds are not as detrimental as once thought. More research is needed, especially to understand the potential beneficial roles of nitrates (52, 54).

until the supplement is discontinued. Skeletal muscle has limitations on how much creatine can be stored, and any excess gets converted to creatinine and is excreted (2, 3, 39, 45, 55).

Creatine is a widely researched sports supplement and the subject of numerous publications in peer-reviewed journals. Substantial data support an ergogenic benefit for maximum isometric strength and both single and repeated bouts of high-intensity exercise lasting less than 150 seconds. More pronounced benefits are seen in those same activities lasting less than 30 seconds. In conjunction with resistance training, creatine supplementation might lead to greater gains in strength, power, and lean body mass. The increased strength is likely caused by the increased ability to train at a higher intensity before fatigue sets in. The reported increased lean body mass should not be confused with increased skeletal muscle mass. Lean body mass is composed of muscle, water, and bone, and it is thought that much of the lean body mass increase is caused by the fluid retention required for creatine storage within the muscle. Glycogen loading, creatine loading, or a combination of both has been shown to change skeletal muscle metabolites, resulting in significant increases in total body water and thus overestimation of changes in lean body mass (56). Some body composition methods are able to detect changes only to lean body mass as a whole, not to skeletal muscle. But other studies have been able to demonstrate the effectiveness of creatine at the level of the muscle, using more sophisticated techniques (3, 39, 45, 55). For more information on creatine and other sports supplements for resistance training, refer to chapter 12.

Creatine does not seem to have an ergogenic benefit for improving maximal aerobic capacity or improving field performance in long-duration aerobic events such as long-distance running. Although scientific support for use of creatine with certain activities is abundant, the results are not unanimous because responses to creatine supplementation are individualized; some people are responders and others are nonresponders (3, 39, 45, 55, 57).

Direct response to creatine cannot be determined without a muscle biopsy or sophisticated medical imaging procedure, so screening for this is not feasible. But because of fluid retention, weight can be accurately measured and used as an indicator of creatine retention. Furthermore, improvements in the weight room or the field can be assessed to help evaluate whether a person is responding to creatine use (3, 39, 45, 55).

Current data indicate no health risks with creatine use up to 4 years, but more research is needed to assess effects with long-term use (over decades) (2). The published literature suggests that short-term use does not result in permanent or adverse effects in kidney, liver, the heart, or muscle in healthy adults (58). Caution should be used with doses greater than 3 to 5 grams per day in people with preexisting renal disease or those with another disease that can affect kidney function, such as diabetes or hypertension (59). Note that weight gain might be an undesirable side effect for those participating in weight-sensitive sports, and GI stress, though rare, is a reported potential side effect from some types of creatine (3, 39).

❓ DO YOU KNOW?

Although creatine supplementation is popular among athletes, it might have a therapeutic application in clinical populations. Creatine supplementation has been shown to be well tolerated and effective in improving skeletal muscle function in those with muscular dystrophy, muscle myopathies and disorders, and neuromuscular and neurometabolic disorders (60, 61). To see a benefit in those populations, higher doses may be needed (21-56 g/day) and therefore should be done under the care of a physician or qualified medical professional (62). Although few physicians are well versed on dietary supplements, they can oversee any medical changes stemming from creatine supplementation.

Supplements Promoted for Pain and Inflammation

Although an adequate training stimulus is required for strength, skeletal muscle hypertrophy, and other physiological gains, sometimes the inflammatory side effects can be unpleasant. Many athletes and active people seek supplementation to ease pain and discomfort posttraining.

> **PUTTING IT INTO PERSPECTIVE**
>
> ### DOES CREATINE SUPPLEMENTATION LEAD TO DEHYDRATION?
>
> A common belief is that creatine can hinder tolerance to exercise in the heat, cause muscle cramps, or compromise hydration status. This belief stems from the fluid retention that accompanies creatine storage and the reports of dehydration in high school football players using creatine. Many athletes, however, start practice in a dehydrated state. Also, a review of the scientific literature examining randomized clinical trials shows no evidence that creatine impairs the body's ability to dissipate heat or contributes to dehydration when recommended doses are used (2, 3, 39, 45, 55).

Creatine and DOMS

In addition to the ergogenic effects of creatine mentioned in the previous section, supplementation offers other potential benefits. Limited research has suggested that creatine supplementation may reduce symptoms of delayed onset muscle soreness (DOMS), improve recovery from immobilization or complete inactivity, improve cognitive function when fatigued from multitasking or sleep deprivation, and hasten recovery from concussion or traumatic brain injury (animal data). More research is needed on these topics before recommendations can be made (2).

Beta-Hydroxy-Beta-Methylbutyrate

Leucine is an essential, branched-chain amino acid that serves as a trigger for skeletal muscle protein synthesis. Beta-hydroxy-beta-methylbutyrate (HMB), a metabolite of leucine, has been reported to have therapeutic effects in people with atrophic conditions and cachexia (wasting) (63-65). Athletes and bodybuilders have expressed an interest in using the compound to increase skeletal muscle strength and hypertrophy.

Early research studies reported that HMB reduces skeletal muscle damage with resistance training. Unfortunately, this area of study has not significantly increased over time, so published research studies are somewhat scarce. The most commonly reported ergogenic effects include reduced muscle damage and increased strength, primarily in novice weightlifters, but minimal data support this claim. No safety concerns or significant side effects have been reported in the literature at this dosage. Based on available research, there does not appear to be an ergogenic benefit in trained persons of all ages with no actual increases in skeletal muscle protein synthesis (66, 67). This supplement might have therapeutic effects in older adults who are confined to bed rest or those with muscle-wasting disease. Any possible benefits of HMB may also be obtained through quality dietary protein sources consumed in proper amounts (2, 63-65).

Glucosamine and Chondroitin

Osteoarthritis is a degenerative joint disease caused by wear and tear of cartilage tissue from excess body weight (one of the top causes), mechanical stress through repetitive motion (running up and down a field for years), and oxidative damage and inflammatory responses from the anabolic-catabolic balance of the joint, synovium, matrix, and chondrocytes (all parts of the working joint). Although some people get this condition later in life as a result of age, many athletes and active people are at risk because of the volume of training and injury history that accompanies many sports (68). Many people seek pain medications, particularly nonsteroidal anti-inflammatory drugs (NSAIDs, such as ibuprofen or aspirin) to decrease their symptoms, but over time NSAIDs can lead to a number of side effects, including stomach pain and ulcers (that might lead to bleeding), heartburn, headaches, and dizziness. For those allergic to NSAIDs, side effects include rashes, throat swelling, and difficulty breathing (69).

Glucosamine and chondroitin sulfate are popular supplements for minimizing the pain of osteoarthritis and delaying progression of the disease. Glucosamine, a naturally occurring amino sugar found in meat, fish, and poultry, is made by cartilage cells. It is used as a building block of the cartilage matrix. Chondroitin sulfate is a type of protein present in cartilage. Research on this topic examines outcomes of reduction in pain and decreased joint space narrowing (more narrow spaces mean less cartilage to cushion joints). Glucosamine sulfate and glucosamine hydrochloride help rebuild the cartilage matrix and decrease activity of an enzyme that damages tissue. Sulfate is a source of the essential nutrient sulfur, which is important for cartilage (70).

Experts disagree about whether glucosamine and chondroitin supplementation may help knee and hip osteoarthritis, the areas of the body most studied. The National Institutes of Health (NIH) conducted a large study called the Glucosamine/Chondroitin Arthritis Intervention Trial (GAIT) in patients with mild knee pain due to osteoarthritis. They compared glucosamine hydrochloride, chondroitin, both supplements together, celecoxib (a prescription drug used to manage osteoarthritis pain), and a placebo (an inactive substance). The participants who took the prescription drug had better pain relief at 6 months than those who received the placebo. Those receiving the supplements had no significant improvement in knee pain. On the other hand, several European studies reported that patients felt better after taking glucosamine sulfate. Until more research is complete, people cannot count on glucosamine or chondroitin to relieve arthritis pain in the knee or any other joint. Other than the negative interaction with blood-thinning drugs, glucosamine and chondroitin appears to be relatively safe. People with diabetes should check for the effect on blood sugar if they take glucosamine regularly (71).

Gelatin, Vitamin C, and Collagen

Although data are very limited, a combination of 5 to 15 grams of gelatin combined with 50 mg of vitamin C or approximately 10 grams per day of collagen hydrolysate may increase collagen production in the body, thicken existing cartilage, and reduce perception of pain. These supplements appear to have little to no side effects, but the functional benefits in athletes for maintenance and recovery are not well established at this time (2).

Curcumin

Curcumin is the main active ingredient in the Indian spice turmeric, which gives curry its vivid yellow color. It has been used in India for thousands of years because of the purported powerful anti-inflammatory and antioxidant effects. Limited but promising research suggests curcumin may help with chronic inflammatory conditions, metabolic syndrome, arthritis, anxiety, and hyperlipidemia. It may play a role in recovery for athletes and active people by decreasing exercise-induced inflammation and muscle soreness. Most of the studies use turmeric extracts composed primarily of curcumin with dosages often exceeding 1 gram of curcumin per day. People turn to supplementation because consuming that level through food is difficult and many do not enjoy the taste of the spice in that dosage. Because curcumin is poorly absorbed, it is often combined with piperine, a compound naturally found in black pepper. Piperine enhances the absorption of curcumin by several hundred percent (72).

Omega-3 Polyunsaturated Fatty Acids

Omega-3 (n-3) polyunsaturated fatty acids (PUFA) have been studied for years regarding protective effects on health, particularly cardiovascular health, and the relationship with whole body inflammation. The prospects of n-3 PUFA use in athletes for health and performance purposes is a newer area of research (73). The most common dietary source of n-3 PUFAs is oily fish. The highest content is found in wild salmon, herring, mackerel, trout, halibut, tuna, shrimp, snapper, cod, anchovies, and sardines. The active n-3 PUFAs in fish oil are eicosapentaenoic acid (EPA) and docosahexaenoic acid (DHA). Alpha linolenic acid (ALA) is found in plant sources such as flaxseed, walnuts, canola oil, soybean oil, soybeans, and tofu. ALA requires conversion to EPA in the body, which is a slow, inefficient process (relatively small amounts of ALA are converted to EPA and even less to DHA). People who want to consume a vegetarian source of EPA and DHA can purchase EPA and DHA derived from marine algae (74).

Specific to sport performance and recovery from training, n-3 PUFAs are thought to possess anti-inflammatory properties by enhancing membrane fluidity of skeletal muscle cells. The studies in this area thus far examine the effects of n-3 PUFAs on promoting skeletal muscle cell adaptation, enhancing energy metabolism, improving skeletal muscle recovery from training, and facilitating recovery from injury. Limited research suggests that n-3 PUFA supplementation may have a beneficial role in improving endurance performance by reducing the oxygen cost of training and in promoting recovery from eccentric contraction skeletal muscle damage. Furthermore, although not well established, some encouraging evidence demonstrates the positive effects of n-3 PUFA intake and maintenance of muscle protein synthesis rates during a period of injury (75). Promising research is examining the role of n-3 PUFAs on improving risk of developing illness and skills such as reaction time. More research is needed in this area (76)

A specific area of research in this area is examining the role, if any, of n-3 PUFAs in the prevention and treatment of traumatic brain injury and sports-related concussions (SRCs). From animal model research, evidence supports the neuroprotective effects of n-3 supplementation for both injury prevention and treatment. In humans we see reduced DHA concentration in the neurons and brain following injury. Human trials are not abundant, however, because of the ethical challenges of conducting such studies and because this area of research is new. Furthermore, SRC is not a one-size-fits-all injury (every brain injury is unique). We need more data to determine the role of n-3 PUFA supplementation for both prevention and treatment of SRCs (77).

Although we do not have enough data to make specific supplement recommendations for n-3 PUFAs for athletes, encouraging a diet rich in these compounds may be prudent for optimal health of athletes.

Supplements Claiming to Enhance Immune Health

Some supplements are clearly marketed toward a particular sport or type of activity, whereas others might have an appeal and application to a broader audience. Many of these supplements claim to improve physical health, and any benefits might also apply to the physically active adult or competitive athlete. Supplements claiming to enhance immune health are examples of products that appeal to many people, active or not. This chapter discusses those that are of particular interest to athletes.

Gut Health Supplements

The human gut provides approximately 70 percent of our immune protection, acting as a physical barrier and interacting with gut-associated lymphoid tissue, which protects the body from invasion of foreign cells (78). Therefore, many athletes and active people seek to optimize their immunity during training. Unfortunately, none of the dietary supplements marketed for this purpose have enough evidence to support claims that they can ensure an optimal immune system with training. Still, a review of the current thinking behind the products is useful.

Probiotics and Prebiotics It is normal to have bacteria in the gastrointestinal tract, called gut flora, and the goal in using probiotics is to modify the gut flora so that the number of beneficial bacteria increases while the number of potentially harmful ones decreases. Probiotics are live microorganisms like bacteria and yeast, which when administered in adequate amounts benefit health. But research is not clear on what constitutes an adequate amount, and the amount may be different for every individual. Furthermore, although gut microbiota compositions appear to be variable among athletes, those who train regularly and consume adequate protein may show even greater differences in composition from their sedentary counterparts, increasing the difficulty in determining what constitutes a healthy gut microbiome (79).

Although probiotics are best known for their role in digestive and immune health, probiotic strains have a wide variety of functions, including promoting nutrient absorption and supporting mental health. But not all probiotics deliver the same benefits. The most common species studied in supplemental probiotics are lactobacillus and bifidobacterium. A probiotic should be nonpathogenic (contain only good, healthy bacteria, not harmful ones), be resistant to processing (gastric juices, bile) so that they survive transit through the gut, colonize intestinal epithelial tissue (increase the number of good bacteria in the gut), and provide measurable benefit as backed by human clinical trials. Also, the probiotic name listed on the label should contain all three parts—genus, strain, species. Probiotics are sold in many forms, including capsules, powders, and fermented (sugars broken down by bacteria and yeast) dairy products (80, 81). Probiotic foods include yogurt, kefir, kombucha, barley, bananas, oats, wheat, soybean, asparagus, leeks, chicory, Jerusalem artichokes, garlic, and onions. Probiotic products should be labeled in CFU, the scientifically accepted unit of measure for probiotics and used to report probiotic quantity in many studies conducted to assess the safety or benefits of probiotics (79).

> **DO YOU KNOW?**
> Probiotics have three parts to their name—genus, species, and strain. Think of it like a first, middle, and last name. As you get to the last name, you are a getting a lot more specific. If you search for your first name on the Internet, chances are you will get a mountain of hits. Now try searching for your complete name in quotation marks, including your middle name. This expression is much more specific and therefore more likely to result in a website that features you rather than someone with only the same first name.

Research is evolving on the effectiveness of probiotics in the general population, so using probiotics may be of interest among athletes. The most well-studied roles for probiotics are supporting digestive health and immune health. But specific strains can support vaginal health, incidence and duration of diarrhea in infants or adults, gut transit time (how fast food moves through the gut), and other functioning. Moderate evidence suggests that certain strains and doses may help reduce upper respiratory symptoms (URS) in athletes and trained people. Although a potential benefit exists for reducing gastrointestinal distress and related issues, more evidence is required in this area. In reviewing the published research, a limiting factor is that several different strains are used in studies in different amounts and for varied lengths of time. This variability makes it difficult to compare studies and make generalizations based on research findings (2, 79, 81, 82).

> **DO YOU KNOW?**
> Probiotics populate your gut and alter the community that lives there. When you stop taking a probiotic, it washes out within a few days. Consider it a temporary houseguest in your gut.

A prebiotic is an ingredient that targets the microbiota (bacteria) already present within the gut, acting as a food for the target microbes. Prebiotics are carbohydrates that are not digested and therefore reach the colon, where they become fermented. Prebiotics are found in some fruits, vegetables, and whole grains. As with probiotics, some research suggests that prebiotic consumption might help athletes reduce their risk of developing respiratory and GI illnesses during periods of heavy training and psychological stress (83).

Many other supplements on the market claim to boost immunity and are targeted toward athletes. Until more research studies are conducted, the efficacy of the following supplements for supporting immune health in athletes is not well established (2):

- Carbohydrate—low to moderate levels of research support
- Bovine colostrum—low to moderate levels of research support
- Polyphenols (e.g., quercetin)—low to moderate levels of research support
- Glutamine—limited research support
- Caffeine—limited research support
- Echinacea—limited research support
- Omega-3 PUFAs—limited research support
- Vitamin E—no research support
- Beta-glucans—no research support

Vitamin D, Vitamin C, and Zinc

Vitamin D insufficiency and deficiency in athletes and active people has been associated with increased URS (upper respiratory symptoms). Until more research data are available, the goal should be to maintain optimal vitamin D status. Vitamin D is discussed in more detail in chapter 6. Vitamin C intake in the range of 0.25 to 1.0 grams per day may be associated with lower incidence of URS if taken at the initial onset of symptoms. Vitamin C does not seem to have an effect in treating symptoms after they are established. Similarly, zinc taken within hours of URS onset may decrease the duration of the illness, but it does not play a role in preventing or treating URS. Caution should be taken with supplementation because high doses can lead to undesirable taste, nausea, and can actually decrease immune function (2).

Supplements Claiming to Alter Body Composition

Effective weight management requires balancing energy intake (not consuming more calories than burned) over time, but many people are looking for a quick fix. Losing or maintaining body fat with diet and exercise is time consuming and both physically and mentally hard for many people. Many supplements claim to ease this burden, promising that fat loss or lean body mass gains can be achieved with consumption of a simple product. In this section we look at the marketing claims made by some of the supplement manufacturers and the currently available scientific evidence examining the efficacy of said promises and claims.

Supplements Claiming to Increase Lean Body Mass

To gain skeletal muscle mass, a training stimulus must be coupled with adequate energy and protein intake. Dietary protein intakes meeting the demands of training (see chapter 5 for more details) is effective in facilitating skeletal muscle protein synthesis (muscle mass gains) in both young and older people. Adequate dietary protein during energy restriction (e.g., 1.2–1.5 g/kg body weight) is warranted to minimize losses of muscle mass during this purposeful fat-loss process (84, 85). Leucine is a branched-chain amino acid that seems to be a trigger for skeletal muscle protein synthesis and plays an important role in protein balance with training. Leucine alone, however, is not sufficient for gaining muscle mass. All essential amino acids are required (3, 84, 85).

Supplements Claiming to Decrease Fat Mass

Athletes commonly seek to achieve an optimal body composition for performance, and sometimes for aesthetic appearance. Losing body fat while maintaining or gaining skeletal muscle mass

---

PUTTING IT INTO PERSPECTIVE

IS NATURAL ALWAYS SAFE?

Many people seek natural food and supplement products, assuming that such items are healthier than their counterparts and safe for consumption—and often this is the case. The FDA does not officially regulate the term "natural," yet in the eyes of the FDA, "natural" means that no artificial or synthetic ingredients have been added (31). But "natural" does not guarantee safety. Natural products will be safe for many people, but they can have side effects and might interact with each other or with over-the-counter or prescription drugs. For example, vitamin K interferes with blood-thinning medications, and St. John's wort can speed the breakdown of many drugs (including antidepressants and birth control pills), thereby reducing their effectiveness (31).

In addition, some products labeled as natural might be contraindicated for people with certain diseases or conditions. For example, a joint health supplement may contain natural ingredients such as glucosamine that should be used with caution by people with diabetes or shellfish allergies, and high doses of caffeine can increase heart rate (31, 32). Manufacturers of supplement products might not include warnings about potential adverse effects or list those persons who should not use the supplement. The general recommendation is not to take any supplement unless you are certain that it will not aggravate a preexisting condition or interact adversely with any other medication or supplement you are already taking. Of course, such certainty is hard to come by. If you feel the need to take a supplement with unknown contraindications or side effects, always start with a small dose and be sure that your physician, RDN, and pharmacist know you are taking it.

is a difficult task involving careful manipulations in energy balance so that enough energy can be consumed to sustain training without taking in excess energy that promotes weight gain. Sometimes athletes turn to dietary supplements for assistance with the process. Unfortunately, no safe and effective weight-loss supplements can achieve this goal. Even so, understanding some of the popular products promoted for body fat loss is important.

> Caffeine: Although some data demonstrate a small effect of caffeine on body weight measures (86), support is insufficient to recommend caffeine as an effective fat-loss or weight-loss strategy (87). Studies often combine caffeine with other compounds, or caffeine appears in multi-ingredient products, making it difficult to draw conclusions about caffeine itself.
> Green tea: Green tea has an insignificant effect on fat loss or weight loss (87, 88). With that said, if people or athletes enjoy the beverage, there is no reason to recommend its discontinuation. Although research is limited and no conclusions can yet be made, there is potential for beneficial effects on some heart disease risk factors, including blood pressure and cholesterol (88).
> Conjugated linoleic acid: Earlier animal research studies demonstrated a benefit, but insignificant effect was found on fat loss or weight loss in humans (2).
> Chitosan: Insignificant effect on fat loss or weight loss (2).
> Glucomannan (konjac fiber): Insignificant effect on fat loss or weight loss (2).
> Chromium picolinate: No effect on fat loss or weight loss (2).

DRUGS COMMONLY USED IN SPORT

Although many dietary supplements are readily available and legal for use and purchase, other substances are not legal. Performance-enhancing drugs (PEDs) are used to achieve drastic alterations of the body's physiological functions in an attempt to improve athletic performance. These PEDs, however, can be extremely dangerous and in some cases even deadly. Organizations such as the U.S. Anti-Doping Agency (USADA) (30) and the World Anti-Doping Agency (WADA) (25) help provide education about PEDs and keep information on prohibited lists (89). In addition to consuming illegal substances, some athletes use alcohol in attempts to improve performance outcomes. These products are not only potentially problematic for competition eligibility but also have negative effects on overall health.

Stimulants

Many stimulants are used under a physician's care to treat conditions such as attention deficit hyperactivity disorder (ADHD), asthma, narcolepsy, and obesity. The most used prohibited stimulant-based drugs are amphetamine and its derivatives, D-methamphetamine and methylphenidate. These drugs are used in medical settings for specific purposes, yet athletes turn to them for their purported ability to increase energy and concentration, and thereby enhance performance. They might also be used in some weight-class sports as a means of decreasing appetite. Prohibited stimulants tend to produce significant side effects in both the central nervous and cardiovascular systems. Use of amphetamines or related compounds, even when prescribed by a doctor and taken as directed, can cause tremors, tachycardia, jitteriness, and insomnia, and more seriously, myocardial infarction, stroke, and even death if taken incorrectly. The side effects from methylphenidate include Raynaud's phenomenon (a rare disorder that causes vasospasm of the arteries in response to cold temperatures or emotional stress, which reduces blood flow, leading to feelings of numbness or cold. Raynaud's typically affects the fingers and toes), profuse perspiration, and reduced appetite (90). Combining stimulants with exercise, or exercise in the heat, can have additional effects that lead to heat illness or heat-illness-related death (89, 91).

Anabolic Androgenic Steroids

In a medical setting, anabolic androgenic steroids (AAS) are used to treat clinical testosterone deficiency. In the world of competitive sport, athletes take these compounds to gain skeletal muscle mass. In addition to being banned or prohibited by sport organizations, AAS have many dangerous physiological and psychological side effects associated with their illegal use (e.g., not prescribed by a physician to treat a medical condition), especially because the doses taken may be well beyond the therapeutic level prescribed to treat medical conditions. The most common undesirable side effects include gynecomastia (growth of breasts), testicular atrophy (reduction in testicle mass), and widespread acne, especially on the chest and back. More significant side effects affect the cardiovascular system, including increases in total cholesterol and LDL cholesterol and reductions in high-density lipoprotein cholesterol. Further, in some instances, illegal or unsupervised use of AAS use can lead to liver damage, accelerated puberty, and stunted growth in young people. Women have additional, sometimes irreversible, side effects including dysfunction in menses, male-pattern hair growth or alopecia, voice deepening, and clitoris enlargement. Some athletes use multiple forms of AAS and a cycling pattern of use to minimize side effects. They might also use other drugs concurrently in an attempt to counteract side effects. Athletes must fully understand the legal implications, competition eligibility issues, and, most important, the many health risks associated with AAS use (89, 91, 92).

Peptide Hormones, Growth Factors, and Related Substances

The primary use of peptide hormones is for various medical conditions, and they are also commonly used to treat cancer or premature birth. Presence of an abnormal concentration of a hormone, its metabolites, or relevant ratios of hormones or markers in a bodily test sample is prohibited unless the athlete can prove that the concentration was due to a diagnosed medical condition. Examples of these substances include human growth hormone (hGH), erythropoietin (EPO), insulin, human chorionic gonadotrophin (HCG), and adrenocorticotrophin (ACTH) (89).

Human growth hormone (hGH) is naturally released in the body, and its highest secretion occurs during the adolescent growth spurt. Deep sleep, heat stress, hypoglycemia, and exercise stimulate endogenous release. Human growth hormone in its natural form requires a prescription and is intended to treat a limited number of medical conditions, including short stature, Turner syndrome, Prader-Willi syndrome, muscle wasting from AIDS, and growth hormone deficiency.

Prescription and distribution of this drug is tightly regulated. Taking hGH for nonlegitimate medical reasons (e.g., to enhance performance or for antiaging benefits) while not under the supervision of a licensed physician or medical practitioner permitted to prescribe these substances might be illegal. Some athletes use hGH in an attempt to improve cardiorespiratory fitness, increase skeletal muscle mass, reduce fat mass, or recover more quickly from injury. The side effects associated with hGH are numerous, including depression, fluid retention, and, with long-term use, acromegaly (chronic elevated levels of hGH in the body). Symptoms of acromegaly include swelling and subsequent abnormal growth of the hands and feet; overgrowth of bone in the face (protruding of the brow and lower jaw, enlargement of the nasal bone, and spacing of the teeth); carpal tunnel syndrome; and enlargement of body organs, including the heart. Still other symptoms might include joint pain; coarse, oily skin; skin tags; enlarged lips, nose, and tongue; voice deepening; sleep apnea; excessive sweating and foul odor; fatigue and weakness; headaches; impaired vision; decreased libido; erectile dysfunction in men; and menstrual cycle abnormalities or breast discharge in women. Many of these symptoms develop with long-term use and elevated hGH levels. Currently, it remains unclear whether higher doses over a shorter time, as used by some athletes, would result in the same level of side effects (55, 89, 91).

Marijuana

Marijuana, which comes from the *cannabis sativa* plant, contains substantial amounts of tetrahydrocannabinol (THC). THC is the major psychoactive component found in marijuana. Marijuana has become more readily available over the years and is available for purchase for recreational use in many states. Although it may be legal in certain places, marijuana is regulated at the state government level and the regulations for purchase and use vary tremendously across the United States. Under the Controlled Substances Act (CSA), Congress classifies marijuana as a schedule 1 drug. This classification means that it has a high potential for abuse, is not currently accepted for medical use in the United States, and lacks accepted safety for use under medical supervision (93). Physiological side effects of marijuana use include increased heart rate, impaired short-term memory, slowed bodily coordination and reaction time, reduced ability to concentrate, distorted sense of time and space, and respiratory complications and diseases. Psychological effects include mood instability and impaired thinking and reading comprehension (89). Self-reported use of marijuana is emerging, especially in athletes seeking help with pain and concussion management (94). Controlled research experiments need to be conducted and published to determine the physiological and psychological effects of marijuana on performance and recovery in athletes.

Cannabidiol (CBD) is a nonintoxicating cannabinoid reported to have psychological and physiological effects that may be beneficial to athletes and their performance and recovery. These purported beneficial effects in animal studies include anti-inflammatory, neuroprotective, and analgesic properties. Early studies suggest that CBD may be beneficial for athletes by reducing anxiety in stressful situations and in those with anxiety disorders. Other preliminary studies do not report CBD being beneficial for sleep, cognitive function, and thermoregulation. More well-controlled studies on CBD use in supporting athletic performance are needed before conclusions can be drawn (93, 95).

Alcohol Use

Athletes choose to use alcohol for a variety of reasons, from the perception of "taking the edge off" to social acceptance and team building. Although prevalence of alcohol consumption is similar in the athletic and general populations, its use is especially popular in the college setting during weekend festivities and celebrations associated with team success. The NCAA has cited alcohol as the most abused drug in collegiate sport. Research suggests that college athletes associate alcohol consumption with an enhanced sense of well-being and that social drinking helps build group identification (96).

Although the research on low to moderate alcohol intake preexercise or during exercise is inconclusive, detrimental effects on athletic performance have been reported (3, 97). For example, alcohol might negatively affect metabolism, thermoregulation, motor skills, and mental concentration. Some of these negative effects might persist for hours after consumption. Alcohol likely impairs endurance performance through impairment of gluconeogenesis, glucose uptake, and glucose use. A recent study examined the effects of alcohol consumption on rates of skeletal muscle protein synthesis after an acute exercise bout and reported reduced rates even when the alcohol was coingested with protein (98). Such consumption would likely result in slowed recovery, repair, and growth of tissue (3, 97, 99).

Overconsumption of alcohol can lead to alcohol-related illness or death. This issue is of increasing concern among college students, because excess alcohol consumption can lead to undesirable consequences. Estimates are that over 1,500 college students die from alcohol-related unintentional injuries each year (100). A relation is also suspected between alcohol use and suicidal tendencies among students (101). In addition, results from a 2019 survey in college students aged 19 to 24 years reported that each year alcohol-related physical assaults have affected about 690,000 people and sexual assaults have affected about 97,000 people (100). Approximately 25 percent of college students report suffering negative academic consequences related to drinking alcohol, such as missing classes, falling behind in class, and doing poorly on exams and papers (100).

Postexercise nutrient intake is critical for optimal recovery for athletes. Although alcohol is not a nutrient, it does contain energy (approximately 7 kcal/g). Postexercise is the time when an athlete should be focusing on rehydration, adequate repletion of glycogen with carbohydrate sources, and maximizing skeletal muscle protein synthesis with dietary protein intake. If time after training is spent consuming alcohol instead of nutrient-rich foods, recovery may be compromised (3, 97, 98, 102).

SUMMARY

Dietary supplements are defined and regulated by the FDA, and advertising is regulated by the FTC. Supplements are regulated differently from food additives and drugs. FDA standards govern Supplement Facts labels and the claims that manufacturers can make about a product. Allowable claims can be categorized into three groups: nutrient content, health, and structure/function claims. Nutrient content claims refer to the amount of a given nutrient in a product, whereas health claims describe a relation between a nutrient and disease. Both types of claims are approved by the FDA. Structure/function claims are not preapproved by the FDA and require a disclaimer that the FDA has not evaluated the claim and the supplement is not intended to "diagnose, treat, cure or prevent any disease."

Some sport organizations have lists of banned substances; other sport groups do not impose such regulations. Several professional organizations or certification programs are available to help people navigate this issue and the process of certifying products that are sold to the consumer. Some dietary supplements may enhance performance or training adaptations such as muscle mass gains, and others do not. Although hundreds of supplements are on the market, the IOC classifies them into categories: (a) those used to provide a practical form of energy and nutrients; (b) those taken to prevent or cure specific nutrient insufficiencies or deficiencies; (c) those with strong evidence of efficacy of performance improvements for specific activities; (d) those claiming to improve training capacity, recovery, muscle soreness, and rehabilitation from injury; (e) those claiming to enhance immune health; and (f) those claiming to alter body composition by increasing lean mass and reducing fat mass.

Supplements presented in this chapter might perform as claimed, but that material does not imply endorsement by this textbook. Athletes or others interested in using supplements should consider safety and eligibility concerns, analyze the cost-to-benefit ratio, and seek professional guidance when needed. The potential physiological benefits or performance gains of a product need to be weighed against potential disadvantages, and the product should then be used only after evaluation for safety, efficacy, and compliance with relevant antidoping codes and legal requirements. When supplements are used, the regimen should be fitted to the individual's needs and goals.

FOR REVIEW

1. Why do athletes choose to use dietary supplements?
2. How are dietary supplements regulated?
3. What are the three categories of claims used on dietary supplements, and how do they differ?
4. What are a few considerations when exploring the use of dietary supplements?
5. What is peer-reviewed scientific evidence?
6. Explain the seals used on supplement labels. What do they mean?
7. Which organizations provide information about banned substances?
8. For the following supplements, list the popular claim, purported mechanism of action for performance improvement, and the overall impression of safety and efficacy:
   - Carbohydrate-containing sports foods
   - Protein supplements
   - Caffeine
   - Sodium bicarbonate
   - Nitrate
   - Creatine
   - Beta-alanine
   - HMB
   - Vitamin D
   - Omega-3 PUFAs
9. Why would athletes use pre- and probiotic supplements?
10. Describe the negative aspects of using stimulants, anabolic androgenic steroids, and alcohol in sport.

PART IV

APPLICATION OF NUTRITION FOR SPORT, EXERCISE, AND HEALTH

The final section of this book includes information on applying sports nutrition principles. This section covers ideal body weight and composition for health and athletic performance and presents various assessment methods to estimate body composition. Nutrition for aerobic training and sport (chapter 11) brings the information conveyed in chapter 2 full circle by giving specific examples of fueling for endurance sports. Chapter 12 covers the principles behind nutrition before, during, and after resistance exercise, as well as overall diet and its effect on training gains. Supplements specific for resistance training are also covered. Chapter 13 outlines strategies to achieve optimal body composition, including decreasing fat and gaining muscle for recreational and competitive athletes. The principles behind these dietary strategies are also discussed. Finally, chapter 14 covers how to work with active people who fall into special populations and have unique nutrition needs.

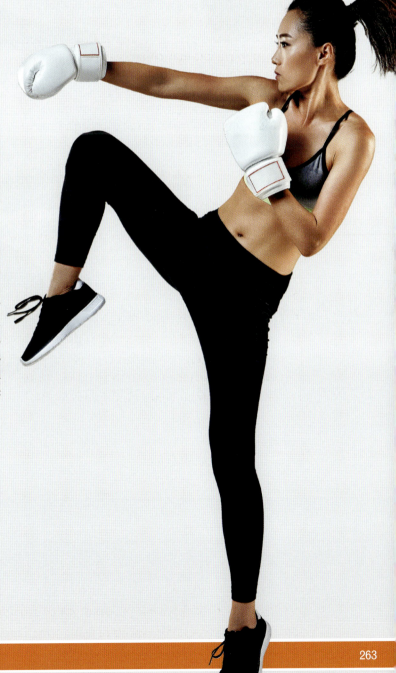

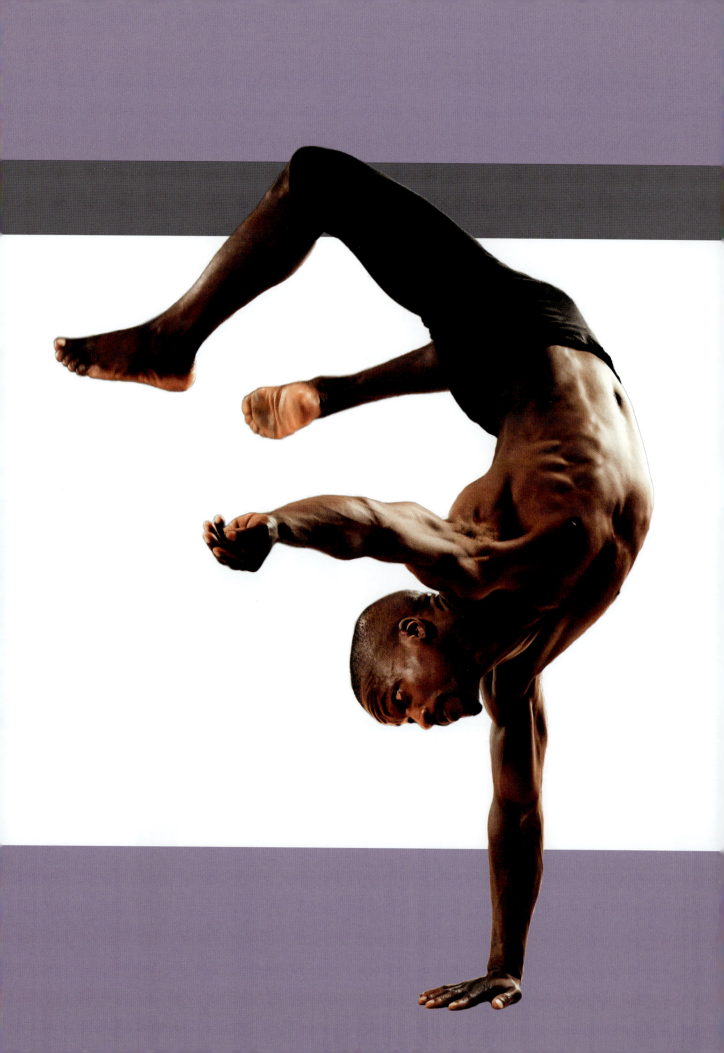

10

Body Weight and Composition

> **▶ CHAPTER OBJECTIVES**
>
> After completing this chapter, you will be able to do the following:
>
> - Explain the difference between body weight and body composition.
> - Explain how body weight and body composition affect sport performance.
> - Describe the compartments of the body as they pertain to body composition.
> - Discuss the genetic and environmental factors that contribute to body composition.
> - Discuss the principles behind the common methods of body composition assessment.
> - Explain how to interpret and communicate body composition estimates.

Health organizations use different terms to describe the composition of the human body. Some terms refer to the absolute size of the body (e.g., body weight or mass), whereas other terms assess the body's composition, or relative amounts of muscle, fat, bone, and water. Distinguishing between the size and the composition of the body is important because they have different effects on human health. Excess body weight, caused by high body fat, is dangerous because it increases disease risk (1). Lean body mass, which is composed primarily of muscle, bone, and water, is healthier than adipose tissue, especially when present in large quantities in the body.

The conditions termed *overweight* and *obesity* increase a person's risk of morbidity from hypertension; dyslipidemia coronary heart disease; gallbladder disease; stroke; type 2 diabetes; sleep apnea; osteoarthritis; respiratory problems; and endometrial, breast, prostate, and colon cancers (2). In fact, the U.S. Centers for Disease Control and Prevention (CDC) has declared modern American culture "obesogenic" in nature, meaning that the normal way of life causes Americans to be fatter and heavier than ideal. American culture promotes excessive intake of unhealthy, **energy-dense foods** that makes it easy to be habitually physically inactive (3). Body weight that is higher than what is considered healthy for a given height is described as overweight or obese (4). More specifically, **overweight** means that a person weighs more on a scale than the healthy reference standard, whereas being obese means that a person is carrying a higher percentage of body fat than what is desirable within the healthy reference standard. Over 70 percent of adults over 20 years of age are overweight or obese. Over 40 percent of adults are obese (5). Weight management is undeniably a challenge for many Americans, including sedentary, moderately active, and even competitive athletes (6, 7).

In 2013 the American Medical Association (AMA) presented a report classifying **obesity** as a disease and basing the diagnosis on having a body mass index (described later in the chapter) above 30 kg/m² (8). Their position is that classifying obesity as a disease will help the way that medical professionals address it with their patients. Other professional groups have published arguments against classifying obesity as a disease because they believe that it is only a risk factor for other diseases and that diagnosing this in the large number of people who are obese could result in more health care costs from drugs and surgeries. Their position is that labeling an obese person as having a diagnosed illness would promote a drug or surgical intervention rather than lifestyle change. Furthermore, using body mass index is an imperfect way to classify a person as obese (9, 10).

FACTORS CONTRIBUTING TO BODY WEIGHT AND COMPOSITION

Both genetic and environmental factors contribute to the accumulation of body fat. Humans are born with a tendency to store body fat in amounts

OBESITY AND INFLAMMATION

Chronic inflammation is an underlying factor in several diseases, including obesity. Fat tissue pumps out inflammatory compounds. There is a theory that as white adipose tissue (WAT, the predominant type of fat in the body) increases, it shifts from an anti-inflammatory or neutral tissue to one that is proinflammatory. WAT secretes proteins called adipokines. It is believed that normal-sized adipocytes secrete anti-inflammatory molecules, whereas full adipocytes (seen with weight gain) secrete proinflammatory molecules. As overweight and obesity increase over time, a shift to an overall proinflammatory state may occur (11). Overweight and obese people may also have altered gut flora, containing more harmful bacteria and less beneficial bacteria as compared with those of normal weight. This condition might also contribute to higher levels of inflammation. Note that this area of research is new. The current evidence suggests that adipose tissue contributes the most to systemic inflammation (11).

that are predetermined by our genetic makeup. Genetics, as well as muscularity, influence where fat is deposited on the body, but this does not mean that our ultimate body shape and size are completely outside our control. We can shape our environment by adopting healthy eating behaviors, exercising regularly, and engaging in activities of daily living. Doing this can be difficult because, as consumers, we are inundated with an abundance of inexpensive, energy-dense foods. In addition, many jobs demand little physical exertion, although they may be mentally exhausting at times. Successfully overcoming the temptation to be physically inactive and to overeat or choose unhealthy food requires a level of discipline that escapes many people. This circumstance is unfortunate because our food selections and level and type of physical training ultimately determine how close to our genetic potential we become. A tiny percent of the population has a genetic condition that makes it extremely challenging to achieve and maintain a body weight and composition that promotes health and well-being (12).

Genetic Factors

Genetics contribute to our height, weight, body fat distribution, and metabolism, regardless of our environment. Identical twins raised in different households have been found to have similar body weights to one another, and children of adopted parents have been shown to resemble the body types of their biological parents more closely than those of their adoptive parents. In addition to inheriting body weight and fat distribution, children also tend to inherit specific body types, such as being tall and thin or short and stout. This tendency is important to remember when setting body composition goals because some ideals might be unattainable no matter how hard a person trains or how disciplined they are about food choices. For example, a very tall and thin person might never be able to put on enough muscle mass to be a bodybuilder, nor may a very muscular, stocky person ever achieve extreme leanness and become an elite runner (12).

Another area of active research that suggests a genetic component to body weight and fatness is known as the **set point theory**, which proposes that the brain, hormones, and enzymes work together to regulate body weight and fat at a genetically predetermined level that solidifies sometime during young adulthood. This theory surmises that any attempt to change body weight voluntarily from the set point initiates a series of physiological and metabolic responses that ultimately result in no further loss of body fat, or a plateau. These responses may include storing fat more efficiently, decreasing metabolism, or stimulating appetite (12).

❓ DO YOU KNOW?

The set point theory may help explain some of those stubborn pounds of body weight that keep coming back after a time spent trying to lose weight.

Environmental Factors

Environment plays a significant role in body weight regulation. Although genetic factors limit what can be accomplished, healthy behaviors and choices, such as choosing the correct foods and portion sizes and getting sufficient quantity and quality of exercise, engaging in activities of daily living, and learning behavioral modification and self-monitoring techniques certainly can help maximize genetic potential. Poor food choices are often learned behaviors that can become lifelong habits. Over time, new habits can be established by building on small, positive changes. Although athletes might seem more disciplined than the general population, they too struggle with food choices because of many factors, including limitations in financial resources, lack of knowledge about nutrition, need for convenience, and preferences for certain foods (12).

BODY WEIGHT AND COMPOSITION CONCERNS IN ACTIVITY AND SPORT

Many competitive athletes are young and do not have long-term health consequences at the forefront of their minds. But athletes should seek to strike a balance between weight for optimal performance and weight for long-term health. Instead, immediate performance outcomes are often the focus. Similarly, some people new to activities such as cycling or running races want to commit to short-term goals that enable them to complete an event. Like the general public, some athletes also face the struggle of needing to decrease or maintain an ideal weight and body composition for optimal performance. Many athletes have **body image** concerns, especially those in sports in which they might be judged on aesthetics and performance, such as gymnastics, figure skating, and physique sports (including bodybuilding, bikini, and fitness competitions).

Most athletes who are concerned about weight management are either overweight or obese and want to reduce their body fat levels to conform to healthy values, or they are already normal weight, or even lean, and want to reduce body fat further and increase lean mass for either aesthetic or performance reasons. Body weight and composition are somewhat easily manipulated and thus tend to be target areas of change when considering certain sports or activities. Many active people place a huge emphasis on body weight, assuming that it is an absolute predictor of athletic performance. Although weight and fat can certainly play a role in athletic success, no one weight or percent fat level is indicative of positive performance outcomes (13). Athletes seeking weight loss or fat loss must do so safely so as not to jeopardize their health or physiological function. Fortunately, the well-established weight-management principles that hold for the general population also apply to athletes and active people (14).

Many athletes fluctuate in weight throughout a year, depending on whether they are in the off-season, training season, or competition period. For most athletes, body fat is lowest during the competition period, but this level might be hard to maintain throughout the other periods. Too much fluctuation is not the best situation for the athlete because extreme measures may be required to obtain and maintain the ideal competition weight. Ideally, an athlete should strive to stay within 3 to 4 percent of their competition weight throughout the calendar year (13). By doing so they need to make only minor adjustments during training and competition periods. Extreme chronic dieting or repeatedly losing and gaining significant amounts of weight can be an indicator that the athlete is trying to achieve an unrealistic body weight (14).

Different sports and activities differ significantly in the body composition that might affect performance outcomes. For some sports or activities, skeletal muscle size and shape might be the target, whereas others might require a balance of strength and power for movement. Many sports have weight classes for competition and require competitors to achieve a delicate balance of the lowest possible body weight while maximizing skeletal mass and power (13).

On the opposite side of the spectrum, being overweight or overfat is disadvantageous in many sports because carrying extra mass is physiologically inefficient. In some sports, such as long-distance running and cycling, lower body mass can contribute positively to efficiency in energy expenditure and improved heat dissipation. For bodybuilders or those in physique competitions, low levels of body fat are required because participants are judged on their aesthetic appearance. Some people, such as gymnasts and acrobatic performers, require a body composition that optimizes biomechanical movement. In contrast, being too thin or too lean might negatively affect both performance and long-term health. For most

---

PUTTING IT INTO PERSPECTIVE

NEGATIVE CONSEQUENCES OF YO-YO DIETING

The term *yo-yo dieting* has been used to describe a situation in which a person goes on a diet to lose weight only to gain that same weight back. Such diets are often fads that call for eliminating key food groups in an attempt to reduce energy (calorie consumption). They usually promote quick weight loss, and many have a defined period of time. After the person completes the diet, they gain the weight back—sometimes even more weight returns than was originally lost. Lean body mass is often lost during these diets, yet primarily fat is gained back. Ultimately, such diets do not maintain a healthy body composition, nor do they teach lifelong healthy eating habits. Competitive athletes, and others, might succumb to such methods with the intention of losing weight for improved performance, but losing weight in an unhealthy fashion can be detrimental to performance.

athletes, having a higher percentage of lean mass with a lower percentage of body fat is desirable. Although some optimal body composition ranges are presented later in the chapter, there is no one ideal body fat target associated with optimal performance in any given sport or activity (13). Chapter 13 provides a detailed discussion on achieving optimal body composition.

Body Mass Index

Body weight is different from **body mass index (BMI)**. **Body weight or body mass** is how much a person weighs on a scale and is usually expressed in pounds or kilograms. With a calibrated scale, weight can be measured with great accuracy. BMI was originally created to assess population-based rates of obesity.

BMI uses both body weight and height to classify people into four subclasses: underweight, normal, overweight, and obese. See table 10.1 for the classification and table 10.2 to determine how to calculate BMI (3, 4, 15, 16). BMI correlates with body fatness in most people, but it is not an actual measure of body fat (17, 18), nor is it a measure of visceral fat, the kind of fat stored in the abdomen and covering internal organs, including the liver, pancreas, and intestines (19). BMI cannot distinguish between excess fat and muscle or bone mass. BMI can overestimate fatness in athletes with higher lean body mass and therefore should not be used with this population (20-22). In thin children, BMI is a better measure of fat mass (23). Age, sex, ethnicity, and muscle mass affect the association between BMI and body fat in both children and adults. BMI can overestimate body fat in athletes and others with muscular builds and underestimate body fat in older persons or those who have lost muscle (24).

A BMI between 18.5 and 24.9 kg/m^2 is considered a normal or healthy body weight. BMI within this range is associated with the lowest risk of developing a chronic disease or death. Those classified as overweight might have an increased risk of disease and death, and those who are obese have the highest risk of developing several diseases, including cardiovascular diseases and type 2 diabetes. BMI is a useful initial screening tool to help identify people who might be overweight or obese. BMI is also used to track population-based rates of overweight and obesity. But BMI should not be used in isolation to determine health, disease, or disease risk (24). A disadvantage of using BMI is that it does not specifically differentiate between body weight and amount of body fat. Thus, BMI overestimates fat in those with high muscle mass. For example, a muscular male athlete with low body fat could have a BMI that classifies him as overweight or obese. His weight would be higher than expected for his height, although he is not overfat and thus not at a higher risk for disease based on body composition. If the BMI is 25 kg/m^2 or greater,

Table 10.1 BMI Classification

BMI (kg/m^2)	Classification
Below 18.5	Underweight
18.5–24.9	Normal or healthy
25.0–29.9	Overweight
30–34.9	Obesity class I
35.0–39.9	Obesity class II
>40	Obesity class III (extremely obese)

Table 10.2 Determining BMI

Measurement units	Formula and sample calculation
Kilograms and meters (or centimeters)	*Formula:* weight (kg) / (height [m])^2 With the metric system, the formula for **BMI** is weight in kilograms divided by height in meters squared. Because height is commonly measured in centimeters, divide height in centimeters by 100 to obtain height in meters. *Example:* weight = 68 kg, height = 165 cm (1.65 m) *Calculation:* 68 ÷ (1.65)^2 = 24.98
Pounds and inches	*Formula:* weight (lb) / [height (in.)]^2 × 703 Calculate BMI by dividing weight in pounds by height in inches squared and multiplying by a conversion factor of 703. *Example:* weight = 150 lb, height = 5 ft 5 in. (65 in.) *Calculation:* [150 ÷ (65)^2] × 703 = 24.96

determining whether weight loss should be the goal is important. Because BMI is associated with increased risk of developing certain chronic diseases, perhaps current body fat levels along with any medical laboratory values can be an indicator as to whether weight loss is warranted. If an athletic person with large, defined musculature has a high BMI value, then BMI may not be the best tool for estimating level of body fatness. In such situations, having body composition (absolute fat and lean mass) measured might be of value, although these techniques require the assistance of a qualified exercise professional (4).

Body Fat Patterns

In addition to body weight, the amount and distribution of body fat can influence health and performance. Levels of body fat can rise because of adipose cell **hyperplasia** (growing more fat cells) or by cell **hypertrophy** (growth of existing cells). Given a state of chronic positive energy balance, the ability to store body fat is limitless. Whether there is a stage in life at which hyperplasia predominates over hypertrophy is debatable, but most agree that both ultimately occur as a result of chronic positive energy balance (25).

People have different body shapes, characterized by three types: ectomorph, mesomorph, and endomorph. Individuals can either be predominately one of the three shapes or fall somewhere between two shapes. In addition to body shape, differences are also seen in body fat patterning. Overweight people who carry most of their weight around the middle fall into the **android** type, or apple shaped. Such people tend to have both subcutaneous (just beneath the skin) and visceral (deep) body fat, and the amount in each area varies from person to person. This shape—specifically, the larger amount of visceral body fat—increases the risk of developing chronic diseases caused by a multitude of factors, one being fat surrounding vital organs. Those who carry weight in their hips, thighs, and buttocks are called **gynoid**, or pear shaped. This fat is usually predominately subcutaneous and not associated with the same risk of developing chronic disease. Although the android shape is more common in men and the gynoid in women, this is not always the case (26). See figure 10.1 for a visual demonstration of android versus gynoid obesity patterns.

Taking a measurement of waist circumference is one way to look more closely at body fat pat-

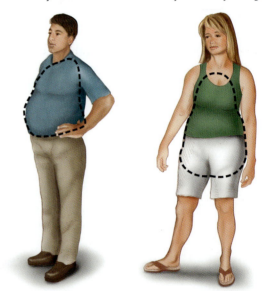

Figure 10.1 The android shape describes people who carry more body fat in their upper body, specifically the abdominal region. The gynoid shape describes people who carry more body fat in the lower part of their body, specifically the hips, buttocks, and thighs.

PUTTING IT INTO PERSPECTIVE

HOW TO ESTIMATE A DESIRED BODY WEIGHT FROM BMI

What should you do if your BMI is higher than the healthy BMI range? First, you need to determine if the BMI is high because of excess body fat or because you are a muscular person. If you think that excess body fat is the culprit, you can use your current BMI to calculate a desired weight that will move you to the healthy BMI range. Simply take your height in inches squared and multiply it by the desired BMI (e.g., 24). Then divide by 703.

Example: A person weighs 180 pounds and is 5 feet 5 inches tall. Current BMI is 30. The desired BMI is 24.
4,225 × 24 = 101,400. 101,400 ÷ 703 = 144 lb

> **PUTTING IT INTO PERSPECTIVE**
>
> ### HOW DO I MEASURE MY WAIST CIRCUMFERENCE?
>
> › In a standing position, place the tape measure horizontally near your belly button, just above your hip bones.
> › Measure at the narrowest portion of your waist.
> › Make sure the tape is snug but not compressing the skin.
> › Take the measurement after you comfortably exhale.
> › For additional information on taking waist circumference, visit the Centers for Disease Control and Prevention website (4).

terns. Waist measures of more than 35 inches (88.9 cm) for women or more than 40 inches (101.6 cm) for men classify people as being at increased risk for developing chronic disease. Use of both BMI and waist circumference can be helpful in determining risk of chronic disease or the need for a weight-management intervention (4).

Body Composition

Body composition refers to the components that make up the body. Although the scientific literature offers a few body composition models, the one most discussed in sports nutrition is the four-compartment model. In this model, the body is compartmentalized into body fat and lean body mass (LBM), sometimes referred to as fat-free mass (FFM). Fat-free mass includes everything except body fat. Organs, muscle, tendons, ligaments, bones, and skin are all part of fat-free mass. While FFM contains no body lipids, LBM contains a small amount of essential body lipids. LBM is further compartmentalized into skeletal muscle mass, total body water, and bone mass. Any of these four components can change through diet or training interventions. Body water changes can occur very rapidly, whereas changes in bone mass take a minimum of several months. Most athletes tend to focus on manipulating their body fat and skeletal muscle mass to achieve a body that is perceived to be more desirable for aesthetics, performance, or both (26).

Some of the different types of body fat are considered essential, and the rest are considered storage. Essential body fat is a component of many tissues and must be maintained to avoid compromising physiological function. Storage fat, however, results from a chronic positive energy balance (too many calories) and can be altered (lost) without a negative effect on physiological function, provided that dietary practices that create unacceptably low energy availability and psychological stress are avoided (13). In fact, a judicious and balanced approach to fat loss will likely improve health if a person is overfat. Essential body fat is approximately 3 percent of body mass for men and 12 percent of body mass for women; body fat percentages lower than these are not optimal for health and physiological functioning. With the rise of obesity in our society, good estimates for average body fat values in the current general population are not available. For most healthy adults, the total body fat percentage is between 12 and 15 percent for young men and between 25 and 28 percent for young women (27). Further classification of body fat percentages is listed in table 10.3 (27, 28).

ESTIMATING BODY COMPOSITION

Although many techniques give a body composition value, all of these are just estimates. Measuring body composition with 100 percent accuracy in a living human body is not possible. All methods used today are based on early research on cadavers (29). Cadaver analysis was used to develop statistically sound prediction equations for body composition, and included in these is a percentage error. If a female athlete has her body composition assessed by one of the techniques with a 4 percent margin of error, and she is assessed to have 15 percent body fat, her body

Table 10.3 Classification of Body Fat Percentages

Males	Females	Classification
2	12	Essential
5–10	8–15	Athletic
11–14	16–23	Good
15–20	24–30	Acceptable
21–24	31–36	Overweight
>24	>36	Obese

Data from Jeukendrup (2010); Lohman and Going (1993).

fat could be anywhere between 11 and 19 percent. Although errors are unavoidable, they can be minimized with proper equipment and technique. For example, the equipment must be calibrated, and a standardized operating protocol must be used. If measuring before and after a program or intervention, the same equipment should be used, and in most cases, the same operator should take the measurements. Valid and reliable equations should be used to calculate body composition. The athlete being tested might need to follow a protocol that involves being in the same state of feeding or fasting and at a consistent hydration level (not after exercise or sweating). For females, time in the menstrual cycle may need to be consistent, depending on the type and purpose of the measurement. When following protocols for each specific measure of body composition, several methods are useful for assessing baseline body composition or examining change with training and intervention. Ideal body composition includes a range of values that is individually determined as appropriate for a given individual. Any normative body composition targets should be set as a range of values rather than one number that might be considered ideal (13).

Understanding Compartment Models

Two-, three-, or four-compartment models may be used to estimate body composition. A two-compartment model assumes the body is separated, or compartmentalized, into fat and LBM. This model, developed in the 1940s, was based on the inverse relation between body density and body fat. If body density can be measured, then body fat can be estimated from the developed prediction equations. This model has a few assumptions that apply to all individuals, and these assumptions may or may not be true. When estimating body fat from body density, it is assumed that the density of all fat tissue and all LBM tissue is the same for all individuals and that the proportions of the water, muscle, and bone of the LBM are constant within and between all persons. This model is useful for detecting changes in total body fat, although it cannot detect the individual components that make up total LBM. If body fat decreases and LBM increases, it cannot be determined if LBM changes were caused by changes in muscle, bone, or water. LBM and muscle might be over- or underestimated if significant shifts occurred in water content caused by hyper- or hypohydration during measurement. Because changes in bone mass occur over a minimum of 6 to 12 months and are relatively minor, changes in bone do not have an appreciable effect on body composition measures (26).

> **? DO YOU KNOW?**
>
> Many nutrition and training studies rely on a two-compartment model to make conclusions about LBM. But this model does not distinguish between LBM changes in LBM components (water, bone, muscle).

Because the total body water (TBW) portion of the LBM can change both drastically and rapidly, to adjust for hydration status of an individual, a three-compartment body composition model was proposed in 1961 (29). In this model, the body can be separated into fat and LBM, and TBW is assessed independently. The methods for assessing TBW with the greatest possible accuracy require a lab setting with radioisotopes in which the hydrogen molecules are labeled. This method requires the collection of saliva, urine, or blood and might require a physician, depending on the isotope used and specimens collected. This method is expensive. Although some bioelectrical impedance devices estimate TBW, they are not as accurate as isotope dilution methods (26).

In a four-compartment model, measurements are made for body density (and hence body fat), TBW, and total body bone mineral. The remaining unmeasured component is assumed to be muscle mass. Like the three-compartment model, this model provides enhanced accuracy, but the measurement of more variables results in increased time and cost. Specialized equipment, laboratories, and personnel are needed, so this method is not used as frequently as the two-compartment model. Although the three- and four-compartment models increase accuracy of body composition estimates, they are usually limited to research settings in sophisticated laboratories. A six-compartment model, called the atomic-level model, is used for validation of some of the common body composition models and techniques, but this model requires extensive research laboratories and is not used outside the research setting (26).

Choosing a Method

Many factors can influence the choice of a body composition method. Although everyone wants to use the most accurate and convenient one, the choice is not that simple. As mentioned, some methods require specialized equipment and skilled operators and can be quite expensive. Some of the simplest and inexpensive methods lack the desired accuracy. When choosing a method, accuracy, cost, portability, ease of use, and subject comfort must be considered.

Recall that all body composition methods are estimates. In the methods described, mathematical equations are used to predict body composition values. The two key statistical methods used in body composition are correlation and regression. Correlation estimates the strength of a relation between two variables, and regression is used to predict one variable from another variable or multiple variables. Population-specific equations have been developed on narrow groups of people with similar physical characteristics.

Generalized equations developed on a wider range of people are better suited for use in settings where people might vary in age, gender, ethnicity, fatness, or athletic condition. Knowing the research behind the published equation can help ensure that the best equation is used for the population being tested, which might require obtaining the original published article and understanding its application for those being measured. Many of the newer automated methods or workplace computer systems may have prediction equations built in and may or may not specify where that equation originated (26).

Using Body Composition Methods

Body composition assessment methods can be categorized as laboratory methods or field methods. Laboratory methods are found in sophisticated research settings. Although they tend to be expensive and sometimes require in-depth techniques, these methods have the greatest accuracy. Some lab techniques also require additional levels of training, such as radiation safety training or a license to operate equipment. A few of the common techniques include hydrometry, hydrodensitometry, air displacement plethysmography, and dual-energy X-ray absorptiometry. These methods may provide some of the reference values for the derivation of equations used in the more common field methods. Field methods such as anthropometric skinfold thickness and bioelectrical impedance analysis are less accurate but are more convenient and not as expensive (26).

Hydrometry

Hydrometry is a measurement of TBW. In this method, the concentration of labeled isotopes of hydrogen or oxygen equilibrate with bodily fluids, and then samples from saliva, urine, or blood can be taken to estimate TBW. This method is costly, requires specialized lab equipment, trained personnel, and sometimes a physician. This method is not commonly used with athletes in field settings but has been used in research settings with both athletes and nonathletes (26).

Hydrodensitometry

Hydrodensitometry is also referred to as hydrostatic weighing or underwater weighing (UWW).

Densitometry is the measurement of body density, and *hydro* means "water." In this method, water is used to estimate the body density of a person. A basic physics principle applies here: Body density = body mass / body volume.

Body mass or weight can be measured with great accuracy. Weighing a person underwater is used to estimate body volume, and thus body density is derived. An established prediction equation is then used to calculate the percent body fat from the body density. Accuracy of the method depends somewhat on using an appropriate prediction equation.

A specialized tank is required to weigh a person who is completely submerged in water. Some tanks use a hanging scale, and some of the better instruments have a scale on the bottom of the tank. The person being assessed must expel as much air as possible from the lungs.

The basic principle behind this technique involves buoyancy. Fat tissue is less dense than water, whereas LBM is denser than water. The more body fat a person has, the more buoyant they are (they float) and the less they weigh underwater. On the contrary, the leaner a person is, the less buoyant they are (they sink) and the more they weigh underwater. The other factor in the body that contributes to buoyancy is air in the lungs. A person is asked to expel that air while underwater, but completely emptying the lungs is not possible. The air that is left after the attempt to exhale is called residual lung volume. This value must also be measured or estimated and factored into the assessment.

One limitation of UWW is the variance in quality of tanks and equipment. A good, accurate system is expensive and requires technical skill to administer. Although underwater weighing can be used on both lean and morbidly obese people (who are mobile), tank dimension can be the limiting factor. Even under the best of practices, the minimum **standard error of the estimate (SEE)** is ± 3.5 percent (30), and the minimal error published about this method demonstrates a 1 to 2 kg body fat error, or a little over 3 percent body fat in an average person. Therefore, as described earlier, for a calculation resulting in a 15 percent body fat value, the range of possible values would be 12 to 18 percent. If lower-quality equipment or an inappropriate prediction equation is used, the error can greatly exceed this estimate (26). Considering the limitations, if this procedure is available, it can provide the athlete and their coaching staff with information about a baseline body fat mass or changes in body fat with training and nutrition intervention.

Air Displacement Plethysmography

Like UWW, **air displacement plethysmography (ADP)** estimates body volume and thus body density. Instead of water displacement, air displacement is used. This procedure usually takes less than 10 minutes and requires the subject to sit quietly. The one discomforting factor of this method is that the person is completely enclosed in the machine (although light is available, and a window is usually provided). Like UWW, this equipment is expensive and usually limited to lab settings. It might not work well for small individuals or children, and because the chamber size cannot be adjusted, some obese persons simply might not fit. If all conditions are ideal, the SEE is approximately ± 2.2 to 3.7 percent (30), which might still lead to an average error of 3 to 4 percent in percent body fat (26). Additional research is needed to establish a more precise SEE, because the current values are not founded on an abundance of published data. Similar to UWW, this procedure can provide athletes and coaches with information about a baseline body fat mass or changes in body fat with training and nutrition intervention.

Dual-Energy X-Ray Absorptiometry

Dual-energy X-ray absorptiometry (DEXA) was first developed to measure bone mineral density, but later it was found to provide quite accurate assessment of soft tissue composition (fat) at the same time. This method requires exposure to radiation, but the dose is relatively low and considered safe for most people (the dose is less than 1/10th the dose of a standard chest X-ray and less than a day's exposure to natural radiation, including that from sunlight exposure). Despite the low dose, this method should not be used on pregnant women (31). In some states, urinary pregnancy tests are required. Subject comfort is relatively high in that the person must lie still on a table for approximately 10 minutes. The dimensions of the table and table weight capacity limit this method. An extremely tall person might exceed the dimensions of the table, thus compromising accuracy. Each machine also has a weight limit because of the sensitive X-ray tubes located within the table. Thus, overweight and obese or very large people might not be able to be tested. Other limitations are the great expense to purchase the machine and provide service calls for required maintenance, the need of a trained operator, and state statutes. In many states, a license is required to operate the machine; in some states, a physician order or prescription is required. With an accurate machine and under ideal conditions, the SEE is ± 1.8 percent (30), and the percent body fat error is thought to be 1 to 2 percent (26), although some studies show higher error rates (32). More research is needed to establish the SEE, because its current values are not founded on sufficient published data. If we consider all methods of body composition assessment, DEXA has the lowest SEE (whereas skinfold thickness has the highest) (13).

In addition to offering relatively good accuracy, DEXA can provide valuable health information in terms of body composition and bone mineral density (BMD) that applies both to the recreational exerciser and the competitive athlete. BMD can be very useful, especially in younger athletes, in whom bone formation is still occurring. Young female athletes with low BMD can be identified, especially in those sports where low body weight is preferred (33). In some of these weight-controlled sports, athletes use weight-control strategies that include eliminating food groups rich in calcium and vitamin D. Poor intake of calcium and vitamin D combined with low energy intake can result in reduced bone formation despite participation in exercise training. Even in women who are past the age of bone formation, knowing their value for BMD is critical. If the BMD is less than optimal, efforts and interventions can still be taken to prevent further BMD loss (33).

Skinfold Thickness

Skinfold thickness has been used in the field for many years and is still used today to estimate percent body fat. In this method, the thickness of a subcutaneous fat fold is measured with a device called a caliper. See figure 10.2 for the skinfold testing sites commonly used. An assumption underlying the method is that subcutaneous fat is proportional to total body fat. Subject comfort varies; for some, the pinch hurts for a few seconds, and for others, it is virtually painless. Subjects might feel self-conscious about having a person pinching their fat folds, so this method

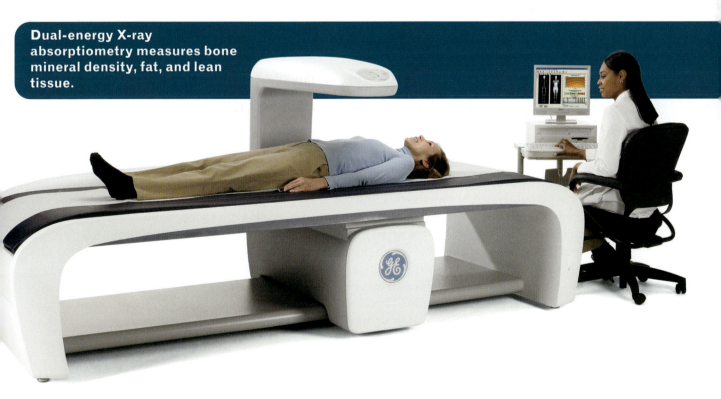

Dual-energy X-ray absorptiometry measures bone mineral density, fat, and lean tissue.

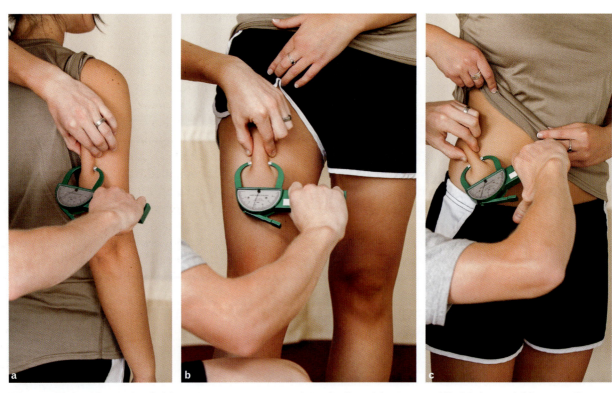

Figure 10.2 Many skinfold testing sites are used, including (*a*) triceps, (*b*) thigh, and (*c*) suprailiac.

should always be done in a private setting. In this technique, skinfold thickness is measured, and prediction equations are used to estimate body density and, from that, body fat. Over 100 different equations are offered in the literature for this purpose, so the operator must fully understand the equation used and its appropriateness for the population being measured. Some equations, called generalized equations, were developed on a nonhomogeneous population with varying characteristics (age, gender, body shape) (34, 35). Other equations are considered population specific, because they were developed on a homogeneous population of similar physical characteristics and should not be used on people outside those parameters. When considering an equation for use, try to choose one that was developed using valid reference methods or multicompartment models.

After an equation is selected, the research literature should be reviewed to determine which sites on the body should be used to take skinfold thickness. Most equations require at least three sites but might include more. This procedure requires much precision, giving careful attention to anatomical landmarks and technique. Resources are available to learn about all possible sites and the exact landmarks and procedure to be used for each fold measurement (26, 36). Skinfold measurement technique takes practice with people of many different body types and shapes. Adhering carefully to the standardized procedures increases both the accuracy and consistency (reliability) of the measurements.

In addition to an appropriate equation, a good skinfold caliper is required. Most of the valid equations use a high-quality metal caliper that produces a constant pressure throughout the measurement. Inexpensive (often plastic) calipers do not produce constant force throughout the measurement and tend to be much less accurate. A high-quality metal caliper can be purchased for less than a few hundred dollars and will last a long time with proper care.

Other factors to consider to improve accuracy when taking measurements include ensuring that the skin is dry, allowing time after a workout for body fluid compartments to normalize (36, 37), and taking each measurement at least twice. If the first two measurements differ by more than

2 millimeters, a third (or fourth) measurement is required. Rotating through all measurement sites and then repeating the process is the best approach, rather than taking two or more sequential measurements from the same site because depression of the skin can reduce the accuracy of repeated back-to-back measures (30). One limitation of skinfold measuring is the difficulty in measuring obese people. Identifying anatomical locations or isolating a single fold can be challenging, and sometimes the jaw of the caliper is not large enough. Also, note that the accuracy of this method is extremely variable because of the vast choice of equations and the precision and skill required for success. Even in the best-case scenario, the SEE is approximately ± 3.5 percent (30) and is often significantly higher, depending on the equation used and operator skill (26). Also, standardization of skinfold sites, measurement techniques, and calipers vary around the world. Still, all things considered, this method remains common because it is inexpensive, convenient, quick, and can be used on athletes by anyone trained in the proper protocol and technique, including team physicians, coaches, trainers, and even teammates. The comfort level of this method for athletes is relatively high.

Bioelectrical Impedance Analysis

Bioelectrical impendence analysis (BIA) is another popular method of estimating body composition, because of its ease of use, high subject comfort, and relatively low cost. This method does not require great technician skill and can be easily used with all individuals, including those who are obese. In this technique, a harmless electrical current is passed through the body and the impedance, or resistance, to that electrical current is measured. The principle behind this method is that LBM conducts electricity well, whereas body fat resists electricity. The higher the percentage body fat, the higher the resistance value. Because LBM contains water, and water conducts electricity, hydration status can affect the reading. The subject should be in a state of euhydration for the most accurate measurement. Timing of eating, drinking, exercise, and menstrual cycle stage must stay consistent when multiple measurements are taken.

Most research-quality machines measure the conduction through the whole body, requiring the placement of electrodes, and are more expensive than other devices. These devices usually give a value for resistance, and the investigator can then choose a prediction equation that ultimately predicts body fat. As with skinfold testing, many equations are available, so careful consideration is needed to increase accuracy. Other BIA machines may be considered, including lower-body analyzers (they look like a scale) and upper-body analyzers (they are handheld devices). Because the machine is measuring the resistance to an electrical current, these devices may introduce more errors. For example, someone with a gynoid fat pattern carries most of their body fat in the hips, buttocks, and thighs. If a handheld device is used, the current runs primarily through the upper body and misses most of the body fat compartments. Similarly, an android obese person carries most of their fat in the upper abdominal region and may get an inaccurate reading from a standing device because the electrical current runs primarily through the legs and lower body. These handheld or standing devices are available at many major retailers, are less expensive, and are easy to use. Many have only one prediction equation and thus offer no option for adjustments. An instant value is given for percent body fat. Although these devices may be somewhat useful for estimating body fat in large population groups, they are less appropriate for estimating body fat in small groups because of individual variances.

In a best-case scenario, when an effective analyzer and an appropriate prediction equation are used, the SEE for this method is ± 3.5 to 5.0 percent, depending on the equipment and equation used for body fat prediction (30). If a lower-quality device is used, the error can be significantly higher. BIA is a relatively inexpensive method that may be portable and can be used for obese persons with great comfort (26).

Interpreting Body Composition Results

As stated earlier, no method can measure body composition in a living human with 100 percent accuracy. In each method, assumptions are made that might not hold true in all people. Furthermore, no one method is better than the others in every case. Different methods measure different variables; for instance, hydrometry measures TBW; UWW and ADP measure body density; and DEXA measures bone mineral mass. Taken together, these methods can give a reasonably accurate value for interpreting body composition results. When using a field method, accuracy can be improved through proper equation selection, equipment, and technique. Even in the best of circumstances, errors can occur in any method of measurement. As discussed, if a person is assessed at 20 percent body fat and the method used has a 3 to 4 percent margin of error, the individual's actual percentage body fat ranges from 16 to 24 percent. Such imprecision might not be an issue if assessments are being used primarily to track change over time, such as during nutrition and exercise intervention. Most of the popular methods can be used in an initial assessment to help determine the overall health of the person being measured and to help determine whether intervention is warranted (26).

As introduced earlier, to minimize the margin of error for each technique, several body composition-testing protocols and guidelines are recommended. For instance, if the goal is to assess body composition outcomes over time with multiple measures, using the same technique and equipment will help maintain acceptable accuracy and precision. Moreover, best practice is to use the same technician for conducting all body composition measures. In addition to following these recommendations, other guidelines can help maintain accuracy and repeatability (test-retest reliability). These include rigorous technician training and documented test-retest reliability training for all technicians before initiating body composition assessments (13). Subjects interested in having their body composition assessed must also do their part to minimize the margin of error. Subjects should attempt to void before every measurement session; maintain consistent training, supplementation, and hydration practices (38); and take note that successive body composition measurements should occur during a fasted state or at least at the same time of day.

Before offering body composition assessment to athletes, practitioners should educate them on broad concepts related to strengths and limitations of the technique used and the importance of observing the established protocols to maximize accuracy. The first educational priority of all involved should be to discuss why body composition measurements have inherent limitations and provide only estimates of fat and fat-free mass. A second priority is to emphasize the importance of following strict preassessment and testing protocols to maximize measurement reliability (39). Educational efforts on how to interpret body composition estimates should also be extended to coaches and health care providers who work with athletes.

After an estimate of body fat is acquired, a person might wish to reduce body fat. A desirable body weight can be calculated as a goal to obtain a certain percentage of body fat. This formula is popular for this estimation:

$$\text{Desirable body weight} = \text{LBM} / (1 - \text{desired percent body fat})$$

Example: A 180-pound (81.6 kg) male who has 20 percent body fat wants to reduce his fat to 15 percent.

$$180 \text{ lb} \times 0.20 \text{ body fat} = 36 \text{ lb fat mass}$$

$$180 \text{ lb} - 36 \text{ lb fat mass} = 144 \text{ lb LBM}$$

$$\text{Desirable body weight} = \text{LBM} / (1 - \text{desired percentage of body fat})$$

$$144 / (1 - 0.15) = 144 / 0.85 = 169$$

An ideal scenario would be to incorporate athlete body composition assessments within an overall schedule that is appropriate to the performance of the sport, the practicality of undertaking assessments, and the sensitivity of the athlete to knowing body fat estimates (13). Note that the technical errors associated with all body composition techniques limit the usefulness of body composition reports for coaches to use for athlete selection or to predict athletic performance. Instead of using the results to set absolute body composition goals or to apply absolute criteria to categorize groups of athletes, body composition results should be compared with acceptable body composition ranges from a similar reference population (e.g., men's basketball 6%–12%) (28, 40). Finally, given that body fat content often varies over the course of the season and over the athlete's career, goal body composition ranges should be established and appropriately tracked at critical times (13).

When facilitating these monitoring programs, the communication of body composition results with coaches, other athletic staff, and athletes should be undertaken judiciously. Limitations in measurement technique should be recognized, and care should be taken to avoid promoting an unhealthy obsession with dieting and weight loss (41, 42).

SUMMARY

Body weight and composition is determined by a combination of genetic and environmental factors. Although people cannot control their genetic makeup, they can control some of their environmental factors. A sound diet and personalized training program can help people maximize their genetic potential to achieve their goals. Body weight is a simple measurement of mass and does not take body compartment or tissues into account. Body composition is the proportion of the body that is fat in relation to lean body mass. Lean body mass can be further subdivided into skeletal muscle, water, and bone. These components of body composition can be estimated in various ways in both the research laboratory and field settings.

FOR REVIEW

1. Describe the components of body composition.
2. Explain the difference between overweight and obesity.
3. Describe the role of genetics in body weight and composition.
4. What is a desirable BMI?
5. What is a limitation to classifying an individual based on BMI?
6. Describe the different body fat patterns and the physiological differences.
7. Can percent body fat ever be too low? Explain your answer.
8. What is a limitation of using two-compartment models to measure body composition?
9. For each of the listed body composition assessment methods (hydrometry, hydrodensitometry, air displacement plethysmography, dual-energy X-ray absorptiometry, skinfold thickness, and bioelectrical impedance), list the physiological principle, strengths, limitations, and error of measurement.

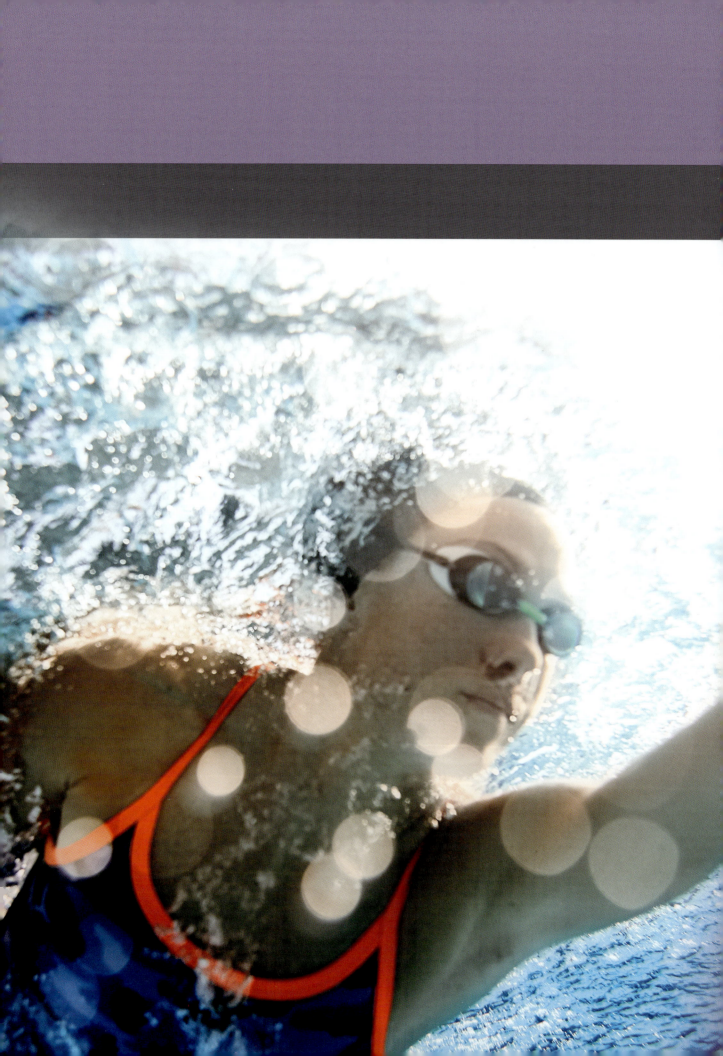

Nutrition for Aerobic Endurance

▶ CHAPTER OBJECTIVES

After completing this chapter, you will be able to do the following:

> Identify the defining characteristics of endurance activities.
> Further understand how ATP is produced from energy-yielding macronutrients during endurance activities.
> Identify nutrient requirements of endurance athletes, including preparation for, participation in, and recovery from competitive events.
> Explain how to select foods to meet nutrient requirements for endurance.
> Discuss unique challenges facing endurance athletes.
> Further understand how endurance training affects macronutrient metabolism.

Many sports and events—running, cycling, swimming, and soccer, among others—are thought of as endurance activities because of the long duration they take to complete. Although some of these events last less than an hour, others continue for many hours, or even days. Each endurance event has its own unique duration and environmental challenges, and thus its own set of nutrition requirements for energy-yielding macronutrients, micronutrients, and fluids (1).

ATP PRODUCTION DURING ENDURANCE ACTIVITIES

The continuous muscle contraction that is characteristic of endurance activities requires a near constant production of ATP at the skeletal muscle site, and stronger and faster movements necessitate greater ATP synthesis to meet the need for more energy. If ATP production cannot keep up with demand, movements will necessarily become slower or weaker (2). As discussed in chapter 2, ATP can be produced from several systems working simultaneously inside the muscle, including

> the ATP-PC system,
> the partial oxidation of glucose (e.g., glycolysis),
> the complete oxidation of glucose,
> the complete oxidation of fatty acids, and, to a limited extent,
> the complete oxidation of carbon skeletons derived from amino acids (2).

The big question is which system is primarily used to supply ATP during endurance exercise?

The answer lies in how quickly oxygen and substrate can be delivered to the working muscle. Metabolic systems are working together at any given time, and the contribution of each system depends on the ATP demand. At rest and during lower-intensity activities, ATP demand is low and fat is the preferred fuel source. With increasing intensity of exercise, skeletal muscle ATP demand increases and carbohydrate becomes the preferred source of fuel. The switch from predominantly fat to predominately carbohydrate is known as the crossover concept (3).

Ideally, the muscle completely oxidizes glucose and fatty acids to produce large quantities of ATP with no metabolic by-products that contribute to fatigue (e.g., hydrogen ions produced from metabolism). In this ideal situation, glucose and fatty acids enter the muscle cell from the bloodstream, where they circulate in free form and are delivered to working muscle, along with plentiful oxygen. This perfect situation occurs when exercise intensity is relatively low (<50% $\dot{V}O_2max$, such as when walking) and will continue in this manner as long as there are sufficient free fatty acids (FFAs) and glucose circulating in blood to meet the ATP demand. When exercise intensity becomes moderate or higher (>50% $\dot{V}O_2max$), the transport of substrates from the bloodstream into contracting muscle cells takes too long to match the demand for ATP. As a result, glucose and FFA are taken from the limited supply of glycogen and triglycerides that are stored within the muscle itself. Average glycogen stores can range from 70 to 500 grams, providing 280 to 2,000 kcal of energy (3-5), and intramuscular triglycerides make up only a small portion of total fat stores in the body, approximating 1 to 2 percent (6, 7). The greater the exercise intensity, the greater the proportion of substrate that comes from intramuscular sources; at near maximal intensity, over 90 percent of substrate comes from within the muscle. Note that this relation between exercise intensity and glycogen use is critical to understanding the cause of substrate fatigue, as discussed later in the chapter (2, 5, 8, 9).

Regardless of their origin (plasma or muscle), the combination of glucose and fatty acid oxidation provides roughly 95 to 98 percent of the total ATP produced during endurance exercise; the remaining 2 to 5 percent comes from amino acids. This ratio remains consistent during exercise of all intensities, except during the later stages of very prolonged endurance exercise, when glycogen reserves are running low and amino acids from the breakdown of skeletal muscle can contribute up to 15 percent of total ATP production. Normally, amino acids are preserved for important functions related to growth, maintenance, and repair, but they are used in increasing amounts to produce ATP as glycogen levels in the body decline during lengthy exercise. Reliance on amino acids for fuel during endurance exercise can be reduced by the common practice of ingesting carbohydrate during activity. The relative percentages of glucose and fatty acids used during exercise depend primarily on exercise intensity; higher intensities favor greater glucose use and lower intensities favor fat use (figure 11.1) (2, 3, 5, 8, 9).

The reason that carbohydrate use increases and fat use decreases with increasing exercise intensity is in part due to the amount of oxygen delivered to the muscle at higher intensities and to the capacity of the muscle to use this oxygen to oxidize substrates completely. Moving faster or more forcefully activates the sympathetic nervous system, resulting in elevated heart rate, blood pressure, and respiration. The overall effect is to enhance oxygen delivery to the working muscle, thereby making it possible to fully oxidize FFA and glucose. If oxygen availability is plentiful and the muscle cell has the capacity to process the oxygen delivered to it, such as during low-intensity exercise (10%–35% $\dot{V}O_2$max), then predominantly FFA will be used because the complete oxidation of FFA produces more ATP than does an equal amount of glucose. As exercise intensity increases to moderate and higher levels (>35% $\dot{V}O_2$max), oxygen uptake at the muscle becomes a limiting factor and begins to prevent some of the FFA and glucose from being completely oxidized; partial oxidation of glucose, however, is unaffected by this shortage of oxygen. The result of all this is that glucose becomes the substrate of choice at intensities greater than approximately 35 percent $\dot{V}O_2$max and is virtually the sole ATP producer at near maximal exercise. Moreover, the amount of glucose that is partially oxidized because of limited oxygen availability with high exercise intensity rises. This circumstance contributes to a buildup of lactic acid. Lactic acid separates into lactate and hydrogen ions. As hydrogen ions build up, muscle pH decreases (acidity increases), leading to metabolic fatigue. The fact that glucose can undergo partial oxidation to produce ATP and fatty acids cannot is just one reason that glucose is considered a more oxygen-efficient fuel than are fatty acids, meaning that glucose will produce more ATP per unit of oxygen than will the same amount of fatty acids (2, 3, 5, 8, 9).

ENERGY-YIELDING MACRONUTRIENT REQUIREMENTS OF ENDURANCE ATHLETES

Endurance athletes who can produce ATP at a rapid rate for long periods have a distinct advantage over competitors who cannot do so as rapidly or for quite as long. Those advantages come from physiological adaptations that result from specific aerobic training. Exercising at high intensities might help a person go faster, but it will also result in progressive glycogen use over time, because glucose is pulled from intramuscular sources. Fatigue resulting from glycogen depletion of skeletal muscles was discussed in chapter 3. Without glucose, virtually all voluntary muscle movements eventually slow down or cease because of the inability to synthesize ATP from *any* source. Athletes experiencing substrate fatigue from lack of carbohydrate stores and the metabolic ability to use them (due to lack of training) will slow down, walk with a stagger, or fall. The rate of glycogen depletion can be blunted by maintaining a constant supply of glucose in the blood through intake of carbohydrate during exercise, but even this method can preserve only a finite amount of muscle glycogen. Maximizing the amount of glycogen in skeletal muscle before the event begins is another way to increase the amount of time the athlete can exercise before running out of glycogen. Finally, glycogen could be spared if more fatty acids were oxidized instead

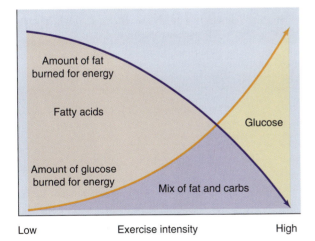

Figure 11.1 The switch from primarily fat for fuel to primarily carbohydrate as the preferred fuel with increasing exercise intensity is known as the crossover concept (3).

of glucose. The drawback to this system is that oxidation of fatty acids requires ample oxygen, which is not as plentiful during intense exercise. So, using fatty acids in place of glucose seems to have a cost, and that cost is the inability to move as fast or as forcefully as possible. If finishing an endurance event is more important than finishing as fast as possible, then training the body to use more fatty acids than glucose might be a good idea. This concept, called training low, involves training for an event by including workouts in a state of lower glycogen stores. This idea is discussed in detail later in the chapter. This section provides recommendations for (2, 3, 5, 9, 10) the consumption of energy-yielding macronutrients (fat, carbohydrate, protein) for optimal ATP production before, during, and after endurance events.

> **? DO YOU KNOW?**
> Extreme glycogen depletion (insufficient glycogen to meet ATP demand) in those who regularly consume carbohydrates (as opposed to those who have adapted to a low-carbohydrate diet or ketogenic diet) results in the inability of skeletal muscle to generate ATP for contraction. The result, known as "bonking" or "hitting the wall," is characterized by the inability to move forward. Performance will be significantly diminished until carbohydrate fuel again becomes available.

Habitual Intake of Energy-Yielding Macronutrients

Ideally, athletes and active people would consume a diet that promotes the following characteristics over a long period (e.g., decades):

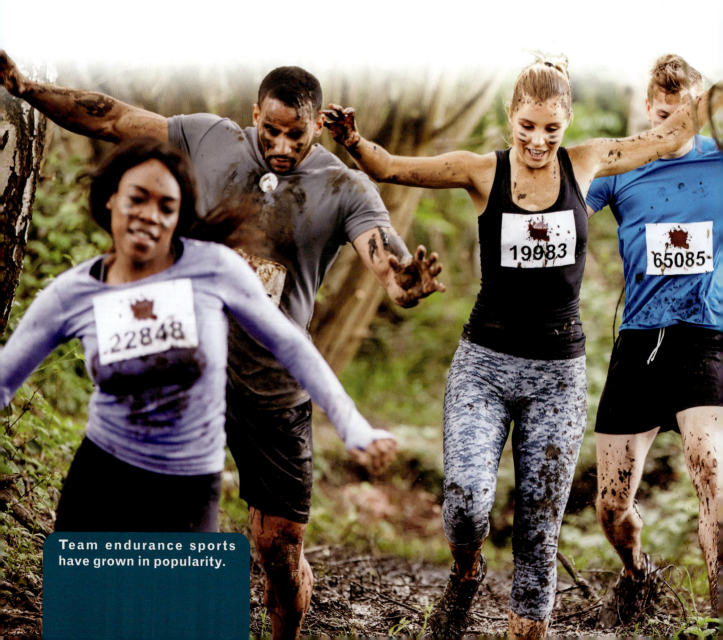

Team endurance sports have grown in popularity.

- Consistently staying within a healthy body weight range ideal for their sport
- Overall health and well-being
- Prevention and management of disease
- Optimal physical performance

The first ideal requires that athletes consume energy in amounts that are consistent with what they expend. Consistently consuming less than adequate energy could have many drawbacks, depending on the total calorie deficit (average amount of calories below average daily calorie needs) and foods consumed. These drawbacks might include nutrient deficiencies, loss of lean tissue (e.g., muscle, particularly if protein intake is not sufficient; see chapter 13), compromised immune and endocrine function, slowed healing of injuries, and impaired sport performance (1, 11-13).

Energy requirements of endurance athletes vary considerably but can be quite high for some sports (table 11.1). Recreational exercisers or novice athletes might require an additional 300 to 500 kcal per day to support their activity, and runners or cyclists training for a long-distance competitive event might need an additional 2,000 or more kcal per day to support their training. Energy expenditure of ultraendurance athletes range from 5,000 to 10,000 kcal per day. Because scientific literature that provides solid estimates of energy expenditure for men and women in different sports is scarce, athletes must pay close attention to their energy balance. If endurance athletes are unintentionally losing weight, they should increase energy intake; if they are unintentionally gaining weight, they should reduce intake. Athletes with high energy expenditures often have trouble consuming adequate energy. To meet those energy demands, such people must often snack continuously throughout the day or consume bigger meals and be selective in choosing energy-dense foods (1).

Recall from chapter 3 that the DRI for carbohydrate for adults is 45 to 65 percent of total energy intake and that added sugar intake is limited to 10 percent of energy or less each day (15, 16). Because athletes' requirements do not always fit these parameters, carbohydrate recommendations

Table 11.1 Energy Demands and Considerations for Different Sports

Energy demand	Sport	Special considerations
Relatively low energy expenditure	- Baseball - Golf	Careful carbohydrate consumption before and during activity, if any, should not lead to energy imbalance.
Generally high energy expenditure	- Basketball - Cycling - Running - Ice hockey - Soccer - Tennis - Swimming - Wrestling* - Rowing*	- Expenditure varies based on body size, training volume, and training or competition duration. Expenditure tends to be greater at the collegiate and professional levels. - Intake and expenditure must be individualized based on performance and body composition goals.
Generally high energy expenditure per kg body weight, but athletes may be small	- Figure skating - Gymnastics	Intake and expenditure must be individualized based on body composition goals. Body weight and composition are emphasized.
Highly variable	- Weightlifting - Track and field events - Football - Martial arts	Intake and expenditure must be individualized based on performance and body composition goals.

*Body weight and body composition are of critical importance.
Based on Karpinski and Rosenbloom (2017).

PUTTING IT INTO PERSPECTIVE

CARBOHYDRATE AVAILABILITY VERSUS HIGH CARBOHYDRATE

The term **energy availability** refers to energy intake minus energy expenditure of exercise divided by fat-free mass. This term has been used, especially for female athletes, to describe the dietary energy remaining for other body functions after exercise training. It can be argued that carbohydrate availability is a preferable way to think about carbohydrate needs in athletes. Intake alone may not be the best measure of physiological status. Carbohydrate availability accounts for the total daily intake and timing throughout the day and whether this intake meets the demand of exercise by adequately supplying glucose for the working skeletal muscle and central nervous system. Intake matched to or exceeding demand would be considered a state of high carbohydrate availability, whereas low carbohydrate availability would mean that carbohydrate intake or stores are too limited to meet the demands of training (13, 14).

are best expressed in absolute quantities (e.g., g or g/kg body weight) rather than as a percentage of total calories consumed. General carbohydrate recommendations for athletes were summarized in chapter 3 (table 3.6), and sample daily carbohydrate gram targets based on body weights were provided in table 3.7.

The AMDR for fat is 20 to 35 percent of total energy intake, an appropriate range for most athletes. Dietary fat recommendations are tricky because, in practice, endurance athletes need to estimate their carbohydrate and protein needs first and then fill in the remaining calories with fat. If an athlete wants to stay in a state of energy balance, it may turn out that fat intake falls at the lower end of the AMDR. Chronic fat intake of less than 20 percent of total calories is discouraged for most athletes who do not have extreme energy expenditures, because consuming less than 20 percent of total calories from fat might impair

? DO YOU KNOW?

Although all food that you eat is digested and metabolized, your body can digest and metabolize only so much food within a given time. For example, during many endurance activities you can burn 500 to 1,000 kcal per hour, but consuming that much energy during a training period would likely cause an upset stomach and impaired performance. The goal during endurance sports is to postpone substrate fatigue, not to replace exact energy expended with food. The bottom line is that your body cannot replenish energy with food as fast as it expends energy.

fat-soluble vitamin absorption and lead to reduced intake of essential fats, such as omega-3 fatty acids (13), and does not lead to improved performance. Lower fat intakes should be reserved for acute periods in preparation for competition or for an actual precompetition meal (13, 15, 16).

Endurance exercise training produces many microscopic injuries within muscle that must be repaired, and it creates the need to replace proteins, particularly in the mitochondria, that tend to undergo significant turnover because of the repetitive stress of lengthy exercise. This process requires a balance between muscle protein synthesis and muscle protein breakdown. Both physical training and dietary protein intake stimulate the anabolic process of muscle protein synthesis. For these reasons, athletes in general need 1.2 to 2.0 g/kg of dietary protein. Although athletes may benefit from a protein intake outside this range under certain training circumstances (17), more research is needed before a generalization can be made to an entire group of athletes. Athletes with larger training volumes leading to extensive skeletal muscle adaptation, repair, and remodeling tend to benefit from consumption at the upper end of the range. Endurance athletes need more dietary protein than their sedentary counterparts, but they typically do not have the most extensive skeletal muscle protein turnover and thus some athletes can consume at the lower end of the range (13). These recommendations are broad, and therefore factors such as body composition and training volume may play a role in pinpointing the recommendation for an individual athlete. Athletes on a lower-calorie diet need more protein

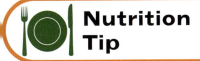

Nutrition Tip: Energy expenditure can be high in some endurance events. Because the body cannot replace all the energy lost in these sessions, the best approach is to use the general sports nutrition principles presented in this chapter rather than consume as much food as possible.

to minimize muscle mass loss during weight loss (see chapters 12 and 13) (1, 11).

Carbohydrate Loading

Maximizing glycogen reserves preceding an endurance event is a common strategy among athletes. The process of **carbohydrate loading** was introduced in 1967 and has been used for years in an attempt to supercompensate glycogen stores (4). The theory is that if a person can deplete glycogen with exercise followed by repletion with a high-carbohydrate diet, then more glycogen will be stored than if the person maintains an exercise routine and consumes a steady amount of carbohydrate. Carbohydrate loading appears to be an effective strategy for endurance events lasting 90 minutes or more if implemented at least 24 hours before an event (13). Athletes who may benefit from this strategy include distance runners, road cyclists, cross-country skiers, and open-water swimmers. Research suggests that performance can be improved by approximately 2 to 3 percent when glycogen stores are supercompensated, as compared with having normal stores (18). Note that because every gram of stored glycogen also retains 3 to 4 grams of water (18, 19), glycogen-loading protocols can induce a gain in body weight of up to 2 kilograms (4.4 lb), which may cause the athlete to feel weighed down before the event (18). Whether an athlete can perform well with the added body water weight is left to them to decide (4).

Carbohydrate loading can be approached in various ways. The goal is to increase carbohydrate availability during the later stages of an event. This objective can be accomplished by tapering training volume about a week before an event and then gradually increasing carbohydrate intake to the goal quantity for the individual event or sport.

Other carbohydrate-loading strategies have been demonstrated as well. For example, an athlete can consume a high-carbohydrate diet for 3 days in concert with tapering exercise the week before competition and resting completely the day before the event. The total diet should provide adequate energy and carbohydrate each day, approximately 8 to 10 g/kg body weight of carbohydrate. This regimen should increase muscle glycogen stores 20 to 40 percent above starting levels (20). But higher intakes of carbohydrate, 10 to 12 g/kg body weight of carbohydrate, have been suggested for marathon runners, road-race cyclists, and some team games during the 36 to 48 hours before the event (21, 22). Although carbohydrate loading appears to be effective for improving performance for some endurance athletes, the research data are mixed because in some studies subjects did not consume an adequate amount of calories each day (23-25). Another potential challenge is in female athletes who have a lower energy requirement (e.g., <2,500 kcal/day) but who might benefit from carbohydrate loading. To be an effective strategy, these athletes may need to exceed daily energy requirements during the loading program to see a beneficial effect on glycogen storage (23-25).

Additional research has suggested that glycogen levels can be enhanced without a depletion stage. Athletes can consume a high-carbohydrate diet (10–12 g/kg body weight) coupled with rest for as little as 36 to 48 hours before an endurance event. Carbohydrate intake before an event should include choices that are low in dietary fiber or residue to prevent excessive or untimely bowel movements. Athletes should experiment with intake during practice or training rather than wait until the week or day of the actual event. Athletes need to determine the optimal training, total carbohydrate intake and food choices that best suit their goals (13, 26, 27).

Day of an Event

Precompetition intake the day of an event can be critical for optimal performance. Athletes should prepare for an event by consuming enough food to avoid hunger, provide adequate fuel and fluids, and top off glycogen stores while minimizing potential for gastrointestinal (GI) distress. No one precompetition meal best suits everyone; carbohydrate and other nutrient intake will vary depending on factors such as type of event, time of event, environmental conditions, physiological training status of the athlete, stress of the athlete, and individual preferences. Many athletes prefer to begin an endurance event with full glycogen stores. Note, however, that other athletes might choose a different approach, which will be discussed later in the chapter (13, 22). Further, some research suggests that consuming carbohydrate just before an event might have additional benefits. Most research has been on endurance athletes whose sport involves continuous movement, but it might also apply to those who participate in sports that include intermittent high-intensity periods, such as soccer. Carbohydrate ingestion before an event will likely be beneficial for prolonged, sustained, or intermittent activities lasting an hour or longer and for those who have not eaten for several hours before an event (13, 26, 28). For events of shorter duration, adequate glycogen stores will likely be enough to supply the needed fuel for ATP synthesis.

The amount of carbohydrate recommended the day of an event depends on the length of time preceding the start of the activity:

> If an event is 3 to 4 hours away, the athlete has time to digest a full meal containing up to 3 to 4 g/kg body weight of carbohydrate. Aerobic endurance athletes who eat within 4 hours before competition should consume approximately 1 to 4 g/kg body weight of carbohydrate and 0.15 to 0.25 g/kg body weight of protein (13).

> If the event is 2 hours away, the carbohydrate recommendation is reduced to 1 to 2 g/kg body weight (13).

> If an event is early in the morning, the athlete might have only about an hour to prepare and consume a meal. The carbohydrate recommendation is then 0.5 to 1 g/kg body weight (table 11.2) (13, 26, 29).

For this meal to be well tolerated by the athlete, it should be low in fat and have low-fiber carbohydrate and perhaps a little protein, depending on the intensity and duration of the event and personal preference. Because fluids are also important, consuming a carbohydrate-containing beverage along with the meal might be desirable if carbohydrate needs cannot be met through food alone. Fluid needs are discussed in chapter 8. Each athlete should experiment with intake amounts before competition. Generally, a small meal or snack with a beverage is sufficient, but all athletes are different and must determine what works best for them. Some athletes need to have a little solid food in the stomach, whereas others do not tolerate anything solid and prefer a beverage only. Precompetition jitters can affect how athletes respond to food and fluids, but this circumstance is difficult to replicate in practice and thus hard to prepare for (1, 26, 29).

Intake of Energy-Yielding Macronutrients During an Event

Consuming carbohydrate immediately before and during exercise lasting longer than 60 minutes appears to have a beneficial effect on endurance performance because it provides additional glucose to the working skeletal muscles and thereby lessens the need for the muscle to tap into its glycogen reserves. The amount of carbohydrate recommended is a wide range of 30 to 90 grams per hour and is meant to provide as much glucose as can be oxidized without causing GI distress

Table 11.2 Carbohydrate Recommendations Before an Endurance Event

Hours before event	Carbohydrate (g/kg BW)	Suggestions
3-4	3-4	Mixed energy-yielding macronutrient meal with carbohydrate beverage
2	1-2	Light meal or snack or carbohydrate beverage
1	0.5-1	Snack or carbohydrate beverage

BW = body weight.
Note: Low-fiber or low-residue foods should be consumed.
Data from Burke et al. (2011); Cermak and van Loon (2013); Thomas, Erdman, and Burke (2016).

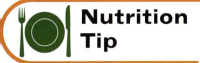

Nutrition Tip Some athletes might decide to try a new food or strategy before an important event. This approach can have undesirable consequences, because the body might respond to one food or supplement differently from others. In addition, some athletes feel pressure or nervousness on the day of an event or game, which can affect digestive function. Therefore, athletes are advised to stick with foods and supplements used during training and save new strategies and foods for practice days.

(figure 11.2). The higher end of the range (60–90 g/hour) is reserved for events lasting longer than 2.5 hours. Although individuals differ in their rate of glucose breakdown, little scientific evidence suggests that requirements differ based on body weight. For this reason, daily training and preevent recommendations are in absolute terms (e.g., g/hour) instead of relative terms (e.g., g/kg body weight/hour) (13, 26, 29-31). Note the research studies examining these higher rates of glucose use were conducted in controlled laboratory studies using cyclists. Whether these findings translate to all endurance athletes is yet to be determined, especially because cycling does not jostle the stomach like running does. This jostling or movement creates another avenue for potential digestive distress during running (32).

In addition to considering the total amount of glucose ingested and used, it is also important to take into consideration the way that different types of carbohydrates are broken down and used at different rates. If glucose alone is consumed, the limiting factor in carbohydrate availability during activity is the intestinal absorption of glucose. Glucose requires one type of transport system to cross the small intestinal wall for absorption. This sodium-dependent transporter can absorb a maximum of 60 grams per hour of glucose. But this is not the case when other forms of carbohydrate are simultaneously consumed. For example, fructose uses a completely different transporter (GLUT5) than does glucose (GLUT4), allowing an opportunity to get more glucose to the working muscle (recall that fructose gets converted

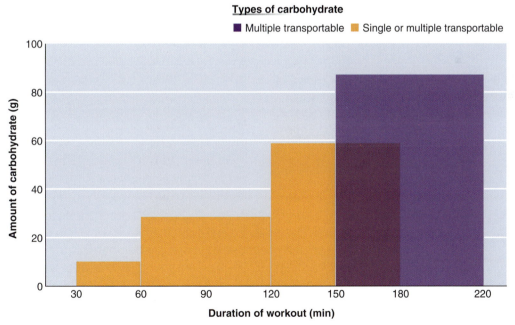

Figure 11.2 Both amount and type of carbohydrate are important to optimize endurance performance. More total carbohydrate and carbohydrate from different sources are needed with increased training time. The higher doses and types are most important for the elite endurance athlete wishing to maximize glucose oxidation. This topic is not applicable to the recreational athlete exercising for an hour or less per day.

to glucose in the liver after absorption) (figure 11.3) (13, 29-31). Think of different intestinal transporters as different cars going down the highway to a destination and different types of carbohydrate (maltodextrin, glucose, fructose, etc.) as your friends. If you have 12 friends and one compact car, you'll need to deliver one group of friends to the destination, go back to pick up more friends and deliver them to the destination, and finally go back a third time to be able to deliver the final group (and yourself) to the destination. This process is slow. Now imagine you have three separate cars. All your friends can hop in the cars and make it to the destination at the same time. From the standpoint of carbohydrate absorption in the small intestine, the different forms can be absorbed simultaneously rather than being absorbed one form at a time.

When glucose is combined with fructose in an approximate 2-to-1 ratio, the carbohydrate mix can be absorbed at a higher rate of up to approximately 90 grams per hour, because both transporters are working simultaneously. Think of it as having two doorways for the carbohydrate to get through rather than one—both doorways are open to welcome the carbohydrate at the same time: Fructose enters through one doorway, and glucose enters through the other. Taking advantage of this concept allows an athlete to maximize the amount of total carbohydrate that can be delivered to working muscle, a concept that can be of great value during extremely long events (e.g., >2.5 hours) but not as useful during relatively shorter events. Many products on the market contain both glucose (and glucose isomers) and fructose (e.g., gels, bars, and liquids), and they all appear to have a similar effect, so individual preference and tolerance should be considered when choosing which to use (13, 29-31).

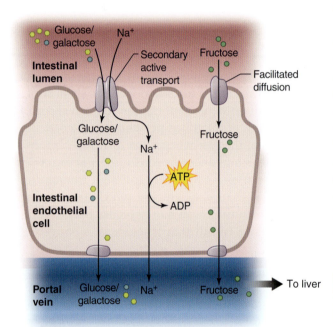

Figure 11.3 Because glucose and fructose use different intestinal transporters into the intestinal cell, they are not competing for entry space. Therefore, more total carbohydrate in the form of glucose can get into the body and to working muscle.

? DO YOU KNOW?

The limiting factor for using glucose as a fuel source is the absorption of dietary carbohydrate. Research shows that athletes who regularly consume carbohydrate can increase the absorptive capacity of the small intestine (and their tolerance)—called "training the gut." This should be practiced well before an important event (31).

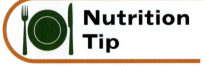

Nutrition Tip

The body can digest and use only so much carbohydrate at a time. Most sports drinks designed for endurance athletes are a 6 to 8 percent carbohydrate solution because solutions greater than this are more likely to result in GI distress (13, 29-31). Consuming juice or another sugary beverage might seem acceptable, but most of these have a carbohydrate concentration well above 6 to 8 percent. Although diluting the beverage to the correct carbohydrate concentration is possible, this process may not be as convenient as using a readily available drink, because mixing and measuring take a bit of time. In addition, these beverages might not contain the correct forms of carbohydrate in ideal proportions and might be missing needed electrolytes.

> **❓ DID YOU KNOW?**
>
> Participating in a lower-intensity activity lasting less than 60 minutes will likely not require any additional carbohydrate consumption during the event or training session, especially if the person is in a fed state from a prior meal or snack.

Most preevent meals focus on carbohydrate content, without guidelines for fat. Although some research shows that a high-fat preexercise meal results in increased plasma-free fatty acid concentration and fatty acid oxidation, whether this translates to an actual performance benefit in humans is unclear. Further, consuming large amounts of fat shortly before exercise can result in GI stress. For this reason, consuming a high-fat meal during the day of competition is not recommended, although taking in small amounts of healthy fats are not contraindicated either (13, 35). More information on manipulation of dietary fat and carbohydrate in attempts to translate metabolic adaptations to better performance is presented later in the chapter.

Research examining the effects of consuming protein during endurance events is limited. Some studies suggest that ingestion of carbohydrate and protein together during endurance activities can promote overall protein accretion and increased time to exhaustion, but other research has not confirmed those findings. Further, critics of this work argue that time to exhaustion is not necessarily an indicator of improved performance because few events go to complete exhaustion and that improvements in event finish time would be a better gauge. In studies that do assess race finish times, coingestion of carbohydrate with protein does not seem to improve finish time over consuming carbohydrate alone. Thus, there is currently little rationale to recommend the consumption of protein during endurance exercise (36, 37).

Macronutrient Intake After an Event

Optimizing glycogen repletion is important for athletes who must train or compete hard on multiple occasions on the same day or on successive days. Glycogen stores replenish at a rate of about 5 to 7 percent per hour, and 20 to 24 hours are needed to reestablish stores when adequate carbohydrate is consumed. Without purposefully modifying dietary patterns, glycogen will eventually replenish with sufficient carbohydrate intake, but this process might take some time and might not maximize glycogen stores between bouts of activity. This protocol is not ideal for the athlete needing to train or perform again within 24 hours. Optimizing glycogen replacement is even more important if subsequent training or an event takes place within several hours of the first activity period. In this case the athlete should begin ingesting carbohydrate as soon after activity as

---

PUTTING IT INTO PERSPECTIVE

CONTINUOUS ENDURANCE SPORTS VERSUS ENDURANCE ACTIVITIES

Some matches in sports, such as tennis, can last for several hours and thereby qualify as endurance events, but they are never continuous in the way that long-distance running is, for example. Sports like tennis and soccer are characterized by high-intensity bouts of activity interspersed with shorter periods at lower intensity or relative rest. These sports require large amounts of carbohydrate for fuel, and the ingested carbohydrate might also improve motor skills, mood, and force production, as well as reduce fatigue and perceived exertion. Although the research on carbohydrate intake in intermittent endurance sports like soccer is not as abundant as it is for continuous endurance sports, carbohydrate intake during prolonged, intermittent activities is recommended for optimal performance. For events lasting 60 to 90 minutes, 60 grams of carbohydrate per hour will likely suffice. Carbohydrate intakes greater than 60 grams will likely be of benefit only if the event stretches to 2 to 3 hours, if the intensity of activity is high for most of the event, or if the athlete does not begin the event in a fed, glycogen-filled state yet relies on glycogen for fuel (i.e., has not adapted to a low-carbohydrate diet and is competing in a lower-intensity event) (13, 26, 29, 33, 34). Keep in mind, however, that intakes greater than 60 grams of carbohydrate per hour have been studied only in cyclists and that tolerance may vary in other sports.

possible to maximize glycogen stores for the next training session (13, 26, 31, 36, 38, 39).

Both glucose and insulin are used to replenish glycogen. Consuming carbohydrate-rich foods provides the glucose needed for glycogen synthesis. Muscle glycogen synthesis occurs in two stages, the first being insulin independent and the second insulin dependent. During the first phase (30 to 60 minutes postexercise), glycogen depletion itself appears to be a stimulus for glycogen resynthesis. Depleted levels of glycogen and skeletal muscle contraction during exercise are thought to act as a stimulus for translocation of the GLUT4 transport protein to the cell membrane of the muscle (figure 11.4). It appears that this enhanced glucose transport declines rapidly if carbohydrate is not consumed within 1 or 2 hours after exercise. In addition, lower levels of glycogen stimulate activity of the enzyme **glycogen synthase**, which is the key enzyme responsible for glycogen synthesis (13, 26, 31, 36, 38, 39).

The second phase of skeletal muscle glycogen synthesis, beginning 1 to 2 hours postexercise and lasting for up to 48 hours, is marked by a period of enhanced insulin sensitivity. Because this period is dependent on carbohydrate intake and its subsequent glycemic response (which increases insulin), it is most ripe for nutrition strategies aimed at maximizing glycogen synthesis. Based on the best available data, the recommendation for immediate carbohydrate intake postexercise ranges from 1.0 to 1.5 g/kg body weight, with 1.2 g/kg considered the optimal amount. A mixture of carbohydrate, namely glucose, glucose polymers, maltodextrin, fructose, and if practical, galactose, appears to provide the best results during this second phase of glycogen resynthesis. Some evidence suggests that fructose ingestion causes a more rapid replenishment of liver glycogen compared with glucose, but fructose alone does not optimally restore muscle glycogen (29). The recommended amount of carbohydrate should be consumed immediately after exercise to maximize the enhanced metabolic window for rapid glycogen replenishment. The best practice is to follow this with repeated consumption at frequent intervals (e.g., 1.0–1.2 g/kg each hour) for the first 4 hours and then resume normal intake until daily targets are met. Delaying carbohydrate intake for as little as 2 hours postexercise might cause the athlete to miss the window of opportunity and not maximize glycogen stores before the next event. Again, this protocol is important for multiple-day or successive-day training or events, but not as important if there is no need to optimize glycogen stores rapidly (13, 26, 31, 36, 38, 39).

The form of carbohydrate might not be as important as the amount. It appears that glycogen can be replenished equally well with both liquid and solid carbohydrates, so the athlete's personal preference should be the primary determinant. It is not clear whether the glycemic index of the carbohydrate makes much of a difference during the second phase of glycogen repletion. Although logic suggests that high-glycemic index foods would induce an elevated insulin response and glycogen synthesis, this phenomenon has not been repeatedly demonstrated in the scientific literature. In fact, some data suggest that any form of carbohydrate, regardless of its glycemic index, ingested immediately postexercise will promote glycogen replenishment. More research is needed before we can recommend a definitive glycemic index pattern postexercise to maximize glycogen synthesis and stores (13, 26, 31, 36, 38-40).

Carbohydrate should be consumed soon after an endurance event has ended, but what guide-

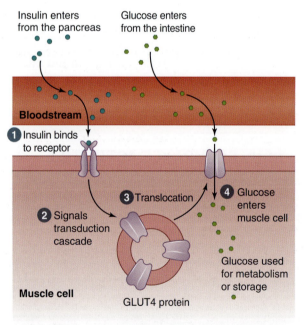

Figure 11.4 To replenish glycogen in the cells of the liver and skeletal muscle, both glucose and insulin are needed. Glucose comes from the ingestion of dietary carbohydrate, and insulin is secreted when blood sugar rises in response to carbohydrate intake.

PUTTING IT INTO PERSPECTIVE

CAFFEINE AND GLYCOGEN REPLENISHMENT

Caffeine is often used as an ergogenic aid for enhanced endurance performance, but some evidence suggests that it might also be helpful during glycogen replenishment during recovery from exercise. Although the mechanism is unclear, caffeine might increase insulin sensitivity during the recovery period and improve intestinal absorption of carbohydrate. Note that some people are sensitive to caffeine and may experience in undesirable side effects such as jitteriness or sleeplessness after ingestion. Given the circumstances, an athlete interested in caffeine as an ergogenic aid should consume the smallest dose that results in the desired effect in order to decrease the risk of undesirable side effects (13, 36).

---

lines should govern the other energy-yielding macronutrients—fat and protein? Specifically, do they influence glycogen replenishment? This topic has been studied for several years, and thus far findings are not conclusive. In theory, protein or certain amino acids might enhance postprandial insulin secretion and thus glucose uptake and glycogen synthesis. But the data suggest that this may occur only when carbohydrate intake immediately after exercise is less than the recommended amount. In fact, when consuming the recommended amount of 1.2 g/kg body weight carbohydrate, adding protein does not enhance glycogen repletion. Although protein may not have a valuable effect on glycogen repletion, it does play an important role in other processes involved with skeletal muscle growth and repair (see chapter 5) and should be included in the immediate post-exercise meal for this reason alone (13, 36, 41).

FOOD SELECTION TO MEET NUTRIENT REQUIREMENTS

Whereas estimating nutrient requirements is a relatively straightforward process, selecting foods and beverages to meet daily nutrient requirements can be a challenge. Many athletes may be unfamiliar with the process of researching the nutrient contents of food products and then taking the next step of combining them in such a fashion to meet their daily nutrient needs. Athletes wanting to consume a target amount of carbohydrate (e.g., 350 g) merely need to read the labels on all the products they plan to eat that day and calculate the number of servings of each that in aggregate will provide the recommended amount of carbohydrate. For example, assume that a male athlete wants to eat 1 cup of the product described by the label in figure 11.5. The label states that one serving of the product is 1/2 cup, so 1 cup of the product is equivalent to two servings (42-44). Figure 11.6 provides a sample list of foods containing about 350 grams of carbohydrate.

Nutrition Facts

8 servings per container
Serving size   1/2 cup (55g)

Amount per 1/2 cup
Calories   **140**

	% Daily Value*
Total Fat 8g	**12%**
Saturated Fat 1g	**5%**
Trans Fat 0g	
Cholesterol 0mg	**0%**
Sodium 160mg	**7%**
Total Carbohydrate 13g	**4%**
Dietary Fiber 3g	**12%**
Total Sugars 3g	
Added Sugars 3g	**1%**
Protein 3g	
Vitamin D 2mcg	10%
Calcium 260mg	20%
Iron 8mg	45%
Potassium 235mg	6%

*The % Daily Value (DV) tells you how much a nutrient in a serving of food contributes to a daily diet. 2,000 calories a day is used for general nutrition advice.

Figure 11.5 Based on the food label of this product, 1 cup is two servings and contains 26 grams of total carbohydrate with 6 grams of sugar and 6 grams of fiber included in that total.

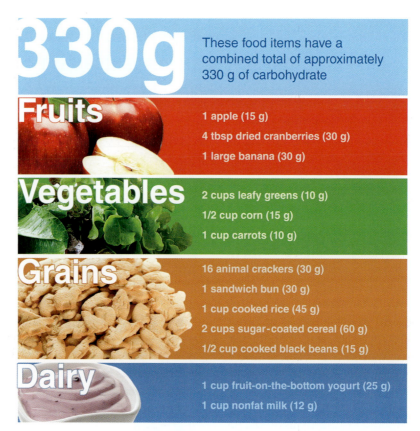

Figure 11.6 These foods should be spread out throughout the day with consideration for training schedule and recovery.

Food labels work great for manufactured products, but many foods do not have labels, such as fruits and vegetables. In this case, we have a couple of choices. Many grocery stores have food composition tables in the produce aisle for reference. Another option is to use a standard food composition table found in many general nutrition textbooks. But the most comprehensive one is provided by the USDA in the form of an extensive database of foods that is available to the public and simple to access by searching for USDA FoodData Central (45). Like the food labels on products, the USDA database provides total carbohydrate, fiber, sugar, fat, and protein contents per serving, but the database also provides much more nutrition information—more than the typical athlete will need.

TYPES OF CARBOHYDRATE AND PERFORMANCE

Traditional sports drinks, gels, and other supplements marketed for endurance athletes usually contain a combination of glucose, sucrose, and maltodextrin (also known as a glucose polymer). All are digested rapidly, providing a quick source of energy immediately before and during exercise. Ingesting these products result in an increased insulin level that facilitates the uptake of glucose into the muscle to be broken down for ATP generation (46).

Some athletes are concerned about glucose and insulin spikes and falls, because an inconsistent level of blood glucose can alter perception of

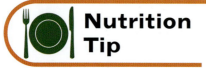

Nutrition Tip Consider whether the serving size on a food label is for a cooked or raw product. For example, oats most commonly report the serving size as dry oats, but when cooked they become engorged with water. Therefore, a cup of cooked oats has far fewer nutrients than a cup of dried oats.

fatigue and negatively affect performance. This concern may be unnecessary because this is not a common occurrence. A few new products have appeared on the market that claim to provide energy without the same amount of instability as glucose, sucrose, and maltodextrin and without the same level of insulin needed for uptake. Carbohydrates with a higher molecular weight than glucose or maltodextrin are made in a laboratory and are absorbed more slowly. These compounds were originally formulated for people with glycogen storage disease and then extended for use by people with diabetes. In the sports nutrition community, the compounds are often referred to as superstarch or waxy maize. The theory and promotion behind their use as a sports supplement is that they do not result in a rapid rise in blood glucose and instead provide steady blood sugar, so effort, whether perceived or real, will be improved. Studies that consistently show favorable changes in blood glucose and insulin responses, glucose uptake and oxidation (use), glycogen resynthesis, or absolute improved performance in the field are lacking. Exercised muscles respond just fine to a rise in blood glucose, so the benefit of using these compounds remains questionable (46-50).

UNIQUE CHALLENGES FACING ENDURANCE ATHLETES

All sports have unique characteristics that often require participants to take certain measures to help them perform or tolerate the activity better. In this section we describe situations in which endurance athletes might want to take such measures.

Inability or Unwillingness to Consume Extra Carbohydrate During Activity

In many cases an athlete cannot or will not consume additional carbohydrate during an endurance activity. For example, some athletes do not have good gastrointestinal tolerance for traditional sports beverages. Some athletes who participate in weight-sensitive sports cannot afford to consume excess calories (e.g., wrestlers, gymnasts). Consuming carbohydrate during activities shorter than 1 hour in duration is not warranted when the goal is to spare glycogen, but there may be other reasons to justify carbohydrate consumption. Some studies show improved performance after subjects simply rinse their mouths with a carbohydrate-containing beverage and spit it out without swallowing. This practice is sometimes referred to as mouth rinsing. The exact mechanism is still being studied, but it appears that the brain can detect the presence of carbohydrate or energy in the mouth, perhaps anticipating carbohydrate delivery into the body, which somehow leads to improved performance. Tasting carbohydrate appears to be more stimulatory than tasting other products because the same level of brain activity is not seen with nonnutritive sweeteners; it is more than just perceived sweet taste that triggers the excitation in the brain. This strategy may allow those athletes to exercise at a greater intensity with less fatigue, or a lower perception of fatigue, without ingesting the unwanted energy (calories) (31, 51).

Research studies examining the effects of carbohydrate mouth rinsing have increased over the last few years, and some positive results have been found with training bouts lasting between 30 and 75 minutes (52, 53). Although a few of these published studies found a small benefit or no benefit at all, most of them reported some significant improvement in performance, especially in endurance activities lasting 25 to 60 minutes (52, 53). There is little support for an ergogenic effect with anaerobic events or resistance training (53). In research trials specific to cycling, the carbohydrate mouth rinse may have the potential to increase mean power output, but it may not improve completion time (52). A few studies reported that carbohydrate mouth rinsing may be more effective in a fasting, somewhat glycogen-depleted state, but this circumstance likely does not represent actual eating schedules of most athletes. The overall picture must be considered with regard to training demand and total carbohydrate needs. More research in this area is warranted before conclusions can be made (53).

Gastrointestinal Distress

Some endurance athletes experience GI stress during training and competition, a condition that certainly can cause impaired performance. The severity of GI distress might vary from mild to

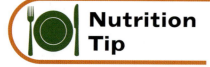

Nutrition Tip

Certain micronutrients are of concern for endurance athletes (13, 54, 55):

- Iron: Intense training may lead to increased iron losses in sweat, urine, feces, and hemolysis caused by compression of the blood vessels in the soles of the feet or with vigorous contraction of the muscles involved in intense activity. Some athletes limit rich food sources such as meat.
- Vitamin D: This vitamin may play a role in muscle function, injury prevention, reduction of inflammation, and immune function. Some athletes may be insufficient or deficient because of limited sun exposure. Food sources are limited, and vitamin D deficiency is a particular concern for those who eliminate dairy from the diet.
- Calcium: This mineral may be low in athletes who restrict total calorie intake or restrict or avoid dairy foods. Over time, bone mineral density may be compromised when calcium intake is consistently inadequate. Specialty testing is needed to measure bone density, and it may not be part of the routine physical exam.
- Antioxidants: Choosing a diet rich in antioxidants is prudent for health and recovery. Because whole foods contain a mixture of antioxidants and phytonutrients, the same health benefits may not be achieved through supplementation. In addition, high supplement doses may be more harmful than helpful, especially if an athlete is consuming quantities exceeding tolerable *upper* intake level (UL). There are no generalized recommendations for micronutrient supplementation for all endurance athletes. Qualified health care professionals should use a baseline nutrition assessment including dietary intake and laboratory tests to determine nutrient adequacy. The first strategy should be to encourage a well-balanced diet containing a variety of foods that meet micronutrient needs. If needs cannot be met with food or if a deficiency is present, supplementation (or in some cases such as B_{12}, an injection) can be used under the recommendation of a qualified health care professional.

---

severe. The most common symptoms are nausea, vomiting, abdominal pain, and diarrhea. Discomfort and unwanted stops at a toilet can be the difference between winning and losing, or for less competitive athletes, between dropping out and finishing a race. The prevalence of GI distress in endurance athletes is unclear, but studies suggest that 30 to 50 percent of all endurance athletes experience GI symptoms and 30 to 90 percent of distance runners experience GI symptoms related to training (32, 56-58).

> **? DO YOU KNOW?**
>
> Some GI problems are transient and associated only with training and competition, but others can be a result of celiac disease, irritable bowel syndrome, inflammatory bowel disease (ulcerative colitis or Crohn's disease), or another medical condition.

Nutrition intake can significantly affect symptoms of GI distress. The traditional culprits are fiber, fat, protein, concentrated carbohydrate drinks, and dehydration. For example, fiber, fat, and protein can delay gastric emptying, and consuming fructose alone (from fruit juice) or a high mixed carbohydrate solution during higher-intensity exercise can cause fluid shifts in the GI tract that may cause GI distress and impaired performance. Because gastrointestinal responses may vary from person to person or within a person from day to day, a wise approach is to experiment with nutrition strategies during practice before implementing them in a competitive environment (56-58).

Desire to Enhance Fatty Acid Oxidation

Carbohydrate is a key fuel source for endurance activity. Because glycogen stores in the body are limited and significantly more fuel is available from fatty acids, many athletes seek to manipulate the diet to force the body to use more fat instead of carbohydrate to fuel their event. Although these strategies have become popular in use, the scientific evidence to support their use is not abundant.

Training in a Glycogen-Depleted State

Success or failure in most endurance activities depends physiologically on the ability to produce ATP at a rapid rate over a long duration, an endeavor that requires large storage reserves of glycogen and the capacity to use fuel sources other than muscle glycogen, specifically fatty acids. A protocol designed to train the body to oxidize fatty acids preferentially over glucose during exercise—called training low, competing high—has gained increased attention. The underlying theory behind this protocol is that by conducting training sessions in a somewhat glycogen-depleted state, the body will learn to prefer fatty acids over glucose as a fuel. Some protocols combine this with a lower-carbohydrate, higher-fat diet, often referred to as fat loading, for a short period before the competitive event, before ultimately switching to a higher-carbohydrate diet right before the event. From a physiological standpoint, this protocol does appear to accomplish its mission; it can result in increased intramuscular triglyceride stores and elicits greater fat oxidation and decreased use of skeletal muscle glycogen during exercise. The problem is that in sporting events success is measured based on performance, not metabolic adaptations or source of fuel. Currently, there is no evidence of improved performance from training low. More field-based research studies are needed to see if metabolic adaptations translate into improved performance. Although training low might result in some physiological adaptations, it might also trigger undesirable side effects, such as fatigue during exercise and inability to train or compete at high intensities, either of which contributes to failure instead of success (10, 13, 22, 59-62).

Training low has been controversial in the sports nutrition literature for quite some time. Some of the earlier studies conducted on this topic were used to promote this protocol. These studies had different study designs, making comparisons difficult, and the sample sizes and total number of studies were small. The research concluded that a low-carbohydrate, high-fat (LCHF) diet resulted in fat being the preferential fuel source and glycogen being spared. The protocols did not match for or consider initial glycogen levels, so the conclusion is not fully accurate. Still, the observed increased use of fat as a fuel source (increased fatty acid oxidation) is worth further examination (22). The earlier research studies did demonstrate some interesting findings, which are summarized here (22):

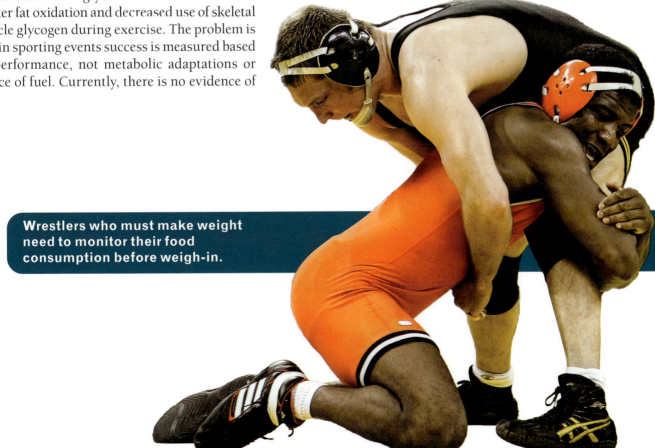

Wrestlers who must make weight need to monitor their food consumption before weigh-in.

› Consuming a LCHF diet for as little as 5 days can cause skeletal muscle adaptations such as increased intramuscular triglyceride stores; increased activity of the enzyme hormone-sensitive lipase, which facilitates fatty acid mobilization from storage; and enhanced cellular metabolic processes that ultimately allow increased oxidation (use) of fat for fuel. As fat oxidation increases, carbohydrate oxidation (breakdown or use) appears to decrease and this reduction seems to be caused by changes in glycogen utilization by skeletal muscle.

› Even after several days of using a LCHF diet and then switching to a higher-carbohydrate regimen, the enhanced fat utilization persists. These fat metabolism adaptations remain even if carbohydrate is introduced closer to an event.

› Despite the metabolic changes that appear to take place with consumption of a LCHF diet, evidence of a translation to an actual performance benefit is lacking. The studies had small sample sizes, and the changes might not apply to all individuals. People who do not respond well or tolerate carbohydrate during exercise would adapt better to this protocol than those who do well with carbohydrate loading and consumption of carbohydrate during exercise. Further, many of these protocols in the research studies were conducted on submaximal exercise in a glycogen-depleted state. This scenario may not be what is actually happening for athletes in the field. In addition to the study methodological limitations, ultraendurance athletes already experience training adaptations that include enhanced fat oxidation, regardless of the specific ratio of carbohydrate to fat intake. LCHF consumption may be useful for some people, but not for all, and it might actually impair performance, particularly in activities requiring higher intensity or power requirement for success (even at the end of a marathon when trying to sprint to the finish). Glycogen utilization is the preferred source of energy in those scenarios (22, 63).

In addition to this research, another angle fitting into this goal of training low includes purposefully withholding dietary carbohydrate replenishment following intense training. The person would go to sleep in a glycogen-depleted state (sleep low) and then perform the next morning. One study reported increased fat oxidation during prolonged submaximal cycling, but researchers did not examine performance in this study (64). The first study of this type to examine real-world endurance performance in trained triathletes reported improved performance with recovery from training sessions in a glycogen-depleted state followed by high carbohydrate availability right before subsequent

PUTTING IT INTO PERSPECTIVE

MINIMIZING GI DISTRESS FOR ATHLETES

The following strategies can be used to prevent or minimize GI distress in endurance athletes. But if an athlete has a diagnosed medical condition, such as celiac disease, irritable bowel syndrome, or Crohn's disease, which requires medical nutrition therapy, then a referral should be made to an RDN familiar with these conditions.

› Avoid high-fiber foods during the day, or even days, before competition. On all other days, consuming a diet with adequate fiber will help keep the bowel regular, thereby helping decrease the likelihood of constipation.

› Use high-fructose foods with caution, particularly drinks that are exclusively fructose; beverages containing both fructose and glucose might be better tolerated.

› Do not eat within 3 hours of competition if you have a sensitive stomach.

› Avoid dehydration by starting the event well hydrated and consuming fluids throughout the event. Avoid overhydration.

› Do not ingest concentrated carbohydrate-containing beverages (e.g., 100% juice).

› Practice new nutrition strategies many times before implementing them during competition.

Reprinted from E.P. de Oliveira, R.C. Burini, and A. Jeukendrup, "Gastrointestinal Complaints During Exercise: Prevalence, Etiology, and Nutritional Recommendations," *Sports Medicine* 44 (Suppl 1) (2014): S79-S85. Distributed under the terms of the Creative Commons Attribution License.

training. More practical application research like this is needed before specific protocols can be recommended as a strategy for endurance athletes.

With the increased use of social media, support for this approach has increased based on anecdotal evidence. It is surprising that only a few additional studies have been completed and published on this topic. Although the topic is popular enough to stimulate conversation, not enough evidence exists to make better conclusions. None have shown a performance benefit to the LCHF diet, and one of the studies did not impose a typical carbohydrate restriction used in the LCHF protocol.

More research needs to be completed that compares nonketogenic LCHF diets versus ketogenic LCHF diets. Some theorize that chronic carbohydrate restriction resulting in ketone production is beneficial because the body can adapt to use these ketones as a fuel source during exercise. This idea sounds nice in theory, but we have no data on the amount of energy that ketones can provide as an exercise substrate (22).

Until more research is available, we need to think critically about the use of LCHF diets and exercise performance. The popular media and anecdotal promotion of this approach imply that it is based on evidence from and applicable to a wide range of athletes. In fact, it might be applicable only to ultraendurance athletes or those undergoing long periods of submaximal exercise, if it is beneficial at all. Although general guidelines for carbohydrate consumption do exist for before, during, and after endurance activities, sports dietitians who are current in their practice work with their athletes to avoid unnecessary, excess carbohydrate intake and to tailor their recommendations for carbohydrate amount and type to the individual. Balance in all nutrition aspects of the diet is an important concept (22).

Ketogenic Diets and Endurance Performance

Another type of LCHF diet is called the ketogenic diet. These ketogenic, or "keto," diets have been popular for years for body fat loss and are generally characterized as consuming less than 50 grams per day of carbohydrate and approximately 60 to 80 percent of calories from fat. Although the previously published LCHF diets categorized as fat adaptation diets or training-low diets failed to show significant performance benefits, popular interest expanded in similar diets that are labeled ketogenic. The theory behind these diets for endurance exercise is that a person can train the body to produce and use ketone bodies for fuel as an alternative source to glucose. Glucose oxidation requires several steps, and it is believed that ketones can provide a consistent and rapid energy supply to working muscles (65). Metabolic ketosis is defined as elevated serum ketone bodies from 0.5 to 3.0 mM, which can be achieved through dietary manipulation of low carbohydrate intake. This condition should not be confused with ketoacidosis, a complication of diabetes, which is defined as serum ketone levels of 3.8 to 25 mM and requires medical attention (66).

Although some studies did demonstrate decreased glucose oxidation and increased fat oxidation with ketogenic diets, little research data demonstrate significant endurance performance enhancement (65-73). Furthermore, most of the research that has been completed has been in a laboratory setting that may or may not translate to performance in the competitive field. Several reasons might explain these mixed research findings:

> Small sample sizes with less-than-ideal study designs
> Heterogeneity across study designs, making comparison difficult
> Questionable adherence to the diet
> Variability in genetic factors and sex of study participants
> Variability in body composition of study participants

Although performance benefits are in question with ketogenic diets, some of the studies in athletes reported body fat loss. More research is needed in athletes of varying body composition, including competitors with an ideal body weight and composition who may be looking to maintain lean body mass rather than lose body fat (68). Although a few studies reported impaired performance while on a ketogenic diet (70, 74), many did not. Additional applied research studies are needed comparing different types of endurance events, specific dietary protocols, and improvement of performance in the actual competitive field.

DO YOU KNOW?

Ketogenic, or "keto," diets have been around for several decades as a nutrition therapy for epilepsy. In recent years keto diets have been promoted for weight loss and improved endurance performance. Traditionally, the physiological state of ketosis is induced by consuming a low-carbohydrate diet for about 3 weeks or more. Using ketone supplements is promoted as a way of rapidly achieving acute ketosis. Currently, not enough research has been completed to support the effectiveness of these supplements in achieving a desired ketogenic state, and even less research has examined their effect on endurance performance. More important, ketone supplements may have several negative consequences, including gastrointestinal distress, headaches, and impaired performance (65, 73, 75).

GENERAL RECOVERY FROM TRAINING

Exercise training for sport and competition is physiologically and psychologically demanding, and achieving proper recovery from such training is crucial for optimal health and performance. Physiological recovery involves rest, sleep, proper nutrition, and possibly medical or related interventions and is critical to preventing mental fatigue and includes cognitive and relaxation techniques (77).

To obtain improvements in performance with training, a degree of functional overreaching (appropriate physiological stress from training) is required, coupled with proper recovery. Functional overreaching may lead to short-term discomfort or disruption in performance without long-term physiological consequences. If excessive training demands are regularly followed by inadequate recovery, worse conditions of nonfunctional overreaching and underrecovery can result. Nonfunctional overreaching is associated with physiological decrements and psychological consequences and is considered a precursor to developing overtraining syndrome (OTS). OTS is characterized by the following (29, 77-79):

> Continuous muscle soreness, strain, or pain
> Overuse injuries
> Fatigue
> Reduced appetite and weight loss
> Decline in performance
> Increased perceived efforts of workouts
> Sleep disturbances
> Decreased immunity or illness
> Psychological burnout and loss of motivation
> Clinical or endocrine disturbances

Recovery from training requires a multifaceted approach in which protocols vary tremendously depending on the training volume and physiological and psychological state of the athlete. A combination of physiological markers such as blood-based variables serving as markers for muscle damage, inflammation, and endocrine disturbances; psychological variables such as the athlete's readiness to perform; and nutritional assessment must be used by qualified practitioners. Proper assessment and recovery plans must be implemented by a multidisciplinary team of experts and must be individualized to the athlete. Standardized protocols, or a one-size-fits-all approach, are not appropriate because of the high intraindividual and interindividual variability with the recovery process. Training loads may vary depending on the stage of training and competition; higher training loads are allowed during preseason and preparation phases and lower training loads should be used before competition. In addition to insisting that the athlete get physical rest and use proper recovery strategies, the practitioner must help them secure a positive view of the recovery process and its relevance. Clear communication about the compliance expectations is needed (29, 77-79).

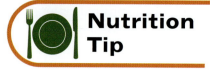

Nutrition Tip Sports nutrition guidelines are evidence based and developed using the current available research. These guidelines are often suited for a wide range of athletes, but they can never replace the individualized approach that is likely necessary for optimal health and performance. Athletes might use these guidelines as a starting point during preparation and training, but they must learn what works best for them through trial and error. Sometimes an athlete might fall outside an established guideline. The certified specialist in sports dietetics (CSSD) (76) uses a modernized, periodized approach to meet the needs of individual athletes.

PUTTING IT INTO PERSPECTIVE

OVERTRAINING SYNDROME

Overtraining syndrome (OTS) is characterized by chronic inadequate energy intake coupled with long periods of inadequate carbohydrate intake and high-volume training. A long-term performance decrement can occur with or without physiological symptoms. Restoration of physiological function and performance can take several weeks to several months and requires an individualized approach. There is no one-size-fits-all recovery protocol. The only "cure" for OTS is reduced training volume, or complete rest, along with the consumption of adequate energy, protein, carbohydrate, and fluids (29, 77-79).

EFFECTS OF ENDURANCE TRAINING ON MACRONUTRIENT METABOLISM

Endurance training elicits numerous physiological adaptations that lead to enhanced performance, including improved delivery, uptake, and oxidation of glucose; larger glycogen stores in skeletal muscle; greater oxygen uptake in working muscle; and a better ability to use lactate as a fuel source. Trained skeletal muscle is also more sensitive to insulin and possesses a greater amount of GLUT4 proteins, thereby allowing enhanced glucose uptake and utilization. Endurance-trained people have larger left ventricle heart volumes, larger blood volume, increased capillary density, and greater myoglobin concentration, all of which contribute to greater oxygen delivery to the muscle, which when coupled with increased mitochondrial density and concentration of metabolic enzymes in muscle cells results in a greater ability to oxidize glucose and fatty acids completely (2).

SUMMARY

Endurance athletes participate in events that have demanding energy requirements and pose unique challenges to the body's main ATP-producing systems, particularly the ability to oxidize glucose completely for lengthy periods without fatigue. Carbohydrates are of primary importance for long-term ATP production, and numerous strategies exist to preserve muscle glycogen by delaying its utilization or increasing its content in muscle. Endurance athletes face distinct and demanding nutrient requirements for energy, fat, carbohydrate, and fluids, and the challenge of translating these requirements into actual food choices can be daunting. Fortunately, tools that assist in the process of selecting foods, beverages, and supplements are readily available, and these significantly help endurance athletes satisfy the unique nutrition requirements of their chosen activity.

FOR REVIEW

1. Explain how carbohydrate and fat are used as fuel sources during exercise of varying intensities.
2. How can an athlete minimize fatigue during prolonged endurance exercise?
3. What are the carbohydrate recommendations before an endurance event? List for 1, 2, 3, and 4 hours preevent. What types of carbohydrate are recommended at each time?
4. What are the carbohydrate recommendations during exercise? Do the recommendations change with time and intensity?
5. What are the carbohydrate recommendations for recovery to maximize glycogen stores, including both quantity and timing?
6. Describe the role of glycemic index in making carbohydrate recommendations before, during, and after endurance exercise.
7. Many endurance-enhancing supplements are marketed specifically toward athletes. Can an endurance athlete obtain the same benefits from typical foods? Give examples.
8. Describe the theory behind training low, competing high. Is this strategy widely recommended? Why or why not?
9. List strategies for minimizing GI distress during endurance training.

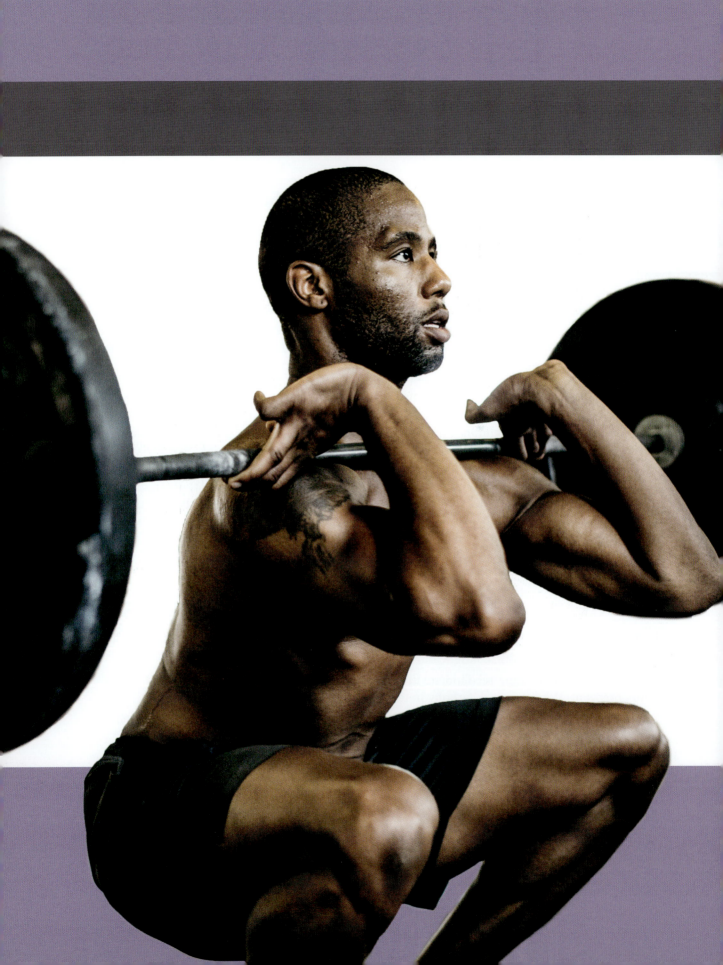

Nutrition for Resistance Training

> **CHAPTER OBJECTIVES**
>
> After completing this chapter, you will be able to do the following:
>
> › Discuss differences in protein needs between children, younger adults, and the elderly for maximizing training adaptations.
> › Discuss protein recommendations for people who are following a lower-calorie diet (below their average daily calorie needs to maintain weight) while following a resistance-training program.
> › Determine if resistance exercise performance is altered by a low-carbohydrate or ketogenic diet.
> › Discuss nutrition before, during, and after resistance training.

Many people include resistance training in their exercise program. In this chapter we discuss nutrition strategies to support resistance training by providing the energy (calories) and nutrients needed to fuel skeletal muscle contraction, support skeletal muscle growth and repair, replenish carbohydrate stores, and minimize muscle soreness. Although research continues to uncover how specific nutrients and supplements affect muscle functioning and acute and chronic training adaptations (gains made from a resistance-training program), interindividual results from incorporating one or more of these strategies may vary considerably based on the training program used, genetic differences in response to training, training status (from untrained to highly trained), age, gender, overall diet, adaptation to diet, and possibly **nutrigenomics** (the interaction between nutrition and genes—a relatively new area of study).

Although a person's overall training diet has a profound effect on improvements made through resistance training, considerable research has focused on the timing of specific nutrients and the influence of supplements during the preexercise, exercise, and postexercise periods on performance, recovery, and changes in muscle mass, strength, and power over time.

> **? DO YOU KNOW?**
>
> Many people recognize the role of muscle mass in strength and athletic performance, but muscle mass also has an important role in reducing risk of obesity, cardiovascular disease, type 2 diabetes, osteoporosis, and **sarcopenia**, the age-related loss of muscle mass and strength (1).

NUTRITION BEFORE RESISTANCE TRAINING

The main purpose of preexercise foods, beverages, or supplements consumed within an hour or less before resistance training is to hydrate the athlete, top off glycogen stores for those who need it, and decrease hunger. In addition, adding protein to a preexercise snack might be advantageous if the athlete has not consumed protein for several hours prior or if their daily protein needs are high and the preexercise meal represents an important opportunity to help them meet their total protein needs. For instance, a 280-pound (127 kg) male athlete who is trying to gain 20 pounds (9 kg) will have substantial daily protein needs and might find it challenging to consume the quantity of food (including protein) necessary to gain weight, particularly if he is training for several hours a day (more time spent training means less time available to eat).

Hydration

Staying hydrated is important for resistance training. Hypohydration compromises resistance-training performance and recovery (2, 3). Methodological considerations in study design, however, make it difficult to distinguish the mechanism through which hypohydration affects strength, power, and high-intensity exercise performance. Cardiovascular strain such as decreases in maximal cardiac output and blood flow to muscle tissue (and thus a decline in the delivery of nutrients and metabolite removal) are plausible contributing factors (2, 4). The studies to date indicate that dehydration of 3 to 4 percent body weight loss reduces muscle strength by approximately 2 percent, muscular power by approximately 3 percent, and high-intensity endurance performance (maximal repeated activities lasting >30 seconds but <2 minutes) by approximately 10 percent (2).

Hypohydration also affects the hormonal response to exercise. In one resistance-training study, increasing levels of hypohydration (from 2.5% of body weight to 5% of body weight; these are high levels of hypohydration) led to progressive increases in the stress hormones cortisol and norepinephrine, and a subsequent increase in blood glucose, presumably to cope with increased physiological demands (the stress response leads to greater energy substrate availability for exercising muscle). In another study, mild dehydration leading to a 0.5 to 0.9 percent decrease in body weight due to fluid restriction did not decrease power. Hypohydration to 2 percent of body weight, however, led to a decrease in power, and acute rehydration did not restore power to normal levels (5). These results suggest that hypohydration significantly enhances stress from resistance exercise and could impair training adaptations. Over time, these changes could decrease training adaptations to resistance training if training is consistently performed in a hypohydrated state (4).

Given the effect of hypohydration on strength, power, and repetitive activity lasting more than 30 seconds but less than 2 minutes (2), athletes engaging in resistance-training sessions would be wise to ensure they are adequately hydrated. The best way to do this is to consume enough fluid over the course of the day to ensure adequate hydration status. Although fluid intake before resistance exercise can help, it may not be enough for those with who are extremely hypohydrated. Although there are no specific preexercise hydration guidelines for resistance exercise, general guidelines for athletes can be followed:

> Drink approximately 5 to 7 ml/kg of fluids with sodium approximately 4 hours before a workout or competition.

> An athlete who cannot urinate or produces dark or scant urine should drink 3 to 5 ml/kg about 2 hours before exercise (6).

Carbohydrate

Carbohydrate from circulating blood sugar and muscle glycogen is the primary source of fuel used during resistance-training session. It is the main fuel used during the active phase of resistance-training session such as lifting a barbell. Carbohydrate is also used between sets when a person is resting, but fat can contribute a substantial amount of energy; estimates range from 20 to 70 percent of total calories expended during the rest period. (7) And although glycogen supplies a large amount of the carbohydrate used during a single resistance-training session, resistance-training workouts generally do not lead to the level of glycogen depletion that would impair performance. Glycogen depletion, however, can occur locally in type 2 muscle fibers after high-volume strength training (7, 8).

❓ DO YOU KNOW?

If you are eating right before a resistance-training session, choose easy-to-digest foods higher in carbohydrate. Fruit, whole-grain crackers, and granola bars are all great options.

The research examining the effect of preworkout carbohydrate intake on resistance-training performance varies based on the total workout volume (7). Acute carbohydrate intake consumed 15 to 120 minutes before exercise is unlikely to affect strength-training performance if the person is in a fed state (not after an overnight fast, for example) and working out up to 10 sets per muscle group. But in studies examining higher-volume workouts (11–17 sets per muscle group), acute carbohydrate intake was more likely to have a positive effect on training performance (7).

Additionally, acute carbohydrate intake may be beneficial for resistance-training performance after overnight fast (7, 8). The research is inconsistent. In one study carbohydrate was beneficial because of a placebo effect or hunger suppression rather than a metabolic advantage. In this study the subjects performed better after eating a carbohydrate-rich breakfast compared with water only. But no difference in performance was found after a carbohydrate-rich breakfast compared with a flavor- and texture-matched placebo breakfast containing 29 kcal (9).

In summary, consuming a carbohydrate-rich meal or snack before doing resistance exercise does not improve strength-training performance except under certain circumstances, such as after fasting or when working out more than 10 sets per muscle group and during two-a-day workouts with a few hours between workouts. Those engaging in a higher-volume workout (>10 sets per muscle group) may benefit from a carbohydrate-rich meal or snack within a few hours before training. Although carbohydrate does not appear to affect resistance-training performance in the fed state, given some uncertainty in the studies to date a general recommendation is to consume at least 15 grams of carbohydrate within 3 hours before exercise (7).

If the athlete has another glycogen-depleting exercise session planned for that day with only a few hours between workouts, then a higher carbohydrate intake may be warranted. The recommendation is to consume 1.2 g/kg per hour during the hours between the first and second training sessions (7). Keep in mind that these recommendations apply to those doing resistance training only, not team sport athletes who may engage in a resistance exercise session followed either immediately or hours later with a sport-specific training session or practice.

> **DO YOU KNOW?**
>
> Muscle size is only one factor that influences muscle strength (10). Several factors other than hypertrophy influence strength, including improving skills (especially for more complex tasks). In those new to resistance training, hypertrophy might contribute to only 2.5 percent of the gain in strength. Most strength gains in novices are due to neural adaptations (modifications in the nervous system) (11). With training, hypertrophy is responsible for a greater percentage of strength gains (12).

Protein and Amino Acids

The only reason that protein is needed in the hours before resistance training is to help meet total daily protein needs. Protein will not improve resistance-training performance. A general recommendation that has been put forth is to consume at least 0.3 grams of protein per kilogram of body weight within 3 hours preworkout (7, 8).

NUTRITION DURING RESISTANCE TRAINING

During resistance training or exercise, athletes have no specific nutritional needs unless they are hungry or are engaging in a high training volume after an overnight fast or an earlier glycogen-depleting workout without a preexercise meal. Although carbohydrate can contribute a significant amount of energy used during resistance training and decreases in glycogen can impair force production and strength while accentuating muscle weakness, resistance-training workouts typically do not deplete glycogen to levels low enough to impair performance. Some studies, however, show critical levels of glycogen depletion in type 2 muscle fibers after high-volume training (more than 10 sets per muscle group), although total muscle glycogen was not depleted to a critical level. In these cases, when an athlete is performing a high volume of strength training, they may benefit from carbohydrate consumed during the exercise session if they are training after fasting for several hours or overnight (7, 8).

Given the effects of higher levels of hypohydration on resistance-training performance, consuming fluid during a training session may be warranted. Data on this topic, however, are lacking.

At this time, no evidence suggests that consuming protein or amino acids during a resistance exercise session is necessary, particularly if protein needs are met at other times of the day.

NUTRITION AFTER RESISTANCE TRAINING

The meal after resistance training is likely more important for those who train more than once per day or those who train once daily but do not meet their daily energy and protein recommendations to support training adaptations.

Replacing Glycogen

Carbohydrate intake after resistance exercise helps facilitate glycogen resynthesis and decrease further muscle breakdown (13-15). After training, the team sport athlete or endurance athlete who relies heavily on carbohydrate to fuel performance should replace glycogen over the period before the next training session. During the first 45 minutes (approximately) after the completion of training, muscles rapidly replenish carbohydrate. After about 45 minutes, the rate of glycogen resynthesis decreases (16, 17). Those who are performing two glycogen-depleting workouts in a day within a few hours of one another should consume 1.2 grams of carbohydrate per kg body weight per hour during the hours between the first and second training sessions (7). People who have more than 8 hours between training sessions or those who do not train every day do not necessarily need to consume carbohydrate immediately after training in an effort to replace glycogen rapidly. Instead, they can fully replenish their carbohydrate stores over 24 hours before their next bout of training if total daily dietary carbohydrate intake is adequate to support training (18). See figure 12.1 for sample meal plans for resistance training.

> **DO YOU KNOW?**
>
> Many factors affect the amount of carbohydrate needed to replenish glycogen stores completely, including glycogen levels before the start of exercise, the intensity and duration of the resistance exercise session, body weight, habitual carbohydrate consumption, and carbohydrate consumption before or during exercise.

SAMPLE 2,200 KCAL DIET

Meal or food

Breakfast
- Two egg sandwiches
  - Five scrambled eggs
  - Two slices of 100% whole-grain bread
- Fruit, chopped, 1 cup

630 kcal
32 g protein

Morning snack
Banana
80 kcal

Lunch
- Burrito bowl
  - 3 oz cooked marinated chicken
  - 1 oz shredded cheese
  - 1/2 cup of fajita-style vegetables
  - 1-1/2 cups cooked brown rice
  - Half avocado, sliced

660 kcal
32 g protein

Afternoon snack
Apple
80 kcal

Dinner
- Pasta with meatballs
  - 1 cup cooked whole-grain pasta
  - 3 oz turkey meatballs
  - 1/2 cup marinara sauce
- Salad with spring greens, chopped carrots, sun-dried tomatoes, and 2 tbsp oil-based dressing
- 1% milk, 8 oz

750 kcal
39 g protein

SAMPLE 6,000 KCAL DIET

Meal or food

Breakfast
- Four slices turkey bacon, thick-sliced, dark-meat turkey
- Steel-cut oats made with raisins, hemp seeds, brown sugar, and milk
  - 1/2 cup (measured dry) steel-cut oats
  - 1-1/4 cup 1% milk
  - 1/4 cup raisins
  - 2 tbsp hemp seeds
  - 1 tbsp brown sugar
- Orange mango shake
  - 8 oz 100% orange juice
  - 1/2 cup frozen mango

990 kcal
48 g protein

Midmorning snack
- Two cashew butter and jelly sandwiches
  - 2 tbsp cashew butter on each
  - 1 tbsp jelly on each
  - Two slices whole-grain bread for each sandwich
- 1% milk, 10 oz
- 1 banana

910 kcal
34 g protein

Lunch
- Side salad with a packet of dressing
- Grilled chicken sandwich
- Large baked potato with 2 tbsp light butter spread
- 1% milk, 8 oz
- Mixed berries, 1 cup

1,070 kcal
43 g protein

Postlift meal
- Chocolate peanut butter shake
  - 10 oz chocolate milk
  - One scoop vanilla or chocolate whey protein (25 g protein)
  - 3 tbsp peanut butter (or another nut butter)
  - One banana
- Salted pretzels, 3 oz

1,000 kcal
53 g protein

Dinner
- Baby carrots (about 10) with hummus (4 tbsp)
- Atlantic salmon, 4 oz cooked
- Sauteed vegetables cooked in 2 tsp oil
- Wild rice, 2 cups cooked with 2 tbsp light butter
- Soy milk, 8 oz

1,086 kcal
56 g protein

Evening snack
- 100% dark berry juice, 8 oz
- Yogurt parfait with
  - 1 cup nonfat vanilla Greek yogurt
  - 2/3 cup granola
  - 1 tbsp chia seeds
  - 1/4 heaping cup raisins
  - 1/4 cup honey-roasted pistachios

944 kcal
32 g protein

Figure 12.1 Sample food plans for maximizing resistance-training outcomes.

Building and Repairing Muscle

A series of steps are involved in building and repairing muscle tissue, as shown in figure 12.2.

Two factors influence net **muscle protein balance**: muscle protein synthesis and muscle protein breakdown. Muscle protein synthesis must

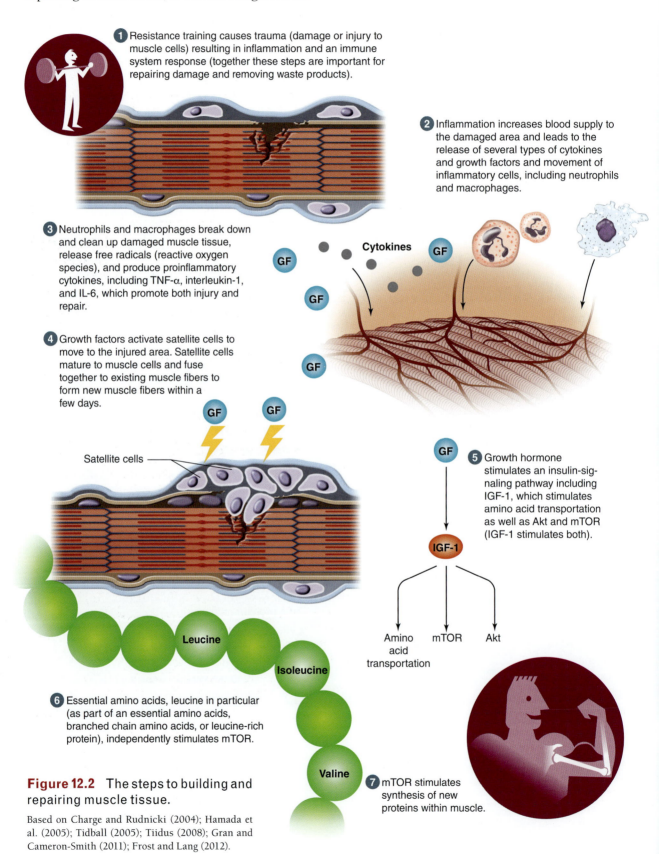

1. Resistance training causes trauma (damage or injury to muscle cells) resulting in inflammation and an immune system response (together these steps are important for repairing damage and removing waste products).

2. Inflammation increases blood supply to the damaged area and leads to the release of several types of cytokines and growth factors and movement of inflammatory cells, including neutrophils and macrophages.

3. Neutrophils and macrophages break down and clean up damaged muscle tissue, release free radicals (reactive oxygen species), and produce proinflammatory cytokines, including TNF-α, interleukin-1, and IL-6, which promote both injury and repair.

4. Growth factors activate satellite cells to move to the injured area. Satellite cells mature to muscle cells and fuse together to existing muscle fibers to form new muscle fibers within a few days.

5. Growth hormone stimulates an insulin-signaling pathway including IGF-1, which stimulates amino acid transportation as well as Akt and mTOR (IGF-1 stimulates both).

6. Essential amino acids, leucine in particular (as part of an essential amino acids, branched chain amino acids, or leucine-rich protein), independently stimulates mTOR.

7. mTOR stimulates synthesis of new proteins within muscle.

Figure 12.2 The steps to building and repairing muscle tissue.

Based on Charge and Rudnicki (2004); Hamada et al. (2005); Tidball (2005); Tiidus (2008); Gran and Cameron-Smith (2011); Frost and Lang (2012).

PUTTING IT INTO PERSPECTIVE

ALCOHOL AND EXERCISE

If you want to get in a good lift before heading out to the bars to throw back a few beers, you might feel as if you are pumping up your muscles. In men, however, alcohol consumed after exercise decreases the effect of dietary protein on muscle protein synthesis and impairs anabolic signaling. Alcohol does not have the same effect in women (24). In addition, high doses of alcohol decrease testosterone in men, and long-term use decreases the androgen receptor activity, so even if you have a lot of testosterone circulating, the ability of your body to use it decreases.

be greater than breakdown for growth to occur (19). Chronic net gains in the muscle protein pool lead to improvements in strength and hypertrophy over time. When muscle protein breakdown chronically exceeds muscle protein synthesis, a net loss occurs in the protein pool (muscle atrophy) over time (20, 21).

❓ DO YOU KNOW?

Muscle protein breakdown is a physiologically important process that helps remove damaged proteins. Think of this process as tearing down part of an old building and rebuilding it with newer, stronger materials. Although breakdown is essential, excess breakdown is not beneficial.

Muscle protein synthesis is suppressed during exercise. Resistance training increases both muscle protein synthesis and muscle protein breakdown. Blood flow to muscle increases after resistance training, enhancing the delivery of the amino acids from protein to muscle (14). The synergistic effect of resistance training combined with greater amino acid availability (from consuming protein or essential amino acids) leads to a greater increase in acute muscle protein synthesis compared with resistance exercise alone, leading to a net gain in muscle protein (outweighing breakdown) postexercise (13, 14, 20). Muscle protein breakdown after resistance training varies, with reported ranges from 31 to 51 percent (13, 14). Relatively small amounts of carbohydrate, between 30 and 100 grams, consumed after resistance training reduce muscle protein breakdown (19, 22). But muscle protein synthesis is considered the most important part of this equation, making up more than 70 percent of improvements in net protein balance through resistance training, whereas muscle protein breakdown has a smaller contribution to net protein balance (19). Net muscle protein balance remains negative if carbohydrate alone is consumed without the addition of essential amino acids or protein (figure 12.3) (19, 22).

For maximum muscle protein synthesis, the idea of an anabolic window of opportunity has been put forth: The athlete must eat anytime within this window of time after training for maximum gains. This theory has largely been based on training in the fasted state after which the body is in a catabolic state until food is consumed. And indeed, consuming protein and carbohydrate soon after training makes practical sense if training is carried out after an overnight fast (23). Under

PUTTING IT INTO PERSPECTIVE

STRENGTH-TRAINING GAINS

Strength increases during the first few months of resistance training are achieved not only through changes in muscle size but also through changes in neural adaptations. Therefore, novices might get stronger before they notice any appreciable increase in muscle size (27). Also, the same strength-training program can elicit a wide range of responses. Some people will show little to no gains, whereas others might have profound changes in muscle size and strength (28-30). The wide variability in response to a well-designed strength-training program might help explain some of the variability observed in response to nutrition interventions (31).

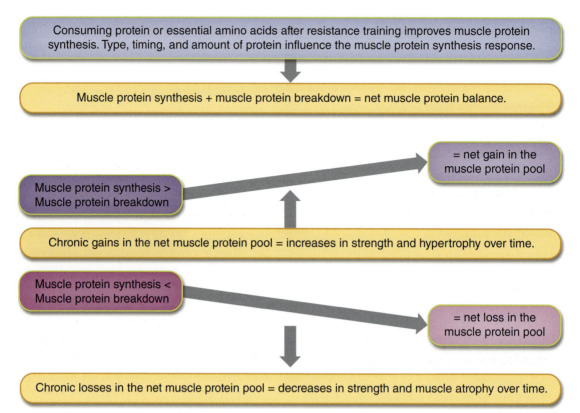

Figure 12.3 The muscle protein balance equation.

fed conditions, however, there is no evidence to suggest that protein must be consumed right away for maximum gains. Instead, consuming a protein-rich meal within a 3- to 4-hour period anytime from before to after resistance exercise is considered sufficient for maximal gains; see figure 12.4 (23).

> **? DO YOU KNOW?**
>
> Invasive procedures are required to examine changes in muscle protein synthesis, so not enough studies have been done in children to make a research-based recommendation for protein intake after resistance training in this age group (25, 26).

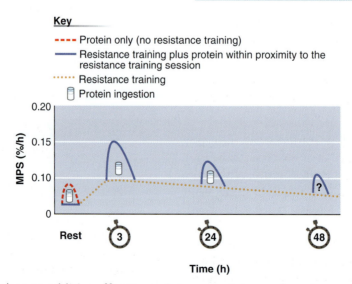

Figure 12.4 Protein has an additive effect to resistance training, enhancing muscle protein synthesis more than resistance training alone.

Effect of Concurrent Training

Concurrent training sessions are those performed back to back. For instance, a coach might choose to have athletes work on speed and perform strength training immediately afterward, or vice versa. Some studies report interference—aerobic training interferes with resistance exercise performance (32). Other studies, however, show that moderate-intensity endurance exercise does not impair acute bouts of resistance exercise, anabolic signaling, or the hypertrophy response (33-37). Physiological and molecular responses to concurrent training depend on the duration and type of exercise:

- Moderate-intensity endurance exercise before or after lifting may enhance strength gains compared with lifting alone (without the endurance work beforehand or afterward).
- Repetitive sprint activity or high-intensity interval training (HIIT) followed by upper-body lifting does not interfere with muscle growth (38).
- Running or repetitive sprint activity followed by lower-body lifting will likely result in interference; cycling has less effect than running (38).
- Cycling HIIT training back to back with lifting can negatively affect lower-body strength gains. Adding a longer rest period between cycling and lifting helps minimize the negative effect of HIIT on lower-body strength gains (32, 38).
- Concurrent running HIIT and lifting does not negatively affect lower-body strength gains.
- Concurrent training (endurance training plus heavy lifting) may improve endurance performance (32, 34, 38-41).

In addition to paying close attention to the type of training and sequence of concurrent training, it is important to examine whether the athlete is in a fed or fasted state, how trained the athlete is, and how adapted they are to concurrent training regimens (42-44).

Scant research has examined the effect of concurrent training and nutrition interventions compared with the many studies examining how pre-, during, and postworkout nutrition alters acute changes after a single training session (45). A concurrent training model seems to lead to greater acute increases in muscle protein synthesis in the fed state compared with resistance exercise alone (33, 34).

Although determining optimal nutrition strategies is difficult because of the sheer number of variables, including different types of concurrent training programs, general recommendations can be made based on the research on concurrent training models, nutrition interventions used in single training studies (endurance, sprint performance, resistance training, etc.), and proposed mechanisms responsible for exercise interference (46, 47).

Some athletes may want to perform endurance exercise in a glycogen-depleted state to promote greater metabolic adaptations in skeletal muscle. Immediately after endurance exercise, they might also delay carbohydrate intake for the same reason. But these strategies need to be carefully considered because they can lead to skeletal muscle breakdown and decreases in glycogen, as well as diminished resistance-training performance, particularly when used in a concurrent model when resistance training is performed immediately after endurance exercise (47). For peak training performance, athletes should consume enough carbohydrate after their first training session before they perform their second session. In addition, over the course of prolonged concurrent sessions, the athlete may want to consider consuming a small amount of dietary protein if their stomach can handle it during aerobic or high-intensity interval training before strength training in addition to consuming a leucine-rich, fast protein soon after resistance training to maximize muscle protein synthesis (33).

HOW DAILY DIETARY INTAKE AFFECTS MUSCLE

Although pre-, during, and postexercise nutrient intake has received considerable attention, the most important factors for optimal resistance-training adaptations include total daily protein intake, per meal amount of protein, and intake of specific nutrients that support muscle function.

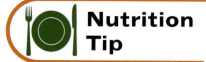

Nutrition Tip: Low total protein intake is associated with a reduction in muscle mass and strength throughout the life cycle (51, 52).

Exercise increases protein needs; athletes engaging in resistance training will benefit from consuming approximately 1.2 to 2.0 grams of protein per kilogram body weight per day to maximize muscle protein synthesis (13, 48, 49).

Studies in children and adolescents suggest that these athletes also need more protein than their sedentary counterparts to meet the demands of growth and training. Although the amount of protein they need per day is unclear, 1.2 to 2.0 grams of protein per kg body weight per day has been put forth as a general recommended range (25, 48).

As the body ages, muscle mass tends to decrease as a result of sarcopenia. This challenge is considerable, but exercise, particularly resistance training, and the consumption of an adequate amount of protein per meal and per day represent promising strategies to delay the onset and progression of sarcopenia. Older adults should aim for 1.2 to 2.0 grams of protein per kilogram body weight daily (50).

Meal Patterns and Muscle Growth

In adults, the initiation of protein synthesis is regulated by leucine, which upregulates the mTORC1 pathway that controls the synthesis of proteins in muscle (53, 54). A high-quality, leucine-rich protein should be a central part of each meal if the goal is to maintain or build muscle. See figure 12.5 for the leucine content of commonly consumed proteins. As noted in figure 12.6, research suggests that younger adults need approximately 2 to 3 grams of leucine per meal or 0.05 grams of leucine per kg body weight, whereas older adults might need 3 to 5 grams of leucine per meal to maximize muscle protein synthesis (55-58). Younger adults can meet this leucine threshold with 20 to 25 grams of high-quality protein (providing about 8.5–10 grams of essential amino acids), such as egg or whey. If opting for a protein source with less leucine per serving, more protein is necessary to meet the leucine threshold of 2 to 3 grams. For instance, approximately 30 grams

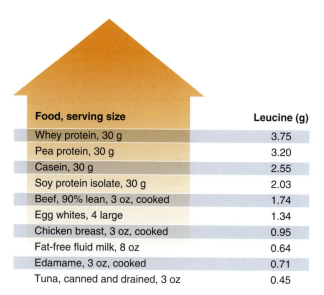

Figure 12.5 Leucine content of common foods and supplements.

Data from Babault et al. (2015); Pennings et al. (2011); U.S. Department of Agriculture (2013).

of soy protein contains approximately 2 grams of leucine. Older adults need more leucine and protein because of age-related decline in muscle sensitivity to amino acids (discussed later in the chapter). They should consume at least 0.4 grams of protein per kg body weight per meal and 1.2 to 2.0 g/kg per day to maximize muscle protein synthesis (50, 59). Although leucine is critical for turning on the machinery underlying protein synthesis, all essential amino acids are necessary for maximal muscle protein synthesis (60).

? DO YOU KNOW?

Although adults need to eat a certain amount of leucine and protein at each meal to maximize stimulation of muscle protein synthesis, children, teens, and young adults (those in their early 20s or under—the exact age is not clear) do not need to follow specific per-meal guidelines for protein. Their drive for protein synthesis is not leucine dependent, so they will grow and get stronger as long as total dietary protein and calorie needs are met.

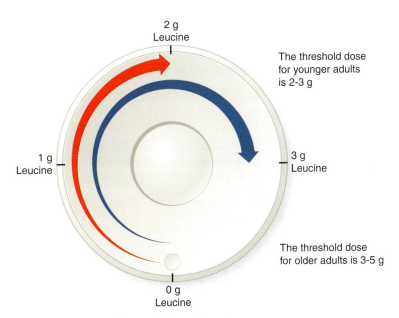

Figure 12.6 Leucine turns on muscle protein synthesis.

The anabolic effect (upregulation in muscle protein synthesis) of a meal lasts approximately 3 to 5 hours.

Therefore, consuming regular meals containing a sufficient amount of protein can help maximally stimulate muscle protein synthesis following each meal and ultimately maximize MPS over a 24-hour period (53, 61-63). Despite this recommendation, many adults eat an uneven pattern of protein. They consume little protein at breakfast, more at lunch (yet still not enough to stimulate MPS maximally), and a sufficient amount of protein at dinner (64). By doing this, only their evening protein intake maximizes MPS. They miss out on earlier opportunities to maximize MPS at breakfast and lunch.

The body does not have a long-term storage site for protein. When more protein is consumed than needed at that time, the gut can retain amino acids and release them later for incorporation into tissues, including muscle (65). But the consumption of a very large amount of protein at one meal does not lead to greater acute muscle protein synthesis compared with a more modest amount of protein (66). In a 7-day crossover feeding study with a 30-day washout period (a period when they went back to their regular diet) after each trial, researchers examined how different patterns of protein intake affected muscle protein synthesis over a 24-hour period. Each of the two study diets provided enough energy for weight maintenance and 1.2 grams of protein per kg body weight per day (90 g of protein). Diet 1 provided an even distribution of protein intake—about 30 grams at breakfast, 30 grams at lunch, and 30 grams at dinner. Diet 2 provided a skewed distribution of protein intake set to mimic a typical American diet (a low-protein breakfast and most protein consumed at dinner)—about 10 grams at breakfast, 15 grams at lunch, and 65 grams at dinner (67). Carbohydrate content at each meal was held constant, while dietary fat content was manipulated to ensure that total daily calorie intake remained similar on each diet and that carbohydrate, fat, and protein intake was not different between the diets. Consuming the same amount of protein at each meal resulted in an approximately 25 percent greater mixed muscle protein synthesis (contractile proteins make up a large part of this) over the 24-hour period, as measured on study day 1, compared with when protein intake was skewed. By day 7, when study subjects were habituated to the diet, a similar muscle protein synthetic response was observed. This study suggests that an even distribution of approximately 30 grams of protein per meal leads to greater muscle protein synthesis compared with a skewed distribution that reflects a typical American diet, even after 7 days of habituation to the pattern of protein intake. Figure 12.7 shows

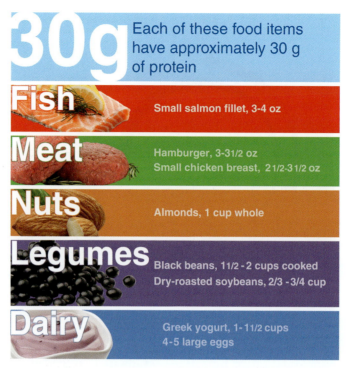

Figure 12.7 What does 30 grams of protein look like?

examples of food with 30 grams of protein. It is not clear from this study if higher per-meal doses of protein would have resulted in greater increases in acute muscle protein synthesis and greater improvements in muscle mass and strength over time (68, 69). Greater quantities of protein may possibly lead to greater net protein gains in some people (65). To maximize gains, some have suggested that protein intake per meal should be 0.4 g/kg per meal across four meals to reach 1.6 g/kg per day. Athletes who need more protein can divide their total protein goal per day in g/kg by the number of meals they plan to eat to get their ideal per-meal protein dose (70).

? DO YOU KNOW?

Athletes and active adults are not the only ones who can benefit from consuming an even distribution of protein per meal (as opposed to a skewed distribution) and following minimum per-meal leucine and protein guidelines. All adults can likely benefit from this approach including but not limited to hospital patients (71), those rehabbing from an injury (72), anyone looking to decrease the progression of sarcopenia (59), and the elderly (66, 73).

Modifying Protein-Poor Meals to Maximize Muscle Protein Synthesis

If the per-meal protein recommendations seem like a lot of food, or if a higher-protein diet is contraindicated, another strategy might increase acute muscle protein synthesis to the same extent as a higher-protein meal. Leucine or EAAs can be added to a lower-protein meal to help increase muscle protein synthesis (53, 74-76). This strategy, however, might not translate to the same long-term results as consuming recommended amounts of high biological value protein at each meal.

In a 2-week study, leucine added to meals low in EAAs improved acute muscle protein synthesis and anabolic signaling in older adults consuming just over the RDA for protein (0.81 ± 0.04 g protein per kg body weight per day) (77). But a longer-term study found that the addition of leucine to meals did not improve muscle mass, strength, or muscle quality in diabetic or healthy older adults who consumed enough protein throughout the day (78).

PUTTING IT INTO PERSPECTIVE

WHAT IS THE MAXIMUM AMOUNT OF PROTEIN YOUR BODY CAN DIGEST AND USE AT ONE TIME?

What is the ideal amount of protein per meal to maximize muscle protein synthesis and satiety (fullness) without wasting food or money? Current studies suggest that 25 to 45 grams per meal might be best for maximizing muscle protein synthesis, although we do not know the upper limit beyond which protein synthesis will not continue increasing to any appreciable extent (69, 79, 80). The ideal amount of protein per meal varies among people based on age, training status, amount of energy consumed each day, amount of protein they consume each day, the quality and leucine (or EAA) content of the protein, other nutrients consumed at mealtime in conjunction with protein, and health status (20, 65, 81, 82). Some researchers suggest that there is a "muscle full" effect, a dose-dependent upper limit of muscle tissue saturation of amino acids beyond which the amino acids are no longer used to increase muscle protein synthesis but instead are oxidized (62). But no studies have examined the maximum amount of protein intake at a meal and how this relates to changes in muscle strength and mass over time (65). In addition, few studies have examined whether consistently higher total daily protein intake (above the recommendations listed in this text) affects measures of resistance-training performance and lean body mass. No studies to date have separated the effect of higher protein intake from higher calorie intake on those variables (comparing diets with the same total amount of energy but considerably higher amounts of protein in one diet). One study in resistance-trained people found that 4.4 grams of protein per kg body weight per day along with more total energy each day did not lead to greater increases in lean body mass compared with 1.8 grams of protein per kg body weight per day and significantly fewer calories per day (83).

In summary, adding amino acids to a lower-protein meal will not help over the long term, and athletes should not use the strategy. Instead, athletes should focus on total daily protein intake and the relatively even distribution of protein intake per meal to maximize MPS.

HOW DIETING AFFECTS MUSCLE

A higher protein intake combined with resistance training can preserve muscle on a lower-calorie diet. But the overall calorie deficit and speed of weight loss are important factors influencing muscle loss when dieting. If the calorie deficit is small, higher amounts of dietary protein and resistance training can counter most of the breakdown in muscle proteins. When the size of the caloric deficit is large, protein alone cannot stop the loss of skeletal muscle mass completely (20).

Even short periods of energy restriction can decrease postmeal increases in muscle protein synthesis. One study found a 27 percent decline in postmeal muscle protein synthesis after 5 days on a reduced-calorie yet higher-protein diet (30 kcal per kg fat-free mass and 1.4–1.6 g of protein per kg body weight), which shows that even when protein intake is twice the RDA, it is not always enough to preserve muscle protein synthesis during times of major caloric restriction.

In another study, 39 adults were randomized to receive 0.8 grams of protein per kg body weight per day (the RDA for protein), 1.6 grams of protein per kg body weight per day (twice the RDA), or 2.4 grams of protein per kg body weight per day (three times the RDA). For the first 10 days of the study, the subjects were placed on a diet for weight maintenance. After this period, they were put on a 21-day diet consuming 40 percent fewer calories than they needed to maintain weight. All groups lost the same amount of weight regardless of dietary protein intake. But the groups consuming two and three times the RDA for protein lost significantly more fat and less fat-free mass than the group consuming the RDA for protein. Also, the anabolic response to a protein-rich meal was significantly lower when subjects were given the RDA for protein on the lower-calorie diet compared with when they consumed the RDA for protein on the regular-weight maintenance diet. The anabolic response to a meal was not different between the weight maintenance and lower-calorie diet phases when subjects consumed two or three times the RDA. Combined, these results suggest consuming two to three times the RDA for protein while consuming significantly less energy preserved muscle mass during weight loss (84).

> **? DO YOU KNOW?**
>
> Gaining muscle when cutting calories is difficult because lower-calorie diets decrease the intracellular signaling necessary for the synthesis of new proteins in muscle, and muscle tissue may be less sensitive to protein when calorie intake is insufficient (85).

Low-Carbohydrate Diets and Resistance Training

Although carbohydrate is the main source of energy used during resistance training and exhaustive bouts of resistance training can reduce glycogen substantially, a longer-term, higher-carbohydrate diet does not seem to offer any advantage for strength-training performance. In a meta-analysis looking at 17 studies that examined longer-term high-carbohydrate diets versus lower-carbohydrate or ketogenic diets, 15 of the 17 studies found no effect of carbohydrate on strength-training performance or strength development. Eight of the studies were isocaloric; those consuming both the higher- and lower-carbohydrate diets ate the same amount of calories per day (7).

Carbohydrate loading is a technique that endurance athletes have used for decades to supercompensate glycogen stores and improve performance. In general, endurance athletes taper their training program for a specified period while consuming a higher-carbohydrate diet, generally between 8 and 12 grams of carbohydrate per kg body weight each day. Endurance athletes with a high training load are on the higher end of this range of carbohydrate intake (86, 87). Few studies have looked at the effect of carbohydrate loading on resistance exercise performance, and the limited research to date does not support carbohydrate loading for improving resistance-training performance. But no published studies in resistance-trained people have examined how following a nonketogenic low-carbohydrate diet affects resistance-training performance parameters such as 1 RM or max number of repetitions performed for a specific lift (how many reps a person can perform at 200 pounds [91 kg] on the bench press, for example). The studies to date on low-carbohydrate diets show that a very low-carbohydrate, high-protein diet (7% carbohydrate, 63% protein, 30% fat) and low-carbohydrate, moderate-protein diet (20% carbohydrate, 50% protein, 30% fat) led to greater total weight and fat mass losses (though not significant) compared with a high-carbohydrate, low-protein diet group (55% carbohydrate, 15% protein, 30% fat) in healthy obese women engaged in a circuit-training program (88).

A bodybuilder's goal is not performance related but instead appearance related. Therefore, bodybuilders might carbohydrate-load before competition to increase muscle size, a practice that makes sense physiologically (particularly if they consume a lower-carbohydrate diet for a few days and then carbohydrate-load), yet there is little research on this practice. In one study examining carbohydrate loading for 24 hours after 3 days of carbohydrate depletion, authors found significant increases in body mass and muscle thickness in those who carbohydrate-loaded versus the bodybuilders who did not. Although carbohydrate loading led to an acute increase in muscle volume and physical appearance, it also resulted in many gastrointestinal side effects, particularly constipation and diarrhea (8). To notice a difference in muscle size, increasing total calorie intake during the carbohydrate-loading period may be warranted (89).

Based on the research to date, bodybuilders, power lifters, and Olympic weightlifters do not necessarily need to consume a higher-carbohydrate diet (>4 or more g of carbohydrate per kg body weight), as is recommended to many athletes, particularly endurance athletes.

Ketogenic Diets and Resistance Training

As discussed in chapter 4, ketogenic diets are very high-fat diets, and although the specific percentages of fat, protein, and carbohydrate vary, the diets are generally about 75 to 90 percent fat, 5 to 20 percent protein, and 5 to 10 percent carbohydrate (90). For more information regarding the rationale and history behind this approach, refer to chapter 4.

A person needs at least 7 days to reach nutritional ketosis and 3 to 4 weeks to adapt fully to relying on ketones to fuel exercise. The diet is not ideal for resistance training because many of the signaling pathways needed for muscle hypertrophy are blunted while following a ketogenic diet. In addition, protein intake must be kept fairly low to stay in a state of ketosis. A lower-protein diet can impair muscle gains. In one study, subjects placed on a ketogenic diet while consuming less than 1.2 grams of protein per kg of ideal body weight per day lost muscle and saw their athletic performance decline. The ketogenic diet is not beneficial for fat loss compared with consuming the same amount of energy from a lower-fat diet. NIH researchers admitted 17 overweight or obese men to a metabolic ward and placed them on a high-carbohydrate baseline diet for 4 weeks followed by 4 weeks on an isocaloric ketogenic diet. (This diet contained the same amount of energy as the high-carbohydrate diet.) The men lost weight and body fat on both diets. The ketogenic diet did not lead to greater fat loss as compared with the high-carbohydrate diet, and in fact body fat loss slowed during the ketogenic diet and subjects lost muscle (91).

Trading carbohydrate for fat may seem like a huge benefit for athletes, particularly endurance athletes who train and compete for several hours at a time (92). In addition to training the body to use body fat, the ketogenic diet contains more fat, which actually produces more energy (ATP) (93). But fat is a slow source of fuel—the human body cannot access it quickly enough to sustain high-intensity exercise—so this diet is really only (potentially) applicable to ultrarunners and triathletes competing at a relatively moderate to slow pace. To date, however, there is no research to suggest that either a ketogenic diet or a carbohydrate diet is superior to a higher-carbohydrate diet for endurance performance.

Some people opt for a modified ketogenic diet, which is really a low-carbohydrate, as opposed to ketogenic, diet. A study in gymnasts found that a very low-carbohydrate diet (<30 g of carbohydrate per day), a so-called modified ketogenic diet (4.5% carbohydrate, 54.8% fat, and 40.7% protein, which equaled approximately 2.8 g of protein per kg/day) for 30 days resulted in significant fat mass losses and the gymnasts were able to maintain their lean body mass. In addition, they maintained power and strength while training 30 hours per week (93).

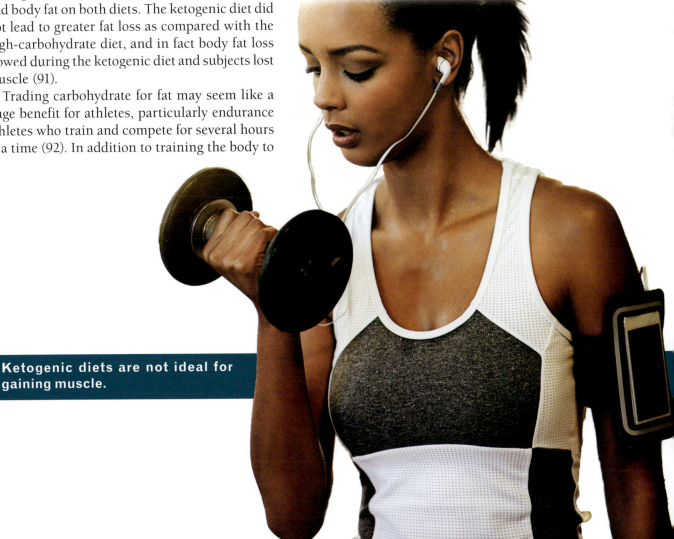

Ketogenic diets are not ideal for gaining muscle.

A ketogenic diet has some nutrition and cardiovascular drawbacks. Studies in epileptic children show soon after the start of the diet, blood cholesterol levels rise and artery stiffness increases (94, 95). High total and LDL cholesterol are risk factors for cardiovascular disease, and artery stiffness decreases the ability of the arteries to expand to accommodate changes in pressure. Increased artery stiffness is an early sign of vascular damage and a risk factor for cardiovascular disease (96). After 6 to 12 months on the diet, or if a patient goes off the diet, blood cholesterol levels dropped back to normal, and artery stiffness returned to normal after 24 months on the diet (94, 95). A high-fat diet may also increase levels of harmful bacteria and decrease levels of beneficial bacteria in the gut (gut bacteria influences many aspects of health, including immune system and gastrointestinal tract functioning) (97). In addition, food choices are limited, which makes it difficult to get enough calcium, vitamin D, potassium, and folate versus folic acid. Ketogenic diets may increase sodium needs because of electrolyte excretion. Potassium and sodium are critical for muscle functioning (including heart functioning), so a ketogenic diet should never be attempted without a physician's guidance. During the first few weeks on the diet, people might suffer headaches and feel fatigued, as if exercise requires more effort (98).

> **DO YOU KNOW?**
>
> A ketogenic diet is always low in carbohydrate, but a low-carbohydrate diet is not necessarily a ketogenic diet. The literature includes a wide variety of definitions for "low carbohydrate." A ketogenic diet is always high in fat; 80 to 90 percent of energy comes from dietary fat.

NUTRIENTS THAT SUPPORT MUSCLE FUNCTIONING

Several nutrients are important for muscle functioning, including magnesium, vitamin D, and zinc. Low levels of magnesium can lead to muscle cell dysfunction and a decrease in muscle cell carbohydrate uptake, whereas magnesium deficiency can lead to muscle cramping, muscular twitching or spasms, muscular fatigue, numbness, and tingling (99, 100).

Vitamin D deficiency can lead to muscle weakness and pain (101, 102). Although vitamin D supplementation to achieve normal vitamin D levels benefits muscle strength and physical performance while helping decrease risk of falls in the elderly (102-104), the research in younger people has not been as promising.

An earlier systematic review found vitamin D had a small but significant positive effect on muscle strength with no effect on muscle mass or muscle power. Supplementation was more effective in people 65 years of age or older, in addition to those who were deficient before the start of the study (105). But a recent systematic review and meta-analysis found that vitamin D supplementation among athletes to achieve normal levels did not lead to improvements in strength (106). This review and meta-analysis included only five studies, and therefore more research needs to be done in this area with athletes from a variety of sports.

Low zinc status can lead to declines in muscle strength and power output, and correcting a zinc deficiency can improve muscle strength (107-109). All vitamins and minerals and their effect on athletic performance are discussed in chapters 6 and 7.

SPORT SUPPLEMENTS FOR RESISTANCE TRAINING

Creatine monohydrate is a supplement that increases body weight, strength, and muscle mass in many healthy younger adults (110-112). In addition, a 2014 meta-analysis in older adults found that creatine supplementation taken in combination with resistance training led to greater increases in lean body mass and some measures of strength, as well as significant improvements in functional performance compared with placebo (113).

Beta-hydroxy-beta-methylbutyrate (HMB) is a metabolite of leucine, although only 5 percent of leucine is converted to HMB during metabolism (114). HMB can help decrease muscle breakdown in frail elderly people who are unable to exercise, as well as those on bedrest (115-117). But HMB does not improve strength, muscle size, or body composition in young adults engaged in a resistance-training program (118, 119).

SUMMARY

Carbohydrate from circulating blood sugar and muscle glycogen is the main source of energy for resistance training. When carbohydrate stores are low, performance suffers, and immune and central nervous system functioning can be acutely suppressed. Adequate carbohydrate after exercise provides energy for the process of muscle building and repair, helps decrease muscle breakdown, and replenishes glycogen so that the athlete has adequate energy for the next training session. In addition to carbohydrate, hydration status affects resistance-training performance by altering the hormonal and metabolic response to resistance exercise and making the heart work harder.

Protein is not necessary for resistance-training performance, although recommended amounts are essential for the repair aspects of muscle recovery and the maximization of training adaptations. Both protein and essential amino acids consumed before or after resistance training will stimulate acute muscle protein synthesis. At least 20 to 40 grams of protein should be consumed after exercise, although more may be necessary in some circumstances. Over time, a sound resistance-training program combined with post-workout protein and protein-rich meals spaced evenly throughout the day will improve strength and muscle hypertrophy in adults. Aging alters the anabolic response to protein intake, so older adults benefit from greater amounts of protein postexercise and at mealtime.

FOR REVIEW

1. Why do those who are cutting calories below their daily needs benefit from consuming more protein each day? How much protein should they aim for?
2. Explain why a ketogenic diet may not be beneficial for those engaging in a resistance-training program.
3. Why do older adults need more protein than younger adults after exercise?
4. How does alcohol affect resistance-training outcomes?
5. What regulates protein synthesis in children?

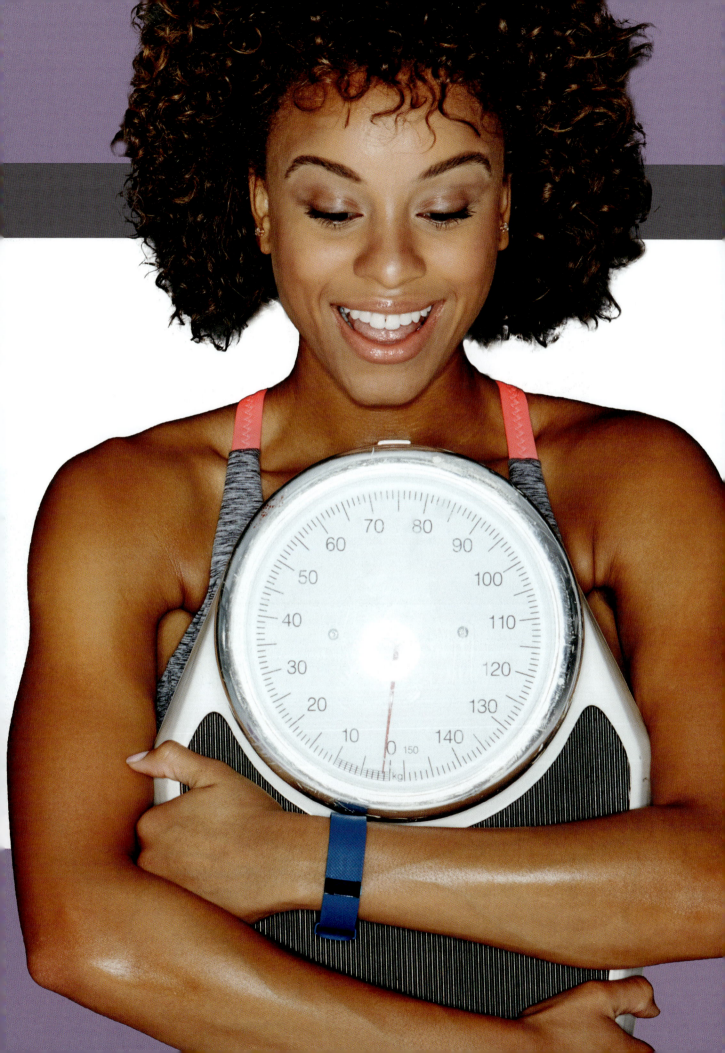

13

Changing Weight and Body Composition

> **▶ CHAPTER OBJECTIVES**
>
> After completing this chapter, you will be able to do the following:
> - Describe the health implications associated with excess body fat, overweight, and obesity.
> - Describe the health implications associated with very low body fat.
> - List strategies that an athlete can use to lose body fat and gain lean body mass (separately or at the same time).
> - Discuss how popular diets promote weight loss.
> - Discuss why higher protein intake is important during weight loss.
> - Discuss how low energy (calorie) intake affects the ability to increase muscle hypertrophy, train, and compete.
> - Describe why people often plateau on their weight-loss journey or regain weight.
> - Outline effective strategies for decreasing weight-loss plateaus and limiting weight regain.

Body composition is often described as the ratio between fat and fat-free mass. As discussed in chapter 10, there is no universal definition for optimal body composition, which is subjective (1). Also, what an athlete considers ideal might differ from what a coach or performance staff member considers ideal. To manipulate body composition, fat and skeletal muscle are altered through training and nutrition. But each person's response to diet modifications and training varies, including how much body fat can be lost or how much muscle can be gained within a particular timeframe. Body composition goals may be adjusted over time based on how the body responds to training and health status (including injuries), and for athletes, how changes in body composition or the effort needed to sustain such changes affects performance. And although focusing on fat and muscle with dietary interventions is more common, bone should not be forgotten.

UNDERSTANDING BODY FAT

The two main types of body fat are essential body fat and storage fat. **Essential fat**, necessary for physiological functioning, is found in bone marrow, the heart, lungs, liver, spleen, kidneys, intestines, muscles, and fat-rich tissues of the central nervous system (2). Essential fat for men and women is approximately 3 percent and 12 percent body fat, respectively (2). In women, essential fat is higher because it includes fat in the breasts, hips, and pelvis for reproduction. Storage fat is energy accumulated for later use and found around internal organs (**visceral fat**) and directly below the skin (**subcutaneous fat**). Storage fat increases over time when excess energy (calories) is consumed and decreases when more energy is burned than is consumed. Visceral fat wraps around organs like a blanket and contributes to inflammation (3). Higher levels of visceral fat are associated with higher risk for several chronic diseases (4, 5). Subcutaneous fat is not associated with the same chronic disease risk as visceral fat, and it may protect the body from collisions (6, 7).

> **❓ DO YOU KNOW?**
> People can be within normal weight yet have high levels of visceral fat (8).

Health Implications of Excess Body Fat

Excess body fat, technically called excess adiposity, takes a toll on the entire body. Obesity increases risk of many health problems and diseases, including

- type 2 diabetes,
- heart disease,
- stroke,
- certain types of cancer,
- sleep apnea,
- osteoarthritis,
- fatty liver disease,
- kidney disease,
- depression,
- chronic inflammation,
- osteoarthritis, and
- complications during pregnancy, such as gestational diabetes; high blood pressure, which can affect the health of the mother and the baby; premature birth; stillborn birth; and neural tube defects.

Based on Arabin and Stupin (2014); Gregor and Hotamisligil (2011); Guffey, Fan, Singh, and Murphy (2013); Marshall and Spong (2012); Pi-Sunyer (2009); Polednak (2008); Roberts, Dive, and Renehan (2010).

Obesity also increases risk of **all-cause mortality** (death from all causes), cancer mortality, and cardiovascular mortality (9). Despite the risk factors associated with being overweight and being obese, both conditions have steadily increased over the past several decades. In 2017 to 2018, 42.5 percent of adults over the age of 20 were obese and another 31.1 percent were overweight, and 19.3 percent of children and adolescents ages 2 to 19 were obese (10, 11). See figure 13.1 for factors contributing to the rise in overweight and obesity.

Excess fat around the waist is associated with increased risk of disease. The waist-to-hip ratio is used as a measure of higher waist circumference and reflects increased visceral fat better than BMI does (figure 13.2) (12, 13).

Blood Vessels, the Heart, and Kidneys

Obesity can increase blood lipids, including cholesterol and triglycerides (blood fats). Lipo-

Changing Weight and Body Composition 323

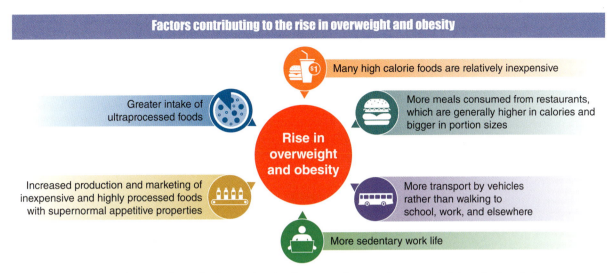

Figure 13.1 What factors have led to a rise in the prevalence of overweight and obesity?

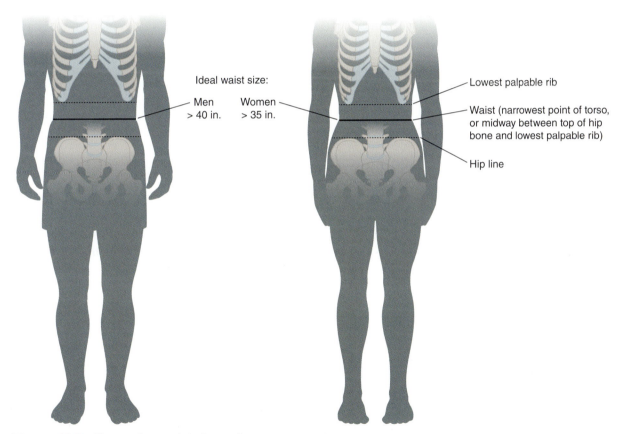

Figure 13.2 Measuring waist circumference.
Based on National Heart Lung and Blood Institute (1998).

proteins transport cholesterol through the body. **Low-density lipoprotein (LDL)** carries cholesterol from the liver to tissues, where it is used for a variety of functions, including incorporation as a structural component in cell membranes and the synthesis of steroid hormones. Although cholesterol is essential, high blood LDL can increase cholesterol buildup in arteries and is associated with increased risk for heart disease (14). **High-density lipoprotein (HDL)** carries

HIGH BLOOD PRESSURE AND PLAQUE BUILDUP ON ARTERY WALLS

Atherosclerosis is similar to the buildup of dirt and debris inside a garden hose. When gunk builds up in a hose, you must turn up the water pressure to continue getting the same amount of water from the hose. Plaque buildup in arteries means that the heart must work harder and generate more force to push blood through the body. That force damages artery walls.

cholesterol back to the liver for excretion or recycling. Thus, HDL is sometimes referred to as good cholesterol and is not associated with increased risk for heart disease. There are various types or subclasses of LDL and HDL, each of which has different effects in the body. Triglycerides do not directly cause clogging of the arteries, although high levels of triglycerides are associated with increased risk of cardiovascular disease (15, 16).

Excess body fat causes the heart to work harder to pump blood, because the heart must overcome resistance in blood vessels to deliver blood throughout the body. Over time, greater force of blood against artery walls leads to an increase in blood pressure (17), a condition called **hypertension**, which can damage and weaken artery walls. Plaque (composed of fat, cholesterol, calcium, and other substances) adheres more easily to damaged artery walls (figure 13.3). Plaque buildup, called **atherosclerosis**, decreases the diameter of arteries, narrowing the space blood travels through. Narrow artery walls decrease the flow of oxygenated blood to tissues and organs and increase risk of blood clots, which can block blood flow partially or completely (18). High blood pressure and atherosclerosis are risk factors for cardiovascular disease, diseases of the heart and blood vessels, and chronic kidney disease. Healthy kidneys help maintain blood pressure by regulating blood volume and electrolytes as well as through hormonal control. Damage to kidneys can impair kidney functioning, which may result in fluid buildup in blood vessels and an even greater increase in blood pressure (19).

? DO YOU KNOW?

Smoking and exposure to secondhand smoke also damages artery walls.

Obesity, Insulin Resistance, and Type 2 Diabetes

Obesity can impair the body's ability to use insulin properly (insulin resistance) through several mechanisms including chronic low-grade inflam-

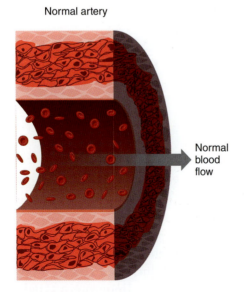
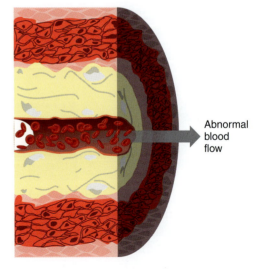

Figure 13.3 Plaque buildup in an artery.

> **PUTTING IT INTO PERSPECTIVE**
>
> ## ATHLETES AND OBESITY
>
> Athletes are not immune to obesity and obesity-related health consequences. A study in 90 Division I college football players found that 21 percent were obese (all were linemen), as defined by 25 percent body fat or greater, as measured by BOD POD; 21 percent had insulin resistance (13 of the 19 players with insulin resistance were linemen); and 9 percent had metabolic syndrome (all linemen) (31).

mation, endoplasmic reticulum (ER) stress, and mitochondrial dysfunction (20). Insulin helps reduce blood sugar (typically referred to as blood glucose) in two ways:

- Insulin reduces glucose production in the liver (from stored glycogen), thereby helping reduce blood sugar.
- Insulin helps muscle, fat, and liver cells take up sugar (glucose) from the bloodstream, which lowers blood sugar.

Insulin also stimulates glucose storage in the form of glycogen in liver and muscle. Stored muscle glycogen is used for energy during exercise. Over time, high blood sugar decreases the body's ability to use insulin effectively, which can lead to insulin resistance (cells become resistant to the action of insulin) and type 2 diabetes (21).

Ninety percent of those with type 2 diabetes are overweight or obese (22). Type 2 diabetes can damage many parts of the body, including nerves, kidneys, eyes, and skin, while also increasing risk of heart attack and stroke (23). Weight loss can attenuate or reverse obesity-induced insulin resistance (24). Even small decreases in body weight can improve metabolic outcomes.

Cancer and Other Health Consequences

Gaining weight increases the risk for several cancers, even if the weight gain does not result in overweight or obesity. Scientists believe that this increased risk might be caused by several factors, including an increase in estrogen produced from fat; increased insulin and insulin-like growth

> **PUTTING IT INTO PERSPECTIVE**
>
> ## IS IT POSSIBLE TO BE FIT AND FAT?
>
> The concept of being fit and fat refers to being healthy despite being overweight or obese (i.e., metabolically healthy obesity) (32). In several studies, those who are metabolically healthy obese do not have insulin resistance, diabetes, high cholesterol, or high blood pressure. This finding is perplexing because obesity is a risk factor for several diseases, yet these studies show that some obese people do not have the level of complications expected from obesity (33, 34). Metabolically healthy obesity suggests that a high level of cardiovascular fitness attenuates some of the metabolic and cardiovascular disease risk factors associated with being overweight or obese (35). As a result, obese people who are fit may be healthier and live a longer life than normal-weight unfit people (36). Indeed, research shows that fitness has a powerful protective effect on health: Unfit people have twice the risk of death from all causes (all-cause mortality) compared with overweight and obese fit people (37).
>
> Despite the protective effect of exercise, this research is not without debate because much of it has been funded by a large soda manufacturer (38). In addition, those who are metabolically healthy and obese have a higher risk of developing type 2 diabetes and cardiovascular disease compared with healthy lean people (39). Also, few people meet the criteria for being fit and fat because "obesity is independently associated with reduced cardiovascular fitness" (35). More important, this state of metabolically healthy obesity is transient. Metabolically healthy obesity is a temporary state that occurs before the onset of metabolic syndrome and increased cardiovascular disease risk. Therefore, metabolically healthy obesity is not a reliable indicator of future disease risk. As a result, weight loss and lifestyle management for disease risk factors should be recommended to all people with obesity (40).

factor-1 (IGF-1), which might fuel the development of some types of tumors; chronic inflammation (fat produces inflammatory compounds); and an increase in hormones produced in fat cells that might affect cell growth (25-27).

Inflammation and excess fat around the neck might make the airway smaller, resulting in sleep apnea (28). Fat buildup in the liver can injure liver tissue, leading to damage, scarring (cirrhosis), and liver failure (29). Also, excess weight puts pressure on weight-bearing joints, increasing wear and tear of cartilage, the cushioning between joints, and risk for osteoarthritis (30).

DECREASING BODY FAT

A person might want to decrease body fat for a variety of reasons, including lowering disease risk and improving health, body image, or athletic performance.

Studies examining weight loss show that numerous dietary approaches can be effective, as long as they create an energy deficit over time (see figure 13.4) (41). Losing weight too quickly and repeatedly, however, can lead to a decrease in muscle and bone mass, a greater drop in metabolic rate (energy burned each day) than predicted by weight loss alone, and less energy available to train and get through each day (42-45). Generally, rapid weight loss should be avoided unless warranted for health reasons.

Health Implications of Low Body Fat

When body fat gets too low, energy levels and tolerance for cold decrease. Athletic performance might also suffer. Body fat below essential fat can compromise health and be associated with **low energy availability**; energy intake may be insufficient to meet physiological needs after meeting the energy needs of exercise. Low energy availability can lead to irregular menstrual cycles or complete cessation of menstruation (46). Irregular menstruation and altered menstrual functioning can compromise bone health and might increase risk of infertility (47).

Determining a Healthy Weight Goal and Daily Energy Needs

The first step in determining a healthy body weight goal is weighing in a euhydrated state and measuring body composition (45). These measures can be used to determine how much body fat people should lose to put them within an optimal range for health or, for athletes, within a sport-specific body fat range.

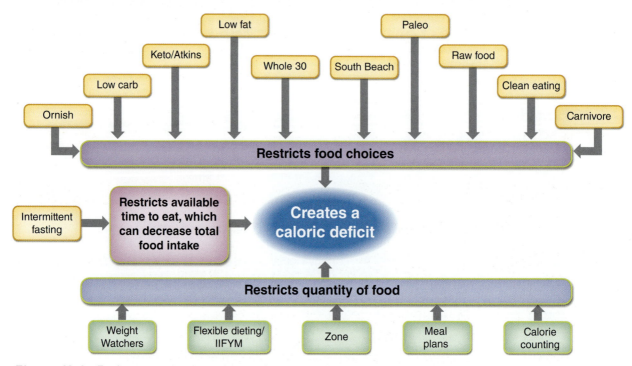

Figure 13.4 Reducing caloric intake is a fundamental component to diets.

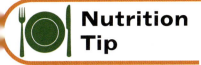

Nutrition Tip: If you are competing in a sport, either recreationally or competitively, you should focus on weight loss during the off-season or base phase of training. If you are working on weight loss in-season or before competition, cut calories as little as possible to preserve muscle mass, prevent a large drop in resting metabolic rate (RMR), and minimize training and performance decrements.

Next, energy needs can be estimated by using one of the following equations.

Harris–Benedict equation

Men BMR = 66.5 + (13.8 × weight [kg]) + (5 × height [cm]) − (6.8 × age)

Female BMR = 655.1 + (9.6 × weight [kg]) + (1.9 × height [cm]) − (4.7 × age)

Cunningham equation

RMR = 500 + (22 × lean body mass [kg])

Mifflin–St. Jeor equation

Men RMR = (10 × weight [kg]) + (6.25 × height [cm]) − (4.92 × age) + 5

Women RMR = (10 × weight [kg]) + (6.25 × height [cm]) − (4.92 × age) − 161

All these equations take body weight into account, and some also consider age, height, and lean body mass to predict **basal metabolic rate (BMR)** or resting metabolic rate (RMR). BMR measures the amount of energy burned at rest in a comfortable temperature at least 12 hours after activity and 10 to 12 hours after eating. RMR is measured at least 3 to 4 hours after activity or strenuous activity. The Cunningham equation considers lean body mass and is thus more applicable to athletes and other active people (49). BMR or RMR can be multiplied by an activity factor, or METs (metabolic equivalents) can be added to estimate total daily energy needs to maintain weight. Table 13.1 shows common activity factor values. Subtract the desired daily caloric deficit from total calories per day for weight loss. Metabolic equivalents are an estimate of energy expenditure during activity (50, 51). When considering number of calories burned each day, be sure to account for activities of daily living (nonathletic activities such as walking, gardening, playing with the kids, etc.) as well as energy burned through restlessness (fidgeting and constant movement) (52). Some people are extremely active outside of their training or athletic endeavors, whereas others tend to be sedentary when not training (53).

? DO YOU KNOW?

A caloric deficit of 500 to 1,000 kcal below estimated daily energy needs is generally recommended for weight loss (54, 55). But people with lower energy needs (women, older adults) and growing children and teens should minimize their total caloric deficit to ensure they are getting enough nutrients for good health (more calories consumed means more opportunities to consume nutrients) and for growth, development, bone health, and reproductive functioning.

PUTTING IT INTO PERSPECTIVE

DETERMINING IF WEIGHT GOALS ARE REALISTIC

A realistic weight goal

- takes weight history, history of family, body weight and shape, and past history of eating disorders, obesity, and disordered eating into account;
- does not compromise health or increase risk of injuries;
- promotes sound eating habits and supports training and performance;
- meets the needs for growth, development, and reproductive functioning; and
- can be maintained without extreme weight control practices or constant dieting (48).

Table 13.1 Average Energy Cost of Physical Activities Expressed in Calories per Minute (kcal/min) and Relative to Body Weight (kcal^{-1} · kg^{-1} · min^{-1})

Activity	Estimated kcal/min (derived from MET values, assuming 1 MET = 1.5 kcal/min)	Relative to body mass (kcal^{-1} · kg^{-1} · min^{-1})
Basketball game	12.0	0.123
Cycling		
Cycling hard uphill	21.0	0.071
Cycling flat terrain (<10.0 mph [16.1 km/h])	6.0	0.107
Cycling flat terrain (>20 mph [32.2 km/h])	24.0	0.343
Running		
7.5 mph (12.1 km/h)	14.0	0.200
10.0 mph (16.1 km/h)	18.0	0.260
Sitting	1.5	0.024
Sleeping	1.0	0.017
Standing	1.8	0.026
Swimming laps, freestyle, hard	15.0	0.285
Tennis, singles	12.0	0.101
Walking, 2.0 mph (3.2 km/h)	3.0	0.071
Resistance training, vigorous	9.0	0.117

Note: Values presented are for a 154-pound (70 kg) person. These values will vary depending on many other factors and should be viewed as estimates that can give athletes and clients a sense of how energy expenditure varies among activities. The energy cost of other activities can be found at https://sites.google.com/site/compendiumofphysicalactivities/ Activity-Categories.

Reprinted by permission from B. Murray and W.L. Kenney, *Practical Guide to Exercise Physiology: The Science of Exercise Training and Performance Nutrition*, 2nd ed. (Champaign, IL: Human Kinetics, 2021), 132.

Weight loss is not simple math, and people do not lose weight in a linear fashion. In 1958 a physician discovered that 1 pound (0.45 kg) of fat stores approximately 3,500 kcal (56). This discovery resulted in thousands of textbooks, articles, websites, and weight-loss programs inaccurately predicting weight loss by dividing 3,500 by the daily calorie deficit to get the number of days it would take to lose a pound. For instance, many would assume that subtracting 500 kcal per day from the amount of energy necessary to maintain weight would lead to a 1-pound (0.45 kg) weight loss in 7 days. But this simple math equation is inaccurate because it makes many assumptions: that we need the exact same number of calories each day to be in a state of energy balance; that calories burned each day through physical activity and activities of daily living remain constant from day to day; that we can calculate exactly how many calories we are eating; and that our bodies do not adapt to dieting and weight loss. Metabolism decreases with weight loss, providing one explanation for less-than-expected weight-loss results (57). Decreased adherence to a particular diet, however, might be the primary factor slowing the rate of weight loss or leading to a plateau in weight (58-60).

Validated weight-loss calculators can be used to predict the approximate amount of time required to lose weight. These calculators take into account decreases in metabolism that occur with weight loss. They are easy to find online. A weight-loss calculator created by Pennington Biomedical Research Center is called Weight Loss Predictor. A second one is Body Weight Planner by the USDA: http://BWplanner.niddk.nih.gov.

? DO YOU KNOW?

Self-reported measurements of dietary intake are notoriously inaccurate because food intake is often underestimated. Measurements may more accurately reflect a dieter's perceived effort to adhere to the intervention rather than their true dietary intake (71).

PUTTING IT INTO PERSPECTIVE

WHAT CAUSES WEIGHT-LOSS PLATEAUS AND WEIGHT REGAIN?

A typical scenario is that early weight loss stalls after a time as the person hits a plateau. Progressive weight regain follows (61). As people continue to lose weight, they fight an increasingly tough battle against biological responses that make it harder to continue losing weight (keep in mind that in much of the weight-loss research, studies were done in overweight and obese people, not active athletes) (62). In a meta-analysis of 29 long-term weight-loss studies (none of which were done in athletes), 80 percent of the weight lost was regained within 5 years (63). What makes weight loss and maintenance so difficult? Three main factors cause weight-loss plateaus and weight regain. As weight is lost, RMR, which accounts for the majority of calories that most people burn each day, decreases; the drive to eat increases; and some people experience an unintentional decrease in NEAT (non-exercise-associated thermogenesis), the energy burned because of activity that does not involve intentional exercise. NEAT includes fidgeting, maintaining posture, moving around during the day, and so on. All three factors can lead to diminishing returns on weight-loss plans over time. Like a domino effect, plateaus can hamper a person's motivation to stick to a diet and exercise plan (64, 65).

When a person loses weight, they expend less energy for movement because fewer calories are required to carry a lower body weight than a higher body weight. Even if muscle mass is preserved, losing weight leads to a drop in metabolism (RMR). Oftentimes this reduction in metabolism is greater than predicted based on the change in body weight and body composition. Furthermore, greater amounts of weight loss seem to lead to even greater decreases in RMR (65). This phenomenon is termed *metabolic adaptation* (42, 44, 66-68). Reasons for this drop in metabolism are not entirely clear, although it is correlated with the degree of energy deficit (the greater the energy decrease, the greater the drop in metabolism) and changes in circulating hormones that affect appetite (44, 69). As metabolism slows with significant weight loss, a person has to drop calories further to maintain their new size. Metabolic adaptation may persist in some people despite significant weight regain. In fact, in the Biggest Loser study, the participants experienced a continued drop in metabolism 6 years after the Biggest Loser competition, despite gaining back a significant amount of their weight. Interestingly, the degree of metabolic adaptation at the end of the Biggest Loser competition was not associated with weight regain; instead, those with greater long-term weight loss also had greater ongoing metabolic slowing. Despite weight regain and metabolic adaptation, the Biggest Loser participants kept off an average of 11.9 ± 16.8 percent of weight compared with baseline, while 57 percent of the participants maintained at least 10 percent weight loss (65).

Not all studies show a continued reduction in RMR following weight regain after weight loss. But unlike the Biggest Loser study, those studies may not have accounted for a person's state of energy balance; overeating or undereating during the period immediately before RMR was tested may influence RMR measurements (65). Interestingly, this metabolic adaptation is not evident in those who have had Roux-en-Y gastric bypass surgery, a restrictive-malabsorptive weight-loss surgery for those with a BMI over 40 or a BMI over 35 with obesity-related comorbidities (several contraindications and risks are associated with this surgery), despite continued weight loss (69, 70).

In addition to a decrease in RMR with weight loss, the concentration of the hormone leptin decreases while ghrelin increases, causing an increase in appetite and a decrease in satiety. These persistent endocrine adaptations make long-term weight maintenance difficult (71, 72). In fact, this adaptation may be the largest contributor to weight regain. In a 52-week trial, researchers found that appetite increased equivalent to approximately 100 kcal per day above baseline per kg of body weight lost, about three times higher than adaptations in energy expenditure, which were about 20 to 30 kcal per day per kg of body-weight loss (71). On the other hand, some people compensate for weight loss, voluntarily or involuntarily, with a decrease in NEAT. More diet-only versus exercise-only or combined diet and exercise trials report a decrease in NEAT with weight loss. In research studies, participants who lost almost twice as much weight as other participants experienced a decrease in NEAT, suggesting that behavioral compensation may occur when a substantial amount of weight is lost (73, 74).

Behavioral and psychological factors also play a role in weight regain after weight loss. These include decreases in physical activity, increases in depressive symptoms, and disinhibition ("the tendency to overeat in response to negative emotional states or the presence of highly palatable food") (75, 76).

>continued

What Causes Weight-Loss Plateaus and Weight Regain? >continued

There is no difference in risk of regaining weight in those who lose a substantial amount of weight compared with people who lose far less weight (65). But long-term weight loss requires long-term lifestyle changes to combat persistent metabolic adaptation and the increase in appetite and decrease in satiety that occurs with weight loss. Some people may need to reevaluate their goal weight and instead focus on a healthy diet and physical activity they can maintain for a lifetime while letting their weight change fall in place based on the lifestyle they can live with (65).

What can be done to help counteract plateaus and weight regain?

1. Have a long-term plan. Persistent intervention and support through interaction with health care providers or group settings can help improve weight maintenance and long-term outcomes.
2. Consider the following factors associated with long-term success: frequent self-monitoring and self-weighing, reduced energy intake, smaller and more frequent meals or snacks throughout the day, increased physical activity, consistent eating of breakfast, more frequent at-home meals compared with restaurant and fast-food meals, reduced screen time, and use of portion-controlled meals or meal substitutes.
3. Support motivation with outcomes. Progress can be marked by reminders of the amount of weight lost or photos of changes that have occurred.
4. Develop cognitive flexibility. Instead of the rigid all-or-nothing thinking associated with many diets, engage in more realistic expectations. Nobody will adhere 100 percent to a plan. Have flexibility when things do not go according to the plan.
5. Find deeper motivation. External motivation such as a reward for weight loss lasts only so long. People tend to stick to a diet or exercise plan better when they have personal significance attached to it or enjoy it. People take ownership when the goal is deeply meaningful or enjoyable. As an example, sticking to a weight-loss diet seems hard, yet many people can follow dietary rules for religious reasons (from Lent and Ramadan to kosher eating, for instance). Shifting focus from weight loss alone to something meaningful can improve outcomes.
6. Manage expectations. Many people have unrealistic expectations for weight loss. Yet research studies show that a 5 to 10 percent weight loss on average is a best-case scenario and few people with significantly high initial weights achieve and maintain an ideal body weight. When a person has unrealistic expectations and does not meet them, demoralization and self-blame can be the result.
7. Get weight maintenance counseling to support healthy behaviors (62).
8. Engage in regular physical activity. People who maintain higher levels of physical activity tend to achieve greater weight loss, whereas decreases in physical activity predict weight regain (76).

Energy-Yielding Macronutrient Requirements for Weight Loss

Many people lose muscle when dieting, which contributes to, yet does not fully account for, the decrease in metabolic rate that occurs with dieting. Several factors affect the amount of muscle mass lost, including physical activity characteristics (type, frequency, and duration); speed of weight loss; total protein intake; total daily energy deficit; gender; baseline level of body fat; and possibly individual differences in hormonal response to dieting. During negative energy balance, muscle mass losses are relatively smaller in obese people as compared with those of "normal" weight (77).

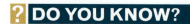

DO YOU KNOW?

Losing weight quickly increases the likelihood of losing muscle during weight loss (42, 43).

A lower-calorie diet that does not contain enough protein will lead to significant muscle loss (78-80). During weight loss, protein intake must be higher to preserve muscle tissue (81-83). A protein intake of at least 1.2 grams per kg body weight (0.55 g of protein per lb body weight) is

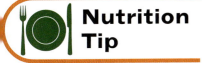

Nutrition Tip: An RD or RDN trained in sports nutrition can help athletes and active people identify a realistic weight goal and create a plan to meet this goal without the use of extreme diets and unsafe weight-loss practices (84, 85).

recommended to maintain muscle during dieting, although more protein, 1.8 to 2.7 grams of protein per kg body weight per day, might be preferable for attenuating the loss of muscle (55). As an example, in one study researchers gave adult volunteers the RDA for protein, 1.6 grams per kg body weight (twice the RDA), or 2.4 grams per kg body weight for 31 days. During the first 10 days, participants were placed on a weight-maintenance diet followed by 21 days of a 40 percent reduction in total calorie intake. Although all three groups lost the same amount of weight, the loss of fat-free mass (which includes muscle) was lower and the loss of fat mass was higher in both those receiving twice the RDA and those receiving three times the RDA for protein. Consuming three times the RDA for protein did not offer an additional advantage over consuming twice the RDA for protein. This study shows that consuming twice the RDA for protein helps not only promote the loss of body fat but also protect lean mass (79). Protein needs depend on many factors, including the amount of the caloric deficit, type of proteins consumed, and training program (type, duration, intensity, and frequency).

Besides meeting recommended guidelines for total daily protein intake, per-meal protein dose matters. The exact amount of protein needed at each meal to stimulate maximal muscle building likely depends on several variables, including the type of protein consumed, total daily energy intake, body weight, and training program. At mealtime, a minimum of 25 to 30 grams of protein containing 2 to 3 grams of leucine for younger adults and at least 3 grams of leucine for older adults is recommended to stimulate maximal muscle protein synthesis (86). Those who are dieting may want to consider consuming a minimum of 20 to 30 grams of a high-quality protein to help them feel satiated longer and ultimately to facilitate weight loss.

PUTTING IT INTO PERSPECTIVE

HOW CAN I FEEL FULL DURING ENERGY BALANCE?

Satiation and satiety help limit overall food intake. **Satiation** is the satisfaction of appetite during a meal, which helps us determine when to stop eating. Satiety is the feeling of fullness after a meal, which affects when we decide to eat again. Satiety decreases over time after eating (87). Several factors influence satiation, including sensory feedback, expectations of feeling full, gastric distension caused by the volume of food consumed, and hormonal feedback to the brain; all these factors help regulate the amount, duration, and frequency of food consumption (88-90). Foods that are higher in volume, such as whole fruits and vegetables, broth-based soups, and whipped shakes can increase satiation.

Protein increases satiety in a dose-dependent manner (the more protein consumed at one time, the fuller we feel, although it is not clear what the upper limit is, beyond which feelings of fullness are not increased). Per-meal doses of at least 30 grams are recommended (91). Habitual consumption of a protein-rich diet, however, might decrease the effect of protein on satiety over time (92). A high-protein breakfast, particularly, appears to be important for improving satiety during the day. Choosing solid as opposed to liquid sources of calories can also enhance satiety (93, 94). Fiber improves satiety, the degree to which depends on the type of fiber consumed. Beta-glucan (from oats and barley), lupin kernel fiber, whole-grain rye, rye bran, and a mixed diet of fiber-containing foods (grains, legumes, vegetables, and fruits) might be best for enhancing satiety (95).

Increases in satiety do not necessarily correspond to a decrease in food intake over the course of a day, because multiple factors affect a person's desire to eat, including the sight or smell of food, habit, and emotional state (we eat when we are bored or stressed, for instance).

In addition to protein, an adequate amount of carbohydrate is important if a training program includes high-intensity exercise. Carbohydrate is the primary source of fuel used during high-intensity exercise because the body can readily access and use it for energy. Fat is a slow source of energy, which means that the body cannot access and use fat quickly enough to sustain high-intensity training (96). If the body lacks an adequate supply of carbohydrate for use as energy, exercise intensity will decrease.

> **? DO YOU KNOW?**
>
> Behavior therapy and support improves weight-loss results and enhances weight maintenance after weight loss. For optimal results, a wise choice is to hire a trained professional with the education and credentials to work in this area. For behavioral strategies that can help facilitate weight loss, see figure 13.5.

Popular Diets and Approaches to Energy Balance

A variety of dietary approaches can lead to weight loss. These methods might include counting calories, cutting down on one macronutrient (as in a low-fat diet or a low-carbohydrate diet), watching portion sizes, taking a nondiet approach, excluding certain foods or food groups, and intermittent fasting or eating only within a certain window of time (e.g., daytime hours between 8 and 5).

Both low-fat and low-carbohydrate diets can lead to weight loss. A meta-analysis of 48 randomized controlled clinical trials examining the effectiveness of popular weight-loss diets—including Atkins, Zone, South Beach (low carbohydrate), LEARN, Jenny Craig, Nutrisystem, Weight Watchers (moderate approaches), Ornish, and Rosemary Conley—for overweight and obese adults (BMI >25) found that most lower-calorie diets result in weight loss as long as participants

---

- Set clear behavioral goals with detailed intervention plans (97).
- Set reasonable goals to achieve long-term success. When possible, tie other outcomes to the goal. For instance, a person may choose to lose 10 pounds (4.5 kg) in an effort to improve their blood lipids. Or an athlete may choose to lose 5 pounds (2.3 kg) in an effort to get faster.
- Do not place blame on the person trying to lose weight if they have not reached their goal because this disapproval is demoralizing. Given the challenges to losing weight and maintaining weight loss, attributing a failure to achieve a certain goal to lack of adherence can stigmatize the person as one who lacks willpower, motivation, or fortitude to lose weight (62).
- Incorporate accountability measures. For the student-athlete, regular check-ins with their sports dietitian on staff may be appropriate.
- Use stimulus control strategies. Stimulus control strategies can help alter the environment for success. For instance, more healthy foods may be placed in the front of the refrigerator or at eye level in cabinets. Exercise clothes can be packed ahead of time for early morning workouts.
- Strategize when eating out:
  - Do not skip meals before eating out.
  - Look at the restaurant menu ahead of time. Limit items that are fried, buttered, creamed, or served with sauce or gravy.
  - When in doubt, ask questions about how the food is prepared.
  - Split higher-calorie items with someone or put them in a to-go box for the next day.
- Limit alcohol intake.
- Seek a specialist for emotional eating.
- Alter the environment by limiting TV and video game time.
- Encourage stress management, which may include breathing exercises, meditation, and more (98).
- If obese, consider seeking the expertise of a registered dietitian and psychological support from a licensed psychologist during weight loss and afterward (99).

Figure 13.5 Behavioral strategies that can help facilitate weight loss.

REFLECTION TIME

DOES CARBOHYDRATE MAKE YOU GAIN WEIGHT?

Carbohydrate does not cause weight gain. In fact, the proportion of carbohydrate or fat in the diet does not affect weight gain or weight loss. Instead, total calorie intake predicts changes in body weight. This axiom is sometimes referred to as "calories in, calories out," or CICO (100).

stay on the diet (78). Research reviews examining popular diets have come to the same conclusion: Most are equally effective for losing weight (although not necessarily keeping the weight off), and evidence is insufficient to recommend one particular dietary approach for all people (101-103).

Research supports the use of a ketogenic diet as an option for losing weight in a wide variety of populations including those who are performing resistance training, (104). In fact, compared with other diets including low-fat diets, a ketogenic diet may be better for glycemic control over a period of 3 to 12 months in those with overweight or obesity and with or without type 2 diabetes (105). But the benefits of carbohydrate restriction on blood sugar control are greatest in the first 3 to 6 months and become less effective over time (106). Also, a ketogenic diet may be difficult to sustain over a longer period. Under isocaloric conditions (both diets contain the same number of calories), however, ketogenic diets are not superior to nonketogenic diet for weight loss or body fat loss in athletic populations or those with obesity. In fact, a well-controlled study conducted in a metabolic ward with overweight and obese men reported that an isocaloric (same amount of calories) ketogenic diet led to small increases in calories expended compared with a low-fat diet but this effect decreased over time and body fat loss slowed on the ketogenic diet (107). A ketogenic diet, however, can lead to a small decrease in appetite and reduced desire to eat when people are left to eat on their own free will (ad libitum eating versus a controlled metabolic ward study) (108). Ketogenic diets may decrease fat-free mass (which includes muscle) even in those who are engaging in resistance training (104).

Many traditional diets such as the Paleo diet and Whole 30 exclude a number of foods, so they represent rigid dietary approaches. Rigid dieting is associated with an on-or-off mentality to dieting, meaning that a person is either on their diet or, if they deviate from it at all, off their diet. Rigid dieting allows little flexibility or variation in food choices. Because adherence to a dietary plan is critical for success, a rigid approach may be more difficult to sustain over a longer period. In fact, rigid dieting is associated with increased overeating, bingeing, and diet setbacks (110).

PUTTING IT INTO PERSPECTIVE

HOW DO I KNOW WHAT DIETARY APPROACH IS BEST FOR ME?

No one diet works for everyone. Research shows that the ability to adhere to a diet is the most important factor in predicting successful weight loss and lack of adherence (not sticking to the plan) is one of the biggest barriers to long-term success (78, 109). People should choose a diet or plan they can adhere to, one that presents the fewest number of challenges and allows them to maintain their health and level of exercise. Instead of following a rigid approach to losing weight, maintaining some flexibility to alter the approach as needed or to switch diets might improve adherence (78). For instance, a person can start by counting calories and then transition to heeding portion sizes and incorporating mindful eating strategies. Mindful eating helps people get in touch with their physiological hunger and satiety cues. In addition, mindful eating helps people examine when they are eating because of stress, boredom, habit, or other reasons not related to hunger. When a person identifies the reason they are eating (e.g., if they are really hungry or using food to cope with something else in life) in addition to their eating cues (i.e., time of day, sight of the vending machine, etc.), they can work on practicing better habits so that they do not turn to food when they are not truly hungry.

Flexible dieting is a more moderate approach to dieting, allowing a person to choose whatever foods they would like as long as it fits within their macronutrient needs or total calorie goals. Although this approach may seem to suggest that a person could eat dessert all day every day, fitting in several calorie-dense foods is difficult because this choice will quickly increase total calorie intake. Research shows that flexible dieting does not lead to the overeating typically associated with rigid dieting. Flexible dieting is positively associated with weight loss, reduced food cravings, and less binge eating (110). Flexible dieting is similar to an approach called "If It Fits Your Macros" (IIFYM). This approach gained traction among bodybuilders and physique athletes as a method to meet their macronutrient goals while allowing a greater variety of foods than permitted by a rigid meal plan. IIFYM means you can eat it as long as it fits into your macronutrient limits (111).

> **? DO YOU KNOW?**
> Dichotomous beliefs about food and eating, such as "good food" versus "bad food," may be linked to a rigid dietary restraint (a tendency to restrict or control food intake consciously), which can interfere with the ability to maintain a healthy weight (112).

Although some people may choose to use a popular diet or to log their food intake in an effort to lose weight, they must be careful to get adequate nutrition for growth, health, performance, and recovery. In particular, performance staff and coaches who are mindful of the signs and symptoms of RED-S (relative energy deficiency in sport) can do a better job screening and treating athletes at risk for or with low EA (energy availability). In addition, athletes who are aware of low EA and RED-S may be better able to voice their concerns about trying to alter their physique in a healthy manner while still being able to perform. RED-S was introduced in chapter 2 and is expanded upon in chapter 14.

Does the Type of Food You Eat Matter?

When people are cutting calories, they have fewer opportunities to get the vitamins, minerals, fiber, and protein necessary for optimal health.

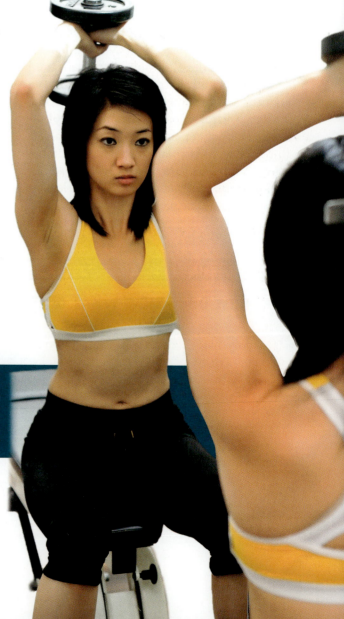

> If you are trying to gain muscle while losing weight at the same time, keep in mind the diet and training information provided in this chapter to help you achieve your goals.

Therefore, they must make their calories count by focusing on nutrient-rich foods. They might also want to choose foods with no (or little) processing as well. The research is limited, but emerging evidence suggests that the body expends more energy digesting foods that are less processed or absorbs fewer calories from the food during digestion, as compared with highly processed foods.

Studies examining intake of whole almonds, pistachios, walnuts, and peanuts suggest incomplete energy absorption from fat. Study subjects absorbed 5 to 21 percent fewer calories than the nuts contained (percentages differed based on the nut). Fewer calories were absorbed from the nuts because of incomplete breakdown of the cell walls within the food (113-115). In addition, some research shows that less dietary fat (and so less calories) is absorbed from peanuts as compared with peanut oil, peanut butter, and peanut flour (116).

In a crossover study in healthy women, study subjects were provided either a sandwich with cheddar cheese on multigrain bread or processed cheese on white bread. Meals contained the same amount of protein, carbohydrate, fat, and calories. Calorie expenditure was significantly greater after consuming the whole food as compared with the processed meal (137 ± 14.1 kcal versus 73.1 ± 10.2 kcal), suggesting that more energy is expended during the digestion of less-processed foods as compared with highly processed foods (117).

Training for Losing Body Fat

Training programs can be tailored to increase calories burned and therefore help with weight loss. Two components make up the total amount of energy burned as a result of exercise:

1. Energy burned during exercise
2. **Excess postexercise oxygen consumption (EPOC)**—the energy burned after exercise

Resistance training is critical for upregulating muscle protein synthesis when dieting (68, 83, 121) to help ensure that muscle mass is maintained (or improved) during weight loss. In addition to burning calories during resistance training and in the period after training through excess postexercise oxygen consumption, the body requires energy (calories) to repair training-induced microscopic damage in muscle while laying down new proteins in muscle. Resistance-training programs designed for weight loss focus on recruiting a greater amount of muscle mass in each session to maximize the amount of calories burned during the session and afterward (excess postexercise oxygen consumption) (122). For example, a program might include more squats instead of calf raises or leg extensions. In addition to focusing on recruiting more muscle mass in each training session, performing supersets

? DO YOU KNOW?

Three main reasons explain why exercise alone (without dietary changes) does not seem to result in the amount of weight loss expected:

- Vigorous exercise can lead to an increase in food consumption. But this circumstance should not be viewed as a reason to avoid exercise or reduce exercise intensity (59). Just be mindful of overall calorie balance.
- People often overestimate how much energy they burn through exercise (59).
- Some, though not all, research studies show that overweight and obese people who increase activity through planned exercise spontaneously decrease NEAT (calories burned through daily movement that does not include exercise) (118-120).

PUTTING IT INTO PERSPECTIVE

WILL BUILDING MUSCLE TURN ME INTO A CALORIE-BURNING MACHINE?

Muscle tissue burns significantly more calories at rest than fat tissue does. Although this difference is statistically significant, it might not translate to a meaningful difference in calories burned over a short period. One pound (0.45 kg) of muscle burns 5.9 kcal per day at rest (RMR), whereas each pound of fat burns 2.0 kcal per day at rest (RMR). Therefore, if a person gains 5 pounds (2.3 kg) of muscle, they will burn approximately 20 more kcal each day (124).

(completing two sets of different exercises back to back before resting, such as a set of squats immediately followed by deadlifts before resting) increases total calories burned during and after exercise (123).

In addition to adding resistance training, incorporating aerobic exercise into a training program can enhance total energy burned during the day. Steady-state (constant intensity) aerobic work sessions can be intermixed with high-intensity interval training (HIIT) to increase total energy burned. Although several studies have suggested that HIIT, which involves repeated bouts of high-intensity exercise followed by low-intensity exercise, increases energy burned during exercise and excess postexercise energy consumption to a greater extent than steady-state exercise (125-128), a systematic review and meta-analysis, including 31 studies, found that HIIT does not lead to greater weight loss than steady-state exercise when matched for total calories burned. But HIIT does lead to greater calories burned in a shorter period, so a person can get more results for a shorter time commitment (159). Note that HIIT can be difficult for people who are very overweight or who have chronic health conditions or injuries.

> **DO YOU KNOW?**
>
> Studies show that changing your diet will lead to greater weight loss than changing your exercise program (129-131). But dieting alone (without exercising) leads to greater decreases in muscle mass compared with combining diet with exercise, particularly with anaerobic exercise (e.g., resistance training) (59). Also, as mentioned previously dieting alone may lead to an increase the likelihood of an unintentional drop in NEAT (73, 74).

A sound training program is an essential component for altering body composition in favor of less fat and more muscle, but overall daily activity is important as well. Research shows that many people compensate for increases in physical activity by being less active the rest of the day. They decrease their activities of daily living, so they burn fewer calories during the rest of the day when they are not working out (53). Activities of daily living include walking to class, cleaning, mowing the lawn, gardening, and washing the car (52, 132).

Training can increase the total amount of calories burned in various ways, but the best exercise for weight loss is the one that a person will stick with over time, both during the weight-loss period and afterward for weight maintenance.

Several strategies can be used to help people decrease calorie intake and thereby lose weight. Research-based nutrition and exercise strategies are shown in figure 13.6.

Sport-Specific Weight and Body Fat Goals

Both obesity and extremely low body fat, defined as below essential body fat levels—less than 5 percent for men and 12 percent for women—come with health consequences (133).

Three categories of sports are most commonly associated with lower body fat (48, 85):

1. Sports in which carrying a lower body weight is advantageous, such as endurance racing, ski jumping, and equestrian events
2. Weight-class sports such as wrestling and judo
3. Aesthetic sports such as gymnastics and figure skating

PUTTING IT INTO PERSPECTIVE

FORGET THE FAT-BURNING ZONE AND RAMP UP THE INTENSITY

As discussed in previous chapters, when you exercise at a lower intensity you burn a greater percentage of calories from fat than when you exercise at a higher intensity. But you also burn fewer total calories per training session compared with training at a higher intensity. If weight loss is the goal, focus on total calories burned in a day rather than worry about burning a greater percentage of fat, as opposed to carbohydrate, during exercise. If you burn more calories during exercise to help create a caloric deficit, your body will tap into fat stores for energy at other times of the day—when you are studying or watching TV, for instance.

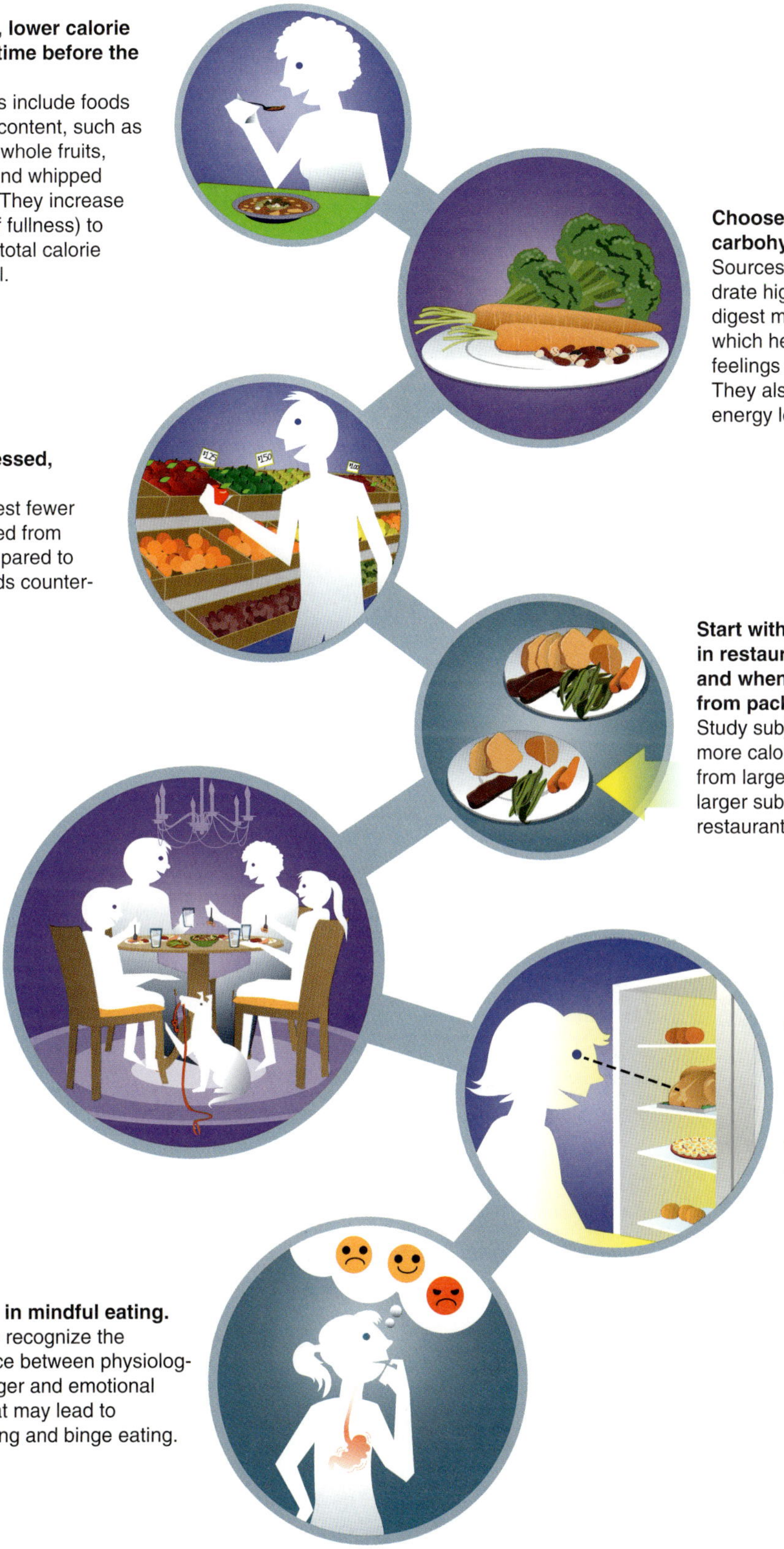

Eat higher volume, lower calorie foods first at mealtime before the rest of your meal.
Higher volume foods include foods with a higher water content, such as broth-based soups, whole fruits, whole vegetables, and whipped low-calorie shakes. They increase satiation (feelings of fullness) to help decrease your total calorie intake during a meal.

Choose high-fiber carbohydrates.
Sources of carbohydrate higher in fiber digest more slowly, which helps increase feelings of fullness. They also help sustain energy levels.

Choose less processed, whole foods.
Some studies suggest fewer calories are absorbed from whole foods as compared to their processed foods counterparts.

Start with smaller portions in restaurants, at home, and when consuming food from packages.
Study subjects consumed more calories when they ate from larger bags of chips, larger sub sandwiches, and restaurant entrées.

Eat at home.
Portion sizes at restaurants have increased and the environmental cues in restaurants encourage overeating. Restaurant meals are often high in calories.

Use environmental cues.
Put less healthy food out of sight, behind closed cabinets, and out of reach. Place healthier food at eye level in the refrigerator, freezer, and inside cabinets.

Engage in mindful eating.
Learn to recognize the difference between physiological hunger and emotional cues that may lead to overeating and binge eating.

Figure 13.6 Effective strategies for consuming fewer calories.

All athletes who must meet weight-class goals should be monitored for use of extreme weight-loss practices that are harmful to health and increase injury risk (134). Athletes who are still growing should also be closely monitored, because severe energy restriction can interfere with growth and development (48).

A wide range of body fat values has been reported in elite athletes, making it difficult to determine ideal ranges for each sport. See table 13.2 for general ranges. Note that body fat measurement techniques, instruments, and equations used vary widely among athletes. In addition, within some sports, quality data on body fat levels are lacking. Furthermore, even less data are available on the relationship between body fat and performance in a variety of sports.

GAINING MUSCLE MASS

Increasing and maintaining muscle mass can help prevent injuries, slow sarcopenia (the age-related decline in muscle mass), and possibly improve athletic performance. Some people also choose to gain muscle mass for aesthetic reasons. Several factors influence the ability to increase muscle size (hypertrophy) and strength, including genetics, current training, previous history of training, and nutrition. The most important modifiable factor necessary for muscle hypertrophy is a well-designed, periodized resistance-training program. A sound diet can improve results obtained from a training program. For muscle hypertrophy, consuming enough total calories and protein is important. Sufficient calories are necessary to provide both the energy to train and the energy necessary for the synthesis of new proteins in muscle.

Energy Needs

Energy needs for weight gain can be estimated by calculating RMR and calories expended through activity and then adding calories on top of this number. The majority of extra calories should come from protein and carbohydrate. At least 44 to 50 kcal per kg body weight is suggested for weight gain (136).

Table 13.2 Body Fat Percentage in Athletes

Sport	Males	Females	Sport	Males	Females
American football (backs) and *nonlineman	9%–12% *14.8% ± 4.1%	No data	Racquetball	8%–13%	15%–22%
American football (linemen)	15%–19%	No data	Rowing	6%–14%	12%–18%
Baseball	12%–15%	12%–15%	Shot-putting	16%–20%	20%–28%
Basketball	6%–12% *12.2% ± 2.0%	20%–27% *23.6% ± 7.5%	Sprinting	8%–10%	12%–20%
Bodybuilding	5%–8%	10%–15%	Softball	No data	*25.1% ± 4.7%
Cycling	5%–15%	15%–20%	Soccer	10%–18% *13.7% ± 2.6%	13%–18% *24.5% ± 3.7%
Cross-country skiing	7%–12%	16%–22%	Swimming	9%–12%	14%–24%
Golf	19.2% ± 3.9%	*30.2% ± 5.3%	Tennis	12%–16%	16%–24%
Gymnastics	5%–12%	10%–16%	Triathlon	5%–12%	10%–15%
High jumping and long jumping	7%–12%	10%–18%	Volleyball	11%–14%	16%–25% *24.8% ± 3.5%
Ice and field hockey	8%–15% *15.2% ± 2.6%	12%–18% *25.0% ± 3.8%	Weightlifting	9%–16%	No data
Marathon running	5%–11%	10%–15%	Wrestling	5%–16% *15.7% ± 4.7%	No data

Values reprinted by permission from A. Jeukendrup and M. Gleeson, *Sport Nutrition*, 2nd ed. (Champaign, IL: Human Kinetics, 2010), 316. Values with an * are from a sample of 337 male and female Division I athletes using DEXA (125).

In well-designed overfeeding studies, participants are given meals to help determine the effect of varying calorie and energy-yielding macronutrient intake on weight, fat, and muscle mass. In these studies, consuming more of the extra calories from protein led to a greater increase in lean body mass. A 10- to 12-week overfeeding study in normal and overweight participants provided 39.4 percent more calories each day than needed for weight maintenance and either 6, 15, or 26 percent of the extra calories as protein. All groups increased body fat, although overfeeding protein led to greater lean body mass gains and an increase in energy expenditure (137). In another study, participants were overfed for 8 weeks and given a diet containing 5, 15, or 25 percent protein. Those given 15 or 25 percent protein stored 45 percent of the extra calories consumed as muscle mass, while those on the low-protein diet stored 95 percent of extra calories as fat (138). Although protein is important for weight gain, individual differences occur in weight gained (fat mass and muscle mass) when calorie intake is increased. People with more fat-free mass may gain less weight when overfed compared with those with less fat-free mass. In addition, the number of calories burned each day increases when overfed, as discussed earlier in the chapter. Thus, weight gain cannot be accurately predicted based on the number of extra calories consumed (139). In other words, adding an extra 3,500 kcal per week will not lead to exactly 1 pound (0.45 kg) of weight gained.

A study in lean and obese men overfed (50% more than calorie needs to maintain weight) carbohydrate or fat found that overfeeding carbohydrate led to an increase in total calories burned and the storage of 75 to 85 percent of excess calories as fat, whereas overfeeding fat had minimal effect on total calories burned and led to the storage of 90 to 95 percent of excess calories as fat (140).

Protein Needs

As noted in chapter 12, it is not entirely clear exactly how much protein is optimal for building muscle; the total amount of protein that should be consumed depends on a person's health status, total calorie intake, and training program. The type of protein consumed might also influence optimal protein intake for hypertrophy; vegetarian proteins may need to be consumed in higher amounts or combined within a 3-hour period to get all essential amino acids in each serving (141). To maximize muscle hypertrophy, a total daily protein intake of approximately 1.2 to 2.0 grams per kg body weight is recommended (142, 143).

Carbohydrate Needs

Carbohydrate is the body's primary source of energy for resistance training; when carbohydrate availability is low, training intensity will drop. Carbohydrate also helps decrease muscle breakdown after a workout and, like the other energy-yielding macronutrients (protein and fat), carbohydrate contributes to total daily caloric needs.

Although fat is the primary source of fuel during moderate-intensity activity (30%-65% of $\dot{V}O_2max$), as intensity increases, carbohydrate use also increases and muscle glycogen becomes an important source of energy (144, 145) (recall the crossover concept, shown in figure 11.1 on page 283). The maximum rate of ATP production from fat is 0.4 mmol/minute, whereas the maximum rate of ATP resynthesis from stored muscle glycogen is 1.0 to 2.3 mmol/minute (146). Thus, ATP is not produced fast enough from stored fat to meet the demand for energy during high-intensity activity (147). Resistance training with low glycogen leads to a decrease in the rate of ATP production (because the body must rely on a slower production of ATP), fatigue, and a decrease in power output (148-150). Studies examining

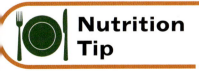

Nutrition Tip When consuming more calories each day, your metabolism will increase, so over time your weight gain might start to plateau and an even greater increase in calories will be needed to continue gaining weight.

various weightlifting protocols reiterate the importance of muscle glycogen; participants used 24 to 45 percent of their glycogen stores after a few sets (151).

Sports Supplements

Protein and creatine are the two most effective supplements for increasing muscle mass. Supplementation with a high-quality protein that provides at least 2 grams of leucine per serving for younger adults and at least 3 grams of leucine per serving for older adults provides a convenient and effective way to consume protein. Although protein supplements can help people meet their essential amino acid needs, whole foods rich in protein also contain nonprotein nutritive components that support muscle protein synthesis. In addition to benefiting skeletal muscle, whole foods contain vitamins, minerals, and other compounds that support overall health (152).

Supplementing with creatine monohydrate may increase body weight, strength, and muscle mass in healthy younger adults and older adults (153-155), although individual responses will vary with creatine supplementation. Some people are considered nonresponders, meaning that they do not see any changes in strength or muscle mass.

> **? DO YOU KNOW?**
>
> Keep in mind that altering fat or muscle mass will not necessarily result in improvements in athletic performance or body image. Simply gaining muscle mass does not automatically translate to improvement on a field or court, in a pool, or on a track. Also, shedding body fat or gaining muscle will not necessarily improve a person's body image. Moreover, some people may be striving for what is unachievable and will never be satisfied with how they look.

LOSING FAT AND GAINING MUSCLE AT THE SAME TIME

In addition to the risk of losing muscle while losing weight, gaining muscle when cutting calories is difficult because lower-calorie diets decrease the intracellular signaling necessary for the synthesis of new proteins in muscle, and muscle tissue might be less sensitive to protein when a person is dieting (80).

Despite these challenges, people can lose body fat and preserve, or even gain, muscle at the same time by combining a higher-protein diet with an intense resistance-training program (156-158). For example, 31 overweight or obese postmenopausal women were put on a reduced-calorie diet of 1,400 kcal per day (with 15%, 65%, and 30% kcal from protein, carbohydrate, and fat, respectively) and randomized to receive either 25 grams of carbohydrate (maltodextrin) or a whey protein supplement twice a day for the 6-month study period. The group receiving the additional protein lost 3.9 percent more weight than the carbohydrate group and preserved more muscle mass (158).

In another intervention study, young, overweight, recreationally active men (before the study they exercised once or twice a week) were placed on an intense 4-week diet and exercise program. Their diet contained 40 percent fewer calories each day than necessary for weight maintenance (providing 15 kcal per pound [0.45 kg] of lean body mass). Half of the men were randomly selected to receive a higher-protein diet (2.4 g of protein per kg body weight [1.09 g of protein per lb body weight]; 35% protein, 50% carbohydrate, and 15% fat). The rest of the men were placed on a lower-protein diet (1.2 g of protein per kg body weight [0.55 g of protein per lb body weight]; 15% protein, 50% carbohydrate, and 35% fat). Although this diet was lower in protein, it provided 50 percent more protein than the RDA for protein (0.8 g/kg body weight per day). Both groups were given enough carbohydrate to sustain a higher-intensity training program. All meals were prepared and provided to participants during the study, which helped control for calories and energy-yielding macronutrients consumed. In addition to their meals, participants were given dairy shakes during the day and immediately postexercise (the lower-protein group was given lower-protein shakes with carbohydrate in them; the higher-protein group received shakes with more protein). Supervised workouts consisted of full-body resistance circuit training three times per week, high-intensity interval training twice per week, and a time trial. In addition to their structured exercise program, all participants were instructed to accumulate at least 10,000 steps per day, as monitored by a pedometer worn on their hip.

Both the lower-protein and higher-protein groups lost weight, and no significant difference between groups was found. Men in the higher-protein group gained 2.6 pounds (1.2 kg) of muscle and lost 10.6 pounds (4.8 kg) of body fat, whereas men in the control group gained very little muscle (0.22 lb [0.1 kg]) and lost 7.7 pounds (93.5 kg) of fat. Both groups improved all but one measure of strength in addition to aerobic and anaerobic capacity. No differences were found between groups in strength, power, aerobic fitness, or performance at the end of the study. In this study, a higher-protein, reduced-calorie diet combined with a high-intensity circuit-training program including interval training and sprints helped participants build muscle. In addition to their total protein intake, participants in the higher-protein group also consumed more protein per meal (approximately 49 g per meal) than those in the lower-protein group (approximately 22 g per meal) (156).

Dieters who want to gain muscle while losing fat may want to consider consuming more than 2 grams of protein per kg body weight (157). Protein intake should be spaced out evenly throughout the day (regular meals containing at least 25–30 g of protein).

SUMMARY

Overweight and obesity result in many health consequences that can be reversed with weight loss. For athletes, decreasing body fat may also be driven by weight requirements of their sport or position, aesthetic demands, performance goals, reduction of injury risk, and joint pain. Losing body weight, especially when done quickly and without adequate dietary protein, can lead to a substantial decrease in muscle mass. To prevent loss of muscle mass when cutting calories, a person must consume more total protein and engage in resistance training. Rapid weight loss, however, can also lead to a more substantial drop in metabolism, so this approach is not recommended unless needed for rapid reversal of obesity-related health consequences. Weight loss is often less than predicted from nutrition and exercise interventions because many people tend to decrease their daily activity after they increase their exercise, adherence to diets drops over time, and metabolism drops with weight loss.

Gaining muscle can improve quality of life in older adults by helping them perform typical daily tasks, such as lifting their groceries or opening a can of food. For athletes, gaining muscle can decrease risk of injuries and improve strength and power. Greater intake of both calories and protein, as well as an effective resistance-training program, is necessary for muscle hypertrophy. People can gain muscle and lose fat at the same time. Doing this requires consuming fewer calories and more protein per day and engaging in a well-designed training program. Like a weight-loss program, a hypertrophy program or a program designed for fat loss and hypertrophy at the same time will result in outcomes that vary among individuals.

FOR REVIEW

1. Why do protein needs increase on a reduced-calorie diet?
2. Describe the health implications that can result from body fat below essential fat levels.
3. Describe the health implications resulting from and associated with excess body fat.
4. Why is carbohydrate essential for high-intensity training?
5. What is low energy availability, and how does it affect health?
6. Why don't people lose weight in a linear fashion? Why don't they lose as much as they predict they would have?
7. What makes popular diets effective?
8. List suggestions for helping people overcome weight-loss plateaus.

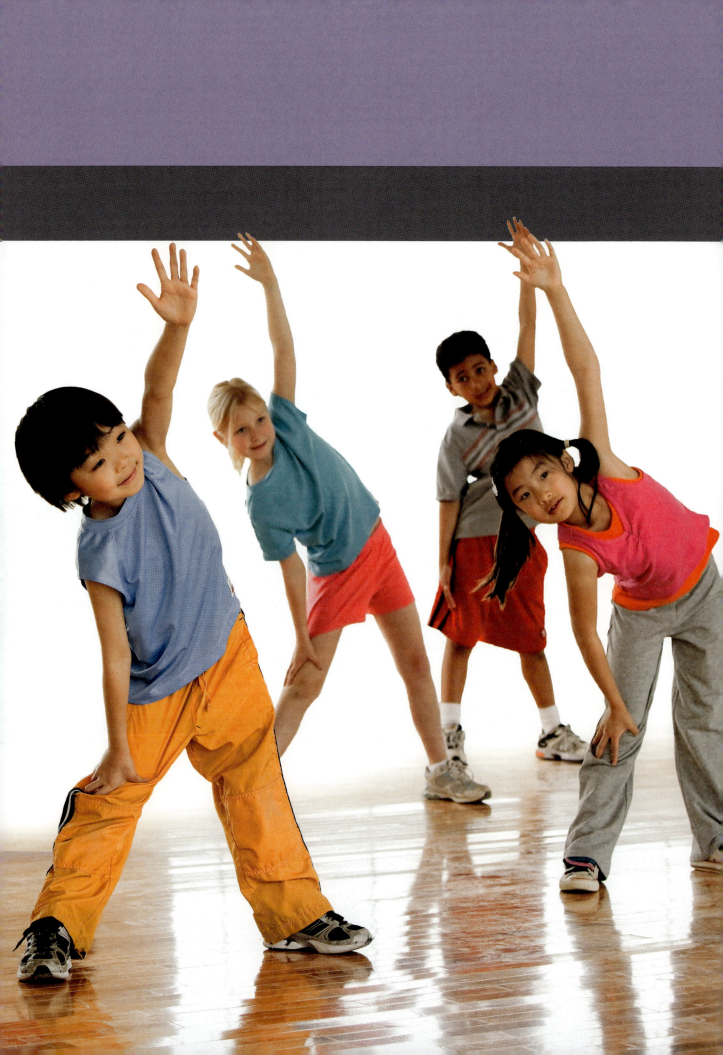

Nutrition Concerns for Special Populations

> **CHAPTER OBJECTIVES**
>
> After completing this chapter, you will be able to do the following:
>
> - Discuss the most important nutrition concerns for active children and adolescents.
> - Discuss the special nutrition needs of masters-level athletes and active older adults.
> - Describe special nutrition concerns for athletes with diabetes.
> - Identify special considerations for athletes who are pregnant.
> - Describe special nutrition concerns for vegetarian athletes.
> - Discuss nutrition challenges associated with disordered eating and eating disorders in physical activity and sport.

Many athletes and other active people face distinct dietary challenges that differ from those of most sedentary people. These differences often have implications for health and exercise performance and might require an individualized approach to meeting nutritional needs. Concerns about the needs of distinct groups, or special populations, differ across the life stages. Nutrition needs of the child athlete, for example, are quite different from those of the masters athlete. When trying to ensure a proper diet that meets all nutritional needs, the considerations of some people, such as vegetarians, people with diabetes, or those with eating disorders, might be far different from those we have discussed in earlier chapters. In this chapter we focus on nutrition for physically active youth, including young athletes; athletes who compete at a masters level; physically active seniors; physically active people and athletes who are pregnant, have diabetes, or are vegetarian; and physically active people and athletes who have eating disorders.

CHILDREN AND ADOLESCENTS

More opportunities than ever before exist for children and adolescents to participate in sport, and children are participating in competitive sporting activities at younger ages. Over 38 million children in the United States participate in team sports, most of them during high school (1). Other trends include increased female participation in sport, increased participation in **extreme sports**, earlier specialization, and year-round training. Some children and adolescents participate in long, intense training several times a week, often without sufficient recovery because of their busy schedules. Such situations call for nutrition plans that meet all needs for growth and development, promote health, enhance athletic performance, and aid in injury prevention. But during periods of rapid growth with accompanying high-energy needs, many children and adolescents, including athletes, fall well short of meeting the standard guidelines for nutrition. Commonly consumed meal patterns are often low in fruits, vegetables, calcium-rich foods, and micronutrients. Excessive saturated fat, sodium, and sugar are often consumed. Unsafe weight-loss practices, low energy availability, disordered eating, and clinically defined eating disorders are of extreme concern in the young, because these issues can have significantly negative effects on overall health, growth, and development (2).

Children and Prepubescent Adolescents Are Not Small Adults

Both benefits and drawbacks are associated with youth participation in sport. Although some of these positives and negatives can also be observed in adults, others are unique to this life stage and can be more significant, having lasting effects into adulthood. Exercise associated with youth sport improves physical fitness, reduces body fat, and decreases risk of chronic disease. Youth participation in sport also enhances bone health, decreases the likelihood of depression and anxiety, improves self-esteem, improves academic achievement, and provides overall improvements in emotional well-being. Risks for both acute physical injury and overuse injury are heightened in the young. Children tend to injure themselves at different anatomic structures than adults. Their bones are weaker than their tendons and ligaments, putting them at risk for fractures throughout the bone and growth plate (3). Some adolescent athletes have decreased flexibility, coordination, and balance, which can increase injury risk while also affecting sport performance and self-esteem, and increasing stress and anxiety. Quick return to sport without appropriate rehabilitation can result in chronic pain, repeated injury, and impaired functioning (4, 5).

In addition to having an immature skeleton, children and adolescents have distinct physiological differences that affect energy expenditure, fuel (substrate) utilization, and thermoregulation during exercise (6, 7). Along with increased demands for energy and many nutrients—as a result of rapid anatomical, physiological, and metabolic changes—children have an immature anaerobic metabolic system before the onset of puberty, which might affect their ability to perform well in high-intensity exercise. Children rely more on fat oxidation and are thus less likely to achieve high rates of ATP generation via the anaerobic pathway (8). They also rely more on carbohydrate consumed during exercise to help them sustain high-intensity exercise.

Nutrition Concerns for Special Populations 345

Children should be cautiously introduced to strenuous activity. Along with limited muscle **glycolytic** activity, children have lower muscle strength related to reduced anaerobic capacity and experience minimal muscle fiber growth in response to exercise. Given the obvious need to avoid child exploitation, data on young athletes are scarce and the available data are fraught with small sample sizes and study designs that indirectly address research questions. An example of this issue is applying research findings from studies conducted in adults to children.

Children should not be thought of as miniadults, and neither should they be grouped collectively when considering their physical development. Many factors, including genetics and environment, affect the individual onset of maturation and must be considered during nutrition planning. Both physiological and psychological differences affect youth's dietary patterns, as well as their perception and receptivity to nutrition information. Many young athletes are most interested in performance and give little thought to the effect of lifestyle choices on long-term health. Consciously or otherwise, they depend on the adults in their lives for guidance. Like their nonathletic peers, young athletes are impressionable and are often up to date with popular trends. Strategic use of infographics and media links designed by credentialed nutrition, health or exercise professionals can be powerful educational tools.

Estimates are that approximately 50 percent of adolescent athletes use dietary supplements (9). Other adolescents may be curious about whether dietary supplements will help their performance

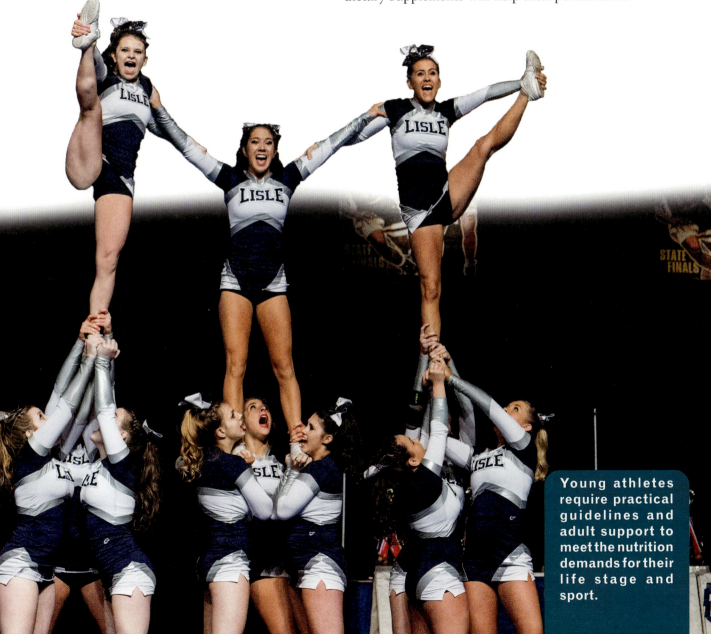

Young athletes require practical guidelines and adult support to meet the nutrition demands for their life stage and sport.

and give them an edge over their competition, particularly if they have witnessed a teammate's or other athlete's success after taking a supplement. Adolescent education on this topic is lacking (9). A first step in addressing this knowledge gap and offering guidance would be talking with physically active adolescents about the benefits and risks of various ergogenic aids, as well as discussing the benefits of food (e.g., carbohydrate, protein, and fat) and what it means to live a healthy lifestyle. Educational programs for active adolescents, especially for those involved in team sports, should include the athlete's friends, athletes, and coaches because they are key influencers for adolescents' use of dietary supplements (9). In addition, discouraging the use of unproven or dangerous dietary supplements can help balance a young athlete's win-at-all-costs mentality (8, 9). Steering young athletes early in the direction of optimal nutrition and harnessing the benefits of whole foods will not deter all of them from experimenting with dangerous and illegal supplements, but it will make a difference and yield long-term benefits for many.

Growth and Development in Childhood

Childhood growth can be erratic, and it is slow compared with adolescent growth. These variable growth patterns result in considerable fluctuations in dietary energy needs. During periods of rapid growth, children might experience unexpected periods of lethargy, poor coordination, and movement inefficiency. Training load itself may be a concern with youth, and little information is available on the effect of intense exercise on growth in children. In many cases, after training load decreases or calorie intake matches calorie output, catch-up growth can occur. An imbalance in energy intake and expenditure (not enough calories to meet the demands of growth and training) can have long-term effects on both performance and health. Chronic low energy availability can lead to short stature, delayed puberty, menstrual irregularities, poor bone health, and increased risk of injury (10). Along with monitoring energy intake and training volume, professionals working with prepubescent athletes should monitor growth by body mass trends and anthropometric variables and not rely solely on growth charts.

Growth charts are used to assess height and weight for age in children. The following guidelines are used to determine weight category for age.

> Underweight: lower than 5th percentile
> Normal weight: 5th to less than 85th percentile
> Overweight: 85th to less than 95th percentile
> Obese: greater than or equal to 95th percentile

Growth and Development in Adolescence

The period of adolescence is a nutritionally vulnerable time of life influenced by peer pressure,

---

PUTTING IT INTO PERSPECTIVE

ENERGY AVAILABILITY

Energy availability equals dietary intake minus exercise energy expenditure (normalized to fat-free mass [FFM]). Energy availability is the amount of energy available to the body to perform all other functions after the energy cost of exercise is subtracted.

Example:

Female is 62 kg (136.4 lb)

2,600 kcal − 600 kcal = 2,000 kcal

2,000 kcal / 62 kg = 32.3 kcal/kg

Having an energy availability below 30 kcal/kg is associated with impairments of a variety of body functions. Energy availability of 45 kcal/kg FFM per day was found to be associated with energy balance and optimal health (11), but more research is needed.

desire for increased autonomy, and significant physical, cognitive, emotional, and social changes. Growth patterns in adolescence are strongly related to genetics but can be influenced by many factors, including energy balance (energy intake and expenditure). Growth spurts tend to occur around 10 to 12 years of age for females and roughly 2 years later for males (figure 14.1). Key body composition changes begin to emerge during this period. Females begin to develop greater fat mass, whereas males begin to acquire more lean body mass and blood volume. Because these physiological changes support power and performance, males may seem more advanced than females on the playing field. As a cumulative result of adolescent growth spurts, adolescents accrue an estimated 15 percent of their final adult height and 45 percent of maximal skeletal mass during adolescence (12, 13). From a measurement standpoint, females add up to 10 inches (25 cm) and 53 pounds (24 kg) and males add 11 inches (27 cm) and 70 pounds (31 kg) during their adolescent years.

As shown in figure 14.2, the appearance of secondary sexual characteristics is a key indicator of pubertal age. For example, a 13-year-old boy who is actively going through puberty has aspects of energy metabolism and muscle physiology that are more advanced than a 15-year-old boy who has not started puberty. In this scenario, the 13-year-old likely has greater glycolytic potential in strength and power sports, is better suited for experiencing muscle metabolic adaptations to training, and has greater capacity to recover from heavy exercise because of the hormonal environment supported by puberty.

Energy Needs

Determining energy needs for children and adolescents is an inexact science in which many of the best estimates for calculating energy needs are extrapolated from adult data (2). Relying on data derived from adults is a flawed approach, however, because children are less metabolically efficient than adults. For instance, energy needs for children during walking and running activities in sport may be as much as 30 percent higher compared with adults (14). Methodology used to predict daily energy needs are further complicated when children compensate for bouts of strenuous physical activity by becoming more sedentary with other physical activities (i.e., less walking, more sitting). Because little guidance has been established for estimating energy needs

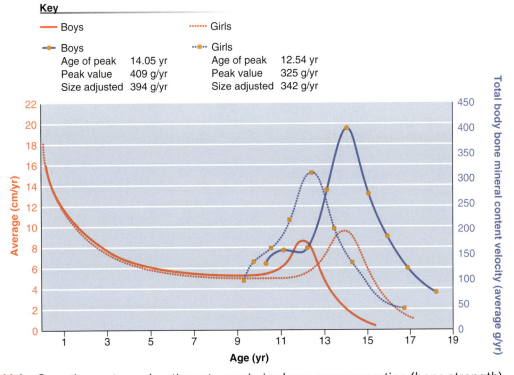

Figure 14.1 Growth spurts are key times to maximize bone mass accretion (bone strength).

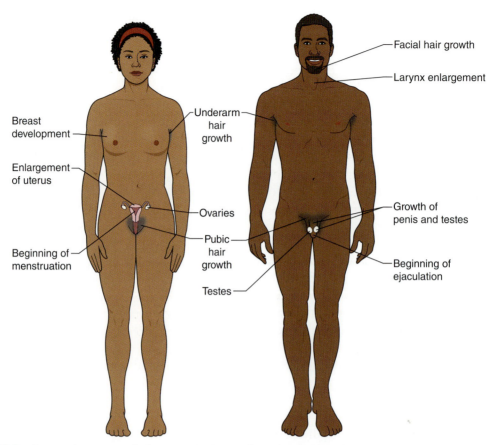

Figure 14.2 Secondary sexual characteristics in females and males.

for children and adolescents, a trial-and-error approach is often implemented.

It can be difficult for active adolescents to support optimal growth and development with adequate energy intake while also meeting the increased energy demands of their sport. Time constraints, travel, and sport-specific eating attitudes can make it challenging to meet energy needs. In addition, high rates of childhood obesity can make energy intake recommendations and strategies to meet them less than clear. Child and adolescent athletes desiring to bulk up could gain excess fat, resulting in reduced speed, endurance, agility, work efficiency, and acclimation to heat, while also potentially increasing their risk of developing obesity. In 2015 to 2016, approximately 18.5 percent of 2- to 19-year-olds were obese (15).

Child and adolescent athletes who are overweight or obese should be encouraged to exercise and follow strategies that promote healthy eating. In this age group, a focus on promoting weight loss is not always recommended. Unless comorbidities are present and weight loss is recommended and monitored by a primary care provider, most professionals agree that promoting weight maintenance and healthy lifestyle changes while waiting for height to increase will lead to a lower BMI and is considered a healthier strategy (16). Strategies to encourage healthy eating include the following (17):

› Choose smaller portions of foods and drinks.
› Place healthy foods and drinks within easy reach.
› Keep less healthy foods out of sight.
› Cut down on fast food.
› Cut down on distractions while eating (TV, phones, the computer, etc.).
› Don't tell children to clean their plate.
› Don't reward children's good behavior with food.

Nutrition Needs

In addition to meeting their energy needs for growth, development, and activity, children and teens need to meet their energy-yielding macronutrient (carbohydrate, protein, fat) needs for health and sport. Specific recommendations in other areas of the diet are also warranted to support performance, health, and overall diet quality. Many recommendations are unique to this age group and are described in the following sections.

Carbohydrate

Carbohydrate needs for optimal athletic performance and recovery are listed in table 14.1. In sporting activities lasting longer than 1 hour or at greater than 70 percent $\dot{V}O_2$max, children and adolescents may be limited by sparse carbohydrate stores and thus rely more on exogenous carbohydrate sources (those they consume before and during activity) and less on glycogen to fuel performance. Strength training in youth can enhance glycolytic activity, but maximal adaptation is not attained until sometime during adolescence when the limited glycolytic activity from childhood is resolved. A diet containing a minimum of 50 percent of energy needs as carbohydrate is a general recommendation for all youth, but carbohydrate utilization in adolescence is similar to that in adulthood and therefore adult recommendations can be used if the training load is high (8, 11). To help meet carbohydrate needs, young athletes can consume carbohydrates in sports foods (drinks, gels, bars) during training and competition (18).

To improve diet quality, child and adolescent athletes would benefit from expanding their palate by consuming a variety of carbohydrate-rich foods, including whole grains, dairy, vegetables, and fruits that provide a wide range of micronutrients, phytonutrients, and fiber.

> **DO YOU KNOW?**
>
> Sugar-sweetened beverages, such as soda, rank among the top five energy sources consumed by people over 2 years of age (19).

Protein

For child and adolescent athletes, protein needs are higher than for nonactive peers, but research suggests that additional needs (above sport amounts) are not required to support growth and development (2). The g/kg body weight recommendations available for adults are considered applicable in adolescence (see chapter 5). Concerns for inadequate protein intake arise with chronic energy restriction, and these concerns are exacerbated if chronic energy restriction is combined with intense physical training. This combination could alter protein metabolism and impair growth and maturation. Child and teen athletes can improve the quality of their diet by making better choices of protein foods to consume. Some children have been found to be more reluctant to add animal-based protein foods to their diet and prefer foods higher in carbohydrate and fat. In adolescence, the quality of protein consumed

Table 14.1 Carbohydrate Intake Guidelines for the Adolescent Athlete

RECOVERY GUIDELINES	
Immediate recovery (0–4 hr)	1–1.2 g · kg^{-1} · hr^{-1} up to 4 hours, then resume daily needs
Daily recovery (low intensity or skill based)	3–5 g · kg^{-1} · d^{-1}
EXERCISE PROGRAM GUIDELINES	
Moderate exercise (1 hr/d)	5–7 g · kg^{-1} · d^{-1}
Endurance (training 1–3 hr/d)	6–10 g · kg^{-1} · d^{-1}
Extreme exercise (training 4–5 hr/d)	8–12 g · kg^{-1} · d^{-1}
DURING SPORT GUIDELINES	
Short duration (0–75 min)	Not required or small amount
Medium or long duration (75 min–2.5 hr)	30–60 g/hr

Based on Desbrow et al. (2014).

could be improved by choosing leaner sources dense with nutrients.

Fat

In recommendations for fat consumption, the minimal absolute grams of fat have not changed much over the years in adults, and research in children and adolescents is limited. Although younger athletes rely more on aerobic metabolism, no evidence currently exists to support a performance benefit from higher fat intake. The most prudent advice for fat intake aligns with following the acceptable macronutrient distribution range (AMDR) of 20 to 35 percent of total energy consumed. For overweight or obese child and teen athletes, a mild reduction in dietary fat (within the AMDR range) is a prudent weight-management strategy. For children and teens, fat intake is strongly associated with increased consumption of cheese, poultry, and snack foods (like chips, cookies, and cakes) and might contribute to intakes above 10 percent of total calories from saturated fatty acids. Many children and teens do not realize that "crispy," "pan fried," and "creamed" are food descriptors associated with increased fat content. Furthermore, child and teen athletes may not know how to make healthy modifications to their diet after reducing consumption of these high-fat foods.

Fluids

Compared with adults, children have a greater ratio of surface area to mass because of their smaller body and lower muscle mass, which may result in greater heat absorption. Children also generate more heat, have a higher body temperature sweat threshold, a lower capacity to produce sweat, and take longer to acclimate to hot environments. Many of these physiological observations begin to resolve during adolescence. Recent recommendations suggest that adolescent athletes should follow the same fluid intake guidelines indicated for adult athletes (2, 20)

It is particularly important for young athletes to begin practice and competition well hydrated. Urine color should be clear or light yellow at the initiation of exercise. Structured hydration protocols for adolescents that can be found elsewhere (8) describe the effects of sweat rates, sport dynamics, availability of fluids, environmental factors, level of fitness, duration, intensity, and fluid preferences on hydration status. Hydration for young athletes is discussed in chapter 8.

> **DO YOU KNOW?**
> Unsafe hypohydration and dehydration practices to lose weight that are commonly practiced in sport include fluid restriction, spitting, use of laxatives and diuretics, rubber suits, steam baths, and saunas.

Micronutrients

Active children and adolescents tend to have greater vitamin and mineral intake than their nonactive peers, and exercise does not appear to increase needs. But suboptimal micronutrient intake may still be an issue, because national and population-based surveys have found that many adolescents fall short in meeting dietary recommendations for several nutrients (vitamin A, folic acid, fiber, iron, calcium, vitamin D, and zinc (21, 22). The most common deficits are iron, calcium, and vitamin D. These deficits can partly be explained by common dietary patterns documented in adolescents that tend to favor foods with a higher fat and added sugar content instead of nutrient-dense foods (21-23). The RDAs for each of these nutrients, consequences of deficiency, and strategies for increasing consumption are discussed in chapters 5 and 6.

> **DO YOU KNOW?**
> About half of the world's children aged 6 months to 5 years have at least one micronutrient deficiency. Most micronutrients cannot be made within the body and must be acquired through the diet. Thus, children and adolescents should be eating well-chosen diets that include a variety of fruits and vegetables, grains, protein, and dairy, as well as other fortified foods to prevent micronutrient deficiencies.

Ergogenic Aids and Dietary Supplements

Some adolescent athletes become vulnerable to the lure of dietary supplements because they are influenced by their peers, sport heroes, and the media. Lay publications, manufacturer claims, and the use of supplements by famous athletes may add to the allure for some adolescent athletes. These factors along with lack of adolescent knowledge and medical guidance predisposes young athletes to significant health risks if supplements are not used safely (24). As described in chapter 9, recommendations for athletes in this age group regarding supplement use are available. When preparing to offer dietary supplement guidance to physically active adolescents, parents, and coaches, professionals must be sure to search for position statements from respected sports nutrition organizations such as Desbrow and colleagues (8) and review reputable research on the dietary supplement practices of athletes in this age group. Another important assignment is to search for position stances on dietary supplement use from respected medical organizations such as the American Academy of Pediatrics. By doing research, professionals will be better prepared to work with young athletes in the future.

MASTERS ATHLETES

Aging brings unique opportunities and experiences. From the standpoint of athletic performance, aging can be detrimental because of its effects on all physiological functions. Exercise, however, is widely accepted as essential for reducing the risk of chronic disease and slowing the loss of physical function associated with aging. Further, given what we know about the importance of physical activity and exercise throughout the lifespan, it is not a surprise that more people are staying involved in exercise and competitive sport in their 50s and beyond. The term *masters athlete* is not universally defined by age and varies by sporting activity, but most masters champions are in their 40s and beyond. Masters-level events are gaining popularity at the local, national, and international level. Many recommendations for masters athletes are extrapolated from recommendations for younger athletes and nutrition needs for the aging, as outlined by the DRIs (25).

Exercise as an Essential Lifestyle Behavior in Aging

The world's population in 2040 will include an estimated 1.3 billion people over age 65, making up 14 percent of the population. This estimation is significantly more than double the approximate 506 million people over age 65 in 2008 (26). Regular physical activity and exercise is essential for keeping the aging population in better health. Exercise is essential for slowing the losses of cardiorespiratory and cardiovascular function, muscle function, and bone mineral density, while helping to control changes in body mass and cognitive function and mitigating insulin resistance.

Cardiovascular and Metabolic Health

Aging athletes who continue to perform endurance exercise

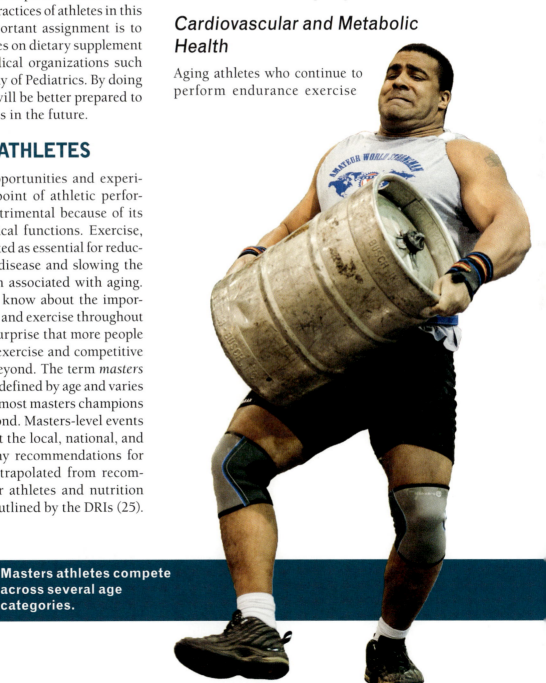

Masters athletes compete across several age categories.

retain greater aerobic capacity than their sedentary age-matched peers (27). Although a decrease in $\dot{V}O_2$max with aging that begins at about age 30 is inevitable, those who begin and maintain endurance exercise can improve their fitness level. Several factors are thought to contribute to this age-related decline in $\dot{V}O_2$max, including social factors such as limited time, commitment to career and family, and less time spent exercising. Physiological changes also contribute and have been explained by changes to exercise economy and lactate thresholds (28). Despite some losses in aerobic performance, one of the benefits of exercise in aging is its effect on maintaining healthy lipid profiles that put masters athletes at lower risk of metabolic and cardiovascular disease (29-31).

In addition to promoting optimal lipid profiles and cardiovascular health, exercise during aging augments overall metabolic health by decreasing risk of insulin resistance. Skeletal muscle helps use blood glucose, and exercise helps improve both insulin signaling and non-insulin-dependent glucose uptake induced by muscle contraction. In the absence of exercise during aging, fasting blood glucose levels commonly rise because of insulin resistance. If unresolved, a series of events may take place involving weight gain, increased inflammation, and increased likelihood of developing type 2 diabetes mellitus. The benefit of regular exercise in staving off diabetes cannot be overstated; the effect appears to be multifactorial, including decreasing risk of obesity (32).

Musculoskeletal Health

Strong bones and muscles are essential to maintaining normal physical functioning and independent living during aging. Usually starting sometime in our 40s, muscle mass starts a slow, progressive decline (33). Some estimates suggest that muscle mass declines 3 to 8 percent each decade, and strength declines approximately 1.5 percent per year and accelerates to 3 percent per year after age 60. At the same time, powerful, fast-acting muscle fibers convert to slower muscle fibers (34-36). This loss of muscle over time is termed *sarcopenia*. Sarcopenia increases a person's risk of falling—a major cause of head injuries, broken bones, and hospitalization in the elderly (37-40). Although muscle loss cannot be completely stopped during aging, it can be blunted through resistance training and eating a well-balanced diet that supports muscle tissue (41, 42). It is never too late to start a resistance-training program; years of evidence suggests that muscle strength can be improved at any age, and this functional benefit can improve gait speed and balance with aging (43, 44). Resistance training also expresses its beneficial effects on bone mass. This outcome is especially important for aging women, who begin to lose bone much earlier than men because of estrogen loss with menopause. Estrogen is important for bone mass accretion.

In addition to resistance training, any exercise has a positive effect on muscle and bone, and these effects can be maximized through high-impact exercise (45). High-impact exercise results in greater stimulation of muscle and mechanical stress on bone, which helps produce stronger tissue. By doing this type of exercise, masters athletes tend to be stronger and have better bone health compared with sedentary counterparts. Even exercise that provides moderate impact can

---

PUTTING IT INTO PERSPECTIVE

PREVENTING OSTEOPOROSIS

Osteoporosis is a silent and increasingly common disease characterized by weak, porous bones. Bone density and quality of bones are reduced during the disease process, and bones commonly become fragile, leading to increased risk of fractures. A simple fall or slip for a person with osteoporosis can lead to a catastrophic bone fracture that can limit physical mobility, contribute additional weakness to muscles and bones, and spark significant functional decline. Although this disease is most associated with aging, it has been identified in younger people because of poor diet, lack of bone-building activity, and amenorrhea. Osteoporosis can be prevented during young adulthood through weight-bearing exercises, a diet with adequate energy intake, and adequate vitamin D and calcium. For the college student, this program can be as simple as taking up weight training or jumping rope while avoiding extreme weight-loss practices and consuming more calcium-rich foods.

improve bone health. These benefits have been documented in physically active adults 65 years of age and older who showed greater bone mineral content from both swimming and running compared with nonactive controls (46).

Body Weight

Obesity is currently estimated to affect over one-third of the adult population, which puts this disease in epidemic status. Overweight, a prerequisite to obesity, is also of concern, and physical inactivity is a major risk factor. Masters athletes are also at risk of weight gain, but exercise is an effective strategy for lessening age-related weight gain. Regular exercise is essential for maintaining a healthy weight, especially after achieving weight loss (47). The absolute amount of exercise recommended for older adults is the same as for all adults—at least 150 minutes (2 hours and 30 minutes) to 300 minutes (5 hours) a week of moderate-intensity aerobic physical activity, or 75 minutes (1 hour and 15 minutes) to 150 minutes (2 hours and 30 minutes) a week of vigorous-intensity aerobic physical activity, or an equivalent combination of moderate- and vigorous-intensity aerobic activity (48). Those who average 60 minutes of moderate physical activity per day appear to gain the least amount of weight (49).

In summary, engaging in regular, moderate-intensity physical activity can help prevent overweight and obesity. This level of physical activity is consistent with the level for most masters athletes.

Cognitive Function

Exercise during aging has multiple positive effects on systemic health, body system function, prevention of weight gain, metabolic disease, and possibly cognitive function. Masters athletes have greater white matter integrity in areas of the brain related to motor control, visuospatial function, and working memory (50). Studies have found that cognitive performance and cerebral blood flow are strongly associated with cardiorespiratory fitness and that the benefits of healthy heart function leading to brain function improvements can be modified by fitness (30, 51). Further, physical activity has proven benefits for overall brain health, function, and neurodegeneration in older adults (29, 52, 53). Just 10 minutes of moderate-intensity physical activity resulted in short-term improvements in cognitive performance, and 3 hours of training or physical activity per week over months to a year revealed improvements in brain structure and function, and cognitive perceptual skills (29).

Energy Needs

The calculation and estimation of energy needs for aging athletes is an inexact science, having many of the same limitations encountered in other life-stage groups. Many energy prediction equations include an age variable that is incorporated into the calculation to reduce the number of calories required for total energy expenditure (TEE). This modification is based on the premise that aging is directly associated with reduced metabolic activity. Although this association is real, reductions in metabolic rate are more likely caused by a reduction of total muscle mass rather than age. An experienced masters-level athlete likely has a higher metabolic rate than an age-matched person who is sedentary.

As discussed in chapter 2, TEE is composed of basal metabolic rate (BMR), **thermic effect of food (TEF)**, and physical activity. All these factors have been independently shown to decrease with age, but physical activity is clearly the most variable. Although many equations to predict TEE are used in practice, if a masters athlete has recent body composition data, the preferred method is to use the Cunningham equation. This equation uses fat-free mass as a variable and has been shown to estimate RMR more accurately than other equations (54).

Nutrition Needs

We know little thus far about the specific nutrition needs of masters-level athletes because data for this population are limited. To date, however, good evidence is available on aging skeletal muscle biology, the physiological benefits of exercise in aging, sports nutrition recommendations for adults, and physiological outcomes of diet and exercise interventions in older recreational athletes. These data are currently being used to extrapolate nutrient recommendations for masters-level athletes. The following sections describe macronutrient, micronutrient, and hydration recommendations for aging athletes.

Macronutrients

Sports nutrition guidelines call for an individualized and periodized approach to carbohydrate and protein needs based on training load and intensity. Carbohydrate needs for both training and acute within- or postexercise scenarios are not age-specific but depend on training and competition demands. A diet consisting of high-carbohydrate, nutrient-dense foods such as whole-grain breads and cereals, fruits and vegetables, and low-fat dairy foods provides quality carbohydrate to meet the masters athlete's needs. Choosing nutrient-dense carbohydrate foods from multiple food groups is also consistent with dietary patterns associated with less cognitive decline. For instance, greater adherence to the Mediterranean, DASH, or MIND (a newer diet similar to a combination of Mediterranean and DASH) diets is associated with less cognitive decline and a lower risk of Alzheimer's disease (55-57).

Given the expected loss of muscle mass in aging, older athletes should strive to meet their daily protein needs and consume protein regularly throughout the day (2). Protein is essential throughout the lifespan because it promotes muscle repair and retention and helps connective tissue recover from exercise, while also bolstering bone health and assisting in the support of metabolic adaptation. Protein sometimes becomes the forgotten nutrient that is essential for bone health. For masters athletes, daily protein needs are consistent with needs of younger adults (1.2–2.0 g/kg per day) with the added goal of consuming at least 0.4 g/kg per meal to combat muscle anabolic resistance seen in aging (2, 11). As with carbohydrate, daily protein needs can be fine-tuned based on changing training intensity and volume of both endurance and resistance exercises. General guidelines for the intake of energy-yielding macronutrients for masters athletes are provided in table 14.2.

Micronutrients

It is generally accepted that as more energy is consumed, more micronutrients are also consumed. Because athletes of all ages tend to consume more energy than their sedentary counterparts do, many athletes also consume more micronutrients. When these athletes also focus on consuming fortified foods and sports foods that contain added micronutrients, they might feel even more assured they are meeting their micronutrient needs. Some studies, however, report that athletes are coming up short on key micronutrients, which could have a negative effect on health and performance. Review chapters 6 and 7 for further discussion.

The need for some micronutrients (vitamin D, vitamin B_6, vitamin B_{12}, and calcium) increases beyond age 50, while the need for iron and chromium decreases (58). When examining studies that report on nutrient intake in aging athletes, the micronutrients of most concern, because of limited intake, were vitamin D, calcium, and vitamin B_{12}. Although both vitamin D and calcium are tied to bone health, both clearly support muscle function and immunity—two important findings for masters athletes. Aging athletes should aim for 1,000 to 1,200 mg of calcium per day from calcium-rich foods. If supplements are used,

Table 14.2 Energy-Yielding Macronutrient Recommendations for Masters Athletes

	Carbohydrate		Protein	Fat	
AMDR	45%–65% of daily calories		10%–35% of daily calories	20%–35% of daily calories	
General sports nutrition guidelines	Light exercise (low intensity)	3–5 g · kg^{-1} · d^{-1}	1.2–2.0 g/kg	Total fat	20%–25%
	Moderate (1 hr/d)	5–7 g · kg^{-1} · d^{-1}			
	High (1–3 hr/d)	6–10 g · kg^{-1} · d^{-1}		Saturated fat	<10%
	Very high (>4–5 hr/d)	8–12 g · kg^{-1} · d^{-1}			

Data from Institute of Medicine (2005); Thomas, Erdman, and Burke (2016).

PUTTING IT INTO PERSPECTIVE

NEGATIVE CONSEQUENCES ASSOCIATED WITH DEHYDRATION

Body fluid deficits that cause a 2 percent or higher drop in weight can impair aerobic performance and cognitive function (64, 65). Dehydration can decrease speed, strength, stamina, and recovery time. It can also raise perceived effort of exertion and lead to an increased body temperature and increased risk for injury. In some scenarios, the heat stress associated with dehydration can contribute to an increased risk of life-threatening exertional heat illness (i.e., heatstroke).

aging athletes should consider using a form that has high bioavailability, such as calcium citrate, and consuming 500 mg or less per serving for greater absorption. For vitamin D, controversy continues over the amount needed in the blood (as 25[OH]D) to signify sufficiency to promote health and athletic performance. Although hotly debated, the IOM defines deficiency when serum 25(OH)D falls below 20ng/ml (59). Using this definition, estimates are that 20 to 100 percent of community-dwelling elderly are vitamin D deficient if not on a vitamin D supplement (60). In the older population, lower vitamin D levels were associated with poor physical performance when subjects were matched by age and gender over a 3-year period (61). Poor vitamin D status is a real concern in aging, and consuming natural food sources of vitamin D is not a reliable way to prevent or reverse a deficiency (60). For this reason, several strategies to improve and maintain vitamin D status may require discussion with a health care provider. These approaches include, but are not limited to, consumption of vitamin D–rich foods, sensible midday sun exposure, maintenance of body weight, and vitamin D supplementation (62, 63).

Fluids

Aging elicits many physiological changes that create challenges in determining hydration needs for masters athletes. With aging comes a decreased response to thirst. The thirst mechanism related to the sensation of thirst is slower to respond both when additional fluid is needed and when fluid needs are met. Further, alcohol and several medications can contribute to a compromised hydration status that might be risky during physical exercise. Masters athletes should not rely solely on thirst to meet fluid needs and should adopt a drinking strategy to maintain adequate fluid intake. See chapter 8 for guidelines on fluid consumption.

PEOPLE WITH DIABETES AND METABOLIC SYNDROME

According to *National Diabetes Statistics Report 2020*, 34.2 million Americans had a diagnosis of diabetes. An estimated 90 to 95 percent of these cases are **type 2 diabetes mellitus**. These numbers are staggering, especially because it is estimated that an additional 2.3 percent of the U.S. population have undiagnosed type 2 diabetes (66). Almost 1.5 million Americans are diagnosed with diabetes every year. At this rate, over the next 25 years the number of Americans with diagnosed and undiagnosed diabetes could nearly double. Many athletes with metabolic diseases such as diabetes are now playing sports, so dietary plans must be designed to meet their metabolic demands and energy needs. Diabetes affects carbohydrate availability and its use by body cells, so specific dietary, exercise, and medication considerations are necessary for athletes with diabetes. With a proper management plan in place, athletes with diabetes can perform just as well as their peers, as evidenced by the Olympics, where athletes with diabetes have won gold.

Diabetes is generally characterized by high blood glucose levels caused by either a lack of insulin or the body's inability to use insulin efficiently. In **type 1 diabetes mellitus** (figure 14.3), **hyperglycemia** results from the pancreas not making insulin. This disease requires insulin injection to normalize blood glucose levels. The loss of insulin production is a result of an autoimmune insult on the pancreas and presents with a quick onset, typically in childhood. In contrast, in type 2 diabetes mellitus (figure 14.4), insulin resistance is the dominant mechanism. **Insulin**

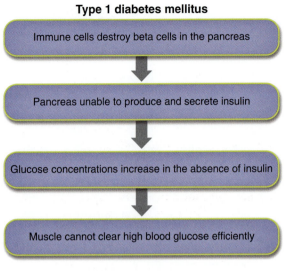

Figure 14.3 Type 1 diabetes.

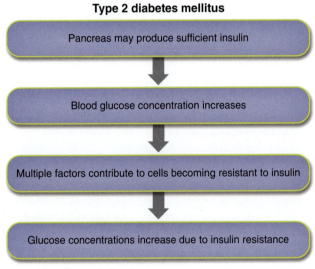

Figure 14.4 Type 2 diabetes.

in the blood, and a diet high in saturated fat are contributing factors to insulin resistance.

When insulin resistance begins, the pancreas makes extra insulin to make up for it. Over time, the pancreas is not able to keep up and cannot make enough insulin to keep blood glucose levels within normal limits. The pancreas wears down and might stop making insulin because of the constant glucose stimulus it receives. Type 2 diabetes mellitus is treated with lifestyle changes (diet and exercise), oral medications, and in some cases insulin.

Type 2 diabetes is associated with **metabolic syndrome** and can lead to permanent organ damage. This syndrome is characterized by high blood pressure, high blood sugar levels, excess body fat around the waist, and abnormal cholesterol levels. When these factors are present together, they increase the risk of heart disease, stroke, and diabetes. Type 2 diabetes is a major cause of morbidity and mortality worldwide and strongly associated with inactivity, obesity, and family history (67). Over 90 percent of those with type 2 diabetes are overweight or obese.

Although type 2 diabetes is typically diagnosed later in life, the rise in obesity and physical inactivity in youth has increased the prevalence of type 2 diabetes in children and teens.

The glucose in the blood stream that has limited capacity to enter cells begins to accumulate in the blood at concentrations higher than normal. Chronic hyperglycemia from diabetes can cause a host of problems due to a change of viscosity of the blood that the added glucose creates and can affect the interaction of glucose with red blood cells as well as small blood vessels in many body tissues.

The poor absorption and disposal of glucose by the body's cells occur as a result of a series of

resistance, a precursor to type 2 diabetes, is the body's inability to respond to and use the insulin it produces. Genetics, obesity, high levels of fat

PUTTING IT INTO PERSPECTIVE

METABOLIC SYNDROME IN ATHLETES

Aggressive lifestyle changes can delay or even prevent the development of serious health problems and help prevent the cluster of conditions associated with metabolic syndrome. Athletes are well positioned to delay the onset of or decrease the severity of metabolic syndrome with frequent exercise and weight control. Although lack of exercise is a strong predictive factor for both diabetes and metabolic syndrome, there is concern about athletes with ongoing interest in weight gain (such as American football linemen). These athletes might become obese, placing them at greater risk for metabolic syndrome when their playing days are over (11).

defective events and create severe alterations to normal energy metabolism. A major component of cellular glucose uptake relies on the action of cellular glucose transporters. These transporters are a large family of proteins that reside in the cell and, upon receiving a signal, translocate to the outer membrane to allow glucose to enter the cell. Without receiving a proper signal, glucose uptake is impaired, which can result in mild to severe rises in blood glucose, depending on the severity of the signal impairment. The signal required to initiate glucose transporter movement comes from insulin. This peptide hormone is secreted from the pancreas in response to very small rises in blood glucose after consuming a meal. Insulin normally binds to receptors on the surface membrane of cells. The docking of insulin to its receptor creates a cascade of intracellular signaling events that stimulate glucose transporter translocation to the cell surface. Normally, this activity results in glucose uptake and a decrease in blood glucose levels. In diabetes, there can be a disruption in insulin release by the pancreas and a decreased response, or insulin resistance of the cells to any insulin that is secreted.

As introduced earlier, complications of diabetes are rooted in two major concerns: cellular starvation, due to the lack of glucose, and hyperglycemia. When the cells are deprived of glucose, the body is fooled into thinking that cells are starving and therefore initiates a series of events that unfortunately does more harm than good. The liver is signaled to release its stored glucose in hopes of providing more fuel for starved cells, but this only results in higher blood glucose concentrations. When blood glucose concentrations get high enough, the kidneys start to respond by filtering the excess glucose into the urine as a means to help manage hyperglycemia. The problem with this response is that it creates additional urine, leading to excessive urination, known as **polyuria**. This condition increases thirst and creates a symptom known as **polydipsia**. Because of these series of events, many people with untreated type 2 diabetes also experience increased hunger, known as **polyphagia**, which can further contribute to hyperglycemia. Although some form of these bodily symptoms may develop in an effort to address the issue of cell starvation, other signals are amplified in response to the ineffectiveness of the previous strategies. Figure 14.5 summarizes the series of events that lead to these metabolic abnormalities and the body symptoms that result.

As the body recognizes that previous attempts to fuel cells have limited effectiveness, it will then turn to using protein and fat as fuel. The body will increase skeletal muscle protein catabolism in order to use amino acids as substrates for gluconeogenesis, as discussed in chapter 2. Fat utilization will also increase in hopes that fat will meet the ATP demands of the cell. Collectively, the result of increased protein and fat utilization is loss of body weight, muscle wasting, and muscle weakness. Although the loss of valuable protein to glucose production has limited effect on solving the metabolic dilemma at hand, increased attempts to use more fat as a fuel source creates additional problems. Without an adequate supply of intracellular glucose, fat cannot be completely oxidized, and intermediate products of fat metabolism can build up, forming ketone bodies. If left unchecked, a significant rise in ketone bodies can lead to a condition known as **ketoacidosis**, which can result in acidification of blood and body fluids that may be life threatening and result in a coma.

? DO YOU KNOW?

One of the most easily observed characteristics of ketoacidosis is fruity-smelling breath. This condition is caused by acetone (a ketone) being produced by organs that are starved of glucose in response to the body's hyperglycemic state. A friend or family member may be able to detect ketoacidosis with just a simple observation.

The treatment regimen for diabetes depends on the type of diabetes diagnosed. Type 1 diabetes mellitus is typically met with a treatment regimen that involves insulin injections combined with regular exercise and a healthy diet to control blood sugar levels. For type 2 diabetes mellitus, cells are not responsive to insulin, resulting in perturbations in glucose uptake. Treatment depends on multiple factors, including average blood glucose levels and amount of endogenous insulin production. Some people with type 2 diabetes mellitus can control their blood glucose levels through healthy eating and physical activity. In addition to diet, exercise, and lifestyle changes,

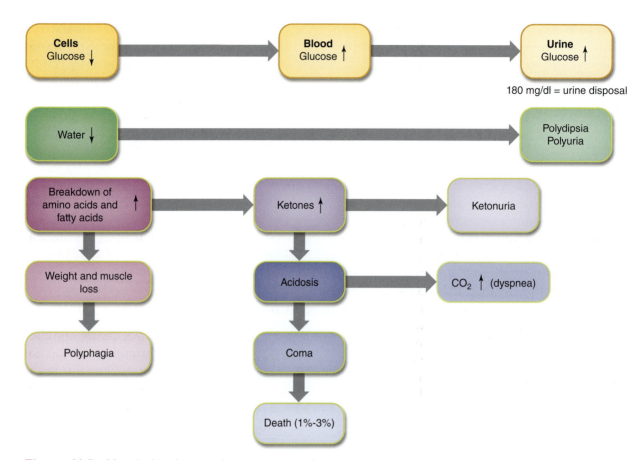

Figure 14.5 Metabolic abnormalities resulting from glucose deficiency in cells.

? DO YOU KNOW?

Because of the direct effect that chronic hyperglycemia has on body tissues, other chronic diseases may develop. Tissues that have very small blood vessels and are vital to the function of a particular organ system are particularly susceptible to chronic high blood glucose levels. The most common complications occur with the eyes, kidneys, nerves, and heart, and may ultimately result in blindness, kidney dysfunction, heart disease, and nerve degeneration.

medications to lower levels of blood glucose are often prescribed to enhance cellular sensitivity to insulin, allowing glucose to be transported more effectively into the cells for energy. Some of the signs and symptoms of diabetes and clinical parameters used to diagnose diabetes appear in table 14.3.

Symptoms of type 1 diabetes
> Polyuria
> Polydipsia
> Polyphagia
> Unusual weight loss
> Extreme fatigue and irritability

Symptoms of type 2 diabetes
> Any of the type 1 symptoms
> Frequent infections
> Blurred vision
> Cuts or bruises that are slow to heal
> Tingling or numbness in the hands or feet

Athletes diagnosed with type 2 diabetes mellitus must understand the effect that training and competition have on their blood glucose levels. To understand and manage this effect, frequent self-monitoring of glucose before and after exercise is necessary to avoid abnormally low levels of blood sugar called **hypoglycemia**. Because muscle contraction provides an additional stimulus for glucose intake and medications are also usually

Table 14.3 Diagnosing Criteria for Diabetes

Diagnosing diabetes	Normal	Prediabetes	Diabetes
Glycohemoglobin test (A1C)	Less than 5.7%	5.7%–6.4%	6.5% or higher
Fasting plasma glucose (FPG)	Less than 100 mg/dl	100–125 mg/dl	126 mg/dl or higher
Oral glucose tolerance test (OGTT)	Less than 140 mg/dl	140–199 mg/dl	200 mg/dl or higher

Based on American Diabetes Association, "Classification and Diagnosis of Diabetes," *Diabetes Care* 39(suppl 1) (2016): S1-S22.

taken to create the same effect, the two stimuli together can sometimes create too much glucose uptake, which limits glucose availability to the central nervous system. The effect of exercise on glucose uptake is strong and can continue for several hours after exercise, with a prolonged effect on blood glucose levels. Although this outcome is thought to be helpful for preventing hyperglycemia, it can be a negative consequence for an athlete with high training demands who is not properly fueled. Monitoring of blood glucose for several hours after exercise may be necessary to monitor for hypoglycemia.

Athletes with type 1 diabetes must be more cautious than athletes with type 2 diabetes. Athletes with type 1 diabetes face a number of challenges in achieving tight blood glucose controls that support athletic performance and devising food and insulin regimens that must adapt quickly to an unpredictable sporting environment. Insulin must be injected at the right times at the right amounts, matched to physical activity level, and paired with carbohydrate intake. Additionally, the mode of exercise that determines whether an activity is more anaerobic or aerobic in nature must be considered because of their different effects on blood sugar management. Aerobic exercise may not cause insulin levels to fall, resulting in a higher risk of hypoglycemia. Furthermore, exercise will increase insulin sensitivity for several hours and may further increase hypoglycemia risk. Anaerobic exercises tend to cause a release of hormones that promote the spilling of additional glucose into the blood that may not be accounted for after insulin is already dosed, resulting in a greater risk of hyperglycemia. To train and compete safely and effectively, athletes with type 1 diabetes must possess good self-management skills to be able to adjust the timing and dose of insulin injections. Proper control of blood glucose will facilitate safe participation in sport and minimize medical complications.

Blood Sugar Management Strategies

Monitoring glucose levels before, during, and after exercise is essential to determining whether an athlete needs to make changes in their diet, exercise program, or medication regimen. Maintaining a blood glucose of 70 to 110 mg/dl on a regular basis is the foundation of controlling diabetes. Portable blood glucose testing devices take a small sample of blood from capillaries at the tips of the fingers, which is placed on a chemically treated test strip and inserted into the testing device. The device provides a quick digital readout of the blood glucose level. Blood glucose is usually tested several times throughout the day. The most important times for testing the athlete are before exercise, immediately after exercise, and several hours after exercise. Decisions on whether to start training or competing or make adjustments to carbohydrate intake or insulin are based on pre-exercise monitoring of blood glucose. If glucose concentrations from the capillary blood test are greater than 250 mg/dl, the athlete should do a urine test for the presence of ketone production in the body. This test is completed by using a different type of chemically treated test strip that interacts with a small amount of urine to change color if ketones are present. Athletes with type 1 diabetes and insulin-dependent type 2 diabetes are more prone to ketone production and should not exercise with a combination of hyperglycemia and urine ketones because of an elevated risk of ketoacidosis. Table 14.4 provides specific considerations for the initiation of exercise related

Table 14.4 Glucose Level Considerations When Initiating Exercise

Preexercise glucose level	Recommendation made by qualified professionals
<100 mg/dl	Ingest additional carbohydrates before initiating exercise: 15-40 g carbohydrates (or more) depending on actual glucose level and the athlete's typical response to added carbohydrates.
>250 mg/dl	Test urine for ketones.
>250 mg/dl, with ketones present	Do not exercise. Make insulin or medication adjustments and then retest glucose and ketones.
>250 mg/dl, without ketones present	Exercise can be initiated.
>300 mg/dl, without ketones present	Exercise with caution.

to blood glucose concentrations for both hypo- and hyperglycemia and the presence of urine ketones.

When hypoglycemia is present before exercise, an athlete must make time to consume carbohydrate and adjust insulin dosage as necessary and should not exercise until hypoglycemia is resolved. The amount of carbohydrate required to help glucose levels rebound to above 100 mg/dl will vary but is generally between 15 and 40 grams. One cup of 100 percent orange juice provides approximately 30 grams of carbohydrate to increase blood sugar concentrations. These are only general guidelines. Remember that treating diabetes with nutrition is considered medical nutrition therapy (MNT), and clients with diabetes may therefore need the guidance of an RDN.

Many athletes with diabetes become accustomed to their training and competition cycles and develop a good feel for what adjustments they need to make for blood sugar control. They should keep in mind, however, that any changes to their training cycle may make their normal regimen inadequate for proper blood sugar control. For instance, any exercise lasting longer than 60 minutes requires additional focus on blood glucose testing. Further, any time the type, intensity, or duration of exercise is modified, the athlete should expect the need for closer monitoring of glucose concentrations and more carbohydrate or insulin adjustments (68).

General Nutrition Recommendations

For athletes with diabetes, the foundation of a healthy diet closely resembles the diet recommendations for the general population. *Dietary Guidelines for Americans 2015-2020* along with the MyPlate food guidance system should form the basis of the foods that make up the diet. The acceptable macronutrient distribution range (AMDR) provides general guidelines for each energy-yielding macronutrient in terms of the percent of total energy that should be consumed, and dosing the daily amount of carbohydrates needed depending on daily activity demand relative to body mass (g/kg body weight) is the most practical approach to get started. With these tools, the athlete with diabetes can begin to build a healthy diet based on cultural food preferences and training and nutrition periodization concepts discussed in other chapters of this text.

Carbohydrate remains the predominant energy for fueling exercise and should make up the bulk of the diet. All carbohydrate foods can fit into a diabetic athlete's diet, but the bulk of the carbohydrates chosen should be nutrient dense, provide fiber, and originate from a variety of food groups. The goal for carbohydrate intake should be to balance intake throughout the day, to support fueling needs of activity, and to support stable blood sugar levels to minimize hypo- and hyperglycemia. Foods high in sugar should be minimized and should not regularly replace nutrient-dense carbohydrate choices.

Protein and fat make up the remaining energy needs of the diabetic athlete's diet. The specific requirements for each generally fall in line with the AMDR recommendations and guidelines set forth by *Dietary Guidelines for Americans*. Additionally, protein needs for recovery and optimal muscle adaptation to training and fat intake guidelines to promote cardiovascular health are similar to those for nondiabetic athletes and the general population. Adjustments in macronutrient composition of the diet may be necessary following consultation with a physician, a **certified diabetes educator** (69), or a registered dietitian nutritionist (70) to personalize recommendations not only to meet the demands of the sport but also to promote euglycemia between the recommended range of 70 to 100 mg/dl and cardiovascular health. Most of the day-to-day monitoring and adjustments to the diet are based on the goal of eating at approximately the same time each day while maintaining consistent intake of carbohydrate throughout the day through meals and snacks.

Specific Nutrition Recommendations

Athletes with type 1 diabetes mellitus should be knowledgeable about estimating the amount of carbohydrate consumed in each meal so that they can match insulin requirements. The key consideration regarding carbohydrate intake during meals is the *quantity* of carbohydrate consumed, not so much the type of carbohydrate or a rigid schedule for carbohydrate intake. These athletes must self-monitor blood glucose levels regularly to learn what affects their blood glucose level (68).

In preparation for training or competition, enough carbohydrate must be available to the body before, during, and postexercise. Likewise, the amount of insulin administered must be tailored to how much carbohydrate has been consumed (64, 71) and adjusted depending on the type, intensity, and time of the exercise. For type 1 diabetes athletes, the glycemic index of foods has not been of much value for athletes with diabetes, and thus the total amount of carbohydrate ingested and the timing of ingestion are the most important variables. Because excessive carbohydrate intake in the days before an event can adversely affect blood sugar control, the practice of carbohydrate loading is often not advised (71).

Carbohydrate should be readily available to consume for exercise or competition lasting more than 30 minutes. Target carbohydrate consumption goals are generally 20 to 30 grams consumed every 30 to 60 minutes of endurance exercise, but the amount can vary greatly based on intensity level of the activity and insulin levels (68). Depending on food preferences and the sport or activity, this goal can be accomplished by drinking most 8-ounce (240 ml) sports drinks, one sports gel, 4 ounces (120 ml) of 100 percent fruit juice mixed with 4 ounces (120 ml) of water, or a cereal-fruit breakfast bar. Athletes with type 1 diabetes participating in explosive, anaerobic events typically do not need additional carbohydrate during the event. During exercise, athletes with type 1 diabetes should be well versed in picking up on the early symptoms of hypoglycemia and recognize that prolonged exertion might make identifying hypoglycemia difficult. If hypoglycemia is evident, immediate access to rapid-acting carbohydrate must be administered to increase circulating glucose levels.

The postexercise goal for athletes with type 1 diabetes is to replenish glycogen stores and prevent hypoglycemia in the postexercise period when insulin sensitivity is enhanced. Carbohydrate intake recommendations for exercise recovery are similar to those for nondiabetic athletes—approximately 1.0 to 1.2 g/kg per hour until normal meals are resumed to meet fueling needs (11).

Specific nutrition recommendations for athletes with type 2 diabetes mellitus are often based on blood glucose response to exercise and adherence to an exercise program. When the etiology of type 2 diabetes mellitus is considered, the value of exercise as the cornerstone of blood sugar control cannot be overstated. Exercise improves insulin sensitivity and, through an insulin-independent mechanism, primes the muscle for increasing the peripheral uptake of glucose (figure 14.6). In fact, exercise has other benefits through promoting carbohydrate oxidation and glycogen storage, metabolic adaptations to burn more fuel more efficiently at higher intensities that can support fat loss, and weight maintenance with improved body composition (72, 73). Just 20 to 30 minutes of any exercise improves insulin sensitivity, and a single bout of endurance exercise can affect insulin sensitivity for 24 to 72 hours (73). The effects of regular resistance exercise are also impressive. Resistance exercise increases muscle mass, which increases the size of the number one organ responsible for glucose uptake and disposal. Bigger engines can burn more energy! A goal for type 2 diabetes athletes is to manage energy intake to promote slow weight loss and to exercise regularly to promote insulin sensitivity.

After an exercise program is initiated, the diet should be modified to reduce energy intake. Over

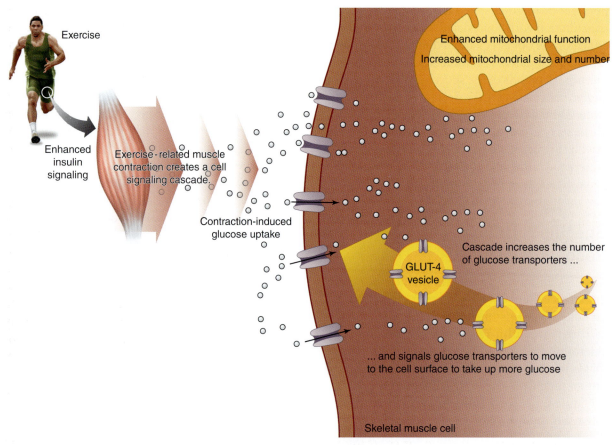

Figure 14.6 Exercise improves muscle sensitivity to glucose.

time, these two strategies will work together to reduce fat mass and improve insulin sensitivity. Immediately before exercise, no additional carbohydrate should be consumed, because the goal is to promote weight loss. During exercise, additional carbohydrate should be avoided (as long as there are no signs of hypoglycemia) to preserve the energy deficit created by the adoption of a healthier diet and to avoid sabotaging progress in weight loss. If carbohydrate must be consumed, a keen awareness of carbohydrate density is important, again to prevent excessive energy intake. During the postexercise timeframe, insulin sensitivity is improved and energy use is amplified, so people with type 2 diabetes mellitus are advised not to consume carbohydrate immediately and instead wait until their next regular meal (74).

Preventing Diabetes Emergencies in Sport

The first step in preventing hypo- and hyperglycemic emergencies in athletes with diabetes is for them to have a track record of consistently managing their diabetes well. Consistent euglycemia coupled with good hemoglobin A1C scores and confidence in the interplay between their training, diet, and medication is essential for building a foundation to reduce emergency risk. Beyond these guidelines, those with diabetes at the greatest risk are those who require insulin. Athletes on oral medications are at a lower risk, and athletes with type 2 diabetes controlled solely with diet and exercise have minimal risk. Hyperglycemia can occur as a result of insulin deficiency during exercise coupled with the actions of other hormones released during exercise that mobilize more glucose into the bloodstream from liver glycogen stores. Maintaining euglycemia before exercise and keeping injectable insulin readily available are important strategies to prevent this emergency. If too much insulin is present during exercise or postexercise recovery, excessive amounts of blood glucose can be taken up by muscle tissue and the liver will stop releasing glucose, resulting in hypoglycemia. Consuming carbohydrate during exercise and exercise recovery and monitoring blood glucose levels for multiple hours postexercise is the best prevention strategy. Additional strategies to prepare for hypoglycemic emergencies include having a food bag on hand with glucose tablets and fruit juice, and making sure that friends, family, teammates, and sporting staff are aware of the location of the food bag and will notice the signs and symptoms of hypo- and hyperglycemia so that they are prepared to act appropriately.

> **? DO YOU KNOW?**
>
> The symptoms of hypoglycemia are individualized and do not normally appear until blood glucose levels reach 70 mg/dl or less. Athletes must know their own signs of hypoglycemia. These include shakiness, nervousness, sweating, irritability, confusion, rapid heartbeat, dizziness, hunger, fatigue, headaches, lack of coordination, and perhaps other symptoms.

PREGNANT WOMEN

Following physician screening for contraindications to exercise, well-chosen exercise programs can safely be incorporated to promote the health of the mother and developing fetus. Although some women may elect to maintain most of their prepregnancy exercise intensity and volume, others strive to remain active but reduce their training load and avoid athletic competition. Guidelines for exercise during pregnancy and the postpartum period can be found elsewhere (75, 76).

Combining exercise with pregnancy creates unique nutrition challenges. Exercise alone increases energy needs and an elevated demand for many nutrients. When pregnancy is added to the equation, energy demands increase again to promote the healthy growth of the fetus. In addition to the increase in energy needs, macronutrient and micronutrient demands also increase and can be nutrition areas of concern for the mother and baby if the diet is not appropriately planned or well chosen.

Physiological Changes Lead to Diet Recommendations

An active lifestyle during pregnancy is linked to several benefits, including an increase in maternal metabolic and cardiopulmonary reserve, normal glucose tolerance, improved psychological well-being, and beneficial fetal and placental adaptations. Physical activity can help prevent excessive weight gain for pregnant athletes and nonathletes. As exercise commences, understanding the normal metabolic changes that affect nutrition needs is important. During pregnancy, the major tenants are making sure that nutrient intake is adequate to meet pregnancy demands while also emphasizing the importance of an active lifestyle. An unhealthy diet and sedentary lifestyle during pregnancy can tip the balance of normal, pregnancy-induced metabolic changes and lead to high or uncontrolled glucose, excessive weight gain, and **gestational diabetes mellitus (GDM)**. You have probably heard people say that pregnant women need to eat for two, but this is far from the truth. Although energy needs increase only marginally during pregnancy, nutrient needs increase substantially. The message should not be eat for two, but eat twice as healthy.

Several physiological changes affect exercise capacity and performance during pregnancy. These changes in turn have an effect on nutrition needs. The cardiovascular system is remodeled by ovarian and placental hormones in early gestation to accommodate the increasing blood volume that comes with pregnancy. Other cardiovascular changes include an increase in resting **cardiac output** during the first trimester and a remodeling of the thoracic cage and diaphragm to a higher position to accommodate placental and fetal growth. Symptoms of shortness of breath are common, caused in part by these mechanical alterations and also by increased sensitivity to carbon dioxide in the blood stream. Thermoregulation steadily improves throughout gestation, including a downward shift in the temperature at which sweating begins. The result is quicker heat loss, which is important because of heat generation by the fetus and fetal dependence on maternal temperature regulation. Metabolic changes support using the mother's blood glucose as a primary energy source for growth of fetus and placenta. To accommodate a greater demand for blood glucose, gluconeogenic pathways in the liver are upregulated and insulin production in the pancreas increases to assist fetal glucose uptake. In the peripheral tissue, there is an increase in skeletal muscle insulin resistance and fat storage.

Although these metabolic changes are considered normal, they can be a significant concern if a mother is living an unhealthy lifestyle that promotes additional insulin resistance and fat storage. An unhealthy lifestyle, combined with normal metabolic adaptations to ensure that a developing fetus has adequate access to glucose, may tip the healthy balance to the development of GDM. Many other factors are thought to play a role in the risk for developing GDM, including, but not limited to, overweight status before pregnancy, family history of GDM, specific ethnicities and ancestry, and pregnancy after the age of 35.

Healthy Weight Gain

Unless directed otherwise by a physician, pregnant women should not be concerned with or initiate efforts to lose weight, but they should also avoid consuming more energy than necessary. The number of daily calories that a pregnant woman needs during pregnancy depends on a host of factors, including her prepregnancy BMI, the rate of body weight change during gestation, age, and level of physical activity (77). Unfortunately, many women start their pregnancy overweight or obese. Others gain more weight than is healthy during their pregnancy. Obesity during pregnancy is a risk factor for both mother and child (in utero, at delivery, and later in life); risks include GDM, gestational hypertension (high blood pressure), cesarean delivery (C-section), birth defects, and even fetal death. If a woman is obese during pregnancy, the chance that her child will be obese later in life increases, and if the mother retains most of the weight gain during pregnancy, she is at greater risk of developing type 2 diabetes mellitus and obesity later in life. Overweight women who retain previous pregnancy weight also tend to start their next pregnancy with a higher early rate of weight gain, which is strongly associated with weight retention at 6 and 12 months postpartum (78). All this considered, recommendations have been published by the Institute of Medicine to provide guidelines for total weight gain and the rate of weight gain recommended for the second and third trimester of pregnancy (table 14.5). The amount of weight gained depends on prepregnancy weight. Research shows that the risk of problems during pregnancy and delivery is lowest when weight gain is kept within a healthy range. The weight recommendations in the table were reaffirmed in 2020 and are presented as a range to guide professionals in giving individualized advice (79). These recommendations serve as a healthy guide during pregnancy and can certainly guide planning of energy intake and energy expenditure to manage healthy weight gain. This information is valuable because exceeding weight-gain recommendations is thought to contribute to fat reserves and weight retention and increases risk of GDM, pregnancy induced hypertension, and a difficult labor and birth. These women are also more likely to have large (for gestational age) babies who are at greater risk for obesity later in life. Proper diet and exercise can go a long way in managing weight gain, preventing GDM, and promoting a healthy pregnancy. Although the subsequent section addresses diet guidelines, physical activity guidelines are important as well. The current recommendation for pregnant women is 30 minutes of moderate exercise on most, if not all, days of the week following a discussion with a doctor before starting or continuing any exercise routine.

Nutrient Needs

Maternal energy needs increase during pregnancy and are a moving target based on the stage of

Table 14.5 BMI and Weight Gain for Second and Third Trimesters

Prepregnancy BMI	Total weight in lb (kg)	Recommended rate for 2nd and 3rd trimesters in lb/wk (kg/wk)
BMI <18.5	28–40 (12.7–18.1)	1–1.3 (0.5–0.6)
BMI 18.5–24.9	25–35 (11.4–15.9)	0.8–1 (0.4–0.5)
BMI 25–29.9	15–25 (6.8–11.4)	0.5–0.7 (0.2–0.3)
BMI >30	11–20 (5.0–9.1)	0.4–0.6 (0.2–0.3)

Adapted from Institute of Medicine (US). Weight Gain During Pregnancy: Reexamining the Guidelines. Washington, DC. National Academies Press; 2009, ©2009 National Academy of Sciences.

PUTTING IT INTO PERSPECTIVE

NUTRITION FOR MULTIPLE BABIES

Women can healthily gain up to twice as much weight (depending on their prepregnancy BMI) when carrying twins compared with carrying a single child. Increased appetite leaves mothers of twins at risk for excessive weight gain during pregnancy, especially during the early months.

Twin pregnancies include increased complications:

> Anemia—twice as likely to occur in women who are pregnant with twins than with a single baby
> Hypertension—more than three times as likely to occur in women who are pregnant with twins than with a single baby

pregnancy, maternal age, and the level of physical activity. In general, pregnant women need between 2,200 and 2,900 kcal a day, but specific recommendations should be individualized. Metabolic rate increases 15 percent during the second and third trimesters of pregnancy without a significant change during the first trimester. This increase during the latter two-thirds of pregnancy is thought to support the growth of the fetus, placenta, and maternal tissues (80). When translating these metabolic changes into energy needs, the general recommendation is that during the first trimester no additional energy beyond resting energy expenditure (REE) adjusted for physical activity is required to support pregnancy. Exceptions are generally recommended for expectant mothers classified as underweight by BMI at the onset of pregnancy. These expectant mothers would benefit from additional energy (calories) to support growth and weight gain. During the second and third trimesters, additional calories required to support weight gain have been translated as approximately an additional 340 kcal and 452 kcal during the second and third trimesters, respectively (77).

❓ DO YOU KNOW?

Additional energy needs during the second and third trimesters of pregnancy can easily be met by eating one extra snack per day. This adjustment is clearly not eating for two!

Simple, commonsense strategies can be employed to prevent excess energy consumption. Extra calories can be avoided by cutting down on foods high in fat and avoiding added sugars. Practical advice includes replacing sugar-sweetened beverages and fried foods with healthy options such as low-fat milk and yogurt, whole fruit, vegetables, and grains. Note that there is not a specific energy estimation equation for pregnancy, and absolute energy needs will vary with exercise during pregnancy by the type of physical activity and the total energy expended. Along with focusing on diet quality, **nutrient density** of foods and meals chosen, and strategically consuming multiple small meals that can help with nausea and heartburn, the most accurate assessment of weight progress is to monitor weight gain while being aware of the weight-gain guidelines based on prepregnancy BMI.

Although supporting a healthy rate of weight gain with proper energy intake is the cornerstone of nutrition recommendations, note that carbohydrate, protein, and fat demands are best met as part of a well-chosen diet built on food variety and nutrient density. Pregnant athletes who maintain their training should not only strive to meet DRI recommendations for carbohydrate, protein, and fat but also consider periodizing their macronutrient choices based on the mode and volume of training to support the energy expenditure of exercise while also supporting healthy weight gain. For example, the RDA for carbohydrate in adult women increases from 130 grams per day to 175 grams per day during pregnancy. When exercise training or an active lifestyle is added to pregnancy, carbohydrate needs can be significantly higher to support increased energy expenditure. The most practical way to determine carbohydrate needs for exercise during pregnancy is to understand that additional carbohydrate is often needed, particularly pre- and postexercise. By assessing fatigue during exercise and monitoring the rate of weight gain, carbohydrate needs can be adjusted accordingly. Note that carbohydrate is the primary source of energy for both mother and fetus, so it should be the predominate macronutrient fuel source (45%-64% of total energy consumed) (77). Carbohydrate foods are also a great vehicle for providing fiber in the diet to aid in preventing hemorrhoids and constipation. According to the Institute of Medicine, the RDA and adequate intake (AI) of fiber for a pregnancy between the ages of 18 and 50 is 28 grams per day (81).

For protein, general pregnancy guidelines suggest an increase to 1.1 grams of protein per kg body weight per day during gestation (77). This recommendation is based on the needs of pregnant women who are primarily sedentary. So pregnant women who participate in regular exercise should use this guidance as a baseline and might require additional protein during times of increased training duration or intensity. As exercise frequency and intensity decline during the third trimester, energy, carbohydrate, and protein needs might to be only slightly elevated beyond sedentary pregnancy needs.

Assuming that energy intake demands are met as part of a well-chosen diet, macronutrient intake is usually directly associated with caloric intake and allows all macronutrient demands to be met (table 14.6). This principle may not be the case if an expectant mother excludes certain food groups from the diet, develops an aversion for a wide range of healthy foods, or begins to follow a fad diet. In these scenarios, protein intake becomes an area of concern. Inadequate protein intake can be harmful for the mother and the baby. Low protein intake can negatively affect a mother's ability to recover from exercise, as well as her normal adaptation to pregnancy. If low protein intake is coupled with low energy intake, body proteins will preferentially be oxidized for fuel and can lead to reduced fitness, lowered immune response, altered fetal development, and increased fatigue.

The metabolic adaptations resulting from exercise combined with pregnancy increase the need for some micronutrients. Meeting energy demands with a sound diet can help an active female meet her micronutrient needs during pregnancy. Pregnant athletes who fail to gain weight, consume poorly chosen diets, or eliminate one or more food groups might be consuming suboptimal amounts of micronutrients.

B Vitamins

An important function of B vitamins is their role in supporting metabolic pathways for energy production. The need for several of the B vitamins—thiamin, riboflavin, niacin—increases during pregnancy. Most B vitamin needs can easily be met by consuming enough energy to gain weight during pregnancy and choosing a wide range of nutrient-dense and fortified foods. The B vitamin of greatest interest during pregnancy is folate (and the synthetic form, folic acid, that is a key component of prenatal vitamins). Folate deficiency can

> **DO YOU KNOW?**
>
> Folate is important for proper DNA synthesis, red blood cell production, and nervous system development. To reduce the risk of neural tube defects, all females of childbearing age who have any chance of becoming pregnant should consume folate-rich foods and fortified foods with folic acid. A folic acid supplement is also strongly recommended.

Table 14.6 Macronutrient Needs for the Nonpregnant, Pregnant, and Pregnant Athlete

Energy-yielding macronutrients	Nonpregnant adult athlete	Pregnancy	Pregnancy plus exercise
Protein	1.2-2.0 g/kg body weight per day	1.1 g/kg body weight per day	>1.1 g/kg body weight per day
Carbohydrates (fiber)	130 (25) g/d minimum; 3-12 g/kg body weight per day	175 (28) g/d minimum; 45%-64% of total energy intake	175 (28) g/d minimum; needs increase to support exercise
Fats	20-35 (% daily calories)	20-35 (% daily calories)	20-35 (% daily calories)

Data from Institute of Medicine (2005).

lead to serious effects for both the mother and her developing fetus. For the mother, megaloblastic anemia can result, causing fatigue and weakness that can contribute to an underlying etiology of depression, irritability, and poor sleep.

For the fetus, folate plays an important role in cell division and the development of the fetal nervous system. The most important stages of neural tube formation occur within the first month of conception, usually before a woman knows she is pregnant. In many cases, weeks of cell division have already taken place when a woman learns she is pregnant, and any defects that have occurred might be too late to address effectively, even if a healthy diet is adopted immediately. Note that folic acid supplementation is recommended for all women of childbearing age to help prevent the risk of folate deficiency and to counter the folate depletion effect of alcohol consumption.

Other Vitamins of Concern

The combined physiological stress of pregnancy and exercise increases the need for both vitamin C and vitamin A. Fortunately, some foods are good sources of both of these vitamins. Vitamin C is a water-soluble vitamin with requirements of 80 to 85 mg during pregnancy to support collagen formation, hormone synthesis, proper immune function, and iron absorption and also increase antioxidant activity (83), all functions important for the pregnant athlete. Note that the increased need for vitamin C to serve as an antioxidant can easily be met through the diet—antioxidant supplementation has not been shown to enhance athletic performance and may decrease training adaptations (84). Pregnant athletes wanting to increase their antioxidant intake should focus on healthy dietary choices instead of relying on antioxidant supplementation.

Vitamin A assists in cell differentiation, proliferation, proper immune function, and development of the spine, heart, eyes, and ears (77). Requirements increase from 700 to 770 micrograms during pregnancy (85, 86). Despite this increase, mothers should seek to increase their vitamin A primarily from plant sources and avoid dietary supplements that contain retinol, unless otherwise directed by a physician. Supplemental forms of retinol can become toxic and unhealthy for the developing fetus (87).

The RDA for vitamin D for pregnant females is 15 micrograms (600 IU) per day of calciferol. Vitamin D deficiency during pregnancy is associated with medical complications such as GDM and decreased bone mineral density. Additionally, vitamin D deficiency can have negative fetal consequences, including low birth weight, neonatal rickets, asthma, or type 1 diabetes (88). Folate and vitamins A, C, and D deserve focus during pregnancy. Increased consumption of these nutrients should begin prior to pregnancy and continue until delivery.

Iron

Iron status can become compromised at the onset of pregnancy because of anatomical and physiological changes that result in expansion of blood volume and increased oxidative tissue demand.

PUTTING IT INTO PERSPECTIVE

WHERE DOES ALL THE WEIGHT GO?

What accounts for the weight gained during pregnancy (82)?

- Baby: 7 to 8 pounds (3.2–3.6 kg)
- Larger breasts: 2 pounds (0.9 kg)
- Larger uterus: 2 pounds (0.9 kg)
- Placenta: 1.5 pounds (0.7 kg)
- Amniotic fluid: 2 pounds (0.9 kg)
- Increased blood volume: 3 to 4 pounds (1.4–1.8 kg)
- Fat stores: 6 to 8 pounds (2.7–3.6 kg)

In active females, iron status can also be compromised because of increased iron losses with exercise. This concern is significant, because iron is involved in fetal development and growth and the needs for red blood cell production and iron nearly double during pregnancy (77). Iron needs during pregnancy are 27 mg per day (58), a level difficult to obtain without careful diet planning or supplementation. A focus on consuming iron-rich foods alongside foods high in vitamin C should be the first strategy to increase iron absorption to help meet iron needs.

VEGETARIAN POPULATIONS

Vegetarian diets vary in the exact foods that are allowed and disallowed (table 14.7). Estimates are that approximately 3.3 percent of the American population choose not to consume meat, fish, or poultry (11, 89). About half of these people do not eat any forms of animal food, including eggs and dairy products. Note that the definitions in table 14.7 are not all-inclusive; new descriptors and definitions of vegetarian eating styles are described elsewhere (90). People choose vegetarian diets for many reasons—from ethnic, religious, moral, or philosophical beliefs to health promotion, food aversions, or financial constraints (11). Vegetarian diets can be nutritionally adequate when well chosen (i.e., include an abundance of fruits, vegetables, whole grains, nuts, soy products, fiber, phytochemicals, and antioxidants) (89). This assertion appears to hold true for vegetarian athletes as well, again as long as the diet is well chosen. Note, however, that some athletes adopt a vegetarian diet to disguise disordered eating (91, 92). The more limited the vegetarian diet, the greater challenge it is to consume an optimal intake of several nutrients. Vegetarians can benefit from comprehensive dietary evaluation and intervention from a sports dietitian to ensure that their diets are nutritionally sound to support training, competition demands, and performance.

The amount of food required to meet the nutrient demands of vegetarians depends on the foods consumed and the energy needs of the athlete. Generally, for all vegetarians, foods rich in iron, calcium, zinc, and protein should be included daily; fortified foods and dietary supplements can be helpful in some scenarios. Vegetarians who consume milk, eggs, cheese, and yogurt can meet their nutrient needs more easily.

Effects on Exercise and Athletic Performance

Research is limited on the long-term effect of vegetarianism on athletic performance (93). At this time, nutrient-rich vegetarian meal patterns are thought to be neither beneficial nor detrimental to athletic performance (94) (95) but can be appropriate for athletes if well chosen (11, 89). Studies are needed to examine elite athletes who habitually consume vegetarian diets. The effect of vegetarian diets on promoting or maintaining changes in athlete body composition also needs to be explored because the achievement of the body composition associated with optimal performance

Table 14.7 Types and Characteristics of Vegetarian Diets

Types of vegetarian diets	Diet characteristics
Vegan	Avoids all animal products and animal-derived foods.
Ovo-vegetarian	Allows eggs but no other animal products.
Lacto-vegetarian	Allows milk and milk products.
Lacto-ovo vegetarian	Allows milk, dairy products, and eggs but no other animal products.
Semivegetarian	Allows some animal-derived foods. Red meat is often the primary animal food not allowed.
Pesco-vegetarian	Allows seafood but no other animal products.
Ovo-pesco vegetarian	Allows seafood and eggs but no other animal products.
Lacto-ovo-pesco vegetarian	Allows dairy products, seafood, and eggs but no other animal products.

is now recognized as a challenging but important goal (11).

Effects on Health

Although data do not support a performance benefit as a result of following vegetarian diet patterns, several reported health-related outcomes are associated with these diet plans. Vegetarian diets have been shown to be lower in saturated fat while providing higher levels of carbohydrate, fiber, magnesium, potassium, carotenoids, and flavonoids (11, 89). Vegetarians have also been reported to have lower death rates from heart disease and associated risk factors such as hypertension and high cholesterol. Vegetarian diets are also endorsed by the American Cancer Association (96) and are associated with a lower risk of prostate and colon cancer (89).

Health benefits associated with a vegetarian diet are multifactorial and likely a result of what a person is both eating and not eating. Increased consumption of phytonutrients, antioxidants, and dietary nitrate are likely key in promoting overall health and might help athletes avoid some of the oxidative stress and immunosuppression effects seen with heavy training (90).

Nutrition Needs

Nutrient concerns for vegetarian athletes can include inadequate intake of energy, protein, fat, and omega-3 fatty acids (figure 14.7) (89). For active people, a vegetarian diet might provide insufficient energy to maintain weight and fuel performance. Often the solution to this problem is to consume higher-energy foods such as nuts, beans, corn, starchy vegetables like peas and potatoes, avocados, dried fruits, and 100 percent fruit juices.

Although vegetarian athletes who include some animal products should be able to meet protein needs easily, vegans should be very aware of protein content of plant foods and consider this in their meal planning. One of the key tenants of vegan diet planning is to choose a variety of

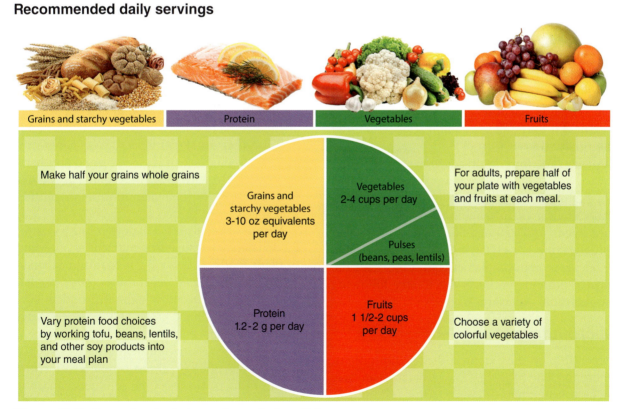

Figure 14.7 Example of a balanced vegetarian diet.

foods to meet energy needs to preserve protein utilization and to consume all essential amino acids in each meal. Fortunately, combining complementary protein foods at every meal is no longer thought to be necessary (97). Nevertheless, complementary foods should be a foundation of the diet plan, along with plant sources that contain all nine essential amino acids. These excellent sources of protein include soy foods such as soybeans, tempeh, and tofu. See figure 14.8 for examples of complementary protein foods.

Although usually not deficient in dietary protein, vegetarian athletes often consume less protein than their nonvegetarian counterparts. In addition, because plant proteins have a lower protein bioavailability, a modest increase in protein intake has been suggested for vegetarian athletes (91). For example, a recent study of vegetarian athletes found that an additional 10 grams of daily protein would be needed to reach the 1.2 g/kg daily target and 22 additional grams would be needed to reach the 1.4 g/kg daily target (11, 98). Meeting daily protein needs to support athletic performance is important, as is supporting muscle protein synthesis by providing an even spread of protein intake across the day and consuming enough energy to support growth and maintenance of lean tissue. Vegetarian athletes should also be reminded that muscle protein synthesis occurs through stimulation of the protein synthetic machinery in response to a rise in leucine concentrations in combination with other essential amino acids from food for incorporation into new proteins (99). In addition to consuming a variety of high-quality plant protein sources, physically active vegetarians should also consume plant foods rich in leucine, such as soybeans, nuts, seeds, and legumes. Studies are still needed to determine the effectiveness of concentrated vegetable protein supplements in stimulating the muscle protein synthesis machinery following various modes of exercise.

Micronutrients

Depending on the extent of dietary limitations, micronutrient concerns for vegetarianism may include iron, zinc, calcium, iodine, vitamin D, and vitamin B_{12} (11, 89). Being a physically active vegetarian is a risk factor for low iron status, mainly because of the low bioavailability of non-heme plant sources. Physically active vegetarians should thus be regularly screened and aim for an iron intake greater that the RDA (i.e., >18 mg for women and >8mg for men) (100, 101). Females might be at greater risk because iron requirements for female athletes can increase up to 70 percent of the EAR (102). Because of the decreased bioavailability of non-heme sources, iron intakes for vegetarians have been recommended as 1.8 higher than for nonvegetarians (103).

Iron deficiency in all athletes can occur with or without anemia and impair athletic performance by decreasing muscle function and limiting work capacity (101, 104). Even in the absence of anemia, a compromised iron status has been shown to have a negative effect on endurance competition times (102). Athletes with clinically diagnosed iron deficiency should follow medical advice that usually includes oral iron supplementation (105), dietary interventions, and follow-up appointments with their care provider. Reversing iron-deficiency anemia can take 3 to 6 months; this delayed response continues to allow side effects that affect health and performance during the treatment timeframe. This consequence highlights the importance of monitoring iron intake from the diet and adopting eating strategies that promote an increased intake of food sources of well-absorbed iron (11). Athletes concerned about iron status or who have iron deficiency without anemia (e.g., low ferritin without IDA) should increase their intake of food sources containing well-absorbed iron (e.g., heme iron and non-heme iron combined with vitamin C foods) as the first line of defense in their plan to promote optimal iron status.

Vegans are also at risk of developing a vitamin B_{12} deficiency because this nutrient is not found in plant foods. Because B_{12} is found in virtually all animal products, vegetarians following less limited plans that allow animal products such as dairy should have no trouble getting enough B_{12}. Vegans must rely on an additional source of B_{12}, including fortified milk alternatives such as soy milk, fortified breakfast cereal, and fortified yeast products. If these food products cannot be consumed regularly, a supplemental form of B_{12} is recommended.

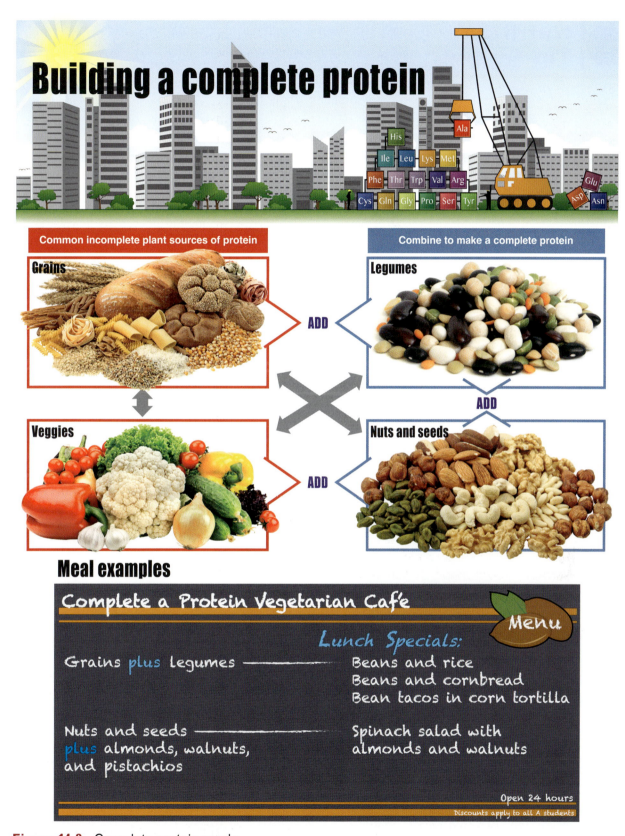

Figure 14.8 Complete protein meals.

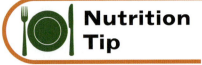

Nutrition Tip

Iron bioavailability in a vegetarian diet can be maximized in several ways. Good sources of non-heme iron such as spinach can provide more absorbable iron by combining spinach with fresh citrus vinaigrette or a fresh squeeze of lemon. Iron bioavailability in green leafy vegetables can also be improved by blanching them in boiling water for 5 to 10 seconds. Cooking vegetarian dishes in cast-iron skillets increases the iron content of food, especially if the food is acidic, such as tomato sauce.

Estimates are that 50 percent of female distance runners consume less than the RDA for zinc, so this mineral is of concern for vegetarian athletes, particularly if a diet is poorly chosen and has low energy intake. Studies have shown that zinc intake and zinc status is highly variable in vegetarian athletes, which is partly explained by GI absorption inhibitors such as phytate and fiber that are abundant in vegetarian diets (106). As with other minerals in the vegetarian diet, zinc-rich foods should be included when planning meals.

Vegetarians who consume dairy take advantage of the most bioavailable source of calcium in the U.S. diet. Vegans, on the other hand, tend to have lower calcium intakes than nonvegetarians and lacto-ovo vegetarians and often fall below the RDA (89). Vegetarian athletes might have an increased risk of lower bone mineral density (107). Foods rich in calcium should be a focus in vegetarian meal planning. In some cases, calcium supplementation is required to meet needs, especially if a vegetarian athlete is restricting energy intake. Calcium needs increase to 1,500 mg per day to optimize bone health in athletes with low energy availability or menstrual dysfunction (11).

Other Concerns

Vegetarian diets might also be low in creatine and carnosine, which can be problematic for athletes who rely on strength, power, and anaerobic performance (108). Dietary creatine is found in animal flesh, and vegetarians have been shown to have a lower body creatine pool than nonvegetarians (109, 110). In both vegetarians and nonvegetarians about 1 gram of creatine is synthesized per day from endogenous body amino acids. Those who consume meat obtain approximately 1 gram

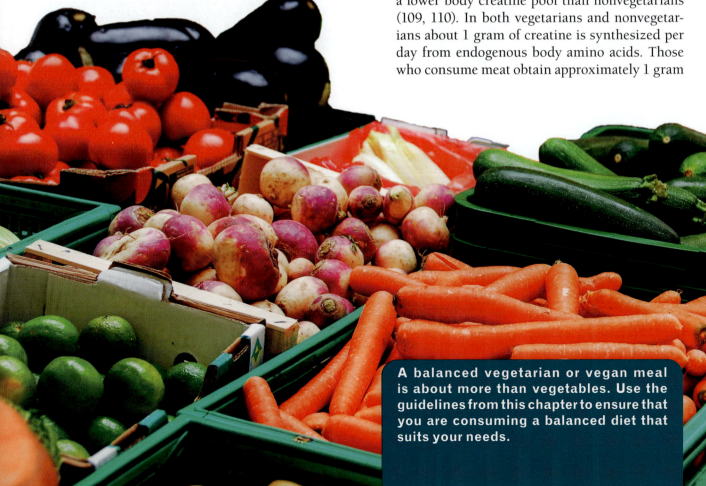

A balanced vegetarian or vegan meal is about more than vegetables. Use the guidelines from this chapter to ensure that you are consuming a balanced diet that suits your needs.

per day of additional creatine. Vegetarians who supplement with creatine tend to have a greater increase in strength, lean body mass accretion, and muscle creatine concentrations, as well as improved work performance (110). Another interesting finding is that a lacto-ovo vegetarian diet does not preserve muscle creatine levels, indicating that dairy products and eggs are not a replacement for meat when attempting to maintain body stores of creatine (111). Vegetarian athletes who rely heavily on strength and power performance can benefit from short-term creatine supplementation. Although anecdotal reports of side effects of creatine supplementation exist, no concerns regarding short-term use have been confirmed. The long-term effects of creatine supplementation are not well described in the scientific literature.

PEOPLE WITH DISORDERED EATING AND EATING DISORDERS

Reports of eating behavior problems have become increasingly prevalent in the past decade, for both athletes and the general population. Athletes face unique challenges; they must deal with the common sociocultural influences as well as the pressure of fitting in and competing at a high level alongside peers and competitors. Many athletes are susceptible to a strong sense of pressure to look and perform a certain way, which might be compounded by coaches, trainers, and family members who have a strong opinion about the ideal body shape and size required to excel. An obsession with obtaining a particular body composition can trigger short- and long-term health problems for both male and female athletes that stem from low energy availability, disordered eating behaviors, and clinically defined eating disorders (EDs).

Disordered Eating Spectrum

Disordered eating (DE) behaviors develop in athletes when they continue to strive for an "ideal" at the expense of health and performance goals, leading to eating disturbances that can cause diagnosable EDs. Those who participate in weight-sensitive sports have the highest risk of developing disordered eating patterns. According to position statements from the International Olympic Committee Medical Commission and the Australian Institute of Sport and National Eating Disorders Collaboration, these sports can be classified into three main groups (112, 113):

1. Gravitational sports in which moving the body against gravity is key to performance (e.g., long-distance running, mountain bike cycling, jumping sports)
2. Weight-class sports such as boxing, martial arts, wrestling, lightweight rowing, and weightlifting
3. Aesthetically judged sports such as figure skating, diving, and gymnastics

DE occurs across a spectrum, starting with eating and exercise behaviors that are appropriate in the short term, such as energy restriction at certain training periods to "lean-up" or "make weight." DE practices often involve a preoccupation with body weight and shape, food restriction, dieting, binge eating, vomiting, or abuse of diuretics, laxatives, and diet pills (114). In contrast, EDs are spectral disorders: They exist on a continuum of severity, have a specific clinical diagnosis, and often become more severe the longer they are present (113).

Normal eating patterns for athletes might include the occasional use of weight-loss methods that are typically short in duration, but for some, this effort can be coupled with strong body dissatisfaction. For some susceptible athletes, these behaviors—often a traditional part of their sport culture—can progress to chronic dieting and frequent weight fluctuation; fasting; passive (e.g., sauna or hot baths) or active dehydration (e.g., exercise with sweat suits) or both; and purging, such as use of laxatives, diuretics, vomiting, and diet pills. These behaviors might occur with or without excessive training (47). These athletes often feel as if they are fat on a daily basis, and their disordered eating behaviors can advance to become a clinically diagnosed ED, in which they succumb to extreme dieting, body image distortion, abnormal eating behaviors, and subsequent decreases in health and athletic performance (114). Failure to meet all criteria for anorexia nervosa or bulimia nervosa should not deter early and comprehensive intervention, because early recognition and intervention can potentially prevent further development of a clinically defined ED (113, 115). Even in the absence of a clinically defined ED, restrictive and purging behaviors are of concern because of their effect on energy availability.

Prevalence, Etiology, and Types

The prevalence of DE in athletes is almost impossible to estimate, but rates seem to continue to increase in many sports, including those that do not promote leanness (116). Prevalence of clinically defined EDs remains difficult to determine because many athletes do not seek diagnosis and treatment. Currently, estimates of the prevalence of DE or EDs in athletes ranges from 0 to 19 percent in males and 6 to 45 percent in females (113). Research on the topic of ED prevalence remains limited; few studies have been done in females, limited research has been done in males, and study designs are poor. Despite these limitations, it is generally agreed that there is a higher prevalence of DE and EDs in athletes compared with nonathletes (113). A large study in Norway compared groups of Olympic athletes with a control group and found that athletes had approximately a three times higher incidence rate of EDs (13.5%) compared with nonathlete controls (117). The presence of EDs is not restricted to female athletes; male athletes are susceptible as well. EDs exist in recreational, high school, and collegiate sports and among personal trainers. These diseases may coexist with other psychological comorbidities such as anxiety, depression, substance use, and obsessive-compulsive tendencies.

EDs go beyond weight dissatisfaction and involve more than abnormal eating patterns and pathogenic weight control behaviors. An ED is not about food per se; it is a mental illness. The best way to understand the significance of an ED diagnosis is to recognize that EDs are underpinned by a psychological pathology with serious nutrition and medical concerns.

EDs were once viewed as disorders of choice, meaning that the person afflicted could easily reverse their condition if they would just eat. This viewpoint did not foster providing guidance to families, and the concept of a genetic etiology was viewed as absurd. Over time etiological theory advanced from choice, to family dysfunction, to complex interactions among genetics, neurobiology, personality characteristics, and environmental factors. Over half of the variance associated with developing an ED is now thought to be attributed to genetic susceptibilities that get "turned on" by a lifetime of environmental exposures (118). In other words, stressful environments may exacerbate EDs, but families or other specific environmental stressors are not independent contributors to ED etiology. Although genetic factors and genetic–environmental interactions (epigenetics) seem to be emerging as the cornerstone for ED etiology, the overall cause is considered multifactorial, involving interacting psychological, neurobiological, genetic, cultural, and social factors. A current prevailing theory is that neurophysiologic and genetic components might set the stage for ED development that could be triggered by weight loss and might be the reason that many psychological symptoms resolve with physical restoration. Therefore, when athletes face a sport culture that pressures them to reduce weight and body fat, support for DE is generated and often maintained. Psychosocial factors identified as contributing factors, which may occur alongside a backdrop of genetic predisposition, include a history of being teased, abuse, low self-esteem, and predisposing psychiatric diagnoses. Personality characteristics that help to cultivate EDs, once developed, include anxiety, perfectionism, low self-directedness, rigidity, emotional avoidance and isolation, and an obsessive evaluation of shape and weight control (113).

EDs are defined by specific physical and mental criteria, as outlined by the American Psychiatric Association's *Diagnostic and Statistical Manual of Mental Disorders, Fifth Edition (DSM-5)* (119). *DSM-5* has designated four categories of eating disorders:

- Anorexia nervosa
- Bulimia nervosa
- Binge eating disorder
- Other specified feeding or eating disorders

Anorexia Nervosa

An anorexia nervosa diagnosis requires three criteria, including the restriction of energy intake below what is required to maintain weight that leads to a significantly low body weight in the context of age, sex, developmental trajectory, and physical health.

A significantly low body weight in adults is defined as a weight that is less than minimally normal. A second requirement for diagnosis is an intense fear of gaining weight or becoming fat, or persistent behavior that interferes with weight gain, even when at a significantly low weight. The final requirement is a disturbance in the way that a person experiences body weight or shape, undue influence of body weight or shape on self-evaluation, or persistent lack of recognition of the seriousness of current low body weight.

The physical effects of anorexia nervosa are shown in figure 14.9. Athletes who meet all the requirements for anorexia nervosa are further classified into one of two subtypes:

> Restricting type: During the last 3 months, the athlete has not engaged in recurrent episodes of binge eating or **purging behavior**.

> Binge eating or purging type: During the last 3 months, the athlete has engaged in episodes of binge eating or purging behavior.

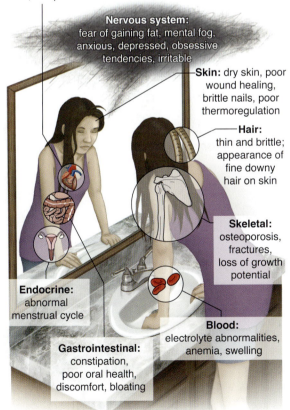

Figure 14.9 Physical effects of anorexia nervosa.

Bulimia Nervosa

A bulimia nervosa diagnosis has four specific criteria, characterized by

> recurrent episodes of binge eating once a week over 3 or more months and

> recurrent inappropriate compensatory behavior to prevent weight gain, such as self-induced vomiting;

> misuse of laxatives, diuretics, or other medications;

> fasting; and

> excessive exercise.

These first two criteria must occur, on average, at least once a week for 3 months. Athletes must also present with

> a self-evaluation that is unduly influenced by body shape and weight, and

> symptoms indicating that the disturbance does not occur exclusively during episodes of anorexia nervosa.

Binge Eating Disorder

The distinct diagnosis of binge eating disorder is newer to *DSM-5* and is intended to increase awareness of the substantial differences with the all-too-common phenomenon of overeating. Binge eating disorder is not just the occasional second helping of food; rather, the disorder includes feeling out of control during the eating episode and feeling distressed about the eating pattern. Binge eating is defined by consuming an amount of food that is definitely larger than most people would eat in a similar period under similar circumstances marked by feelings of lack of control during the eating episode. For an athlete to receive a binge eating disorder diagnosis, key criteria must be met, including recurrent episodes of binge eating that are associated with three or more of the following:

> Eating much more rapidly than normal

> Eating until feeling uncomfortably full

> Eating large amounts of food when not feeling physically hungry

> Eating alone because of embarrassment by how much one is eating

> Feeling disgusted with oneself, depressed, or guilty after eating

Three additional criteria must also be met:

> Binge eating is accompanied by a marked level of distress.
> The binge eating occurs, on average, at least once a week for 3 months.
> The binge eating is not associated with the recurrent use of inappropriate compensatory behavior and does not occur exclusively during the course of bulimia nervosa or anorexia nervosa.

Although disproportionately more females than males develop anorexia and bulimia, with binge eating disorder the ratio is less disparate, at an approximate 3-to-2 female-to-male ratio. Although overeating is a challenge for many Americans, a recurrent binge eating pathology is much less common, far more severe, and associated with significant physical and psychological problems.

Other Specified Feeding or Eating Disorders

At one time, the most frequent eating disorder diagnosis among athletes was eating disorder not otherwise specified (EDNOS), because relatively few patients met the strict criteria for the diagnosis of bulimia nervosa or anorexia nervosa. Those who develop disordered eating behaviors that advance to an eating disorder clinical diagnosis most often first meet the criteria for a newly defined diagnosis called other specified feeding or eating disorders (OSFED) (120, 121). Generally, OSFED is defined as a feeding or eating disorder that causes significant distress or impairment but does not meet the criteria for another feeding or eating disorder. OSFED is a new addition to eating disorder diagnoses found in *DSM-5*. The diagnosis of OSFED is still serious; patients have significant concerns about eating and body image, and health risks are similar to those for the other eating disorders. For example, an athlete who shows almost all of the symptoms of anorexia nervosa but who has retained a normal body mass index can be diagnosed with OSFED.

According to *DSM-5*, OSFED has five subtypes that are atypical of other eating disorder diagnoses:

1. Atypical anorexia nervosa—restrictive behaviors without meeting low weight criteria
2. Bulimia nervosa—lower frequency or limited duration of bingeing and purging
3. Binge eating disorder at a lower frequency or limited duration
4. Purging disorder—recurrent purging of calories through self-induced vomiting, misuse of laxatives and diuretics, or excessive exercising without binge eating behaviors
5. Night eating syndrome—recurrent episodes of night eating, as manifested by eating after awakening from sleep or by excessive food consumption after the evening meal

In the OSFED eating disorder category is also the diagnosis of unspecified feeding or eating disorder. This category serves as a preliminary diagnosis when insufficient information is available to make a specific diagnosis. Symptoms may include any of the disordered eating patterns that cause significant distress or impairment.

? DO YOU KNOW?

Chew and spit (CHSP) is a compensatory behavior sometimes seen in those with ED. It involves chewing typically calorie-dense food and spitting it out before it is swallowed in an attempt not to ingest unwanted calories. CHSP leads to psychological and emotional distress and potential physiological issues such as damage to teeth, stomach ulcers, and alterations in hormones leading to a subsequent increase in hunger (122).

Effect of Disordered Eating on Health and Performance

Although some sports are more associated with eating disorders than others, athletes in any sport can develop an eating disorder. Also, athletes might show signs of short-term disordered eating patterns without developing a clinically defined eating disorder. Any sustained disordered eating pattern is a risk factor for both health and performance concerns.

Health Concerns

Before we look at health concerns associated with disordered eating and eating disorders, remember that these conditions occur along a continuum and may affect different athletes in different ways. An athlete with an eating disorder may appear normal and physically healthy while maintaining their training load and volume. On the other hand, an athlete with disordered patterns or OSFED may have health problems as significant as some cases of anorexia or bulimia nervosa. Initial weight changes might not affect health in ways that can be observed by peers. Behavioral changes such as social withdrawal, teammate conflict, reduced self-esteem or self-confidence, a loss of competitiveness, or an onset of depression and anxiety are not unusual.

Historically, the concept of low energy availability and its effect on health emerged (11) from the study of the female athlete triad (often shortened to triad) (figure 14.10). The triad is formed by the interconversion of three clinical conditions typically observed in young female athletes: disordered eating, menstrual irregularities, and low bone mineral content or density. Each of these three components occurs along a continuum, and at any one time each component could independently present as being mild, moderate, or severe. For instance, a female athlete with a disordered eating pattern might not meet the criteria for an eating disorder but might restrict energy intake enough to produce low energy availability during heavy training. The occurrence of oligomenorrhea or amenorrhea is believed to be induced by some degree of low energy availability and is detrimental to bone mineral density when female athletes present with low energy availability and dysmenorrheic tendencies. Some female athletes with dysmenorrhea have been found to have low bone mineral density in the lumbar spine, hip, and whole body and have an increased risk of bone stress injuries (123, 124). Obtaining a history of disordered eating behaviors is valuable because the effects of low energy availability on bone are cumulative (125).

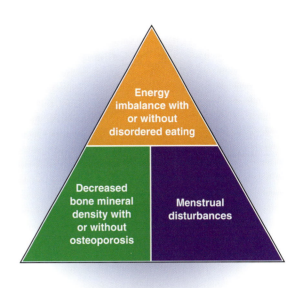

Figure 14.10 Female athlete triad.

Our understanding of the triad has evolved into a broader understanding of the concerns associated with any movement along the spectra away from optimal energy availability, menstrual status, and bone health (4). We now know that other physiological consequences can result from one of the components of the triad in active females, such as endocrine, gastrointestinal, renal, neuropsychiatric, musculoskeletal, or cardiovascular dysfunction (11). Further, this long list of physiological concerns also affects the health of male athletes, leading to an extension of the triad termed relative energy deficiency in sport (RED-S) and recent discussion of making the male athlete triad an official entity in the near future (126). RED-S encompasses several physiological complications observed in males and females involved in sport who consume energy intakes insufficient to meet the needs for optimal body function after the energy cost of exercise has been removed (127). Health and performance consequences of RED-S are shown in figures 14.11 and 14.12.

Performance Problems

Exercise performance might not always be altered by disordered eating or in the early stages of an eating disorder, but as an eating disorder becomes more severe, the downfall of performance is

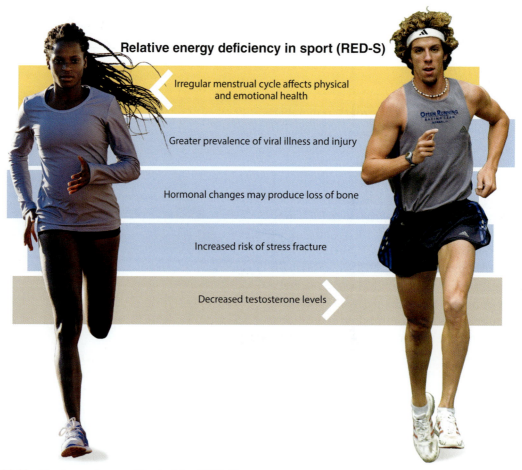

Figure 14.11 Body systems affected by RED-S.

inevitable. In some cases this decline will present as a physical injury that sidelines the athlete from training and competition. In other cases, the onset of performance decline is more gradual and might be a direct result of nutrition deficiencies, low energy intake, the direct physical stress of purging behaviors, or interrupted and less effective training (113).

A significant and chronic reduction in energy intake directly leads to reduced carbohydrate intake, which creates a greater reliance on body proteins to meet energy demands of the sport. The result will ultimately be reduced muscle mass, decreased performance, and increased risk of injury. Energy intake is also strongly linked to micronutrient intake, so active people with an eating disorder will be at greater risk of inadequate consumption of calcium, iron, and other important nutrients. To simplify, the direct effect of inadequate nutrition on performance with eating disorders is most associated with low energy availability. Low energy availability can occur from calorie restriction, excessive energy expenditure from exercise, or a combination of the two. People with an eating disorder and low energy availability will lack the energy necessary to sustain high levels of exercise intensity and might also experience significant bone loss and iron depletion that impair performance. Low energy availability also disrupts normal hormonal responses, which can negatively influence adaptation to training and, for females, promote menstrual dysfunction. Other direct effects of low energy availability resulting from an eating disorder that negatively affect performance include decreased endurance, impaired judgment, decreased coordination, decreased concentration, irritability, depression, decreased glycogen stores, and decreased muscle strength (127). Similar to other aspects of medical complications that result from disordered eating and eating disorders, impairments of health and performance

Nutrition Concerns for Special Populations

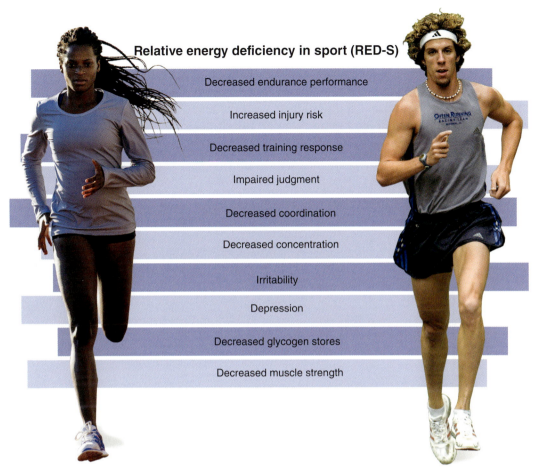

Figure 14.12 RED-S impairs exercise performance in many ways.

occur across a continuum of reductions in energy availability and do not occur at one specific energy availability value or threshold. Note that low energy availability is not synonymous with negative energy balance or weight loss, because chronic low energy availability might reset and lower the athlete's metabolic rate in such a way that low energy intake does not result in weight loss. Low energy availability in male and female athletes can clearly compromise athletic performance in both the short and long term (11).

Prevention and Management

As with most medical conditions, the best defense against eating disorders is prevention. Education is the best evidence-based method and driving force behind prevention. Education can be used to raise nutrition literacy to prevent an unhealthy relationship with food, medical problems, and poor performance. Education should also target elements related to increasing awareness of the problem and its risk factors and safe strategies

PUTTING IT INTO PERSPECTIVE

HELP FOR EATING DISORDERS

Athletes are at increased pressure to perform and have their body shaped in a specific way. Their appearance, as well as their athletic performance, is analyzed. These pressures could trigger an eating disorder or disordered eating in the athlete. If you know someone with an eating disorder or disordered eating, contact the Helpline at 800-931-2237 or seek online resources at www.nationaleatingdisorders.org.

to improve body composition (113). Being able to identify athletes at risk sooner rather than later requires basic knowledge of the signs and symptoms of disordered eating. To address this subject, all athletes, coaches, and athletics staff members should ideally complete a comprehensive education program and pursue continuing education opportunities. Physical, medical, psychological, and behavioral characteristics of the eating disorder spectrum are provided in table 14.8. Prevention of eating disorders occurs on three levels: primary, secondary, and tertiary. Each level is distinctly designed to prevent development and progression to the next level to keep the clinical condition from becoming chronic and debilitating.

Table 14.8 Three Prevention Levels of Eating Disorders

Prevention category	Goals	Targeted intervention
Primary	Protect individuals' predisposing risk factors	Education and instruction • Begins as early as puberty • Focuses on healthy eating, healthy lifestyle patterns, and positive self-image
Secondary	Early identification of those at risk, low energy availability, and the provision of early treatment	Screening and measurement • Eating disorders inventory (EDI) • Eating attitudes test (EAT) • DSM-5
Tertiary	Treatment of clinically defined eating disorders	Multidisciplinary interventions • Medical care • Psychological care • Nutritional care

Based on Maughan (2013).

SUMMARY

This chapter addressed many of the nutrition concerns in exercise, physical activity, and sport that are seen at different life stages (child, adolescent, masters, pregnant), in the vegetarian lifestyle, and in pathological conditions including diabetes mellitus, metabolic syndrome, disordered eating, and eating disorders. For the child and adolescent, the importance of understanding their key physiological differences as compared with adults was emphasized. Nutrition recommendations were presented for this life-stage group. Energy expenditure, substrate utilization, and thermoregulation during exercise are all physiologically different in children. Adolescents have increased requirements for energy and many nutrients as a result of rapid anatomical, physiological, and metabolic changes. In terms of their nutrition needs, children and adolescents should not be considered small adults. At the other end of the lifespan, masters athletes have their own unique nutrition challenges. In aging, a stronger focus is placed on the physiological benefits of exercise and the way in which nutrition can augment those effects. Unfortunately, data are insufficient on the specific nutrition needs of masters athletes, but we have good evidence of the importance of hydration, protein intake, and several key micronutrients.

Disease processes and lifestyle choices can also create unique nutrition concerns. Diabetes mellitus provides unique challenges for athletes and the peers and staff who work with them. A good understanding of the physiological processes involved in blood glucose response to exercise, diet, and medication is necessary to promote exercise performance and long-term health and safety. Knowledgeable and careful planning of dietary strategies that work in parallel with medication regimens to promote euglycemia before, during, and postexercise can support successful exercise and competition.

The vegetarian lifestyle can effectively support exercise and athletic performance. Vegetarian and vegan female athletes, however, are at increased risk for nonanemic iron deficiency, which may limit endurance performance. Vegans should follow a carefully chosen diet to obtain adequate intakes of iron, calcium, zinc, and vitamin B_{12}. If selected properly, vegetarian and nonvegetarian diets are fully capable of providing all the nutrients necessary for the physically active person.

The diagnosis of an eating disorder is not easy. Athletes and nonathletes alike can exhibit disordered eating patterns, even if they do not meet the threshold for an eating disorder diagnosis. Conversely, not every athlete with a low body weight who occasionally exhibits disordered eating behavior has an eating disorder. An eating disorder diagnosis must encompass an identified psychological pathology associated with intense fear of gaining weight or of becoming fat, along with persistent behaviors that interfere with normal weight gain. Participating in exercise or sport and pursuing a well-chosen diet are generally healthy behaviors, but menstrual status, nutrition behaviors, energy availability, and exercise volume should also be assessed. Education on the prevalence, etiology, and clinical manifestations associated with eating disorders should be widespread in environments that are likely to cultivate such disorders, including many sport settings and situations.

FOR REVIEW

1. Describe how a child's anaerobic energy system is different from an adult's.
2. What is much more important than chronological age when evaluating a young athlete's nutrition needs and potential for athletic improvement?
3. What is the best strategy to prevent osteoporosis?
4. Which four micronutrients are needed at increased levels beyond the age of 50?
5. Explain the key differences between type 1 and type 2 diabetes mellitus.
6. For athletes with type 1 diabetes mellitus, what is the carbohydrate consumption goal during prolonged competition lasting 2 hours?
7. Why are vegans at an increased risk for anemia?
8. List some of the benefits of a vegetarian diet. What nutrients are of most concern for the vegetarian athlete?
9. Explain the difference between disordered eating and eating disorders.
10. What is meant by energy availability? How is this related to RED-S?

GLOSSARY

acetyl-CoA—An important molecule in the metabolism of carbohydrates, fats, and protein. Acetyl-CoA provides carbon atoms to the TCA cycle for energy production.

active transport—Movement of molecules across a cell membrane from a region typically of lower concentration to a region of higher concentration.

adenosine diphosphate (ADP)—Composed of adenosine and two phosphate groups; during glycolysis, ADP loses a phosphate group and energy is released.

adenosine monophosphate (AMP)—Composed of adenosine and one phosphate group; involved in energy metabolism.

adenosine triphosphate (ATP)—A molecule that stores the potential energy used to power many cellular activities. Composed of adenosine and three phosphate groups, ATP is created in cells from the breakdown of foods and is used when the cell needs energy to do something active, such as when a muscle cell contracts.

adipocytes—Fat cells.

adipose tissue—Body fat. Adipose tissue is found in subcutaneous (under the skin) locations and surrounding vital organs.

aerobic capacity—A measure of fitness demonstrating the maximal amount of oxygen that can be used by active muscles during physical activity.

aerobic physical activity—Exercise involving large muscle groups moved in a rhythmic manner for an extended time. Swimming, biking, and running are examples. Also termed endurance activity or aerobic exercise.

aerobic system—One of the body's energy systems; it has a large capacity to generate ATP but requires oxygen to function efficiently.

air displacement plethysmography (ADP)—A method to estimate body volume and thus body density. Instead of water displacement, air displacement is used. BOD POD is an example.

albumin—A simple form of protein that is soluble in water, such as that found in egg white, milk, and (in particular) blood serum, in which this protein serves as a transporter (carrying hormones, fatty acids, and more).

all-cause mortality—Death from all causes.

alpha bond—Connects two monosaccharides together within a disaccharide or polysaccharide. These bonds are digested readily in the human digestive system.

alpha-linolenic acid (ALA)—An omega-3 fatty acid found in plants, including flaxseeds and walnuts. ALA is an essential fat, the human body cannot make it, so it must be consumed in the diet.

amenorrhea—The absence of three or more menstrual periods in a row.

amylopectin—The branched chain form of starch representing about 75 percent of the total carbohydrate in plants.

amylose—The straight chain form of starch; amylose is composed of hundreds to thousands of glucose molecules and represents about 25 percent of the total carbohydrate in plants.

anabolism—Metabolic processes involving the synthesis of new molecules.

anaerobic activity—Intense activity performed without relying on oxygen over a short time. Sprinting is an example.

anaerobic system—An important energy system of the body that does not require oxygen. This system can produce ATP faster than the aerobic system can but is limited by carbohydrate availability and lactate production.

android—A body fat pattern representing accumulation of fat primarily in the abdominal region; often referred to as the apple shape.

anemia—A general term used to describe a deficiency of red blood cells or decreased capacity of red blood cells to carry oxygen. There are several types of anemia.

angiogenesis—The growth of new blood vessels.

antibodies—Proteins that make up the immune system and protect the body from foreign pathogens or substances perceived as threats (food allergies, for instance).

antioxidants—Compounds that protect plants from pests and disease and, in some cases, protect cells in the human body from damage caused by free radicals.

atherosclerosis—A disease characterized by plaque buildup in arteries that decreases the diameter of arteries, narrowing the space for blood to travel through. Atherosclerosis can increase risk for heart attack, stroke, and death.

ATP—A high-energy molecule used in all cells of the body and during exercise.

ATP synthase—A protein complex in the ETC that is responsible for regenerating ATP from ADP and inorganic phosphate.

Banned Substances Control Group (BSCG)—A group that tests supplements for banned substances and provides third-party certification.

basal metabolic rate (BMR)—A measure of energy expenditure accounting for basic metabolic demands (living) during rest. BMR is measured in a temperate environment after a 10- to 12-hour fast and refrainment from exercise for 10 to 12 hours.

beta bond—Connects two monosaccharides together within a disaccharide or polysaccharide. Carbohydrates with beta bonds cannot be digested in the human digestive tract.

beta cells—Insulin producing cells within the pancreas.

bile—Substance synthesized by the liver, stored in the gall bladder, and secreted into the small intestine to help digest dietary fat. A primary constituent of bile is cholesterol.

bioelectrical impedance analysis (BIA)—A method for estimating body composition based on the resistance (impedance) of an electrical current running through the body.

body composition—The composition of the body that is fat mass compared with fat-free mass (lean body mass). Body composition can be further divided into fat, muscle, water, and bone (a four-compartment model of measuring body composition).

body image—A subjective view of one's own body.

body mass index (BMI)—A person's weight in kilograms (kg) divided by height in meters squared.

body weight or body mass—How much a person weighs on a scale, usually expressed in pounds or kilograms.

branched chain amino acids (BCAAs)—Nonaromatic amino acids with a branch (a central carbon atom bound to three or more carbon atoms). The three BCAAs—leucine, isoleucine, and valine—are all proteinogenic.

calcitriol (1,25-dihydroxyvitamin D)—The active form of vitamin D in the body. Calcitriol is a steroid hormone that promotes calcium absorption, helps maintain blood calcium and phosphorus levels for normal bone mineralization, and has important physiological effects on cell growth, muscle, and immune system functioning while also reducing inflammation.

calorimetry—The act of measuring energy expenditure by observing changes in thermodynamic variables.

carbohydrate—An organic compound containing the elements carbon, hydrogen, and water. Carbohydrate is a major energy-yielding macronutrient in the human diet. The smallest carbohydrates are monosaccharides such as glucose, fructose, and galactose; the largest are polysaccharides such as starch and fiber.

carbohydrate loading—A nutrition strategy designed to avoid glycogen depletion during endurance activities by maximizing the storage of glycogen in muscles and liver through the consumption of a high-carbohydrate diet for a few days before an event.

carboxyl group—A weak acid group on a molecule characterized by having a carbonyl and hydroxyl group attached to the same terminal carbon atom.

cardiac output—The amount of blood that the heart pumps in 1 minute and equal to the product of the stroke volume and heart rate.

carnitine shuttle—Shuttle located in the mitochondria that is responsible for transferring long-chain fatty acids across the inner mitochondrial membrane to proceed toward beta-oxidation.

catabolism—The breakdown of molecules to generate usable energy.

celiac disease—An autoimmune digestive disease, leading to an abnormal immune response when the protein gluten is ingested.

cell membrane—The outer covering of a cell that controls the exchange of materials between the cell and its environment.

certified diabetes educator (CDE)—Health professional who possesses comprehensive knowledge of and experience in prediabetes, diabetes prevention, and management. A CDE educates people with diabetes and helps the medical team and patient with the management of the condition.

cheilosis—Inflammation and cracking of the lips at the corners of the mouth.

chelated—Attached to another compound; chelated minerals are often attached to an amino acid.

chemical digestion—The breakdown of food in the mouth, stomach, and intestines through the use of acids and enzyme-catalyzed reactions.

chemical energy—Energy released from food during metabolic processing.

chemiosmotic coupling—The continuous flow of hydrogen ions through the ETC protein channels driven by an electrochemical gradient that produces proton motive force to drive ATP synthase.

cholecystokinin (CCK)—Peptide hormone of the gastrointestinal system responsible for stimulating the digestion of fat and protein.

cholesterol—A lipid-like substance found in all cells in the body and incorporated into many hormones, vitamins, and substances used to help digest food. Cholesterol moves in the bloodstream in transport vesicles called lipoproteins. Cholesterol, a component of all animal tissues, is found only in animal-based foods including eggs, red meat, poultry, cheese, and milk. In the human body cholesterol is a structural component of cell membranes, helps repair and form new cells, and is necessary for synthesizing steroid hormones (such as testosterone, androgen, and estrogen) and bile acids.

chylomicron—Lipoprotein particles that transport dietary lipids from the intestines to other locations in the body; they consist primarily of triglycerides but also contain phospholipids, cholesterol, and other proteins.

chyme—The semifluid, pulpy acidic mass that passes from the stomach to the small intestine, consisting of gastric juices and partly digested food.

cis configuration—Unsaturated fatty acids with hydrogen ions on the same side of the double bond.

coenzyme A—Derived from pantothenic acid, a B-vitamin, and functions in metabolic reactions.

collagen—The main structural protein found in human connective tissue, including tendons, ligaments, and cartilage.

colon—The part of the digestive tract that extends from the end of the small intestine to the anus. It absorbs water, minerals, and vitamins from the intestinal contents and eliminates undigested material during defecation. Also called the large intestine.

complex carbohydrates (polysaccharides)—Longer chains of sugar molecules. Starch and fiber are examples. Plant and grain foods, such as peas, beans, breads, and vegetables, containing abundant strands of complex carbohydrates. Complex carbohydrates also have vitamins, minerals, and fiber important to human health.

concurrent training—Two training sessions performed back-to-back, such as speed training immediately followed by strength training or vice versa.

Cori cycle—Metabolic pathway in which lactate produced by the anaerobic energy system in muscle cells moves to the liver and is converted to glucose, which then returns to the muscles and serves as a fuel source.

crossover concept—Describes fat and carbohydrate utilization as fuel sources during exercise. Fat is the primary fuel source used during low intensity while carbohydrate is the primary source of fuel used during high-intensity exercise. The crossover point occurs when carbohydrate utilization exceeds fat utilization; the point at which this happens is determined by exercise intensity and aerobic fitness.

current good manufacturing practices (GMPs)—Manufacturing processes established and enforced by the U.S. Food and Drug Administration (FDA). GMPs provide systems and processes ensuring proper design, monitoring, and control of manufacturing processes and facilities.

cytoplasm—The entire contents of a cell except for the nucleus.

cytosol—A component of the cytoplasm where a variety of metabolic reactions occur.

daily value (DV)—An indicator of how much of one serving of a particular food contributes to a person's nutritional needs; the DV is based on a 2,000 kcal diet.

dehydration—The process of losing body water.

denature—A process through which proteins lose the quaternary structure, tertiary structure, and secondary structure because of exposure to a stimulus that changes protein structure. Common examples are strong acid (such as HCL in the stomach) and heat (cooking).

deoxyribonucleic acid (DNA)—A molecule that carries the genetic instructions used in the growth, development, functioning, and reproduction of all known living organisms.

dietary fat—The kind of fat found in foods and beverages.

dietary fiber—Material in plants, mostly nonstarch polysaccharides, that is not digested by human digestive enzymes and instead passes through the digestive tract relatively unchanged before being eliminated.

dietary reference intakes (DRIs)—Reference values for macro- and micronutrients aimed at preventing or reducing the risk of chronic disease and promoting optimal health.

dietary supplement—A product taken by mouth that contains a dietary ingredient intended to supplement the diet. The dietary ingredients in these products may include vitamins, minerals, herbs or other botanicals, amino acids, and substances such as enzymes and metabolites. Dietary supplements can also be extracts or concentrates and may be found in many forms such as tablets, capsules, soft gels, gel caps, liquids, and powders.

digestion—The breakdown of food into its constituent parts using mechanical and chemical methods.

digestive elimination—The elimination of undigested food content and waste products from the digestive tract.

digestive tract—A term for the entire gastrointestinal tract from the mouth to the anus.

direct calorimetry—Measures heat production by the body, using carbon dioxide, oxygen, and temperature measurements to determine energy expenditure.

disaccharide—Sugars composed of two monosaccharide units. In the human diet, the most common disaccharides are maltose, lactose, and sucrose.

diverticulitis—Inflammation or infection of the small pouches, called diverticula, that bulge outward from the center of the colon (large intestine).

diverticulosis—A condition in which the large intestine contains small pouches, called diverticula, that bulge outward from the center of the colon. Diverticula themselves are not problematic and people having diverticulosis are often asymptomatic.

docosahexaenoic acid (DHA)—An omega-3 fatty acid synthesized by microalgae and present in fish, fish oil, krill oil and algal oils. DHA is the major fat found in the brain and important for brain development and function. DHA is also used to form signaling molecules called eicosanoids and an important structural component of cell membranes.

Drug Free Sport International—A provider of drug-use prevention services for many athletic organizations; delivers strategic alternatives to traditional drug-use prevention programs.

dual-energy X-ray absorptiometry (DEXA)—A laboratory method used to measure bone mineral density and soft-tissue composition (percent body fat).

duodenum—The first part of the small intestine immediately beyond the stomach, leading to the jejunum.

dyslipidemia—Total cholesterol or triglyceride levels above the reference standard, or levels of high-density lipoprotein (HDL) cholesterol below a reference standard.

eccentric contractions—A movement where the skeletal muscle is lengthening. The downward phase of a biceps curl is an example.

eicosanoids—The physiologically active substances that are primarily derived from arachidonic acid; they are involved in intracellular signaling.

eicosapentaenoic acid (EPA)—An omega-3 fatty acid synthesized by microalgae and present in fish, fish oil, krill oil and some algal oils. EPA is used to form signaling molecules called eicosanoids and an important structural component of cell membranes.

electrolytes—Minerals that conduct electricity in the body. Electrolytes affect fluid balance, muscle pH, and muscle functioning. Sodium, chloride, potassium, calcium, magnesium, and phosphorus are electrolytes.

electron transport chain (ETC)—A series of protein complexes that transfers electrons from electron donors as a result of oxidation and reduction reactions while also transferring hydrogen ions within the mitochondria.

endoplasmic reticulum—A type of organelle in eukaryotic cells that is involved in protein synthesis.

endurance training—A regimen of physical activities designed to improve exercise endurance.

energy availability—The amount of energy available for body functions after the calories used during exercise is subtracted from the energy consumed in the diet.

energy-dense food—A food that has a high amount of energy (calories) per gram or portion of the food item.

energy dense—A substance that has a high amount of energy (calories) for a given mass or volume.

energy-yielding macronutrients—Nutrients that supply the body with energy; carbohydrates, fats, and proteins are the energy-yielding macronutrients. (Other macronutrients are water and lipids.)

enrichment—The addition of vitamins and minerals lost during food processing.

enterocytes—Epithelial cells found in the small intestine that contain digestive enzymes and microvilli on its surface.

enterokinases—Enzymes produced by cells of the duodenum and involved in human digestive processes.

enzymes—Protein-containing biological catalysts that accelerate or catalyze chemical reactions.

ergogenic—A term commonly used in sport as something intended to enhance physical performance or recovery from training.

essential amino acids—Amino acids that cannot be made by the human body and must be consumed in the diet.

essential fat—The amount of body fat necessary for physiological functioning. Essential fat is found in bone marrow, the heart, lungs, liver, spleen, kidneys, intestines, muscles, and fat-rich tissues of the central nervous system.

euglycemic—A normal concentration of glucose in the circulating blood.

euhydration—A state of hydration balance or normal water content.

excess postexercise oxygen consumption (EPOC)—Calories burned after exercise has ended.

exercise physiology—The study of the body's responses to exercise, from acute bouts to chronic adaptations with repeated activity and long-term training.

extreme sport—Any sport perceived as having a high level of inherent danger.

FADH$_2$—The reduced form of FAD used for metabolic reactions and derived from the B-vitamin riboflavin.

fat-free mass (FFM)—Anything that is not fat tissue. This includes muscle, connective tissue, bones, organs, and water.

fat soluble—Vitamins stored in the body's fat tissues and more easily absorbed when consumed with dietary fat. Vitamins A, D, E, and K are fat soluble.

fatty acid—A molecule consisting of a long chain of carbon and hydrogen atoms connected to a single acid group at its end. The long carbon chain can be any length, but the ones found in the human diet tend to have between 12 and 22 carbon atoms.

Federal Trade Commission (FTC)—The FTC protects American consumers by preventing fraud, deception, and unfair business practices and ensuring competition in the marketplace.

feedback inhibition—A control mechanism that catalyzes a reaction to produce a specific compound that can reduce the rate of a metabolic reaction when the compound reaches high concentrations.

female athlete triad (triad)—Syndrome of three interrelated conditions that exist on a continuum of severity, including energy deficiency with or without disordered eating, menstrual disturbances or amenorrhea, and low bone mineral density

fermentation—Anaerobic breakdown of sugars by microorganisms in the gut.

fiber—Nondigestible soluble and insoluble carbohydrates that have beneficial physiological effects to human health. Fiber can be naturally occurring parts from plants or synthetic.

food—The plants and animals that humans ingest.

fortification—The addition of nutrients to a food or beverage.

free radicals—Highly unstable reactive oxygen and nitrogen species that are naturally generated in the body during exercise and through metabolism. We are also exposed to free radicals through environmental sources such as cigarette smoke, environmental pollution and sunlight.

fructose—A monosaccharide carbohydrate found in many plant foods and some nutritive sweeteners.

galactose—A monosaccharide found in milk, usually bound to glucose as a disaccharide called lactose.

generally recognized as safe (GRAS)—A designation by the FDA that the substance intentionally added to a food is generally considered safe by experts under the intended conditions of use.

gestational diabetes mellitus (GDM)—High blood glucose levels during pregnancy in women who have never had diabetes. Diagnosis and management are important to protect the mother and baby's health.

glucagon—Hormone secreted by the alpha islet cells of the pancreas in response to hypoglycemia. Glucagon increases blood glucose concentration by stimulating glycogenolysis in the liver.

gluconeogenesis—Synthesis of glucose from noncarbohydrate sources in the liver and kidneys whenever the supply of carbohydrate is insufficient to meet the body's immediate requirements.

glucose—A monosaccharide found in plants primarily in the form of starch and also found in some nutritive sweeteners.

GLUT4—A protein found in cells that helps transport glucose across the cell membrane into the cytoplasm.

gluten—A protein found in foods made from wheat. Gluten gives dough it's elasticity, chewy texture and helps dough rise. Barley, rye and other grains contain proteins related to gluten (though all of these proteins are typically referred to as gluten).

glycemic index—A ranking of carbohydrates according to how quickly they are digested and absorbed, and therefore raise blood glucose levels in the 2-hour time period after a meal, compared with the same amount (by weight in grams) of a reference food, typically white bread or glucose, which is given a GI of 100.

glycemic load—An indicator of the glycemic effect of a food that takes into consideration both the glycemic index and carbohydrate content, in grams, of the food. Glycemic load is computed as the product of a food's glycemic index and its total available carbohydrate content: glycemic load = [GI × carbohydrate (g)]/100].

glycemic response—Change in blood glucose after consuming food.

glycogen—A branched polymer of glucose monosaccharides that serves as the storage form of carbohydrate in the liver and muscles of animals and humans.

glycogenesis—The synthesis of glycogen from glucose subunits for glycogen storage.

glycogenolysis—The metabolic breakdown of glycogen to glucose in the liver and skeletal muscle to maintain blood glucose levels or maintain energy for muscle contraction.

glycogen synthase—Key enzyme responsible for glycogen synthesis in liver and skeletal muscle.

glycolysis—Aerobic or anaerobic process that converts glucose into pyruvate and 2 ATP for cellular energy.

glycolytic—Involving glycolysis.

gynoid—A body fat pattern typically representing accumulation of body fat in the lower half of the body—in the hips, buttocks, and thighs. This pattern is often referred to as the pear shape.

health claims—Describes the relationship between a food, food component supplement ingredient, and decreased risk of a disease or health-related condition.

high-density lipoprotein (HDL)—Carries cholesterol back to the liver for excretion or recycling; HDL is sometimes referred to as "good cholesterol" and is not associated with an increased risk for heart disease.

high-fructose corn syrup (HFCS)—A manufactured nutritive sweetener commonly added to food to improve palatability and shelf life. HFCS is similar in sweetness to table sugar and contains roughly the same amount of fructose as glucose.

homeostasis—A state of balance or equilibrium.

hormones—Chemical messengers secreted directly into the blood to interact with organs and tissues of the body to exert their functions. There are many types of hormones, some of which are complex protein structures.

hydrodensitometry—In this reference method, water is used to estimate the body density and body fat of a person; also called hydrostatic weighing or underwater weighing (UWW).

hydrometry—A laboratory measurement of total body water (TBW).

hydroxyapatite—The storage form of calcium and phosphate in bones and teeth.

hypercalcemia—High blood calcium.

hyperglycemic—An abnormally high concentration of glucose in the circulating blood.

hyperhydration—Overhydration.

hyperphosphatemia—High blood phosphate.

hyperplasia—Growth of more cells.

hypertension—Long-term medical condition in which the blood pressure in the arteries is persistently elevated. Hypertension damages and weakens artery walls.

hypertrophy—Growth of existing cells.

hypoglycemia—An abnormally low concentration of glucose in the circulating blood.

hypohydration—The uncompensated loss of body water.

hyponatremia—Dangerously low blood sodium.

hypophosphatemia—Low blood phosphate.

indirect calorimetry—General energy expenditure measurement technique involving the measurement of oxygen and carbon dioxide gas exchange.

inflammation—The body's normal acute response to injury or attack from foreign invaders, involving localized heat, swelling, and pain. Ideally, inflammation is limited to what is required to counteract the present threat, but many chronic conditions are believed to be related to chronic inflammation (ongoing inflammation).

Informed Choice—A global quality assurance program and third-party supplement testing program designed to minimize the risks of dietary supplement products from being inadvertently contaminated with prohibited and potentially harmful substances.

insensible perspiration—Fluid that evaporates through pores in the skin by sweat glands before the body recognizes it as moisture on the skin.

insoluble fiber—Portion of dietary fiber that is not soluble in water and adds bulk to the stool for easier elimination.

insulin—Hormone secreted by the beta islet cells of the pancreas in response to hyperglycemia (high blood sugar). Insulin promotes glucose uptake and storage, amino acid uptake, protein synthesis, and lipid synthesis and fat storage.

insulin-dependent glucose transport (IDGT)—Process of transporting glucose into a cell that requires the involvement of insulin.

insulin resistance—A condition in which cells fail to respond to the normal actions of insulin.

interesterified fats—Fats that have had fatty acids rearranged, chemically or enzymatically, along the glycerol backbone.

isotopes—Element variations that have the same proton number but different neutron numbers.

ketoacidosis—A metabolic state associated with high concentrations of ketone bodies, formed by the breakdown of fatty acids and the deamination of amino acids. This is associated with a pathological metabolic state in which the body fails to regulate ketone production adequately, causing an accumulation of ketoacids and resulting in a decrease in the pH of the blood. In extreme cases, ketoacidosis can be fatal and is most common in those with untreated type 1 diabetes mellitus. Ketoacidosis should not be confused with ketone production and subsequent ketosis resulting from a ketogenic diet. Ketones produced from a ketogenic diet are managed by the body and do not result in ketoacidosis.

kilocalorie—A calorie. A unit of energy also called a kcal or large calorie. Refers to the amount of heat needed to raise the temperature of 1 kilogram (2.2 lb) of water by 1 degree Celsius (1.8 degrees Fahrenheit).

lactase—An enzyme that catalyzes the breakdown of lactose to glucose and galactose.

lactate—The molecule that remains when one hydrogen ion disassociates itself from a lactic acid molecule. Lactate serves as a fuel source that can be oxidized directly by many cells in the body, including brain, heart, and skeletal muscle. Lactate can also be converted back to pyruvate and glucose and oxidized in those forms.

lactate dehydrogenase (LDH)—The enzyme that catalyzes the reaction from pyruvate to lactate.

lactic acid—A substance produced when pyruvate, the end product of glycolysis, binds with two additional hydrogen ions. Normally, one of the hydrogen ions immediately disassociates itself from the molecule and causes its surrounding environment to become more acidic.

lactose—A disaccharide containing glucose and galactose. Commonly known as milk sugar because it is present in many dairy products.

lactose intolerance—A condition marked by incomplete digestion of lactose. Consumption of milk and other dairy products containing lactose may lead to symptoms including diarrhea, gas, and bloating in those with lactose intolerance. Dairy products vary in the amount of lactose they contain with some containing no lactose.

large intestine—The colon. The part of the digestive tract that extends from the end of the small intestine to the anus. It absorbs water, minerals, and vitamins from the intestinal contents and eliminates undigested material during defecation.

lean body mass (LBM)—The percentage of the body that is not fat. In a four-compartment model, LBM is composed of water, skeletal muscle, and bone.

linoleic acid (LA)—An omega-6 fatty acid that is an essential fat. The human body cannot make it, so it must be consumed in the diet.

lipids—A category of macronutrients that are insoluble in water and have various biological functions in the body. The three main types of lipids are triglycerides, sterols, and phospholipids.

lipogenesis—The metabolic process by which excess acetyl-CoA is converted into body fat.

lipoprotein—Any group of soluble proteins that combine with and transport fat or other lipids in the blood plasma.

liver—Glandular organ that has many functions in the body related to digestion and metabolism, including bile synthesis and secretion, gluconeogenesis, glycogen synthesis and storage, lipolysis, and transamination.

low-density lipoprotein (LDL)—A transport protein. LDL carries cholesterol from the liver to tissues. LDL is often referred to as "bad cholesterol" as high levels of LDL are associated with cardiovascular disease.

low energy availability—Energy intake that is insufficient to meet energy expenditure and physiological needs. Low energy availability can lead to detrimental effects on health and performance.

luminal brush border—Microvilli-covered surface of simple epithelium where nutrient absorption takes place. The microvilli that constitute the brush border have enzymes for digestion anchored into their plasma membrane as integral membrane proteins. These enzymes are found near transporters that allow absorption of the digested nutrients.

macronutrients—Nutrients required in the diet in larger amounts: carbohydrate, protein, and fat.

maltase—An enzyme that catalyzes the breakdown of maltose to glucose.

maltose—A disaccharide containing two glucose molecules. Maltose does not occur naturally in foods but rather during the enzymatic breakdown of starch during digestion.

mechanical digestion—Involves physically breaking the food into smaller pieces. Mechanical digestion begins in the mouth as food is chewed and continues in the stomach as it churns.

medical nutrition therapy (MNT)—An evidence-based application of the nutrition care process, usually including nutrition assessment, nutrition diagnosis, nutrition intervention, and nutrition monitoring and evaluation that typically results in the prevention, delay, or management of diseases or conditions.

medium chain triglycerides (MCTs)—A type of fat made up of a shorter carbon chain that allows it to bypass complex digestion and absorption processes and instead be absorbed directly into the blood.

messenger RNA (mRNA)—The form of RNA in which genetic information transcribed from DNA as a sequence of bases is transferred to a ribosome.

metabolic fatigue—A situation that occurs when exercise intensity rises to a level that prevents glucose from being aerobically oxidized, thereby causing lactate to accumulate in the cell.

metabolic syndrome—The name for a group of risk factors that raises one's risk for developing heart disease, diabetes, and stroke. The risk factors include abdominal obesity, high triglycerides, low HDL cholesterol, hypertension, and high fasting blood sugar.

metabolism—A collection of chemical reactions for bodily processes that consist of anabolic or catabolic reactions.

micronutrients—Nutrients required in small amounts, including vitamins and minerals.

microvilli—Folds and projections on enterocytes that serve to increase the surface area for the digestion and transport of nutrients from inside the intestine into the enterocyte.

mitochondria—The powerhouse of a cell where ATP production and respiration occurs.

modeling—The process through which new bone is formed or old bone is removed. Modeling occurs during childhood and adolescence and shapes bone size and strength.

monounsaturated fatty acids (MUFA)—A type of unsaturated fatty acid that contains one double bond.

mouth—Initial part of digestive tract. Mechanical digestion from chewing and chemical digestion from the action of salivary amylase occurs in the mouth.

muscle protein balance—The difference between skeletal muscle protein synthesis (MPS) and breakdown (MPB).

muscular endurance—The ability to perform repeated skeletal muscle contractions or to hold a contraction over a period of time.

muscular flexibility—The ability to move through the joint's range of motion.

muscular power—Rate at which the work (contraction) is performed.

muscular strength—The maximal force that a skeletal muscle or group of muscles can produce.

NADH (nicotinamide adenine dinucleotide)—The reduced form of NAD used for metabolic reactions. A key component of NADH is the B vitamin niacin.

NADPH (nicotinamide adenine dinucleotide phosphate)—A reduced form of NADP that is formed in the pentose phosphate pathway and used in anabolic reactions.

nonessential amino acids—Amino acids that can be synthesized by the human body and therefore do not need to be consumed.

nonexercise activity thermogenesis (NEAT)—The energy expended by the body for all activities not including exercise, sleeping, or eating.

nonnutritive sweeteners (NNS)—Sweeteners that do not contain a significant amount of energy.

NSF International—NSF International provides third-party certification, which is an independent analysis of a manufacturer's product with standards for safety, quality, and performance.

nucleus—Present in eukaryotic cells; the control center of the cell that contains genetic material.

nutrient absorption—The process of absorbing or assimilating digested substances into cells through diffusion or osmosis.

nutrient content claim—Statement about the level of a nutrient in a product. These are approved and regulated by the FDA and can be used on both foods and dietary supplements.

nutrient density—The relationship of nutrients contained in a food to the amount of energy or calories the food provides. Foods considered nutrient dense provide a lot of nutrients with relatively little energy (calories). This term generally refers to health promoting nutrients.

nutrients—Specific substances that elicit a biochemical or physiological function in the body.

nutrigenomics—The interaction between nutrition and genes.

nutrition periodization—A principle in which nutritional guidelines are adjusted depending on the state of training.

nutrition—As a scientific discipline, the study of how food supplies nutrients to the body and influences health and life.

nutritive sweeteners—Sweeteners that also contain energy.

obesity—A disease in which body weight is greater than what is considered normal or healthy for a certain height due to extra body fat. For adults, "obesity" is defined as a BMI range of 30 to 34.9. A score of 35 or above is "severely obese."

oligomenorrhea—Light or infrequent menstrual periods occurring in women of childbearing age; often defined as a woman who regularly goes more than 35 days without menstruating.

oligosaccharide—Carbohydrates composed of 3 to 10 monosaccharide units.

oral glucose tolerance test (OGTT)—A screening test for diabetes mellitus, in which plasma glucose levels are measured in a person after consuming an oral glucose load. An OGTT reveals type 2 diabetes mellitus or impaired glucose tolerance when plasma glucose levels exceed defined thresholds after consuming the glucose load.

organelles—Found in eukaryotic cells; they have specialized functions within a cell (e.g., nucleus, chloroplast, mitochondria, etc.).

osmolarity—The concentration of solutes, particularly sodium, in the blood.

osteoporosis—A disease characterized by low bone mass and structural deterioration of bone tissue leading to fragile bones and greater risk of fractures; usually of the hip, spine, or wrist.

overload—Gradual increase of stress placed on the body during training.

overreaching—An increase in exercise volume as part of a training program. Overreaching can lead to temporary fatigue and short-term performance decrement, but the athlete quickly returns to normal or even slightly increased function. With long-term overreaching, the body's functional capabilities may be suppressed for several days. However, they rebound (i.e., increase beyond pretraining values) dramatically when the overreaching stimulus is removed.

overtraining—The volumes and intensities of the training being performed that contribute to the inability of the human body to adequately recover. The net result is the overtraining syndrome, a myriad of symptoms and conditions that collectively contribute to impaired performances.

overweight—Body weight that is greater than what is considered normal or healthy for a certain height. For adults, "overweight" is defined as a BMI of 25 to 29.9.

oxaloacetate—A four-carbon compound that combines with acetyl-CoA to initiate the TCA cycle to form citrate. It is also involved in gluconeogenesis, the urea cycle, amino acid synthesis, and fatty acid synthesis.

oxidative decarboxylation—Forms carbon dioxide from the splitting of a carbon-carbon bond.

oxidative phosphorylation—The use of the aerobic energy system to use macronutrient fuel sources (carbohydrate, protein, fat) to phosphorylate ADP to form ATP.

oxidative stress—An imbalance between free radicals and the body's antioxidant defenses.

pancreas—Glandular organ that secretes enzymes for the digestion of carbohydrates, proteins, and fats; also secretes the hormones glucagon and insulin that regulate the metabolism of carbohydrates, proteins, and fats.

pancreatic amylase—An enzyme secreted from the pancreas into the small intestine during digestion that catalyzes the breakdown of starch into sugars.

peak bone mass—Maximum bone strength and density.

pepsin—A protease enzyme that breaks down food proteins into smaller peptides. Produced in the stomach, pepsin is one of the main digestive enzymes in the digestive systems of humans.

pepsinogen—The proenzyme of pepsin, made and released by chief cells in the stomach wall.

peptide bonds—Chemical attachment formed between two molecules, usually involving two amino acids. A carboxyl group of one molecule reacts with an amino group of another molecule releasing a molecule of water.

phosphocreatine (PCr)—A fuel substrate that can rapidly donate its phosphorous group to ADP to form ATP.

phosphagen system (ATP-PC system)—A one-step, anaerobic pathway that uses creatine phosphate to generate ATP.

phospholipids—Structural components of cell membranes and lipoproteins. Phospholipids are necessary for the absorption, transport, and storage of lipids and aid in the digestion and absorption of dietary fat.

photosynthesis—As it relates specifically to human nutrition, photosynthesis is the process through which plants use energy from the sun to convert carbon dioxide and water into glucose plus oxygen.

physical activity level (PAL)—A factor used to express daily physical activity, typically used to estimate a person's total energy expenditure. PAL is often used in combination with the basal metabolic rate to compute the amount of food energy a person needs to consume to maintain a particular lifestyle.

polydipsia—Excessive thirst or excess drinking often associated with uncontrolled diabetes mellitus.

polypeptide—Chains of amino acids linked by a peptide bond that serve as components of proteins.

polyphagia—Excessive hunger or increased appetite that may be caused by medical disorders such as diabetes mellitus.

polysaccharide—Carbohydrate composed of long chains of monosaccharides linked by glycosidic bonds (e.g., cellulose, starch, and glycogen).

polyunsaturated fatty acids (PUFA)—A type of unsaturated fatty acid that contains more than one double bond. Polyunsaturated fatty acids are identified based on the location of their first double bond. Omega-3 and omega-6 fatty acids are examples.

polyuria—Excessive or abnormally large production or passage of urine; often associated with uncontrolled diabetes mellitus.

portal vein—A blood vessel that carries blood from the gastrointestinal tract, gallbladder, pancreas, and spleen to the liver.

postprandial hypoglycemia—Low blood sugar that occurs soon after consuming a meal, usually containing carbohydrate. Also called reactive hypoglycemia.

preformed vitamin A—The active form of vitamin A in the body; preformed vitamin A is found in animal liver, whole milk, and some fortified foods.

principle of detraining—Involves the loss of physiological training responses when exercise is discontinued.

principle of periodization—Training for a particular sport or event into scheduled into smaller periods or blocks that each have specific training goals.

principle of specificity—The training routine must induce a physical stress specific to the system needed for performance enhancements.

proenzyme—A biologically inactive protein that is metabolized into an active enzyme.

proprietary blends—A list of ingredients that are part of a product formula specific to a particular dietary supplement manufacturer. The names and quantities of the individual ingredients in the blend are not disclosed.

protease activation cascade—A series of enzymatic events that lead to the activation of several digestive enzymes.

proteinogenic—Amino acids that are precursors to proteins and are incorporated into proteins during translation.

proton motive force—The electrochemical force generated by the electron transport chain that drives ATP synthase to create ATP.

provitamin A carotenoids—Dark-colored pigments found in some vegetables, oily fruits, and red palm oil. Provitamin A carotenoids include beta-carotene, alpha-carotene, and beta-cryptoxanthin and must be converted to the active form of vitamin A in the body.

purging behavior—Self-induced vomiting or misuse of laxatives, diuretics, or enemas. Purging behaviors are present in many eating disorders.

pyrophosphate—The free phosphate group used to form ADP and ATP; sometimes referred to as inorganic phosphate.

pyruvate dehydrogenase complex (PDC)—A formation of three enzymes that act to convert pyruvate to acetyl-CoA.

quackery—An unproven or unsupported intervention usually promoted for the purpose of financial gain.

reactive hypoglycemia—Low blood sugar that occurs soon after consuming a meal, usually containing carbohydrate. Also called postprandial hypoglycemia.

refined carbohydrate—Carbohydrates that have been processed to remove portions of the whole grain, usually to make the final product more palatable.

registered dietitian nutritionist (RDN or RD)—A credential issued by the Commission on Dietetic Registration of the Academy of Nutrition and Dietetics to people who have expertise in food, nutrition, and dietetics. A college education in nutrition, supervised practice experience, and passing of a national exam is required.

relative energy deficiency in sport (RED-S)—A syndrome of impaired physiological function including, but not limited to, metabolic rate, menstrual function, bone health, immunity, protein synthesis, and cardiovascular health. Encompasses a cluster of health complications that occur in males and females when energy intake may be sufficient to fuel physical activity but not sufficient to maintain the health of many body systems.

rephosphorylate—To add or introduce a phosphate group to a molecule or compound that has previously been dephosphorylated.

resorption—Bone breakdown.

resting energy expenditure (REE)—The amount of energy from food calories required during resting conditions of the body.

resting metabolic rate (RMR)—The amount of energy, usually expressed in kilocalories, required for a 24-hour period by the body at rest. It is closely related to, but not identical to, basal metabolic rate (BMR). RMR tends to be slightly higher than BMR.

reversibility—The reversal of metabolic and physical benefits achieved from training when a person stops training.

rhabdomyolysis—Serious skeletal muscle injury that leads to the release of intracellular muscle constituents into the circulation. Rhabdomyolysis is potentially life threatening.

ribonucleic acid (RNA)—Molecule that plays various biological roles in coding, decoding, regulation, and expression of genes.

rule of five—A guideline used to help select whole grains and cereals that are deemed healthy. The rule refers to selecting grains that have 5 grams or more of fiber and less than 5 grams of sugar per serving.

salivary amylase—An enzyme found in human saliva that catalyzes the breakdown of starch into sugars.

sarcopenia—Age-related loss of muscle mass and strength.

satiation—The physiological satisfaction of appetite during a meal; satiation helps determine when to stop eating.

satiety—The sensation of fullness or absence of hunger after a meal.

saturated fatty acids—Fatty acids that have only single bonds between adjacent carbon atoms so that they can stack tightly on top of one another. Fats containing more saturated fatty acids are solid at room temperature.

secretin—Digestive hormone secreted by the wall of the duodenum; influences the environment of the duodenum by regulating secretions in the stomach, pancreas, and liver.

set point theory—A theory that any attempt to change body weight voluntarily from an established weight in adulthood initiates a series of physiological and metabolic responses that ultimately result in no further loss of body fat, or a plateau. These responses might include storing fat more efficiently, decreasing metabolism, or stimulating appetite.

simple carbohydrate—A monosaccharide; simple sugar.

simple sugar—A monosaccharide.

skinfold thickness—A method for estimating body composition based on the thickness of a fold of skin and underlying subcutaneous fat. The measurement is made using calipers.

small intestine—The part of the intestine that runs between the stomach and the large intestine and where the majority of digestion and absorption of food takes place.

soluble fiber—Portion of dietary fiber that is soluble in water to form a gel-like substance in the stool.

specificity—Targeting a specific energy system to initiate the desired effect of physical training.

sports nutrition—A specialty discipline that examines the role of nutrition in exercise metabolism and the translation to nutrient and supplement guidelines for optimal training, performance, and recovery from exercise.

standard error of estimate (SEE)—A measure of the accuracy of predictions using statistical regression lines.

starch—The form of polysaccharide carbohydrate stored in most plants, which makes it a major source of carbohydrate in the human diet.

stearidonic acid (SDA)—An omega-3 fatty acid found in some seed oils; some fish, including sardines and herring; algae; and GMO (genetically modified organisms) soybeans.

sterols—A type of lipid with a multiple ring structure. Cholesterol is the most well-recognized sterol.

stroke volume—The volume of blood pumped out of the heart's left ventricle during each systolic cardiac contraction.

structure/function claim—The role of a nutrient or dietary ingredient intended to affect the normal structure or function of the human body. Structure and function claims may also characterize the means by which a nutrient or dietary ingredient acts to maintain such structure or function. An example of a structure/function claim is "calcium builds strong bones."

subcutaneous fat—A type of storage fat found directly below the skin.

substrate fatigue—A theory that attributes fatigue during long-duration exercise to skeletal muscle glycogen depletion.

sucrase—An enzyme that catalyzes the breakdown of sucrose to glucose and fructose.

sucrose—A disaccharide containing glucose and fructose. Commonly known as table sugar.

thermic effect of activity (TEA)—Energy expenditure to support the demands of physical activity.

thermic effect of food (TEF)—Energy expenditure from food absorption, metabolism, and storage of food ingested accounting for about 10 percent of total daily energy expenditure.

total energy expenditure (TEE)—The sum of all energy expended over a set period (usually 24 hours).

trans fatty acids—Fatty acids that have hydrogen molecules on opposite sides of the double bond. Man-made trans fatty acids are harmful for heart health.

transfer RNA (tRNA)—RNA consisting of folded molecules that transport amino acids from the cytoplasm of a cell to a ribosome.

tricarboxylic acid cycle (TCA cycle)—Aerobic pathway also known as Krebs cycle or citric acid cycle; uses acetyl-CoA in a series of reactions to create carbon dioxide and ATP.

triglycerides—A type of fat composed of one glycerol molecule and three fatty acid molecules. Triglycerides are the most common type of fat in the body. They are found in cooking oils, butter, animal fat, nuts, seeds, avocado, and olives and made by the body.

trypsin—A protease important in protein digestion by serving to break (cleave) peptide chains. A proenzyme of trypsin, trypsinogen, is produced in the pancreas and found in pancreatic juice.

type 1 diabetes mellitus—A condition in which the pancreas no longer produces enough insulin. Without insulin, glucose in the blood cannot be absorbed into cells of the body.

type 2 diabetes mellitus—A condition in which the body does not make or use insulin effectively. Left untreated, blood sugar remains high.

unsaturated fatty acids—Fatty acids with kinks in their double bonds so that they do not stack neatly on top of one another; fats containing more unsaturated fatty acids, as opposed to saturated fatty acids, are liquid at room temperature.

urea cycle—A cycle of biochemical reactions occurring in many animals that produces urea from ammonia (NH_3).

U.S. Anti-Doping Agency (USADA)—The national anti-doping organization for Olympic, Paralympic, Pan American, and Parapan American sport that has a mission to "Preserve the integrity of competition—Inspire true sport—Protect the rights of U.S. athletes" and the vision "to be the guardian of the values and life lessons learned through true sport."

U.S. Food and Drug Administration (FDA)—The consumer protection agency of the U.S. government that monitors all products classified as foods sold in the United States.

U.S. Pharmacopeial Convention (USP)—An independent scientific, worldwide, nonprofit organization that sets standards for the identity, strength, quality, and purity of medicines, food ingredients, and dietary supplements manufactured and distributed for sale.

villi—Projections on the mucous membrane of the small intestine that increases its surface area, thus facilitating absorption of nutrients.

visceral fat—A type of storage fat found wrapped around the internal organs.

vitamins—Compounds necessary for metabolism, proper growth and development, vision, organ and immune functioning, energy production, muscle contraction and relaxation, oxygen transport, building and maintaining bone and cartilage, building and repairing muscle tissue, and protecting the body's cells from damage.

$\dot{V}O_2$max—A measure of the maximum volume of oxygen that an athlete can use, measured in milliliters per kilogram of body weight per minute.

WADA (World Anti-Doping Agency)—Established in 1999 as an international independent agency to lead a collaborative worldwide movement for doping-free sport.

wellness—A multidimensional concept that includes spiritual, emotional, social, and occupational health as well as physical health.

whole grain—Grain that has been minimally refined or processed; usually eaten in its whole native state.

REFERENCES

Chapter 1

1. U.S. National Library of Medicine. Nutrition. U.S. Department of Health and Human Services, National Institutes of Health. Accessed December 2022. www.nlm.nih.gov/medlineplus/definitions/nutritiondefinitions.html
2. Whitney E, Rady Rolfes S. *Understanding Nutrition*. 16th ed. Cengage; 2022.
3. Sports and Human Performance Nutrition. CSSD. Academy of Nutrition & Dietetics. Accessed December 2022. www.shpndpg.org/shpn/professional-resources/cssd
4. National Institutes of Health. Nutrient recommendations: Dietary reference intakes. National Institutes of Health. Accessed December 2022. https://ods.od.nih.gov/HealthInformation/Dietary_Reference_Intakes.aspx
5. National Academy of Sciences. *Dietary Reference Intakes for Energy, Carbohydrate, Fiber, Fat, Fatty Acids, Cholesterol, Protein, and Amino Acids (Macronutrients)*. 2005. www.nap.edu
6. Academy of Nutrition and Dietetics. *Sports Nutrition*. 6th ed. The Academy of Nutrition and Dietetics; 2017.
7. Paddon-Jones D, Rasmussen BB. Dietary protein recommendations and the prevention of sarcopenia: Protein, amino acid metabolism and therapy. *Current Opinion in Clinical Nutrition and Metabolic Care*. 2009;12(1):86-90. doi:10.1097/MCO.0b013e32831cef8b
8. Phillips SM. Dietary protein requirements and adaptive advantages in athletes. *Br J Nutr*. 2012;108(Suppl 2):S158-67. doi:10.1017/s0007114512002516
9. Lukaski HC. Vitamin and mineral status: Effects on physical performance. *Nutrition*. 2004;20(7-8):632-44. doi:10.1016/j.nut.2004.04.001
10. National Academy of Sciences. *Dietary Reference Intakes: Guiding Principles for Nutrition Labeling and Fortification*. 2003.
11. Phillips SM. A brief review of higher dietary protein diets in weight loss: A focus on athletes. *Sports Medicine (Auckland, NZ)*. 2014;44(Suppl 2):149-153. doi:10.1007/s40279-014-0254-y
12. Henry YM, Fatayerji D, Eastell R. Attainment of peak bone mass at the lumbar spine, femoral neck and radius in men and women: Relative contributions of bone size and volumetric bone mineral density. *Osteoporosis International*. 2004;15(4):263-273. doi:10.1007/s00198-003-1542-9
13. National Academy of Sciences. *Dietary Reference Intakes for Water, Potassium, Sodium, Chloride, and Sulfate*. 2005.
14. Riebl SK, Davy BM. The hydration equation: Update on water balance and cognitive performance. *ACSMs Health Fit J*. 2013;17(6):21-28. doi:10.1249/FIT.0b013e3182a9570f
15. Academy of Nutrition and Dietetics. Medical nutrition therapy. Academy of Nutrition and Dietetics. Accessed December 2022. www.eatrightpro.org/career/payment/medical-nutrition-therapy
16. Thomas DT, Erdman KA, Burke LM. Position of the Academy of Nutrition and Dietetics, Dietitians of Canada, and the American College of Sports Medicine: Nutrition and athletic performance. *J Acad Nutr Diet*. 2016;116(3):501-28. doi:10.1016/j.jand.2015.12.006
17. Centers for Disease Control and Prevention. Control of infectious diseases. *MMWR Morb Mortal Wkly Rep*. 1999;48(29):621-9.
18. Centers for Disease Control and Prevention. Overweight & obesity. Centers for Disease Control and Prevention. Accessed December 2022. www.cdc.gov/obesity/index.html
19. U.S. Department of Health and Human Services and U.S. Department of Agriculture. 2020-2025 Dietary Guidelines for Americans. U.S. Department of Health and Human Services. Accessed December 2022. https://health.gov/our-work/nutrition-physical-activity/dietary-guidelines
20. U.S. Food and Drug Administration. Changes to the nutrition facts label. U.S. Food and Drug Administration. Accessed December 2022. www.fda.gov/Food/GuidanceRegulation/GuidanceDocumentsRegulatoryInformation/LabelingNutrition/ucm385663.htm
21. U.S. Food and Drug Administration. How to understand and use the nutrition facts label. U.S. Food and Drug Administration. Accessed December 2022. www.fda.gov/Food/IngredientsPackagingLabeling/LabelingNutrition/ucm274593.htm#overview
22. U.S. Food and Drug Administration. Label claims for conventional foods and dietary supplements. U.S. Food and Drug Administration. Accessed December 2022. www.fda.gov/food/food-labeling-nutrition/label-claims-food-dietary-supplements
23. U.S. Department of Agriculture. USDA Choose MyPlate. Accessed December 2022. http://www.choosemyplate.gov
24. U.S. Department of Agriculture. MyPlate plan. United States Department of Agriculture. Accessed December 2022. www.choosemyplate.gov/resources/MyPlatePlan
25. U.S. Department of Agriculture. Online tools. United States Department of Agriculture. Accessed December 2022. https://www.nutrition.gov/topics/basic-nutrition/online-tools
26. Churchward-Venne TA, Tieland M, Verdijk LB, et al. There are no nonresponders to resistance-type exercise training in older men and women. *J Am Med Dir Assoc*. 2015;16(5):400-11. doi:10.1016/j.jamda.2015.01.071

27. Leenders M, Verdijk LB, van der Hoeven L, van Kranenburg J, Nilwik R, van Loon LJ. Elderly men and women benefit equally from prolonged resistance-type exercise training. *J Gerontol A Biol Sci Med Sci.* 2013;68(7):769-79. doi:10.1093/gerona/gls241

28. U.S. Department of Health and Human Services. Physical activity guidelines for Americans. U.S. Department of Health and Human Services, Office of Disease Prevention and Health Promotion. Accessed December 2022. https://health.gov/our-work/nutrition-physical-activity/physical-activity-guidelines

29. U.S. Department of Health and Human Services OoDPaHP. *2018 Physical Activity Guidelines Advisory Committee scientific report.* 2018. https://health.gov/paguidelines/second-edition/report

30. Poole DC, Wilkerson DP, Jones AM. Validity of criteria for establishing maximal O2 uptake during ramp exercise tests. *Eur J Appl Physiol.* 2008;102(4):403-10. doi:10.1007/s00421-007-0596-3

31. Fleg JL, Morrell CH, Bos AG, et al. Accelerated longitudinal decline of aerobic capacity in healthy older adults. *Circulation.* 2005;112(5):674-82. doi:10.1161/circulationaha.105.545459

32. Kenney WL, Wilmore JH, Costill DL. *Physiology of Sport and Exercise.* 8th ed. Human Kinetics; 2022.

33. Gormley SE, Swain DP, High R, et al. Effect of intensity of aerobic training on VO2max. *Med Sci Sports Exerc.* 2008;40(7):1336-43. doi:10.1249/MSS.0b013e31816c4839

34. Scribbans TD, Vecsey S, Hankinson PB, Foster WS, Gurd BJ. The effect of training intensity on VO(2) max in young healthy adults: A meta-regression and meta-analysis. *International Journal of Exercise Science.* 2016;9(2):230-247.

35. Xi B, Chandak GR, Shen Y, Wang Q, Zhou D. Association between common polymorphism near the MC4R gene and obesity risk: A systematic review and meta-analysis. *PLoS One.* 2012;7(9):e45731. doi:10.1371/journal.pone.0045731

36. Andreasen CH, Stender-Petersen KL, Mogensen MS, et al. Low physical activity accentuates the effect of the FTO rs9939609 polymorphism on body fat accumulation. *Diabetes.* 2008;57(1):95-101. doi:10.2337/db07-0910

37. Dina C, Meyre D, Gallina S, et al. Variation in FTO contributes to childhood obesity and severe adult obesity. *Nat Genet.* 2007;39(6):724-6. doi:10.1038/ng2048

38. Qi Q, Chu AY, Kang JH, et al. Fried food consumption, genetic risk, and body mass index: Gene-diet interaction analysis in three US cohort studies. 10.1136/bmj.g1610. *BMJ: British Medical Journal.* 2014;348.

39. Ruiz JR, Labayen I, Ortega FB, et al. Attenuation of the effect of the FTO rs9939609 polymorphism on total and central body fat by physical activity in adolescents: The HELENA study. *Arch Pediatr Adolesc Med.* 2010;164(4):328-33. doi:10.1001/archpediatrics.2010.29

40. Santoro N, Perrone L, Cirillo G, et al. Weight loss in obese children carrying the proopiomelanocortin R236G variant. *J Endocrinol Invest.* 2006;29(3):226-30. doi:10.1007/bf03345544

41. Xiang L, Wu H, Pan A, et al. FTO genotype and weight loss in diet and lifestyle interventions: A systematic review and meta-analysis. *Am J Clin Nutr.* 2016;103(4):1162-70. doi:10.3945/ajcn.115.123448

42. Morton RW, Colenso-Semple L, Phillips SM. Training for strength and hypertrophy: An evidence-based approach. *Current Opinion in Physiology.* 2019;10:90-95. doi:10.1016/j.cophys.2019.04.006

43. Burke LM, Castell LM, Casa DJ, et al. International Association of Athletics Federations Consensus Statement 2019: Nutrition for athletics. *Int J Sport Nutr Exerc Metab.* 2019;29(2):73-84. doi:10.1123/ijsnem.2019-0065

44. Issurin VB. New horizons for the methodology and physiology of training periodization. *Sports Med.* 2010;40(3):189-206. doi:10.2165/11319770-000000000-00000

45. Neufer PD. The effect of detraining and reduced training on the physiological adaptations to aerobic exercise training. *Sports Med.* 1989;8(5):302-20.

46. Coyle EF, Martin WH, 3rd, Sinacore DR, Joyner MJ, Hagberg JM, Holloszy JO. Time course of loss of adaptations after stopping prolonged intense endurance training. *J Appl Physiol Respir Environ Exerc Physiol.* 1984;57(6):1857-64.

47. Lemmer JT, Hurlbut DE, Martel GF, et al. Age and gender responses to strength training and detraining. *Med Sci Sports Exerc.* 2000;32(8):1505-12.

48. Manore MM. Weight management for athletes and active individuals: A brief review. *Sports Med.* 2015;45(Suppl 1):83-92. doi:10.1007/s40279-015-0401-0

49. Meeusen R, Duclos M, Foster C, et al. Prevention, diagnosis, and treatment of the overtraining syndrome: Joint consensus statement of the European College of Sports Medicine and the American College of Sports Medicine. *Med Sci Sports Exerc.* 2013;45(1):186-205.

50. Academy of Nutrition and Dietetics. Evidence-based nutrition practice guidelines. Academy of Nutrition and Dietetics. Accessed December 2022. www.eatrightpro.org/practice/guidelines-and-positions/evidence-based-nutrition-practice-guidelines

51. Commission on Dietetic Registration. Accessed December 2022. www.cdrnet.org

52. American College of Sports Medicine. Accessed December 2022. www.acsm.org

53. National Strength and Conditioning Association. Accessed December 2022. www.nsca.com

54. American Council on Exercise. Accessed December 2022. www.acefitness.org

55. National Commission for Health Certifying Agencies. NCCA accreditation. Accessed December 2022. www.credentialingexcellence.org/Accreditation/Earn-Accreditation/NCCA

56. American College of Sports Medicine. Get certified. Accessed December 2022. www.acsm.org/get-stay-certified/get-certified
57. National Strength and Conditioning Association. Certification overview. Accessed December 2022. www.nsca.com/certification-overview
58. American Council on Exercise. Certifications. Accessed December 2022. www.acefitness.org
59. Academy of Nutrition and Dietetics. Sports, cardiovascular, and wellness nutrition. Accessed September 7, 2016. www.scandpg.org
60. Professionals in Nutrition for Exercise and Sport. Accessed December 2022. https://pinesnutrition.org
61. Academy of Nutrition and Dietetics. Accessed December 2022. www.eatright.org
62. Accreditation Council for Education in Nutrition and Dietetics of the Academy of Nutrition and Dietetics. Accessed December 2022. www.eatrightpro.org/acend
63. Academy of Nutrition and Dietetics. Licensure and professional regulation of dietitians. Accessed December 2022. www.eatrightpro.org/advocacy/licensure/professional-regulation-of-dietitians
64. Academy of Nutrition and Dietetics. Nutrition care process. Accessed September 29, 2020. www.eatrightpro.org/practice/quality-management/nutrition-care-process
65. Kruskall L, Manore M, Eikhoff-Shemek J, Ehrman J. Understanding the scope of practice among registered dietitian nutritionists and exercise professionals. *ACSMs Health Fit J*. 2017;21(1):23-32.
66. Academy of Nutrition and Dietetics. Scope of practice. Accessed December 2022. www.eatrightpro.org/practice/dietetics-resources/scope-and-standards-of-practice

Chapter 2

1. Stipanuk MH. *Biochemical and Physiological Aspects of Human Nutrition*. W.B. Saunders; 2000.
2. Burke DG, Chilibeck PD, Parise G, Candow DG, Mahoney D, Tarnopolsky M. Effect of creatine and weight training on muscle creatine and performance in vegetarians. *Med Sci Sports Exerc*. 2003;35(11):1946-55. doi:10.1249/01.mss.0000093614.17517.79
3. Jagim A, Stecker R, Harty P, Erickson J, Kerksick C. Safety of creatine supplementation in active adolescents and youth: A brief review. *Frontiers in Nutrition*. 2018:1-13. doi:10.3389/fnut.2018.00115
4. de Guingand D, Palmer K, Snow R, Davies-Tuck M, Ellery S. Risk of adverse outcomes in females taking oral creatine monohydrate: A systematic review and meta-analysis. *Nutrients*. 2020;12:1780. doi:10.3390/nu12061780
5. Kreider RB, Kalman D, Antonio J, et al. International Society of Sports Nutrition position stand: Safety and efficacy of creatine supplementation in exercise, sport, and medicine. *Journal of the International Society of Sports Nutrition*. 2017;14:18. doi:10.1186/s12970-017-0173-z
6. LaBotz M, Griesemer B. Clinical report: Use of performance enhancing substances. *Pediatrics*. 2016;138(1):e20161300.
7. Previs SF, Fatica R, Chandramouli V, Alexander JC, Brunengraber H, Landau BR. Quantifying rates of protein synthesis in humans by use of 2H2O: Application to patients with end-stage renal disease. *Am J Physiol Endocrinol Metab*. 2004;286(4):E665-72. doi:10.1152/ajpendo.00271.2003
8. Campbell MK. *Biochemistry*. 3rd ed. Saunders golden sunburst series. Saunders; 1999.
9. Pooyandjoo M, Nouhi M, Shab-Bidar S, Djafarian K, Olyaeemanesh A. The effect of (L-)carnitine on weight loss in adults: A systematic review and meta-analysis of randomized controlled trials. *Obes Rev*. 2016;17(10):970-6. doi:10.1111/obr.12436
10. Thomas DT, Erdman KA, Burke LM. American College of Sports Medicine joint position statement: Nutrition and athletic performance. *Med Sci Sports Exerc*. 2016;48(3):543-68. doi:10.1249/mss.0000000000000852
11. Peeling P, Binnie M, Goods P, Sim M, Burke L. Evidence-based supplements for the enhancement of athletic performance. *International Journal of Sport Nutrition and Exercise Metabolism*. 2018;28:178-187. doi:10.1123/ijsnem.2017-0343
12. Koeth RA, Wang Z, Levison BS, et al. Intestinal microbiota metabolism of L-carnitine, a nutrient in red meat, promotes atherosclerosis. *Nat Med*. 2013;19(5):576-85. doi:10.1038/nm.3145
13. Egan B, D'Agostino DP. Fueling performance: Ketones enter the mix. *Cell Metab*. 2016;24:373. doi:10.1016/j.cmet.2016.08.021
14. Lourenco S, Oliveira A, Lopes C. The effect of current and lifetime alcohol consumption on overall and central obesity. *Eur J Clin Nutr*. 2012;66(7):813-8. doi:10.1038/ejcn.2012.20
15. Barnes MJ. Alcohol: Impact on sports performance and recovery in male athletes. *Sports Med*. 2014;44(7):909-19. doi:10.1007/s40279-014-0192-8
16. Burke LM, Collier GR, Broad EM, et al. Effect of alcohol intake on muscle glycogen storage after prolonged exercise. *J Appl Physiol*. 2003;95(3):983-90. doi:10.1152/japplphysiol.00115.2003
17. Hobson RM, Maughan RJ. Hydration status and the diuretic action of a small dose of alcohol. *Alcohol*. 2010;45(4):366-73. doi:10.1093/alcalc/agq029
18. Parr EB, Camera DM, Areta JL, et al. Alcohol ingestion impairs maximal post-exercise rates of myofibrillar protein synthesis following a single bout of concurrent training. *PLoS One*. 2014;9(2):e88384. doi:10.1371/journal.pone.0088384
19. Burke LM, Read RS. A study of dietary patterns of elite Australian football players. *Can J Sport Sci*. 1988;13(1):15-9.
20. Verster JC. The alcohol hangover—a puzzling phenomenon. *Alcohol Alcohol*. 2008;43(2):124-6. doi:10.1093/alcalc/agm163

21. Mujika I, Padilla S. Detraining: Loss of training-induced physiological and performance adaptations. Part II. *Sports Medicine*. 2000;30(3):145-154. doi:10.2165/00007256-200030030-00001
22. Maughan RJ, Burke L, Dvorak J, et al. IOC consensus statement: Dietary supplements and the high-performance athlete. *Br J Sports Med*. 2018;52:439-455. doi:10.1136/bjsports- 2018-099199
23. Gerich JE, Meyer C, Woerle HJ, Stumvoll M. Renal gluconeogenesis: Its importance in human glucose homeostasis. *Diabetes Care*. 2001;24(2):382-91.
24. Widmaier EP, Raff H, Strang KT. *Vander's Human Physiology: The Mechanisms of Body Function*. 10th ed. McGraw-Hill; 2006.
25. Berg JM, Tymoczko JL, Stryer L. *Biochemistry*. 7th ed. W.H. Freeman; 2012.
26. Stryer L. *Biochemistry*. 4th ed. W.H. Freeman; 1995.
27. Deakin V. Energy requirements of the athlete: Assessment and evidence of energy efficiency. In: Burke L, Deakin V, eds. *Clinical Sports Nutrition*. McGraw Hill Australia; 2015:27-53.
28. Manore MM, Thompson JL. Energy requirements of the athlete: Assessment and evidence of energy efficiency. In: Burke L, Deakin V, eds. *Clinical Sports Nutrition*. McGraw Hill Australia; 2015:114-139.
29. Spriet LL. New insights into the interaction of carbohydrate and fat metabolism during exercise. *Sports Med*. 2014;44(Suppl 1):S87-96. doi:10.1007/s40279-014-0154-1
30. Manini TM. Energy expenditure and aging. *Ageing Res Rev*. 2010;9(1):1-11. doi:10.1016/j.arr.2009.08.002
31. St-Onge MP, Gallagher D. Body composition changes with aging: The cause or the result of alterations in metabolic rate and macronutrient oxidation? *Nutrition*. 2010;26(2):152-5. doi:10.1016/j.nut.2009.07.004
32. von Loeffelholz C. The role of non-exercise activity thermogenesis in human obesity. In: De Groot LJ, Chrousos G, Dungan K, et al., eds. *Endotext*. MDText.com; 2000.
33. Ainsworth BE, Haskell WL, Whitt MC, et al. Compendium of physical activities: An update of activity codes and MET intensities. *Med Sci Sports Exerc*. 2000;32(9 Suppl):S498-S504.
34. Guebels CP, Kam LC, Maddalozzo GF, Manore MM. Active women before/after an intervention designed to restore menstrual function: Resting metabolic rate and comparison of four methods to quantify energy expenditure and energy availability. *Int J Sport Nutr Exerc Metab*. 2014;24(1):37-46. doi:10.1123/ijsnem.2012-0165
35. U.S. Department of Agriculture and U.S. Department of Health & Human Services. *Dietary Guidelines for Americans, 2015-2020*. 8th ed. Wise Age Books; 2015.
36. Insel PM. *Nutrition*. 5th ed. Jones & Bartlett Learning; 2014.
37. Cunningham JJ. A reanalysis of the factors influencing basal metabolic rate in normal adults. *Am J Clin Nutr*. 1980;33(11):2372-4.
38. Roza AM, Shizgal HM. The Harris Benedict equation reevaluated: Resting energy requirements and the body cell mass. *Am J Clin Nutr*. 1984;40(1):168-82.
39. Westerterp KR. Reliable assessment of physical activity in disease: An update on activity monitors. *Curr Opin Clin Nutr Metab Care*. 2014;17(5):401-6. doi:10.1097/mco.0000000000000080
40. Slootmaker SM, Chinapaw MJ, Seidell JC, van Mechelen W, Schuit AJ. Accelerometers and Internet for physical activity promotion in youth? Feasibility and effectiveness of a minimal intervention [ISRCTN93896459]. *Prev Med*. 2010;51(1):31-36. doi:10.1016/j.ypmed.2010.03.015
41. Lee JM, Kim Y, Welk GJ. Validity of consumer-based physical activity monitors. *Med Sci Sports Exerc*. 2014;46(9):1840-8. doi:10.1249/mss.0000000000000287
42. Loucks AB. Energy balance and energy availability. *The Encyclopaedia of Sports Medicine*. John Wiley & Sons; 2013:72-87.
43. Joy E, De Souza MJ, Nattiv A, et al. 2014 Female Athlete Triad Coalition consensus statement on treatment and return to play of the female athlete triad. *Curr Sports Med Rep*. 2014;13(4):219-32. doi:10.1249/jsr.0000000000000077
44. Mountjoy M, Sundgot-Borgen J, Burke L, et al. The IOC consensus statement: Beyond the female athlete triad—relative energy deficiency in sport (RED-S). *Br J Sports Med*. 2014;48(7):491-7. doi:10.1136/bjsports-2014-093502
45. McCarthy O, Schmidt S, Christensen MB, Bain SC, Nørgaard K, Bracken R. The endocrine pancreas during exercise in people with and without type 1 diabetes: Beyond the beta-cell. *Front Endocrinol (Lausanne)*. 2022;6(13):981723. doi: 10.3389/fendo.2022.981723

Chapter 3

1. Whitney E, Rady Rolfes S. *Understanding Nutrition*. 16th ed. Cengage; 2022.
2. Kenney WL, Wilmore JH, Costill DL. *Physiology of Sport and Exercise*. 8th ed. Human Kinetics; 2022.
3. Ross CA, Caballero B, Cousins RJ, Tucker KL, Ziegler TR. *Modern Nutrition in Health and Disease*. 11th ed. Lippincott Williams & Wilkins; 2014.
4. National Academy of Sciences. *Dietary Reference Intakes for Energy, Carbohydrate, Fiber, Fat, Fatty Acids, Cholesterol, Protein, and Amino Acids (Macronutrients)*. 2005. www.nap.edu
5. U.S. Food and Drug Administration. Guidance for industry: Questions and answers on FDA's fortification policy. U.S. Food and Drug Administration. Accessed December 2022. www.fda.gov/Food/GuidanceRegulation/GuidanceDocumentsRegulatoryInformation/ucm470756.htm
6. Slavin JL. Position of the American Dietetic Association: Health implications of dietary fiber. *J Am Diet Assoc*. 2008;108(10):1716-1731.
7. Kreitzman SN, Coxon AY, Szaz KF. Glycogen storage: Illusions of easy weight loss, excessive weight regain,

and distortions in estimates of body composition. *Am J Clin Nutr*. 1992;56(1 Suppl):292s-293s.

8. Immonen K, Ruusunen M, Hissa K, Puolanne E. Bovine muscle glycogen concentration in relation to finishing diet, slaughter and ultimate pH. *Meat Sci*. 2000;55(1):25-31.

9. U.S. Food and Drug Administration. CFR—Code of Federal Regulations Title 21. U.S. Food and Drug Administration. Accessed December 2022. www.accessdata.fda.gov/scripts/cdrh/cfdocs/cfcfr/CFR-Search.cfm?fr=137.165

10. Whole Grains Council. Whole grain stamp. Accessed December 2022. https://wholegrainscouncil.org/whole-grain-stamp

11. Thompson JL, Manore MM, Vaughan LA. *The Science of Nutrition*. 5th ed. Pearson Education; 2020.

12. Ivy JL. Muscle glycogen synthesis before and after exercise. *Sports Med*. 1991;11(1):6-19.

13. Jensen J, Rustad PI, Kolnes AJ, Lai Y-C. The role of skeletal muscle glycogen breakdown for regulation of insulin sensitivity by exercise. *Front Physiol*. 2011;2:112. doi:10.3389/fphys.2011.00112

14. Karpinski C, Rosenbloom C. *Sports Nutrition: A Handbook for Professionals*. 6th ed. Academy of Nutrition and Dietetics; 2017.

15. Monro J, Shaw M. Glycemic impact, glycemic glucose equivalents, glycemic index, and glycemic load: Definitions, distinctions, and implications. *Am J Clin Nutr*. 2008;87(suppl):237S-243S.

16. Astrup A, Raben A, Geiker N. The role of higher protein diets in weight control and obesity-related comorbidities. *Int J Obes (Lond)*. 2015;39(5):721-6. doi:10.1038/ijo.2014.216

17. Chiu C, Liu S, Willett W, et al. Informing food choices and health outcomes by use of the dietary glycemic index. *Nutrition Reviews*. 2011;69:231-242.

18. Chiu YT, Stewart ML. Effect of variety and cooking method on resistant starch content of white rice and subsequent postprandial glucose response and appetite in humans. *Asia Pac J Clin Nutr*. 2013;22(3):372-9. doi:10.6133/apjcn.2013.22.3.08

19. Hermansen K, Rasmussen O, Gregersen S, Larsen S. Influence of ripeness of banana on the blood glucose and insulin response in type 2 diabetic subjects. *Diabet Med*. 1992;9(8):739-43.

20. Chiu C, Liu S, Willett W, et al. Informing food choices and health outcomes by use of the dietary glycemic index. *Nutr Rev*. 2011;69:231-242.

21. Cummings J, Stephen A. Carbohydrate terminology and classification. *European Journal of Clinical Nutrition*. 2007;61(suppl 1):S5-S18.

22. Bennett CB, Chilibeck PD, Barss T, Vatanparast H, Vandenberg A, Zello GA. Metabolism and performance during extended high-intensity intermittent exercise after consumption of low- and high-glycaemic index pre-exercise meals. *Br J Nutr*. 2012;108 Suppl 1:S81-90. doi:10.1017/s0007114512000840

23. Tarnopolsky MA, Gibala M, Jeukendrup AE, Phillips SM. Nutritional needs of elite endurance athletes. Part I: Carbohydrate and fluid requirements. *European Journal of Sport Science*. 2005;5(1):3-14. doi:10.1080/17461390500076741

24. Marmy-Conus N, Fabris S, Proietto J, Hargreaves M. Preexercise glucose ingestion and glucose kinetics during exercise. *J Appl Physiol (1985)*. 1996;81(2):853-7.

25. Burke LM, Hawley JA, Wong SHS, Jeukendrup AE. Carbohydrates for training and competition. *J Sports Sci*. 2011;29(S1):S17-S27.

26. McArdle WD, Katch FI, Katch VL. Macronutrient metabolism in exercise and training. *Sports and Exercise Nutrition*. 4th ed. Wolters Kluwer; 2013:167-178.

27. National Institutes of Health. Nutrient recommendations: Dietary reference intakes. Accessed December 2022. https://ods.od.nih.gov/HealthInformation/Dietary_Reference_Intakes.aspx

28. U.S. Department of Health and Human Services and U.S. Department of Agriculture. 2020-2025 Dietary Guidelines for Americans. U.S. Department of Health and Human Services. Accessed December 2022. https://health.gov/our-work/nutrition-physical-activity/dietary-guidelines

29. Institute of Medicine. *Dietary Reference Intakes for Energy, Carbohydrate, Fiber, Fat, Fatty Acids, Cholesterol, Protein, and Amino Acids (Macronutrients)*. National Academies Press; 2005.

30. Thomas DT, Erdman KA, Burke LM. Position of the Academy of Nutrition and Dietetics, Dietitians of Canada, and the American College of Sports Medicine: Nutrition and athletic performance. *J Acad Nutr Diet*. 2016;116(3):501-28. doi:10.1016/j.jand.2015.12.006

31. Sports and Human Performance Nutrition. CSSD. Academy of Nutrition & Dietetics. Accessed December 2022. www.shpndpg.org/shpn/professional-resources/cssd

32. U.S. Food and Drug Administration. Guidance for industry: A food labeling guide. Accessed December 2022. www.fda.gov/food/guidanceregulation/guidancedocumentsregulatoryinformation/labelingnutrition/ucm2006828.htm

33. Burton-Freeman B. Dietary fiber and energy regulation. *J Nutr*. 2000;130(2S Suppl):272s-275s.

34. Clark MJ, Slavin JL. The effect of fiber on satiety and food intake: A systematic review. *J Am Coll Nutr*. 2013;32(3):200-11. doi:10.1080/07315724.2013.791194

35. Zijlstra N, de Wijk RA, Mars M, Stafleu A, de Graaf C. Effect of bite size and oral processing time of a semisolid food on satiation. *Am J Clin Nutr*. 2009;90(2):269-75. doi:10.3945/ajcn.2009.27694

36. Cleveland Clinic. Lactose intolerance. Cleveland Clinic. Accessed December 2022. http://my.clevelandclinic.org/health/diseases_conditions/hic_Lactose_Intolerance

37. Commission on Dietetic Registration. Accessed December 2022. www.cdrnet.org

38. Marsh A, Eslick EM, Eslick GD. Does a diet low in FODMAPs reduce symptoms associated with functional gastrointestinal disorders? A comprehensive systematic review and meta-analysis. *Eur J Nutr.* 2016;55(3):897-906. doi:10.1007/s00394-015-0922-1

39. Hu FB. Resolved: There is sufficient scientific evidence that decreasing sugar-sweetened beverage consumption will reduce the prevalence of obesity and obesity-related diseases. *Obes Rev.* 2013;14(8):606-619. doi:10.1111/obr.12040

40. Fitch C, Keim KS. Position of the Academy of Nutrition and Dietetics: Use of nutritive and nonnutritive sweeteners. *Journal of the Academy of Nutrition and Dietetics.* 2012;112(5):739-758. doi:10.1016/j.jand.2012.03.009

41. Fritsche KL. The science of fatty acids and inflammation. *Adv Nutr.* 2015;6(3):293s-301s. doi:10.3945/an.114.006940

42. Minihane AM, Vinoy S, Russell WR, et al. Low-grade inflammation, diet composition and health: Current research evidence and its translation. *Br J Nutr.* 2015;114(7):999-1012. doi:10.1017/s0007114515002093

43. Massougbodji J, Le Bodo Y, Fratu R, De Wals P. Reviews examining sugar-sweetened beverages and body weight: Correlates of their quality and conclusions. *The American Journal of Clinical Nutrition.* 2014;99(5):1096-1104. doi:10.3945/ajcn.113.063776

44. Te Morenga L, Mallard S, Mann J. Dietary sugars and body weight: Systematic review and meta-analyses of randomised controlled trials and cohort studies. *BMJ.* 2013;346:e7492. doi:10.1136/bmj.e7492

45. U.S. Food and Drug Administration. "Natural" on food labeling. U.S. Food and Drug Administration. Accessed December 2022. www.fda.gov/Food/GuidanceRegulation/GuidanceDocumentsRegulatoryInformation/LabelingNutrition/ucm456090.htm

46. Rolls BJ, Meengs JS, Roe LS. Variations in cereal volume affect the amount selected and eaten for breakfast. *J Acad Nutr Diet.* 2014;114(9):1411-6. doi:10.1016/j.jand.2014.01.014

47. International Food Information Council Foundation. Background on carbohydrates & sugars. September 20, 2016. Accessed December 2022. www.foodinsight.org/Background_on_Carbohydrates_Sugars

48. U.S. Food and Drug Administration. Additional information about high-intensity sweeteners permitted for use in food in the United States. www.fda.gov/Food/IngredientsPackagingLabeling/FoodAdditivesIngredients/ucm397725.htm#Advantame

49. U.S. Food and Drug Administration. High intensity sweeteners. www.fda.gov/Food/IngredientsPackagingLabeling/FoodAdditivesIngredients/ucm397716.htm

50. Greyling A, Appleton KM, Raben A, Mela DJ. Acute glycemic and insulinemic effects of low-energy sweeteners: A systematic review and meta-analysis of randomized controlled trials. *Am J Clin Nutr.* 2020;112(4):1002-1014. doi:10.1093/ajcn/nqaa167

51. Walbolt J, Koh Y. Non-nutritive sweeteners and their associations with obesity and type 2 diabetes. *J Obes Metab Syndr.* 2020;29(2):114-123. doi:10.7570/jomes19079

52. Laviada-Molina H, Molina-Segui F, Pérez-Gaxiola G, et al. Effects of nonnutritive sweeteners on body weight and BMI in diverse clinical contexts: Systematic review and meta-analysis. *Obes Rev.* 2020;21(7):e13020. doi:10.1111/obr.13020

53. Plaza-Diaz J, Pastor-Villaescusa B, Rueda-Robles A, Abadia-Molina F, Ruiz-Ojeda FJ. Plausible biological interactions of low- and non-calorie sweeteners with the intestinal microbiota: An update of recent studies. *Nutrients.* 2020;12(4):1153. doi:10.3390/nu12041153

54. U.S. Food and Drug Administration. Additional information about high-intensity sweeteners permitted for use in food in the United States. Accessed December 2022. www.fda.gov/food/food-additives-petitions/additional-information-about-high-intensity-sweeteners-permitted-use-food-united-states#Advantame

55. U.S. Department of Agriculture. Nutritive and non-nutritive sweetener resources. Accessed December 2022. www.nal.usda.gov/fnic/nutritive-and-nonnutritive-sweetener-resources

56. U.S. Food and Drug Administration. How sweet it is: All about sugar substitutes. Accessed December 2022. www.fda.gov/ForConsumers/ConsumerUpdates/ucm397711.htm

Chapter 4

1. Hussain MM. A proposed model for the assembly of chylomicrons. *Atherosclerosis.* 2000;148(1):1-15.

2. Verkijk M, Vecht J, Gielkens HA, Lamers CB, Masclee AA. Effects of medium-chain and long-chain triglycerides on antroduodenal motility and small bowel transit time in man. *Dig Dis Sci.* 1997;42(9):1933-9.

3. Liu YM. Medium-chain triglyceride (MCT) ketogenic therapy. *Epilepsia.* 2008;49(Suppl 8):33-6. doi:10.1111/j.1528-1167.2008.01830.x

4. Ferrier D. *Biochemistry.* 6th ed. Lippincott, Williams & Wilkins; 2014:522.

5. Schrauwen-Hinderling VB, Hesselink MK, Schrauwen P, Kooi ME. Intramyocellular lipid content in human skeletal muscle. *Obesity (Silver Spring).* 2006;14(3):357-67. doi:10.1038/oby.2006.47

6. Horton TJ, Drougas H, Brachey A, Reed GW, Peters JC, Hill JO. Fat and carbohydrate overfeeding in humans: Different effects on energy storage. *Am J Clin Nutr.* 1995;62(1):19-29.

7. Dirlewanger M, di Vetta V, Guenat E, et al. Effects of short-term carbohydrate or fat overfeeding on energy expenditure and plasma leptin concentrations in healthy female subjects. *Int J Obes Relat Metab Disord.* 2000;24(11):1413-8.

8. Frost E. Effect of dietary protein intake on diet-induced thermogenesis during overfeeding. Presented at Obesity Society Annual Meeting; November 2-7, 2014.

9. Leaf A, Antonio J. The effects of overfeeding on body composition: The role of macronutrient composition—a narrative review. *Int J Exerc Sci.* 2017;10(8):1275-1296.

10. Hawley JA, Schabort EJ, Noakes TD, Dennis SC. Carbohydrate-loading and exercise performance: An update. *Sports Med.* 1997;24(2):73-81.

11. Hall KD. What is the required energy deficit per unit weight loss? *Int J Obes (Lond).* 2008;32(3):573-6. doi:10.1038/sj.ijo.0803720

12. Romijn JA, Coyle EF, Sidossis LS, et al. Regulation of endogenous fat and carbohydrate metabolism in relation to exercise intensity and duration. *Am J Physiol.* 1993;265(3 Pt 1):E380-91.

13. Pendergast DR, Horvath PJ, Leddy JJ, Venkatraman JT. The role of dietary fat on performance, metabolism, and health. *Am J Sports Med.* 1996;24(6 Suppl):S53-8.

14. Jeukendrup AE. Regulation of fat metabolism in skeletal muscle. *Ann N Y Acad Sci.* 2002;967:217-35.

15. Helge JW, Watt PW, Richter EA, Rennie MJ, Kiens B. Fat utilization during exercise: adaptation to a fat-rich diet increases utilization of plasma fatty acids and very low density lipoprotein-triacylglycerol in humans. *J Physiol.* 2001;537(Pt 3):1009-20.

16. Hulston CJ, Venables MC, Mann CH, et al. Training with low muscle glycogen enhances fat metabolism in well-trained cyclists. *Med Sci Sports Exerc.* 2010;42(11):2046-55. doi:10.1249/MSS.0b013e3181dd5070

17. Pitsiladis YP, Duignan C, Maughan RJ. Effects of alterations in dietary carbohydrate intake on running performance during a 10 km treadmill time trial. *Br J Sports Med.* 1996;30(3):226-31.

18. Robins AL, Davies DM, Jones GE. The effect of nutritional manipulation on ultra-endurance performance: A case study. *Res Sports Med.* 2005;13(3):199-215. doi:10.1080/15438620500222505

19. Rowlands DS, Hopkins WG. Effects of high-fat and high-carbohydrate diets on metabolism and performance in cycling. *Metabolism.* 2002;51(6):678-90.

20. Burke LM. Fueling strategies to optimize performance: Training high or training low? *Scand J Med Sci Sports.* 2010;20(Suppl 2):48-58. doi:10.1111/j.1600-0838.2010.01185.x

21. American College of Sports Medicine. Joint position statement: Nutrition and athletic performance. *Med Sci Sports Exerc.* 2000;32(12):2130-45.

22. Rodriguez N, DiMarco N, Langley S. Position of the American Dietetic Association, Dietitians of Canada, and the American College of Sports Medicine: Nutrition and athletic performance. *J Am Diet Assoc.* 2000;100(12):1543-56. doi:10.1016/S0002-8223(00)00428-4

23. U.S. Department of Agriculture. USDA National Nutrient Database for Standard Reference, release 26. www.ars.usda.gov/ba/bhnrc/ndl

24. Otten J, Hellwig J, Meyers L. *Dietary Reference Intakes: The Essential Guide to Nutrient Requirements.* National Academies Press; 2006.

25. U.S. Institute of Medicine. *Dietary Reference Intakes for Energy, Carbohydrate, Fiber, Fat, Fatty Acids, Cholesterol, Protein and Amino Acids.* National Academies Press; 2002.

26. Vannice G, Rasmussen H. Position of the Academy of Nutrition and Dietetics: Dietary fatty acids for healthy adults. *J Acad Nutr Diet.* 2014;114(1):136-53. doi:10.1016/j.jand.2013.11.001

27. IUPAC-IUB Commission on Biochemical Nomenclature. The nomenclature of lipids (Recommendations 1976) *Biochem J.* 1978;171(1):21-35.

28. Bettelheim FA, Brown WH, Campbell MK, Farrell SO. *Introduction to General, Organic, and Biochemistry.* 9th ed. Brooks/Cole, Cengage Learning.

29. U.S. Food and Drug Administration. Title 21: Food and drugs—Subpart I: Multipurpose additives. *Code of Federal Regulations.* 2015;3.

30. U.S. Department of Agriculture. Glycerin: Handling/processing. www.ams.usda.gov/sites/default/files/media/Glycerin%20Petition%20to%20remove%20TR%202013.pdf

31. Sanclemente T, Marques-Lopes I, Puzo J, Garcia-Otin AL. Role of naturally-occurring plant sterols on intestinal cholesterol absorption and plasmatic levels. *J Physiol Biochem.* 2009;65(1):87-98.

32. Chowdhury R, Warnakula S, Kunutsor S, et al. Association of dietary, circulating, and supplement fatty acids with coronary risk: A systematic review and meta-analysis. *Ann Intern Med.* 2014;160(6):398-406. doi:10.7326/M13-1788

33. Liu AG, Ford NA, Hu FB, Zelman KM, Mozaffarian D, Kris-Etherton PM. A healthy approach to dietary fats: Understanding the science and taking action to reduce consumer confusion. *Nutr J.* 2017;16(1):53. doi:10.1186/s12937-017-0271-4

34. Craig M, Yarrarapu SNS, Dimri M. Biochemistry, cholesterol. StatPearls. 2022.

35. Wang DD, Li Y, Chiuve SE, et al. Association of specific dietary fats with total and cause-specific mortality. *JAMA Intern Med.* 2016;176(8):1134-45. doi:10.1001/jamainternmed.2016.2417

36. Kopylov AT, Malsagova KA, Stepanov AA, Kaysheva AL. Diversity of plant sterols metabolism: The impact on human health, sport, and accumulation of contaminating sterols. *Nutrients.* 2021;13(5):1623. doi:10.3390/nu13051623

37. Baumgartner S, Ras RT, Trautwein EA, Mensink RP, Plat J. Plasma fat-soluble vitamin and carotenoid concentrations after plant sterol and plant stanol consumption: A meta-analysis of randomized controlled trials. *Eur J Nutr.* 2017;56(3):909-923. doi:10.1007/s00394-016-1289-7

38. National Research Council. *Diet and Health: Implications for Reducing Chronic Disease Risk.* National Academies Press; 1989.

39. Wang TY, Liu M, Portincasa P, Wang DQ. New insights into the molecular mechanism of intestinal fatty acid absorption. *Eur J Clin Invest.* 2013;43(11):1203-23. doi:10.1111/eci.12161

40. de Oliveira Otto MC, Mozaffarian D, Kromhout D, et al. Dietary intake of saturated fat by food source and incident cardiovascular disease: The Multi-Ethnic Study of Atherosclerosis. *Am J Clin Nutr.* 2012;96(2):397-404. doi:10.3945/ajcn.112.037770

41. U.S. Department of Agriculture. 2015-2020 Dietary Guidelines for Americans. http://health.gov/dietaryguidelines/2015/guidelines
42. Siri-Tarino PW, Sun Q, Hu FB, Krauss RM. Saturated fat, carbohydrate, and cardiovascular disease. *Am J Clin Nutr*. 2010;91(3):502-9. doi:10.3945/ajcn.2008.26285
43. Siri-Tarino PW, Sun Q, Hu FB, Krauss RM. Meta-analysis of prospective cohort studies evaluating the association of saturated fat with cardiovascular disease. *Am J Clin Nutr*. 2010;91(3):535-46. doi:10.3945/ajcn.2009.27725
44. Thompson FE, Subar AF, Loria CM, Reedy JL, Baranowski T. Need for technological innovation in dietary assessment. *J Am Diet Assoc*. 2010;110(1):48-51. doi:10.1016/j.jada.2009.10.008
45. Hunter JE, Zhang J, Kris-Etherton PM. Cardiovascular disease risk of dietary stearic acid compared with trans, other saturated, and unsaturated fatty acids: A systematic review. *Am J Clin Nutr*. 2010;91(1):46-63. doi:10.3945/ajcn.2009.27661
46. Soerensen KV, Thorning TK, Astrup A, Kristensen M, Lorenzen JK. Effect of dairy calcium from cheese and milk on fecal fat excretion, blood lipids, and appetite in young men. *Am J Clin Nutr*. 2014;99(5):984-91. doi:10.3945/ajcn.113.077735
47. de Goede J, Geleijnse JM, Ding EL, Soedamah-Muthu SS. Effect of cheese consumption on blood lipids: A systematic review and meta-analysis of randomized controlled trials. *Nutr Rev*. 2015;73(5):259-75. doi:10.1093/nutrit/nuu060
48. Savaiano DA, Hutkins RW. Yogurt, cultured fermented milk, and health: A systematic review. *Nutr Rev*. 2021;79(5):599-614. doi:10.1093/nutrit/nuaa013
49. Sacks FM, Katan M. Randomized clinical trials on the effects of dietary fat and carbohydrate on plasma lipoproteins and cardiovascular disease. *Am J Med*. 2002;113(Suppl 9B):13S-24S. doi:10.1016/s0002-9343(01)00987-1
50. Sachdeva A, Cannon CP, Deedwania PC, et al. Lipid levels in patients hospitalized with coronary artery disease: An analysis of 136,905 hospitalizations in Get With the Guidelines. *Am Heart J*. 2009;157(1):111-117 e2. doi:10.1016/j.ahj.2008.08.010
51. Biong AS, Muller H, Seljeflot I, Veierod MB, Pedersen JI. A comparison of the effects of cheese and butter on serum lipids, haemostatic variables and homocysteine. *Br J Nutr*. 2004;92(5):791-7.
52. Tholstrup T, Hoy CE, Andersen LN, Christensen RD, Sandstrom B. Does fat in milk, butter and cheese affect blood lipids and cholesterol differently? *J Am Coll Nutr*. 2004;23(2):169-76.
53. Hjerpsted J, Leedo E, Tholstrup T. Cheese intake in large amounts lowers LDL-cholesterol concentrations compared with butter intake of equal fat content. *Am J Clin Nutr*. 2011;94(6):1479-84. doi:10.3945/ajcn.111.022426
54. McNamara DJ, Lowell AE, Sabb JE. Effect of yogurt intake on plasma lipid and lipoprotein levels in normolipidemic males. *Atherosclerosis*. 1989;79(2-3):167-71.
55. Kiessling G, Schneider J, Jahreis G. Long-term consumption of fermented dairy products over 6 months increases HDL cholesterol. *Eur J Clin Nutr*. 2002;56(9):843-9. doi:10.1038/sj.ejcn.1601399
56. Pourrajab B, Fatahi S, Dehnad A, Kord Varkaneh H, Shidfar F. The impact of probiotic yogurt consumption on lipid profiles in subjects with mild to moderate hypercholesterolemia: A systematic review and meta-analysis of randomized controlled trials. *Nutr Metab Cardiovasc Dis*. 2020;30(1):11-22. doi:10.1016/j.numecd.2019.10.001
57. Mozaffarian D, Micha R, Wallace S. Effects on coronary heart disease of increasing polyunsaturated fat in place of saturated fat: A systematic review and meta-analysis of randomized controlled trials. *PLoS Med*. 2010;7(3):e1000252. doi:10.1371/journal.pmed.1000252
58. Summers LK, Fielding BA, Bradshaw HA, et al. Substituting dietary saturated fat with polyunsaturated fat changes abdominal fat distribution and improves insulin sensitivity. *Diabetologia*. 2002;45(3):369-77. doi:10.1007/s00125-001-0768-3
59. Rosqvist F, Iggman D, Kullberg J, et al. Overfeeding polyunsaturated and saturated fat causes distinct effects on liver and visceral fat accumulation in humans. *Diabetes*. 2014;63(7):2356-68. doi:10.2337/db13-1622
60. Beynen AC, Katan MB, Van Zutphen LF. Hypo- and hyperresponders: Individual differences in the response of serum cholesterol concentration to changes in diet. *Adv Lipid Res*. 1987;22:115-71.
61. Katan MB, van Gastel AC, de Rover CM, van Montfort MA, Knuiman JT. Differences in individual responsiveness of serum cholesterol to fat-modified diets in man. *Eur J Clin Invest*. 1988;18(6):644-7.
62. Ordovas JM. Nutrigenetics, plasma lipids, and cardiovascular risk. *J Am Diet Assoc*. 2006;106(7):1074-81. doi:10.1016/j.jada.2006.04.016
63. Li Y, Hruby A, Bernstein AM, et al. Saturated fats compared with unsaturated fats and sources of carbohydrates in relation to risk of coronary heart disease: A prospective cohort study. *J Am Coll Cardiol*. 2015;66(14):1538-48. doi:10.1016/j.jacc.2015.07.055
64. Dowis K, Banga S. The potential health benefits of the ketogenic diet: A narrative review. *Nutrients*. 2021;13(5):1654. doi:10.3390/nu13051654
65. D'Andrea Meira I, Romao TT, Pires do Prado HJ, Kruger LT, Pires MEP, da Conceicao PO. Ketogenic diet and epilepsy: What we know so far. *Front Neurosci*. 2019;13:5. doi:10.3389/fnins.2019.00005
66. Phinney SD. Ketogenic diets and physical performance. *Nutr Metab (Lond)*. 2004;1(1):2. doi:10.1186/1743-7075-1-2
67. Ozdemir R, Guzel O, Kucuk M, et al. The effect of the ketogenic diet on the vascular structure and functions in children with intractable epilepsy. *Pediatr Neurol*. 2016;56:30-34. doi:10.1016/j.pediatrneurol.2015.10.017

68. Kapetanakis M, Liuba P, Odermarsky M, Lundgren J, Hallbook T. Effects of ketogenic diet on vascular function. *Eur J Paediatr Neurol.* 2014;18(4):489-94. doi:10.1016/j.ejpn.2014.03.006

69. Doksoz O, Guzel O, Yilmaz U, et al. The short-term effect of ketogenic diet on carotid intima-media thickness and elastic properties of the carotid artery and the aorta in epileptic children. *J Child Neurol.* 2015;30(12):1646-50. doi:10.1177/0883073815576793

70. Kosinski C, Jornayvaz FR. Effects of ketogenic diets on cardiovascular risk factors: Evidence from animal and human studies. *Nutrients.* 2017;9(5):517. doi:10.3390/nu9050517

71. Poobalan A, Aucott L, Smith WC, et al. Effects of weight loss in overweight/obese individuals and long-term lipid outcomes—a systematic review. *Obes Rev.* 2004;5(1):43-50. doi:10.1111/j.1467-789x.2004.00127.x

72. Brown JD, Buscemi J, Milsom V, Malcolm R, O'Neil PM. Effects on cardiovascular risk factors of weight losses limited to 5-10. *Transl Behav Med.* 2016;6(3):339-46. doi:10.1007/s13142-015-0353-9

73. Motard-Belanger A, Charest A, Grenier G, et al. Study of the effect of trans fatty acids from ruminants on blood lipids and other risk factors for cardiovascular disease. *Am J Clin Nutr.* 2008;87(3):593-9.

74. Rees K, Takeda A, Martin N, et al. Mediterranean-style diet for the primary and secondary prevention of cardiovascular disease. *Cochrane Database Syst Rev.* 2019;3:CD009825. doi:10.1002/14651858.CD009825.pub3

75. Mensink RP, Zock PL, Kester AD, Katan MB. Effects of dietary fatty acids and carbohydrates on the ratio of serum total to HDL cholesterol and on serum lipids and apolipoproteins: A meta-analysis of 60 controlled trials. *Am J Clin Nutr.* 2003;77(5):1146-55.

76. Kris-Etherton PM. AHA science advisory: Monounsaturated fatty acids and risk of cardiovascular disease. *J Nutr.* 1999;129(12):2280-4.

77. Schwingshackl L, Hoffmann G. Monounsaturated fatty acids and risk of cardiovascular disease: Synopsis of the evidence available from systematic reviews and meta-analyses. *Nutrients.* 2012;4(12):1989-2007. doi:10.3390/nu4121989

78. U.S. Department of Agriculture. Nutrient intakes from food: Mean amounts consumed per individual, by gender and age: What we eat in America, NHANES 2009-2010. www.ars.usda.gov/ba/bhnrc/fsrg

79. Ander BP, Dupasquier CM, Prociuk MA, Pierce GN. Polyunsaturated fatty acids and their effects on cardiovascular disease. *Exp Clin Cardiol.* 2003;8(4):164-72.

80. Kapoor B, Kapoor D, Gautam S, Singh R, Bhardwaj S. Dietary polyunsaturated fatty acids (PUFAs): Uses and potential health benefits. *Curr Nutr Rep.* 2021;10(3):232-242. doi:10.1007/s13668-021-00363-3

81. Harayama T, Shimizu T. Roles of polyunsaturated fatty acids, from mediators to membranes. *J Lipid Res.* 2020;61(8):1150-1160. doi:10.1194/jlr.R120000800

82. Lands B. Omega-3 PUFAs lower the propensity for arachidonic acid cascade overreactions. *Biomed Res Int.* 2015;2015:285135. doi:10.1155/2015/285135

83. U.S. Food and Drug Administration. GRAS notices: GRN no. 283. www.accessdata.fda.gov/scripts/fdcc/index.cfm?set=GRASNotices&id=283

84. Walker CG, Jebb SA, Calder PC. Stearidonic acid as a supplemental source of omega-3 polyunsaturated fatty acids to enhance status for improved human health. *Nutrition.* 2013;29(2):363-9. doi:10.1016/j.nut.2012.06.003

85. Lemke SL, Maki KC, Hughes G, et al. Consumption of stearidonic acid-rich oil in foods increases red blood cell eicosapentaenoic acid. *J Acad Nutr Diet.* 2013;113(8):1044-56. doi:10.1016/j.jand.2013.04.020

86. Harris WS, Lemke SL, Hansen SN, et al. Stearidonic acid-enriched soybean oil increased the omega-3 index, an emerging cardiovascular risk marker. *Lipids.* 2008;43(9):805-11. doi:10.1007/s11745-008-3215-0

87. James MJ, Ursin VM, Cleland LG. Metabolism of stearidonic acid in human subjects: Comparison with the metabolism of other n-3 fatty acids. *Am J Clin Nutr.* 2003;77(5):1140-5.

88. Anderson BM, Ma DW. Are all n-3 polyunsaturated fatty acids created equal? *Lipids Health Dis.* 2009;8:33. doi:10.1186/1476-511X-8-33

89. Fleming JA, Kris-Etherton PM. The evidence for alpha-linolenic acid and cardiovascular disease benefits: Comparisons with eicosapentaenoic acid and docosahexaenoic acid. *Adv Nutr.* 2014;5(6):863S-76S. doi:10.3945/an.114.005850

90. Mozaffarian D. Does alpha-linolenic acid intake reduce the risk of coronary heart disease? A review of the evidence. *Altern Ther Health Med.* 2005;11(3):24-30.

91. Plourde M, Cunnane SC. Extremely limited synthesis of long chain polyunsaturates in adults: Implications for their dietary essentiality and use as supplements. *Appl Physiol Nutr Metab.* 2007;32(4):619-34. doi:10.1139/H07-034

92. Burdge GC, Wootton SA. Conversion of alpha-linolenic acid to eicosapentaenoic, docosapentaenoic and docosahexaenoic acids in young women. *Br J Nutr.* 2002;88(4):411-20. doi:10.1079/BJN2002689

93. U.S. Food and Drug Administration. What you need to know about mercury in fish and shellfish. www.fda.gov/food/resourcesforyou/consumers/ucm110591.htm

94. Innes JK, Calder PC. The differential effects of eicosapentaenoic acid and docosahexaenoic acid on cardiometabolic risk factors: A systematic review. *Int J Mol Sci.* 2018;19(2):532. doi:10.3390/ijms19020532

95. Egert S, Stehle P. Impact of n-3 fatty acids on endothelial function: Results from human interventions studies. *Curr Opin Clin Nutr Metab Care.* 2011;14(2):121-31. doi:10.1097/MCO.0b013e3283439622

96. Zehr KR, Walker MK. Omega-3 polyunsaturated fatty acids improve endothelial function in humans at risk for atherosclerosis: A review. *Prostaglandins Other Lipid Mediat.* 2018;134:131-140. doi:10.1016/j.prostaglandins.2017.07.005

97. Li K, Huang T, Zheng J, Wu K, Li D. Effect of marine-derived n-3 polyunsaturated fatty acids on C-reactive protein, interleukin 6 and tumor necrosis factor alpha: A meta-analysis. *PLoS One.* 2014;9(2):e88103. doi:10.1371/journal.pone.0088103

98. Miller PE, Van Elswyk M, Alexander DD. Long-chain omega-3 fatty acids eicosapentaenoic acid and docosahexaenoic acid and blood pressure: A meta-analysis of randomized controlled trials. *Am J Hypertens.* 2014;27(7):885-96. doi:10.1093/ajh/hpu024

99. Konig A, Bouzan C, Cohen JT, et al. A quantitative analysis of fish consumption and coronary heart disease mortality. *Am J Prev Med.* 2005;29(4):335-46. doi:10.1016/j.amepre.2005.07.001

100. Wang C, Harris WS, Chung M, et al. N-3 fatty acids from fish or fish-oil supplements, but not alpha-linolenic acid, benefit cardiovascular disease outcomes in primary- and secondary-prevention studies: A systematic review. *Am J Clin Nutr.* 2006;84(1):5-17.

101. He K, Song Y, Daviglus ML, et al. Accumulated evidence on fish consumption and coronary heart disease mortality: A meta-analysis of cohort studies. *Circulation.* 2004;109(22):2705-11. doi:10.1161/01.CIR.0000132503.19410.6B

102. Mozaffarian D. Fish and n-3 fatty acids for the prevention of fatal coronary heart disease and sudden cardiac death. *Am J Clin Nutr.* 2008;87(6):1991S-6S.

103. Mozaffarian D, Rimm EB. Fish intake, contaminants, and human health: Evaluating the risks and the benefits. *JAMA.* 2006;296(15):1885-99. doi:10.1001/jama.296.15.1885

104. Burr ML, Fehily AM, Gilbert JF, et al. Effects of changes in fat, fish, and fibre intakes on death and myocardial reinfarction: Diet and reinfarction trial (DART). *Lancet.* 1989;2(8666):757-61.

105. GISSI-Prevenzione Investigators. Dietary supplementation with n-3 polyunsaturated fatty acids and vitamin E after myocardial infarction: Results of the GISSI-Prevenzione trial. *Lancet.* 1999;354(9177):447-55.

106. Tavazzi L, Maggioni AP, Marchioli R, et al. Effect of n-3 polyunsaturated fatty acids in patients with chronic heart failure (the GISSI-HF trial): A randomised, double-blind, placebo-controlled trial. *Lancet.* 2008;372(9645):1223-30. doi:10.1016/S0140-6736(08)61239-8

107. Bosch J, Gerstein HC, Dagenais GR, et al. N-3 fatty acids and cardiovascular outcomes in patients with dysglycemia. *N Engl J Med.* 2012;367(4):309-18. doi:10.1056/NEJMoa1203859

108. Rauch B, Schiele R, Schneider S, et al. OMEGA, a randomized, placebo-controlled trial to test the effect of highly purified omega-3 fatty acids on top of modern guideline-adjusted therapy after myocardial infarction. *Circulation.* 2010;122(21):2152-9. doi:10.1161/CIRCULATIONAHA.110.948562

109. Kromhout D, Giltay EJ, Geleijnse JM. N-3 fatty acids and cardiovascular events after myocardial infarction. *N Engl J Med.* 2010;363(21):2015-26. doi:10.1056/NEJMoa1003603

110. Harris WS. Are n-3 fatty acids still cardioprotective? *Curr Opin Clin Nutr Metab Care.* 2013;16(2):141-9. doi:10.1097/MCO.0b013e32835bf380

111. James MJ, Sullivan TR, Metcalf RG, Cleland LG. Pitfalls in the use of randomised controlled trials for fish oil studies with cardiac patients. *Br J Nutr.* 2014;112(5):812-20. doi:10.1017/S0007114514001408

112. von Schacky C. Omega-3 fatty acids in cardiovascular disease—an uphill battle. *Prostaglandins Leukot Essent Fatty Acids.* 2015;92:41-7. doi:10.1016/j.plefa.2014.05.004

113. Marchioli R, Levantesi G. N-3 PUFAs in cardiovascular disease. *Int J Cardiol.* 2013;170(2 Suppl 1):S33-8. doi:10.1016/j.ijcard.2013.06.042

114. Wu JH, Mozaffarian D. Omega-3 fatty acids, atherosclerosis progression and cardiovascular outcomes in recent trials: New pieces in a complex puzzle. *Heart.* 2014;100(7):530-3. doi:10.1136/heartjnl-2013-305257

115. Lembke P, Capodice J, Hebert K, Swenson T. Influence of omega-3 (n3) index on performance and well-being in young adults after heavy eccentric exercise. *J Sports Sci Med.* 2014;13(1):151-6.

116. Heaton LE, Davis JK, Rawson ES, et al. Selected in-season nutritional strategies to enhance recovery for team sport athletes: A practical overview. *Sports Med.* 2017;47(11):2201-2218. doi:10.1007/s40279-017-0759-2

117. Goldberg RJ, Katz J. A meta-analysis of the analgesic effects of omega-3 polyunsaturated fatty acid supplementation for inflammatory joint pain. *Pain.* 2007;129(1-2):210-23. doi:10.1016/j.pain.2007.01.020

118. Miles EA, Calder PC. Influence of marine n-3 polyunsaturated fatty acids on immune function and a systematic review of their effects on clinical outcomes in rheumatoid arthritis. *Br J Nutr.* 2012;107(Suppl 2):S171-S184. doi:10.1017/S0007114512001560

119. Salem N, Jr., Litman B, Kim HY, Gawrisch K. Mechanisms of action of docosahexaenoic acid in the nervous system. *Lipids.* 2001;36(9):945-59.

120. Meier TB, Bellgowan PS, Singh R, Kuplicki R, Polanski DW, Mayer AR. Recovery of cerebral blood flow following sports-related concussion. *JAMA Neurol.* 2015;72(5):530-8. doi:10.1001/jamaneurol.2014.4778

121. Mills JD, Hadley K, Bailes JE. Dietary supplementation with the omega-3 fatty acid docosahexaenoic acid in traumatic brain injury. *Neurosurgery.* 2011;68(2):474-81. doi:10.1227/NEU.0b013e3181ff692b

122. Wu A, Ying Z, Gomez-Pinilla F. Omega-3 fatty acids supplementation restores mechanisms that maintain brain homeostasis in traumatic brain injury. *J Neurotrauma.* 2007;24(10):1587-95. doi:10.1089/neu.2007.0313

123. Wu A, Ying Z, Gomez-Pinilla F. Dietary omega-3 fatty acids normalize BDNF levels, reduce oxidative damage, and counteract learning disability after traumatic brain injury in rats. *J Neurotrauma*. 2004;21(10):1457-67. doi:10.1089/neu.2004.21.1457

124. Wang T, Van KC, Gavitt BJ, et al. Effect of fish oil supplementation in a rat model of multiple mild traumatic brain injuries. *Restor Neurol Neurosci*. 2013;31(5):647-59. doi:10.3233/RNN-130316

125. Mills JD, Bailes JE, Sedney CL, Hutchins H, Sears B. Omega-3 fatty acid supplementation and reduction of traumatic axonal injury in a rodent head injury model. *J Neurosurg*. 2011;114(1):77-84. doi:10.3171/2010.5.JNS08914

126. Wu A, Ying Z, Gomez-Pinilla F. The salutary effects of DHA dietary supplementation on cognition, neuroplasticity, and membrane homeostasis after brain trauma. *J Neurotrauma*. 2011;28(10):2113-22. doi:10.1089/neu.2011.1872

127. Wu A, Ying Z, Gomez-Pinilla F. Exercise facilitates the action of dietary DHA on functional recovery after brain trauma. *Neuroscience*. 2013;248:655-63. doi:10.1016/j.neuroscience.2013.06.041

128. Desai A, Kevala K, Kim HY. Depletion of brain docosahexaenoic acid impairs recovery from traumatic brain injury. *PLoS One*. 2014;9(1):e86472. doi:10.1371/journal.pone.0086472

129. Pu H, Guo Y, Zhang W, et al. Omega-3 polyunsaturated fatty acid supplementation improves neurologic recovery and attenuates white matter injury after experimental traumatic brain injury. *J Cereb Blood Flow Metab*. 2013;33(9):1474-84. doi:10.1038/jcbfm.2013.108

130. Heileson JL, Anzalone AJ, Carbuhn AF, et al. The effect of omega-3 fatty acids on a biomarker of head trauma in NCAA football athletes: A multi-site, non-randomized study. *J Int Soc Sports Nutr*. 2021;18(1):65. doi:10.1186/s12970-021-00461-1

131. Rossato LT, Schoenfeld BJ, de Oliveira EP. Is there sufficient evidence to supplement omega-3 fatty acids to increase muscle mass and strength in young and older adults? *Clin Nutr*. 2020;39(1):23-32. doi:10.1016/j.clnu.2019.01.001

132. Visconti LM, Cotter JA, Schick EE, et al. Impact of varying doses of omega-3 supplementation on muscle damage and recovery after eccentric resistance exercise. *Metabol Open*. 2021;12:100133. doi:10.1016/j.metop.2021.100133

133. McGlory C, Gorissen SHM, Kamal M, et al. Omega-3 fatty acid supplementation attenuates skeletal muscle disuse atrophy during two weeks of unilateral leg immobilization in healthy young women. *FASEB J*. 2019;33(3):4586-4597. doi:10.1096/fj.201801857RRR

134. U.S. Food and Drug Administration. Title 21: Food and drugs—part 184: Direct food substances affirmed as generally recognized as safe. *Code of Federal Regulations*. 1997.

135. Wachira JK, Larson MK, Harris WS. N-3 Fatty acids affect haemostasis but do not increase the risk of bleeding: Clinical observations and mechanistic insights. *Br J Nutr*. 2014;111(9):1652-62. doi:10.1017/S000711451300425X

136. Wang C, Chung M, Lichtenstein A, et al. *Effects of Omega-3 Fatty Acids on Cardiovascular Disease: Evidence Report/Technology Assessment No. 94*. Agency for Healthcare Research and Quality; 2004.

137. Aro A, Antoine J, Pizzoferrato L, Reykdala O, van Poppel G. Trans fatty acids and dairy and meat products from 14 European countries: The TRANSFAIR study. *J Food Compost Anal*. 1998;11:150-160.

138. O'Donnell-Megaro AM, Barbano DM, Bauman DE. Survey of the fatty acid composition of retail milk in the United States including regional and seasonal variations. *J Dairy Sci*. 2011;94(1):59-65. doi:10.3168/jds.2010-3571

139. Dhaka V, Gulia N, Ahlawat KS, Khatkar BS. Trans fats—sources, health risks and alternative approach: A review. *J Food Sci Technol*. 2011;48(5):534-41. doi:10.1007/s13197-010-0225-8

140. Mozaffarian D, Aro A, Willett WC. Health effects of trans-fatty acids: Experimental and observational evidence. *Eur J Clin Nutr*. 2009;63 Suppl 2:S5-S21. doi:10.1038/sj.ejcn.1602973

141. Mozaffarian D, Katan MB, Ascherio A, Stampfer MJ, Willett WC. Trans fatty acids and cardiovascular disease. *N Engl J Med*. 2006;354(15):1601-13. doi:10.1056/NEJMra054035

142. Aro A, Jauhiainen M, Partanen R, Salminen I, Mutanen M. Stearic acid, trans fatty acids, and dairy fat: Effects on serum and lipoprotein lipids, apolipoproteins, lipoprotein(a), and lipid transfer proteins in healthy subjects. *Am J Clin Nutr*. 1997;65(5):1419-26.

143. Judd JT, Clevidence BA, Muesing RA, Wittes J, Sunkin ME, Podczasy JJ. Dietary trans fatty acids: Effects on plasma lipids and lipoproteins of healthy men and women. *Am J Clin Nutr*. 1994;59(4):861-8.

144. Lichtenstein AH, Ausman LM, Jalbert SM, Schaefer EJ. Effects of different forms of dietary hydrogenated fats on serum lipoprotein cholesterol levels. *N Engl J Med*. 1999;340(25):1933-40. doi:10.1056/NEJM199906243402501

145. Bendsen NT, Chabanova E, Thomsen HS, et al. Effect of trans fatty acid intake on abdominal and liver fat deposition and blood lipids: A randomized trial in overweight postmenopausal women. *Nutr Diabetes*. 2011;1:e4. doi:10.1038/nutd.2010.4

146. Aronis KN, Khan SM, Mantzoros CS. Effects of trans fatty acids on glucose homeostasis: A meta-analysis of randomized, placebo-controlled clinical trials. *Am J Clin Nutr*. 2012;96(5):1093-9. doi:10.3945/ajcn.112.040576

147. Bendsen NT, Stender S, Szecsi PB, et al. Effect of industrially produced trans fat on markers of systemic inflammation: Evidence from a randomized trial in women. *J Lipid Res*. 2011;52(10):1821-8. doi:10.1194/jlr.M014738

148. U.S. Food and Drug Administration. Final determination regarding partially hydrogenated oils. *Federal Register*. 2018:23358-23359.

149. Precht D. Variation of trans fatty acids in milk fats. *Z Ernahrungswiss*. 1995;34(1):27-9.

150. Turpeinen AM, Mutanen M, Aro A, et al. Bioconversion of vaccenic acid to conjugated linoleic acid in humans. *Am J Clin Nutr*. 2002;76(3):504-10.

151. Adlof RO, Duval S, Emken EA. Biosynthesis of conjugated linoleic acid in humans. *Lipids*. 2000;35(2):131-5.

152. Mosley EE, McGuire MK, Williams JE, McGuire MA. Cis-9, trans-11 conjugated linoleic acid is synthesized from vaccenic acid in lactating women. *J Nutr*. 2006;136(9):2297-301.

153. Field CJ, Blewett HH, Proctor S, Vine D. Human health benefits of vaccenic acid. *Appl Physiol Nutr Metab*. 2009;34(5):979-91. doi:10.1139/H09-079

154. Gebauer SK, Chardigny JM, Jakobsen MU, et al. Effects of ruminant trans fatty acids on cardiovascular disease and cancer: A comprehensive review of epidemiological, clinical, and mechanistic studies. *Adv Nutr*. 2011;2(4):332-54. doi:10.3945/an.111.000521

155. Nishida C, Uauy R. WHO scientific update on health consequences of trans fatty acids: Introduction. *Eur J Clin Nutr*. 2009;63(Suppl 2):S1-S4. doi:10.1038/ejcn.2009.13

156. Zevenbergen H, de Bree A, Zeelenberg M, Laitinen K, van Duijn G, Floter E. Foods with a high fat quality are essential for healthy diets. *Ann Nutr Metab*. 2009;54(Suppl 1):15-24. doi:10.1159/000220823

157. Tarrago-Trani MT, Phillips KM, Lemar LE, Holden JM. New and existing oils and fats used in products with reduced trans-fatty acid content. *J Am Diet Assoc*. 2006;106(6):867-80. doi:10.1016/j.jada.2006.03.010

158. Berry SE. Triacylglycerol structure and interesterification of palmitic and stearic acid-rich fats: An overview and implications for cardiovascular disease. *Nutr Res Rev*. 2009;22(1):3-17. doi:10.1017/S0954422409369267

159. Hunter JE. Studies on effects of dietary fatty acids as related to their position on triglycerides. *Lipids*. 2001;36(7):655-68.

160. Noakes M, Clifton PM. Oil blends containing partially hydrogenated or interesterified fats: Differential effects on plasma lipids. *Am J Clin Nutr*. 1998;68(2):242-7.

161. Meijer GW, Weststrate JA. Interesterification of fats in margarine: Effect on blood lipids, blood enzymes, and hemostasis parameters. *Eur J Clin Nutr*. 1997;51(8):527-34.

162. Hayes KC. Synthetic and modified glycerides: Effects on plasma lipids. *Curr Opin Lipidol*. 2001;12(1):55-60.

163. Robinson DM, Martin NC, Robinson LE, Ahmadi L, Marangoni AG, Wright AJ. Influence of interesterification of a stearic acid-rich spreadable fat on acute metabolic risk factors. *Lipids*. 2009;44(1):17-26. doi:10.1007/s11745-008-3253-7

164. Sundram K, Karupaiah T, Hayes KC. Stearic acid-rich interesterified fat and trans-rich fat raise the LDL/HDL ratio and plasma glucose relative to palm olein in humans. *Nutr Metab (Lond)*. 2007;4:3. doi:10.1186/1743-7075-4-3

165. Filippou A, Teng KT, Berry SE, Sanders TA. Palmitic acid in the sn-2 position of dietary triacylglycerols does not affect insulin secretion or glucose homeostasis in healthy men and women. *Eur J Clin Nutr*. 2014;68(9):1036-41. doi:10.1038/ejcn.2014.141

166. Mills CE, Hall WL, Berry SEE. What are interesterified fats and should we be worried about them in our diet? *Nutr Bull*. 2017;42(2):153-158. doi:10.1111/nbu.12264

167. U.S. Institute of Medicine. *Dietary Reference Intakes for Energy, Carbohydrate, Fiber, Fat, Fatty Acids, Cholesterol, Protein, and Amino Acids*. National Academies Press; 2005.

168. U.S. Department of Health and Human Services and U.S. Department of Agriculture. *Dietary Guidelines for Americans, 2020-2025*. 9th ed. 2020.

169. Joint FAO/WHO Expert Consultation on Fats and Fatty Acids in Human Nutrition. *Interim Summary of Conclusions and Dietary Recommendations on Total Fat & Fatty Acids*. 2008.

Chapter 5

1. Dai Z, Wu Z, Jia S, Wu G. Analysis of amino acid composition in proteins of animal tissues and foods as pre-column o-phthaldialdehyde derivatives by HPLC with fluorescence detection. *J Chromatogr B Analyt Technol Biomed Life Sci*. 2014;964:116-27. doi:10.1016/j.jchromb.2014.03.025

2. Matthews DE. Proteins and amino acids. In: Ross AC, ed. *Modern Nutrition in Health and Disease*. 11th ed. Wolters Kluwer Health/Lippincott Williams & Wilkins; 2014.

3. Escott-Stump S. *Nutrition and Diagnosis-Related Care*. 8th ed. Wolters Kluwer; 2015.

4. National Center for Health Statistics. National health and nutrition examination survey data. October 28, 2016. http://www.cdc.gov/nchs/nhanes/about_nhanes.htm

5. U.S. Food and Drug Administration. Guidance for industry: A food labeling guide (Appendix B: Additional requirements for nutrient content claims). http://www.fda.gov/Food/GuidanceRegulation/GuidanceDocumentsRegulatoryInformation/LabelingNutrition/ucm064916.htm

6. Brocchieri L, Karlin S. Protein length in eukaryotic and prokaryotic proteomes. *Nucleic Acids Res*. 2005;33(10):3390-400. doi:10.1093/nar/gki615

7. Mitchell HH, Hamilton TS, Steggerda FR, Bean HW. The chemical composition of the adult human body and its bearing on the biochemistry of growth. *J Biol Chem*. 1945;158(3):625-637.

8. Kato H, Suzuki K, Bannai M, Moore DR. Protein requirements are elevated in endurance athletes after exercise as determined by the indicator amino acid oxidation method. *PLoS One*. 2016;11(6):e0157406. doi:10.1371/journal.pone.0157406

9. Thomas DT, Erdman KA, Burke LM. American College of Sports Medicine joint position statement: Nutrition and athletic performance. *Med Sci Sports Exerc*. 2016;48(3):543-68. doi:10.1249/mss.0000000000000852

10. Burke L, Castell L, Casa D, Close G. International Association of Athletics Federations consensus statement 2019: Nutrition for athletics. *International Journal of Sport Nutrition and Exercise Metabolism*. 2019;29:73-84. doi:10.1123/ijsnem.2019-0065

11. Klionsky DJ, Abdelmohsen K, Abe A, et al. Guidelines for the use and interpretation of assays for monitoring autophagy (3rd edition). *Autophagy*. 2016;12(1):1-222. doi:10.1080/15548627.2015.1100356

12. World Health Organization. *Protein and Amino Acid Requirements in Human Nutrition*. WHO technical report series. World Health Organization; 2007.

13. Phillips SM. Dietary protein requirements and adaptive advantages in athletes. *Br J Nutr*. 2012;108(Suppl 2):S158-S167. doi:10.1017/s0007114512002516

14. Rand WM, Pellett PL, Young VR. Meta-analysis of nitrogen balance studies for estimating protein requirements in healthy adults. *Am J Clin Nutr*. 2003;77(1):109-27.

15. Phillips SM, Chevalier S, Leidy HJ. Protein "requirements" beyond the RDA: Implications for optimizing health. *Appl Physiol Nutr Metab*. 2016;41(5):565-72. doi:10.1139/apnm-2015-0550

16. Layman DK. Dietary Guidelines should reflect new understandings about adult protein needs. *Nutr Metab (Lond)*. 2009;6:12. doi:10.1186/1743-7075-6-12

17. Institute of Medicine. *Dietary Reference Intakes for Energy, Carbohydrate, Fiber, Fat, Fatty Acids, Cholesterol, Protein, and Amino Acids (Macronutrients)*. National Academies Press; 2005:1357.

18. Center for Disease Control and Prevention. FastStats: Diet/nutrition. Center for Disease Control and Prevention. https://www.cdc.gov/nchs/fastats/diet.htm

19. Manore MM. Exercise and the Institute of Medicine recommendations for nutrition. *Curr Sports Med Rep*. 2005;4(4):193-8.

20. Morton RW, McGlory C, Phillips SM. Nutritional interventions to augment resistance training-induced skeletal muscle hypertrophy. *Front Physiol*. 2015;6:245. doi:10.3389/fphys.2015.00245

21. Pennings B, Boirie Y, Senden JM, Gijsen AP, Kuipers H, van Loon LJ. Whey protein stimulates postprandial muscle protein accretion more effectively than do casein and casein hydrolysate in older men. *Am J Clin Nutr*. 2011;93(5):997-1005. doi:10.3945/ajcn.110.008102

22. Sarwar G, McDonough FE. Evaluation of protein digestibility-corrected amino acid score method for assessing protein quality of foods. *J Assoc Off Anal Chem*. 1990;73(3):347-56.

23. Witard OC, Garthe I, Phillips SM. Dietary protein for training adaptation and body composition manipulation in track and field athletes. *Int J Sport Nutr Exerc Metab*. 2019;29:165-174. doi:10.1123/ijsnem.2018-0267

24. Morton R, Murphy K, McKellar S, et al. A systematic review, meta-analysis and metaregression of the effect of protein supplementation on resistance training-induced gains in muscle mass and strength in healthy adults. *Br J Sports Med*. 2018;52:376-388.

25. Jager R, Kerksick C, Campbell B, et al. International Society of Sports Nutrition Position Stand: protein and exercise. *J Int Soc Sports Nutr*. 2017;14(20). doi:10.1186/s12970-017-0177-8

26. Rosenbloom CA, Coleman EJ. *Sports Nutrition: A Practice Manual for Professionals*. Academy of Nutrition and Dietetics; 2012.

27. Areta JL, Burke LM, Camera DM, et al. Reduced resting skeletal muscle protein synthesis is rescued by resistance exercise and protein ingestion following short-term energy deficit. *Am J Physiol Endocrinol Metab*. 2014;306(8):E989-97. doi:10.1152/ajpendo.00590.2013

28. Rodriguez NR, Vislocky LM, Gaine PC. Dietary protein, endurance exercise, and human skeletal-muscle protein turnover. *Curr Opin Clin Nutr Metab Care*. 2007;10(1):40-45. doi:10.1097/MCO.0b013e3280115e3b

29. Mettler S, Mitchell N, Tipton KD. Increased protein intake reduces lean body mass loss during weight loss in athletes. *Med Sci Sports Exerc*. 2010;42(2):326-37. doi:10.1249/MSS.0b013e3181b2ef8e

30. Wall BT, Morton JP, van Loon LJ. Strategies to maintain skeletal muscle mass in the injured athlete: Nutritional considerations and exercise mimetics. *Eur J Sport Sci*. 2015;15(1):53-62. doi:10.1080/17461391.2014.936326

31. Shiffman S, Stone AA, Hufford MR. Ecological momentary assessment. *Annu Rev Clin Psychol*. 2008;4:1-32.

32. Phillips SM, Van Loon LJ. Dietary protein for athletes: From requirements to optimum adaptation. *J Sports Sci*. 2011;29(Suppl 1):S29-S38. doi:10.1080/02640414.2011.619204

33. Moore DR. Maximizing post-exercise anabolism: The case for relative protein intakes. *Frontiers in Nutrition*. 2019;6:147. doi:10.3389/fnut.2019.00147

34. Kerksick C, Arent S, Schoenfeld B, et al. International Society of Sports Nutrition position stand: Nutrient timing. *J Int Soc Sports Nutr*. 2017;14:33. doi:10.1186/s12970-017-0189-4

35. Tipton KD. Nutritional support for exercise-induced injuries. *Sports Med*. 2015;45(Suppl 1):S93-104. doi:10.1007/s40279-015-0398-4

36. Churchward-Venne TA, Burd NA, Mitchell CJ, et al. Supplementation of a suboptimal protein dose with leucine or essential amino acids: Effects on myofibrillar protein synthesis at rest and following resistance exercise in men. *J Physiol*. 2012;590(11):2751-65. doi:10.1113/jphysiol.2012.228833

37. Bonaldo P, Sandri M. Cellular and molecular mechanisms of muscle atrophy. *Dis Model Mech*. 2013;6(1):25-39. doi:10.1242/dmm.010389

38. Abbatecola AM, Chiodini P, Gallo C, et al. Pulse wave velocity is associated with muscle mass

decline: Health ABC study. *Age*. 2012;34(2):469-78. doi:10.1007/s11357-011-9238-0

39. Burd N, Beals J, Martinez I, AF. S, Skinner S. Food-first approach to enhance the regulation of post-exercise skeletal muscle protein synthesis and remodeling. *Sports Medicine*. 2019;49(Suppl 1):S59-S68. doi:10.1007/s40279-018-1009-y

40. Tipton KD, Elliott TA, Cree MG, Aarsland AA, Sanford AP, Wolfe RR. Stimulation of net muscle protein synthesis by whey protein ingestion before and after exercise. *Am J Physiol Endocrinol Metab*. 2007;292(1):E71-E76. doi:10.1152/ajpendo.00166.2006

41. Josse AR, Tang JE, Tarnopolsky MA, Phillips SM. Body composition and strength changes in women with milk and resistance exercise. *Med Sci Sports Exerc*. 2010;42(6):1122-30. doi:10.1249/MSS.0b013e3181c854f6

42. Hartman JW, Tang JE, Wilkinson SB, et al. Consumption of fat-free fluid milk after resistance exercise promotes greater lean mass accretion than does consumption of soy or carbohydrate in young, novice, male weightlifters. *Am J Clin Nutr*. 2007;86(2):373-81.

43. Josse AR, Atkinson SA, Tarnopolsky MA, Phillips SM. Increased consumption of dairy foods and protein during diet- and exercise-induced weight loss promotes fat mass loss and lean mass gain in overweight and obese premenopausal women. *J Nutr*. 2011;141(9):1626-34. doi:10.3945/jn.111.141028

44. Messina M, Lynch H, Dickinson JM, Reed KE. No difference between the effects of supplementing with soy protein versus animal protein on gains in muscle mass and strength in response to resistance exercise. *Int J Sport Nutr Exerc Metab*. 2018;28(6):674-685. doi:10.1123/ijsnem.2018-0071

45. Leaf A, Antonio J. The effects of overfeeding on body composition: The role of macronutrient composition—a narrative review. *International Journal of Exercise Science*. 2017;10(8):1275-1296.

46. Wentz L, Liu PY, Ilich JZ, Haymes EM. Dietary and training predictors of stress fractures in female runners. *Int J Sport Nutr Exerc Metab*. Oct 2012;22(5):374-82.

47. Moore DR, Slater G. Protein. In: Burke L, Deakin V, eds. *Clinical Sports Nutrition*. McGraw-Hill Education; 2015.

48. Devries M, Sithamparapillai A, Brimble K, Banfield L, Morton R, Phillips S. Changes in kidney function do not differ between healthy adults consuming higher- compared with lower- or normal-protein diets: A systematic review and meta-analysis. *Journal of Nutrition* 2018;148(11):1760-1775. doi:10.1093/jn/nxy197

49. Van Elswyk M, Weatherford C, McNeill S. A systematic review of renal health in healthy individuals associated with protein intake above the US recommended daily allowance in randomized controlled trials and observational studies. *Adv Nutr*. 2018;9(4):404-418. doi:10.1093/advances/nmy026

Chapter 6

1. Lukaski HC. Vitamin and mineral status: Effects on physical performance. *Nutrition*. 2004;20(7-8):632-44. doi:10.1016/j.nut.2004.04.001

2. U.S. Institute of Medicine. *Dietary Reference Intakes for Vitamin A, Vitamin K, Arsenic, Boron, Chromium, Copper, Iodine, Iron, Manganese, Molybdenum, Nickel, Silicon, Vanadium, and Zinc*. National Academies Press; 2001.

3. Harrison EH. Mechanisms involved in the intestinal absorption of dietary vitamin A and provitamin A carotenoids. *Biochim Biophys Acta*. 2012;1821(1):70-77. doi:10.1016/j.bbalip.2011.06.002

4. Tang G. Bioconversion of dietary provitamin A carotenoids to vitamin A in humans. *Am J Clin Nutr*. 2010;91(5):1468S-1473S. doi:10.3945/ajcn.2010.28674G

5. Lobo GP, Amengual J, Baus D, Shivdasani RA, Taylor D, von Lintig J. Genetics and diet regulate vitamin A production via the homeobox transcription factor ISX. *J Biol Chem*. 2013;288(13):9017-27. doi:10.1074/jbc.M112.444240

6. U.S. Department of Agriculture. USDA National Nutrient Database for Standard Reference, release 26. www.ars.usda.gov/ba/bhnrc/ndl

7. Mashurabad PC, Palika R, Jyrwa YW, Bhaskarachary K, Pullakhandam R. Dietary fat composition, food matrix and relative polarity modulate the micellarization and intestinal uptake of carotenoids from vegetables and fruits. *J Food Sci Technol*. 2017;54(2):333-341. doi:10.1007/s13197-016-2466-7

8. War AR, Paulraj MG, Ahmad T, et al. Mechanisms of plant defense against insect herbivores. *Plant Signal Behav*. 2012;7(10):1306-20. doi:10.4161/psb.21663

9. Williamson JD, Scandalios JG. Plant antioxidant gene responses to fungal pathogens. *Trends Microbiol*. 1993;1(6):239-45.

10. Ginter E, Simko V, Panakova V. Antioxidants in health and disease. *Bratisl Lek Listy*. 2014;115(10):603-6.

11. Lobo V, Patil A, Phatak A, Chandra N. Free radicals, antioxidants and functional foods: Impact on human health. *Pharmacogn Rev*. 2010;4(8):118-26. doi:10.4103/0973-7847.70902

12. Dijkhuizen MA, Wieringa FT, West CE, Muherdiyantiningsih, Muhilal. Concurrent micronutrient deficiencies in lactating mothers and their infants in Indonesia. *Am J Clin Nutr*. 2001;73(4):786-91.

13. Sanjoaquin MA, Molyneux ME. Malaria and vitamin A deficiency in African children: A vicious circle? *Malar J*. 2009;8:134. doi:10.1186/1475-2875-8-134

14. Akhtar S, Ahmed A, Randhawa MA, et al. Prevalence of vitamin A deficiency in South Asia: Causes, outcomes, and possible remedies. *J Health Popul Nutr*. 2013;31(4):413-23.

15. Khan MA, Gilbert C, Khan MD, Qureshi MB, Ahmad K. Incidence of blinding vitamin A deficiency in North West Frontier Province and its adjoining Federally Administered Tribal Areas,

Pakistan. *Ophthalmic Epidemiol.* 2009;16(1):2-7. doi:10.1080/09286580802573185

16. World Health Organization. *Global Prevalence of Vitamin A Deficiency in Populations at Risk 1995-2005: WHO Global Database on Vitamin A Deficiency.* 2009. http://apps.who.int/iris/bitstream/10665/44110/1/9789241598019_eng.pdf

17. Sommer A. Vitamin a deficiency and clinical disease: An historical overview. *J Nutr.* 2008;138(10):1835-9.

18. Oliveira-Menegozzo JM, Bergamaschi DP, Middleton P, East CE. Vitamin A supplementation for postpartum women. *Cochrane Database Syst Rev.* 2010;(10):CD005944. doi:10.1002/14651858.CD005944.pub2

19. Borowitz D, Baker RD, Stallings V. Consensus report on nutrition for pediatric patients with cystic fibrosis. *J Pediatr Gastroenterol Nutr.* 2002;35(3):246-59.

20. Olson JA. Adverse effects of large doses of vitamin A and retinoids. *Semin Oncol.* 1983;10(3):290-3.

21. Zimmerman H. Vitamin A (retinol): Drugs used in dermatotherapy. In: Zimmerman H, ed. *Hepatotoxicity: The Adverse Effects of Drugs and Other Chemicals on the Liver.* Lippincott; 1999:727-9.

22. Blumberg J, Block G. The alpha-tocopherol, beta-carotene cancer prevention study in Finland. *Nutr Rev.* 1994;52(7):242-5.

23. Goodman GE, Thornquist MD, Balmes J, et al. The Beta-Carotene and Retinol Efficacy Trial: Incidence of lung cancer and cardiovascular disease mortality during 6-year follow-up after stopping beta-carotene and retinol supplements. *J Natl Cancer Inst.* 2004;96(23):1743-50. doi:10.1093/jnci/djh320

24. Virtamo J, Pietinen P, Huttunen JK, et al. Incidence of cancer and mortality following alpha-tocopherol and beta-carotene supplementation: A postintervention follow-up. *JAMA.* 2003;290(4):476-85. doi:10.1001/jama.290.4.476

25. Leppala JM, Virtamo J, Fogelholm R, et al. Controlled trial of alpha-tocopherol and beta-carotene supplements on stroke incidence and mortality in male smokers. *Arterioscler Thromb Vasc Biol.* 2000;20(1):230-5.

26. Lips P, van Schoor NM, de Jongh RT. Diet, sun, and lifestyle as determinants of vitamin D status. *Ann N Y Acad Sci.* 2014;1317:92-98. doi:10.1111/nyas.12443

27. DeLuca HF. The transformation of a vitamin into a hormone: The vitamin D story. *Harvey Lect.* 1979;75:333-79.

28. Deluca HF, Cantorna MT. Vitamin D: Its role and uses in immunology. *FASEB J.* 2001;15(14):2579-85. doi:10.1096/fj.01-0433rev

29. Moran DS, McClung JP, Kohen T, Lieberman HR. Vitamin D and physical performance. *Sports Med.* 2013;43(7):601-11. doi:10.1007/s40279-013-0036-y

30. Cantorna MT, Mahon BD. D-hormone and the immune system. *J Rheumatol Suppl.* 2005;76:11-20.

31. van Etten E, Mathieu C. Immunoregulation by 1,25-dihydroxyvitamin D3: Basic concepts. *J Steroid Biochem Mol Biol.* 2005;97(1-2):93-101. doi:10.1016/j.jsbmb.2005.06.002

32. Feldmeyer L, Shojaati G, Spanaus KS, et al. Phototherapy with UVB narrowband, UVA/UVBnb, and UVA1 differentially impacts serum 25-hydroxyvitamin-D3. *J Am Acad Dermatol.* 2013;69(4):530-6. doi:10.1016/j.jaad.2013.04.058

33. Sallander E, Wester U, Bengtsson E, Wiegleb Edstrom D. Vitamin D levels after UVB radiation: Effects by UVA additions in a randomized controlled trial. *Photodermatol Photoimmunol Photomed.* 2013;29(6):323-9. doi:10.1111/phpp.12076

34. U.S. Food and Drug Administration. Tanning products. Accessed July 12, 2016. www.fda.gov/Radiation-EmittingProducts/RadiationEmittingProductsandProcedures/Tanning/ucm116434.htm

35. Boniol M, Autier P, Boyle P, Gandini S. Cutaneous melanoma attributable to sunbed use: Systematic review and meta-analysis. *BMJ.* 2012;345:e4757. doi:10.1136/bmj.e4757

36. Colantonio S, Bracken MB, Beecker J. The association of indoor tanning and melanoma in adults: Systematic review and meta-analysis. *J Am Acad Dermatol.* 2014;70(5):847-57. doi:10.1016/j.jaad.2013.11.050

37. Centers for Disease Control and Prevention. Indoor tanning is not safe. Accessed July 12, 2016. www.cdc.gov/cancer/skin/basic_info/indoor_tanning.htm

38. Bikle DD. Vitamin D metabolism, mechanism of action, and clinical applications. *Chem Biol.* 2014;21(3):319-29. doi:10.1016/j.chembiol.2013.12.016

39. Liu N, Sun J, Wang X, Zhang T, Zhao M, Li H. Low vitamin D status is associated with coronavirus disease 2019 outcomes: A systematic review and meta-analysis. *Int J Infect Dis.* 2021;104:58-64. doi:10.1016/j.ijid.2020.12.077

40. Teshome A, Adane A, Girma B, Mekonnen ZA. The impact of vitamin D level on COVID-19 infection: Systematic review and meta-analysis. *Front Public Health.* 2021;9:624559. doi:10.3389/fpubh.2021.624559

41. Phillips KM, Ruggio DM, Horst RL, et al. Vitamin D and sterol composition of 10 types of mushrooms from retail suppliers in the United States. *J Agric Food Chem.* 2011;59(14):7841-53. doi:10.1021/jf104246z

42. Holick MF. Vitamin D status: Measurement, interpretation, and clinical application. *Ann Epidemiol.* 2009;19(2):73-78. doi:10.1016/j.annepidem.2007.12.001

43. U.S. Food and Drug Administration. Title 21: Food and drugs. *Code of Federal Regulations.* 2015;

44. U.S. Institute of Medicine. *Dietary Reference Intakes: Guiding Principles for Nutrition Labeling and Fortification.* National Academies Press; 2003.

45. Trang H, Cole D, Rubin L, Pierratos A, Siu S, Vieth R. Evidence that vitamin D3 increases serum 25-hydroxyvitamin D more efficiently than does vitamin D2. *Am J Clin Nutr.* 1998;68(4):854-8.

46. Armas L, Hollis B, Heaney RP. Vitamin D2 is much less effective than vitamin D3 in humans. *J Clin Endocrinol Metab.* 2004;89(11):5387-91.

47. Dawson-Hughes B, Harris SS, Lichtenstein AH, Dolnikowski G, Palermo NJ, Rasmussen H. Dietary fat increases vitamin D-3 absorption. *J Acad Nutr Diet.* 2015;115(2):225-30. doi:10.1016/j.jand.2014.09.014

48. Mangin M, Sinha R, Fincher K. Inflammation and vitamin D: The infection connection. *Inflamm Res.* 2014;63(10):803-19. doi:10.1007/s00011-014-0755-z

49. Owens DJ, Allison R, Close GL. Vitamin D and the athlete: Current perspectives and new challenges. *Sports Med.* 2018;48(Suppl 1):3-16. doi:10.1007/s40279-017-0841-9

50. Dai Q, Zhu X, Manson JE, et al. Magnesium status and supplementation influence vitamin D status and metabolism: Results from a randomized trial. *Am J Clin Nutr.* 2018;108(6):1249-1258. doi:10.1093/ajcn/nqy274

51. Holick MF, Binkley NC, Bischoff-Ferrari HA, et al. Evaluation, treatment, and prevention of vitamin D deficiency: An Endocrine Society clinical practice guideline. *J Clin Endocrinol Metab.* 2011;96(7):1911-30. doi:10.1210/jc.2011-0385

52. U.S. Institute of Medicine. *Dietary Reference Intakes for Thiamin, Riboflavin, Niacin, Vitamin B6, Folate, Vitamin B12, Pantothenic Acid, Biotin, and Choline.* National Academies Press; 1998.

53. Herrick KA, Storandt RJ, Afful J, et al. Vitamin D status in the United States, 2011-2014. *Am J Clin Nutr.* 2019;110(1):150-157. doi:10.1093/ajcn/nqz037

54. Parva NR, Tadepalli S, Singh P, et al. Prevalence of vitamin D deficiency and associated risk factors in the US population (2011-2012). *Cureus.* 2018;10(6):e2741. doi:10.7759/cureus.2741

55. Close GL, Russell J, Cobley JN, et al. Assessment of vitamin D concentration in non-supplemented professional athletes and healthy adults during the winter months in the UK: Implications for skeletal muscle function. *J Sports Sci.* 2013;31(4):344-53. doi:10.1080/02640414.2012.733822

56. Wicinski M, Adamkiewicz D, Adamkiewicz M, et al. Impact of vitamin D on physical efficiency and exercise performance: A review. *Nutrients.* 2019;11(11):2826. doi:10.3390/nu11112826

57. Maroon JC, Mathyssek CM, Bost JW, et al. Vitamin D profile in National Football League players. *Am J Sports Med.* 2015;43(5):1241-5. doi:10.1177/0363546514567297

58. He CS, Handzlik M, Fraser WD, et al. Influence of vitamin D status on respiratory infection incidence and immune function during 4 months of winter training in endurance sport athletes. *Exerc Immunol Rev.* 2013;19:86-101.

59. Willis KS, Smith DT, Broughton KS, Larson-Meyer DE. Vitamin D status and biomarkers of inflammation in runners. *Open Access J Sports Med.* 2012;3:35-42. doi:10.2147/OAJSM.S31022

60. Hamilton B, Grantham J, Racinais S, Chalabi H. Vitamin D deficiency is endemic in Middle Eastern sportsmen. *Public Health Nutr.* 2010;13(10):1528-34. doi:10.1017/S136898000999320X

61. Shindle M, Voos J, Gulotta L, et al. Vitamin D status in a professional American football team.

62. Fishman MP, Lombardo SJ, Kharrazi FD. Vitamin D deficiency among professional basketball players. *Orthop J Sports Med.* 2016;4(7):2325967116655742. doi:10.1177/2325967116655742

63. de la Puente Yague M, Collado Yurrita L, Ciudad Cabanas MJ, Cuadrado Cenzual MA. Role of vitamin D in athletes and their performance: current concepts and new trends. *Nutrients.* 2020;12(2). doi:10.3390/nu12020579

64. Halliday TM, Peterson NJ, Thomas JJ, Kleppinger K, Hollis BW, Larson-Meyer DE. Vitamin D status relative to diet, lifestyle, injury, and illness in college athletes. *Med Sci Sports Exerc.* 2011;43(2):335-43. doi:10.1249/MSS.0b013e3181eb9d4d

65. U.S. Institute of Medicine. *Dietary Reference Intakes for Calcium and Vitamin D.* National Academies Press; 2011.

66. Yao Y, Zhu L, He L, et al. A meta-analysis of the relationship between vitamin D deficiency and obesity. *Int J Clin Exp Med.* 2015;8(9):14977-14984.

67. Matsuoka LY, Ide L, Wortsman J, MacLaughlin JA, Holick MF. Sunscreens suppress cutaneous vitamin D3 synthesis. *J Clin Endocrinol Metab.* 1987;64(6):1165-8. doi:10.1210/jcem-64-6-1165

68. Forrest KY, Stuhldreher WL. Prevalence and correlates of vitamin D deficiency in US adults. *Nutr Res.* 2011;31(1):48-54. doi:10.1016/j.nutres.2010.12.001

69. Ziegler PJ, Nelson JA, Jonnalagadda SS. Nutritional and physiological status of U.S. national figure skaters. *Int J Sport Nutr.* 1999;9(4):345-60.

70. Bergen-Cico DK, Short SH. Dietary intakes, energy expenditures, and anthropometric characteristics of adolescent female cross-country runners. *J Am Diet Assoc.* 1992;92(5):611-2.

71. Bescos Garcia R, Rodriguez Guisado F. Low levels of vitamin D in professional basketball players after wintertime: Relationship with dietary intake of vitamin D and calcium. *Nutr Hosp.* 2011;26:945-951.

72. Clark M, Reed DB, Crouse SF, Armstrong RB. Pre- and post-season dietary intake, body composition, and performance indices of NCAA division I female soccer players. *Int J Sport Nutr Exerc Metab.* 2003;13(3):303-19.

73. Fulgoni VL, 3rd, Keast DR, Bailey RL, Dwyer J. Foods, fortificants, and supplements: Where do Americans get their nutrients? *J Nutr.* 2011;141(10):1847-54. doi:10.3945/jn.111.142257

74. Heaney RP, Holick MF. Why the IOM recommendations for vitamin D are deficient. *J Bone Miner Res.* 2011;26(3):455-7. doi:10.1002/jbmr.328

75. Trivedi DP, Doll R, Khaw KT. Effect of four monthly oral vitamin D3 (cholecalciferol) supplementation on fractures and mortality in men and women living in the community: Randomised double blind controlled trial. *BMJ.* 2003;326(7387):469. doi:10.1136/bmj.326.7387.469

76. Bischoff-Ferrari HA. Vitamin D and fracture prevention. *Endocrinol Metab Clin North Am*. 2010;39(2):347-53. doi:10.1016/j.ecl.2010.02.009
77. Bischoff-Ferrari HA, Shao A, Dawson-Hughes B, Hathcock J, Giovannucci E, Willett WC. Benefit-risk assessment of vitamin D supplementation. *Osteoporos Int*. 2010;21(7):1121-32. doi:10.1007/s00198-009-1119-3
78. Veugelers PJ, Ekwaru JP. A statistical error in the estimation of the recommended dietary allowance for vitamin D. *Nutrients*. 2014;6(10):4472-5. doi:10.3390/nu6104472
79. Miller JR, Dunn KW, Ciliberti LJ, Jr., Patel RD, Swanson BA. Association of vitamin D with stress fractures: A retrospective cohort study. *J Foot Ankle Surg*. 2015;55(1):117-20. doi:10.1053/j.jfas.2015.08.002
80. Wharton B, Bishop N. Rickets. *Lancet*. 2003;362(9393):1389-400. doi:10.1016/S0140-6736(03)14636-3
81. Reginato AJ, Coquia JA. Musculoskeletal manifestations of osteomalacia and rickets. *Best Pract Res Clin Rheumatol*. 2003;17(6):1063-80. doi:10.1016/j.berh.2003.09.004
82. Abrams GD, Feldman D, Safran MR. Effects of vitamin D on skeletal muscle and athletic performance. *J Am Acad Orthop Surg*. 2018;26(8):278-285. doi:10.5435/JAAOS-D-16-00464
83. Lotfi A, Abdel-Nasser AM, Hamdy A, Omran AA, El-Rehany MA. Hypovitaminosis D in female patients with chronic low back pain. *Clin Rheumatol*. 2007;26(11):1895-901. doi:10.1007/s10067-007-0603-4
84. Rkain H, Bouaddi I, Ibrahimi A, et al. Relationship between vitamin D deficiency and chronic low back pain in postmenopausal women. *Curr Rheumatol Rev*. 2013;9(1):63-67.
85. Schwalfenberg G. Improvement of chronic back pain or failed back surgery with vitamin D repletion: A case series. *J Am Board Fam Med*. 2009;22(1):69-74. doi:10.3122/jabfm.2009.01.080026
86. LeBlanc ES, Zakher B, Daeges M, Pappas M, Chou R. Screening for vitamin D deficiency: A systematic review for the U.S. Preventive Services Task Force. *Ann Intern Med*. 2015;162(2):109-22. doi:10.7326/M14-1659
87. Grober U, Kisters K. Influence of drugs on vitamin D and calcium metabolism. *Dermatoendocrinol*. 2012;4(2):158-66. doi:10.4161/derm.20731
88. Holick MF. Vitamin D deficiency. *N Engl J Med*. 2007;357(3):266-81. doi:10.1056/NEJMra070553
89. Owens DJ, Tang JC, Bradley WJ, et al. Efficacy of high-dose vitamin D supplements for elite athletes. *Med Sci Sports Exerc*. 2017;49(2):349-356. doi:10.1249/MSS.0000000000001105
90. Tomei S, Singh P, Mathew R, et al. The role of polymorphisms in vitamin D-related genes in response to vitamin D supplementation. *Nutrients*. 2020;12(9):E2608. doi:10.3390/nu12092608
91. Zhang M, Zhao LJ, Zhou Y, et al. SNP rs11185644 of RXRA gene is identified for dose-response variability to vitamin D3 supplementation: A randomized clinical trial. *Sci Rep*. 2017;7:40593. doi:10.1038/srep40593
92. Maughan RJ, Watson P, Cordery PAA, et al. Sucrose and sodium but not caffeine content influence the retention of beverages in humans under euhydrated conditions. *Int J Sport Nutr Exerc Metab*. 2019;29(1):51-60. doi:10.1123/ijsnem.2018-0047
93. Holick MF. Environmental factors that influence the cutaneous production of vitamin D. *Am J Clin Nutr*. 1995;61(3 Suppl):638S-645S.
94. Vieth R. Vitamin D supplementation, 25-hydroxyvitamin D concentrations, and safety. *Am J Clin Nutr*. 1999;69(5):842-56.
95. Beer TM, Myrthue A. Calcitriol in cancer treatment: From the lab to the clinic. *Mol Cancer Ther*. 2004;3(3):373-81.
96. Ross AC, Manson JE, Abrams SA, et al. The 2011 report on Dietary Reference Intakes for calcium and vitamin D from the Institute of Medicine: What clinicians need to know. *J Clin Endocrinol Metab*. 2011;96(1):53-58. doi:10.1210/jc.2010-2704
97. Birge SJ, Haddad JG. 25-hydroxycholecalciferol stimulation of muscle metabolism. *J Clin Invest*. 1975;56(5):1100-7. doi:10.1172/JCI108184
98. Pfeifer M, Begerow B, Minne HW. Vitamin D and muscle function. *Osteoporos Int*. 2002;13(3):187-94. doi:10.1007/s001980200012
99. Grant WB, Lahore H, Rockwell MS. The benefits of vitamin D supplementation for athletes: Better performance and reduced risk of COVID-19. *Nutrients*. 2020;12(12):3741. doi:10.3390/nu12123741
100. Ribbans WJ, Aujla R, Dalton S, Nunley JA. Vitamin D and the athlete-patient: State of the art. *J ISAKOS*. 2021;6(1):46-60. doi:10.1136/jisakos-2020-000435
101. Koundourakis NE, Androulakis NE, Malliaraki N, Margioris AN. Vitamin D and exercise performance in professional soccer players. *PLoS One*. 2014;9(7):e101659. doi:10.1371/journal.pone.0101659
102. Ward KA, Das G, Berry JL, et al. Vitamin D status and muscle function in post-menarchal adolescent girls. *J Clin Endocrinol Metab*. 2009;94(2):559-63. doi:10.1210/jc.2008-1284
103. Barker T, Henriksen VT, Martins TB, et al. Higher serum 25-hydroxyvitamin D concentrations associate with a faster recovery of skeletal muscle strength after muscular injury. *Nutrients*. 2013;5(4):1253-75. doi:10.3390/nu5041253
104. Barker T, Schneider ED, Dixon BM, Henriksen VT, Weaver LK. Supplemental vitamin D enhances the recovery in peak isometric force shortly after intense exercise. *Nutr Metab (Lond)*. 2013;10(1):69. doi:10.1186/1743-7075-10-69
105. Beaudart C, Buckinx F, Rabenda V, et al. The effects of vitamin D on skeletal muscle strength, muscle mass, and muscle power: A systematic review and meta-analysis of randomized controlled trials. *J Clin Endocrinol Metab*. 2014;99(11):4336-45. doi:10.1210/jc.2014-1742

106. Savolainen L, Timpmann S, Mooses M, et al. Vitamin D supplementation does not enhance resistance training-induced gains in muscle strength and lean body mass in vitamin D deficient young men. *Eur J Appl Physiol.* 2021;doi:10.1007/s00421-021-04674-9

107. Ardestani A, Parker B, Mathur S, et al. Relation of vitamin D level to maximal oxygen uptake in adults. *Am J Cardiol.* 2011;107(8):1246-9. doi:10.1016/j.amjcard.2010.12.022

108. Sabetta JR, DePetrillo P, Cipriani RJ, Smardin J, Burns LA, Landry ML. Serum 25-hydroxyvitamin d and the incidence of acute viral respiratory tract infections in healthy adults. *PLoS One.* 2010;5(6):e11088. doi:10.1371/journal.pone.0011088

109. Ginde AA, Mansbach JM, Camargo CA, Jr. Association between serum 25-hydroxyvitamin D level and upper respiratory tract infection in the Third National Health and Nutrition Examination Survey. *Arch Intern Med.* 2009;169(4):384-90. doi:10.1001/archinternmed.2008.560

110. Wyon MA, Wolman R, Nevill AM, et al. Acute effects of vitamin D3 supplementation on muscle strength in judoka athletes: A randomized placebo-controlled, double-blind trial. *Clin J Sport Med.* 2016;26(4):279-84. doi:10.1097/JSM.0000000000000264

111. Han Q, Li X, Tan Q, Shao J, Yi M. Effects of vitamin D3 supplementation on serum 25(OH)D concentration and strength in athletes: A systematic review and meta-analysis of randomized controlled trials. *J Int Soc Sports Nutr.* 2019;16(1):55. doi:10.1186/s12970-019-0323-6

112. U.S. Department of Agriculture. Nutrient intakes from food: Mean amounts consumed per individual, by gender and age: What we eat in America, NHANES 2009-2010. www.ars.usda.gov/ba/bhnrc/fsrg

113. Short SH, Short WR. Four-year study of university athletes' dietary intake. *J Am Diet Assoc.* 1983;82(6):632-45.

114. Loosli AR, Benson J. Nutritional intake in adolescent athletes. *Pediatr Clin North Am.* 1990;37(5):1143-52.

115. Economos CD, Bortz SS, Nelson ME. Nutritional practices of elite athletes: Practical recommendations. *Sports Med.* 1993;16(6):381-99.

116. Berry DJ, Hesketh K, Power C, Hypponen E. Vitamin D status has a linear association with seasonal infections and lung function in British adults. *Br J Nutr.* 2011;106(9):1433-40. doi:10.1017/S0007114511001991

117. Davey T, Lanham-New SA, Shaw AM, et al. Low serum 25-hydroxyvitamin D is associated with increased risk of stress fracture during Royal Marine recruit training. *Osteoporos Int.* 2016;27(1):171-9. doi:10.1007/s00198-015-3228-5

118. Millward D, Root AD, Dubois J, et al. Association of serum vitamin D levels and stress fractures in collegiate athletes. *Orthop J Sports Med.* 2020;8(12):2325967120966967. doi:10.1177/2325967120966967

119. Rebolledo BJ, Bernard JA, Werner BC, et al. The association of vitamin D status in lower extremity muscle strains and core muscle injuries at the National Football League combine. *Arthroscopy.* 2018;34(4):1280-1285. doi:10.1016/j.arthro.2017.10.005

120. Barker T, Martins T, Hill H, et al. Low vitamin D impairs strength recovery after anterior cruciate ligament surgery. *JEBCAM.* 2011;16(3):201-209. doi:10.1177/2156587211413768

121. Di Luigi L, Antinozzi C, Piantanida E, Sgro P. Vitamin D, sport and health: A still unresolved clinical issue. *J Endocrinol Invest.* 2020;43(12):1689-1702. doi:10.1007/s40618-020-01347-w

122. U.S. Institute of Medicine. *Dietary Reference Intakes for Vitamin C, Vitamin E, Selenium, and Carotenoids.* National Academies Press; 2000.

123. Valko M, Rhodes CJ, Moncol J, Izakovic M, Mazur M. Free radicals, metals and antioxidants in oxidative stress-induced cancer. *Chem Biol Interact.* 2006;160(1):1-40. doi:10.1016/j.cbi.2005.12.009

124. Kukreja RC, Hess ML. The oxygen free radical system: From equations through membrane-protein interactions to cardiovascular injury and protection. *Cardiovasc Res.* 1992;26(7):641-55.

125. Pellegrini N, Serafini M, Colombi B, et al. Total antioxidant capacity of plant foods, beverages and oils consumed in Italy assessed by three different in vitro assays. *J Nutr.* 2003;133(9):2812-9.

126. Moshfegh A, Goldman J, Cleveland L. *Usual Intakes From Food and Water Compared to 1997 Dietary Reference Intakes: What We Eat in America, NHANES 2005-2006.* 2005.

127. Klein EA, Thompson IM, Jr., Tangen CM, et al. Vitamin E and the risk of prostate cancer: The Selenium and Vitamin E Cancer Prevention Trial (SELECT). *JAMA.* 2011;306(14):1549-56. doi:10.1001/jama.2011.1437

128. Powers SK, Jackson MJ. Exercise-induced oxidative stress: Cellular mechanisms and impact on muscle force production. *Physiol Rev.* 2008;88(4):1243-76. doi:10.1152/physrev.00031.2007

129. Kim J, Lee J. A review of nutritional intervention on delayed onset muscle soreness. Part I. *J Exerc Rehabil.* 2014;10(6):349-56. doi:10.12965/jer.140179

130. Gaeini AA, Rahnama N, Hamedinia MR. Effects of vitamin E supplementation on oxidative stress at rest and after exercise to exhaustion in athletic students. *J Sports Med Phys Fitness.* 2006;46(3):458-61.

131. Sharman IM, Down MG, Norgan NG. The effects of vitamin E on physiological function and athletic performance of trained swimmers. *J Sports Med Phys Fitness.* 1976;16(3):215-25.

132. Ciocoiu M, Badescu M, Paduraru I. Protecting antioxidative effects of vitamins E and C in experimental physical stress. *J Physiol Biochem.* 2007;63(3):187-94.

133. Taghiyar M, Ghiasvand R, Askari G, et al. The effect of vitamins C and E supplementation on muscle damage, performance, and body composition in athlete women: A clinical trial. *Int J Prev Med.* 2013;4(Suppl 1):S24-S30.

134. Wang Y, Hodge AM, Wluka AE, et al. Effect of antioxidants on knee cartilage and bone in healthy,

middle-aged subjects: A cross-sectional study. *Arthritis Res Ther.* 2007;9(4):R66. doi:10.1186/ar2225

135. Yamaguchi M. Role of carotenoid beta-cryptoxanthin in bone homeostasis. *J Biomed Sci.* 2012;19:36. doi:10.1186/1423-0127-19-36

136. De Roos AJ, Arab L, Renner JB, et al. Serum carotenoids and radiographic knee osteoarthritis: The Johnston County Osteoarthritis Project. *Public Health Nutr.* 2001;4(5):935-42.

137. McAlindon TE, Jacques P, Zhang Y, et al. Do antioxidant micronutrients protect against the development and progression of knee osteoarthritis? *Arthritis Rheum.* 1996;39(4):648-56.

138. Hartley L, Clar C, Ghannam O, Flowers N, Stranges S, Rees K. Vitamin K for the primary prevention of cardiovascular disease. *Cochrane Database Syst Rev.* 2015;(9):CD011148. doi:10.1002/14651858. CD011148.pub2

139. Schurgers LJ. Vitamin K: Key vitamin in controlling vascular calcification in chronic kidney disease. *Kidney Int.* 2013;83(5):782-4. doi:10.1038/ki.2013.26

140. Traber MG. Vitamin E and K interactions—a 50-year-old problem. *Nutr Rev.* 2008;66(11):624-9. doi:10.1111/j.1753-4887.2008.00123.x

141. U.S. Food and Drug Administration. How to understand and use the nutrition facts label. Accessed March 23, 2016. www.fda.gov/Food/IngredientsPackagingLabeling/LabelingNutrition/ucm274593. htm#percent_daily_value

142. U.S. Food and Drug Administration. Title 21: Food and drugs—chapter 1: Food and Drug Administration—subchapter B: Food for human consumption—part 101: Food labeling. *Code of Federal Regulations.*

143. van der Beek EJ, van Dokkum W, Wedel M, Schrijver J, van den Berg H. Thiamin, riboflavin and vitamin B6: Impact of restricted intake on physical performance in man. *J Am Coll Nutr.* 1994;13(6):629-40.

144. Hickson JF, Jr., Schrader J, Trischler LC. Dietary intakes of female basketball and gymnastics athletes. *J Am Diet Assoc.* 1986;86(2):251-3.

145. Deuster PA, Kyle SB, Moser PB, Vigersky RA, Singh A, Schoomaker EB. Nutritional survey of highly trained women runners. *Am J Clin Nutr.* 1986;44(6):954-62.

146. Zempleni J, Hassan YI, Wijeratne SS. Biotin and biotinidase deficiency. *Expert Rev Endocrinol Metab.* 2008;3(6):715-724. doi:10.1586/17446651.3.6.715

147. Chester D, Goldman J, Ahuja J, Moshfegh A. *Dietary intakes of choline: What we eat in America, NHANES 2007-2008.* 2011.

148. Sanders LM, Zeisel SH. Choline: Dietary requirements and role in brain development. *Nutr Today.* 2007;42(4):181-186. doi:10.1097/01. NT.0000286155.55343.fa

149. Fischer LM, daCosta KA, Kwock L, et al. Sex and menopausal status influence human dietary requirements for the nutrient choline. *Am J Clin Nutr.* 2007;85(5):1275-85.

150. Zeisel SH, Da Costa KA, Franklin PD, et al. Choline, an essential nutrient for humans. *FASEB J.* 1991;5(7):2093-8.

151. Spector SA, Jackman MR, Sabounjian LA, Sakkas C, Landers DM, Willis WT. Effect of choline supplementation on fatigue in trained cyclists. *Med Sci Sports Exerc.* 1995;27(5):668-73.

152. Bailey RL, Dodd KW, Gahche JJ, et al. Total folate and folic acid intake from foods and dietary supplements in the United States: 2003-2006. *Am J Clin Nutr.* 2010;91(1):231-7. doi:10.3945/ajcn.2009.28427

153. Woolf K, Manore MM. B-vitamins and exercise: Does exercise alter requirements? *Int J Sport Nutr Exerc Metab.* 2006;16(5):453-84.

154. Beals KA, Manore MM. Nutritional status of female athletes with subclinical eating disorders. *J Am Diet Assoc.* 1998;98(4):419-25. doi:10.1016/S0002-8223(98)00096-0

155. Matter M, Stittfall T, Graves J, et al. The effect of iron and folate therapy on maximal exercise performance in female marathon runners with iron and folate deficiency. *Clin Sci (Lond).* 1987;72(4):415-22.

156. Faber M, Benade AJ. Mineral and vitamin intake in field athletes (discus-, hammer-, javelin-throwers and shotputters). *Int J Sports Med.* 1991;12(3):324-7. doi:10.1055/s-2007-1024690

157. Sullivan G, Wells KB, Leake B. Clinical factors associated with better quality of life in a seriously mentally ill population. *Hosp Community Psychiatry.* 1992;43(8):794-8.

158. Olson JE, Hamilton GC, Angelos MG, Singer JI, Eilers ME, Gaddis M. Objectives to direct the training of emergency medicine residents on off-service rotations: research. *J Emerg Med.* 1992;10(5):631-6.

159. Bergstrom J, Hultman E, Jorfeldt L, Pernow B, Wahren J. Effect of nicotinic acid on physical working capacity and on metabolism of muscle glycogen in man. *J Appl Physiol.* 1969;26(2):170-6.

160. Webster MJ. Physiological and performance responses to supplementation with thiamin and pantothenic acid derivatives. *Eur J Appl Physiol Occup Physiol.* 1998;77(6):486-91. doi:10.1007/s004210050364

161. McCormick DB. Vitamin/mineral supplements: of questionable benefit for the general population. *Nutr Rev.* 2010;68(4):207-13. doi:10.1111/j.1753-4887.2010.00279.x

162. Belko AZ, Meredith MP, Kalkwarf HJ, et al. Effects of exercise on riboflavin requirements: Biological validation in weight reducing women. *Am J Clin Nutr.* 1985;41(2):270-7.

163. Manore MM. Effect of physical activity on thiamine, riboflavin, and vitamin B-6 requirements. *Am J Clin Nutr.* 2000;72(2 Suppl):598S-606S.

164. Fogelholm M, Ruokonen I, Laakso JT, Vuorimaa T, Himberg JJ. Lack of association between indices of vitamin B1, B2, and B6 status and exercise-induced blood lactate in young adults. *Int J Sport Nutr.* 1993;3(2):165-76.

165. Suboticanec K, Stavljenic A, Schalch W, Buzina R. Effects of pyridoxine and riboflavin supplementation on physical fitness in young adolescents. *Int J Vitam Nutr Res.* 1990;60(1):81-88.

166. Kimura M, Itokawa Y, Fujiwara M. Cooking losses of thiamin in food and its nutritional significance. *J Nutr Sci Vitaminol (Tokyo)*. 1990;36(Suppl 1):S17-S24.
167. Hoyumpa AM, Jr. Mechanisms of thiamin deficiency in chronic alcoholism. *Am J Clin Nutr*. 1980;33(12):2750-61.
168. Vognar L, Stoukides J. The role of low plasma thiamin levels in cognitively impaired elderly patients presenting with acute behavioral disturbances. *J Am Geriatr Soc*. 2009;57(11):2166-8. doi:10.1111/j.1532-5415.2009.02542.x
169. Wilkinson TJ, Hanger HC, George PM, Sainsbury R. Is thiamine deficiency in elderly people related to age or co-morbidity? *Age Ageing*. 2000;29(2):111-6.
170. Boldorini R, Vago L, Lechi A, Tedeschi F, Trabattoni GR. Wernicke's encephalopathy: Occurrence and pathological aspects in a series of 400 AIDS patients. *Acta Biomed Ateneo Parmense*. 1992;63(1-2):43-49.
171. Jermendy G. Evaluating thiamine deficiency in patients with diabetes. *Diab Vasc Dis Res*. 2006;3(2):120-1. doi:10.3132/dvdr.2006.014
172. Saito N, Kimura M, Kuchiba A, Itokawa Y. Blood thiamine levels in outpatients with diabetes mellitus. *J Nutr Sci Vitaminol (Tokyo)*. 1987;33(6):421-30.
173. Xanthakos SA. Nutritional deficiencies in obesity and after bariatric surgery. *Pediatr Clin North Am*. 2009;56(5):1105-21. doi:10.1016/j.pcl.2009.07.002
174. Wood B, Gijsbers A, Goode A, Davis S, Mulholland J, Breen K. A study of partial thiamin restriction in human volunteers. *Am J Clin Nutr*. 1980;33(4):848-61.
175. Doyle MR, Webster MJ, Erdmann LD. Allithiamine ingestion does not enhance isokinetic parameters of muscle performance. *Int J Sport Nutr*. 1997;7(1):39-47.
176. Simpson JL, Bailey LB, Pietrzik K, Shane B, Holzgreve W. Micronutrients and women of reproductive potential: Required dietary intake and consequences of dietary deficiency or excess. Part I—folate, vitamin B12, vitamin B6. *J Matern Fetal Neonatal Med*. 2010;23(12):1323-43. doi:10.3109/14767051003678234
177. Gdynia HJ, Muller T, Sperfeld AD, et al. Severe sensorimotor neuropathy after intake of highest dosages of vitamin B6. *Neuromuscul Disord*. 2008;18(2):156-8. doi:10.1016/j.nmd.2007.09.009
178. Bendich A, Cohen M. Vitamin B6 safety issues. *Ann N Y Acad Sci*. 1990;585:321-30.
179. Manore MN, Leklem JE, Walter MC. Vitamin B-6 metabolism as affected by exercise in trained and untrained women fed diets differing in carbohydrate and vitamin B-6 content. *Am J Clin Nutr*. 1987;46(6):995-1004.
180. Leonard SW, Leklem JE. Plasma B-6 vitamer changes following a 50-km ultra-marathon. *Int J Sport Nutr Exerc Metab*. 2000;10(3):302-14.
181. Rokitzki L, Sagredos AN, Reuss F, Buchner M, Keul J. Acute changes in vitamin B6 status in endurance athletes before and after a marathon. *Int J Sport Nutr*. 1994;4(2):154-65.
182. Pawlak R, Lester SE, Babatunde T. The prevalence of cobalamin deficiency among vegetarians assessed by serum vitamin B12: A review of literature. *Eur J Clin Nutr*. 2014;68(5):541-8. doi:10.1038/ejcn.2014.46
183. Gueant JL, Safi A, Aimone-Gastin I, et al. Autoantibodies in pernicious anemia type I patients recognize sequence 251-256 in human intrinsic factor. *Proc Assoc Am Physicians*. 1997;109(5):462-9.
184. Allen LH. How common is vitamin B-12 deficiency? *Am J Clin Nutr*. 2009;89(2):693S-6S. doi:10.3945/ajcn.2008.26947A
185. Carmel R. Malabsorption of food cobalamin. *Baillieres Clin Haematol*. 1995;8(3):639-55.
186. Lindenbaum J, Rosenberg IH, Wilson PW, Stabler SP, Allen RH. Prevalence of cobalamin deficiency in the Framingham elderly population. *Am J Clin Nutr*. 1994;60(1):2-11.
187. Bailey RL, Carmel R, Green R, et al. Monitoring of vitamin B-12 nutritional status in the United States by using plasma methylmalonic acid and serum vitamin B-12. *Am J Clin Nutr*. 2011;94(2):552-61. doi:10.3945/ajcn.111.015222
188. National Institutes of Health. *Your Guide to Anemia*. NIH Publication No. 11-7629.
189. Read MH, McGuffin SL. The effect of B-complex supplementation on endurance performance. *J Sports Med Phys Fitness*. 1983;23(2):178-84.
190. Carr AC, Frei B. Toward a new recommended dietary allowance for vitamin C based on antioxidant and health effects in humans. *Am J Clin Nutr*. 1999;69(6):1086-107.
191. Krause R, Patruta S, Daxbock F, Fladerer P, Biegelmayer C, Wenisch C. Effect of vitamin C on neutrophil function after high-intensity exercise. *Eur J Clin Invest*. 2001;31(3):258-63.
192. Nieman DC, Henson DA, Butterworth DE, et al. Vitamin C supplementation does not alter the immune response to 2.5 hours of running. *Int J Sport Nutr*. 1997;7(3):173-84.
193. Nieman DC, Henson DA, McAnulty SR, et al. Influence of vitamin C supplementation on oxidative and immune changes after an ultramarathon. *J Appl Physiol (1985)*. 2002;92(5):1970-7. doi:10.1152/japplphysiol.00961.2001
194. Peters EM, Goetzsche JM, Grobbelaar B, Noakes TD. Vitamin C supplementation reduces the incidence of postrace symptoms of upper-respiratory-tract infection in ultramarathon runners. *Am J Clin Nutr*. 1993;57(2):170-4.
195. Carrillo AE, Murphy RJ, Cheung SS. Vitamin C supplementation and salivary immune function following exercise-heat stress. *Int J Sports Physiol Perform*. 2008;3(4):516-30.
196. Hemila H, Chalker E. Vitamin C for preventing and treating the common cold. *Cochrane Database Syst Rev*. 2013;(1):CD000980. doi:10.1002/14651858.CD000980.pub4
197. Gerster H. The role of vitamin C in athletic performance. *J Am Coll Nutr*. 1989;8(6):636-43.

198. Johnston CS, Swan PD, Corte C. Substrate utilization and work efficiency during submaximal exercise in vitamin C depleted-repleted adults. *Int J Vitam Nutr Res.* 1999;69(1):41-44. doi:10.1024/0300-9831.69.1.41

199. Dutra MT, Martins WR, Ribeiro ALA, Bottaro M. The effects of strength training combined with vitamin C and E supplementation on skeletal muscle mass and strength: A systematic review and meta-analysis. *J Sports Med (Hindawi Publ Corp).* 2020;2020:3505209. doi:10.1155/2020/3505209

200. Walsh NP, Gleeson M, Pyne DB, et al. Position statement. Part two: Maintaining immune health. *Exerc Immunol Rev.* 2011;17:64-103.

201. Braakhuis AJ. Effect of vitamin C supplements on physical performance. *Curr Sports Med Rep.* 2012;11(4):180-4. doi:10.1249/JSR.0b013e31825e19cd

202. Gomez-Cabrera MC, Salvador-Pascual A, Cabo H, Ferrando B, Vina J. Redox modulation of mitochondriogenesis in exercise: Does antioxidant supplementation blunt the benefits of exercise training? *Free Radic Biol Med.* 2015;86:37-46. doi:10.1016/j.freeradbiomed.2015.04.006

203. Nikolaidis MG, Kerksick CM, Lamprecht M, McAnulty SR. Does vitamin C and E supplementation impair the favorable adaptations of regular exercise? *Oxid Med Cell Longev.* 2012;2012:707941. doi:10.1155/2012/707941

204. Morrison D, Hughes J, Della Gatta PA, et al. Vitamin C and E supplementation prevents some of the cellular adaptations to endurance-training in humans. *Free Radic Biol Med.* 2015;89:852-62. doi:10.1016/j.freeradbiomed.2015.10.412

205. Paulsen G, Cumming KT, Hamarsland H, Borsheim E, Berntsen S, Raastad T. Can supplementation with vitamin C and E alter physiological adaptations to strength training? *BMC Sports Sci Med Rehabil.* 2014;6:28. doi:10.1186/2052-1847-6-28

206. Paulsen G, Cumming KT, Holden G, et al. Vitamin C and E supplementation hampers cellular adaptation to endurance training in humans: A double-blind, randomised, controlled trial. *J Physiol.* 2014;592(Pt 8):1887-901. doi:10.1113/jphysiol.2013.267419

207. Braakhuis AJ, Hopkins WG. Impact of dietary antioxidants on sport performance: A review. *Sports Med.* 2015;45(7):939-55. doi:10.1007/s40279-015-0323-x

Chapter 7

1. Henry YM, Fatayerji D, Eastell R. Attainment of peak bone mass at the lumbar spine, femoral neck and radius in men and women: Relative contributions of bone size and volumetric bone mineral density. *Osteoporos Int.* 2004;15(4):263-73. doi:10.1007/s00198-003-1542-9

2. Sawka MN, Burke LM, Eichner ER, Maughan RJ, Montain SJ, Stachenfeld NS. American College of Sports Medicine position stand: Exercise and fluid replacement. *Med Sci Sports Exerc.* 2007;39(2):377-90. doi:10.1249/mss.0b013e31802ca597

3. Lukaski HC. Vitamin and mineral status: Effects on physical performance. *Nutrition.* 2004;20(7-8):632-44. doi:10.1016/j.nut.2004.04.001

4. Otten J, Hellwig J, Meyers L. *Dietary Reference Intakes: The Essential Guide to Nutrient Requirements.* National Academies Press; 2006.

5. Leone K. Calcium, magnesium, and phosphorus. In: Adams J, ed. *Emergency Medicine: Clinical Essentials.* 2nd ed. Elsevier Saunders; 2013.

6. Ross AC, Manson JE, Abrams SA, et al. The 2011 report on Dietary Reference Intakes for calcium and vitamin D from the Institute of Medicine: What clinicians need to know. *J Clin Endocrinol Metab.* 2011;96(1):53-58. doi:10.1210/jc.2010-2704

7. U.S. Department of Health and Human Services. *Bone Health and Osteoporosis: A Report of the Surgeon General.* U.S. Department of Health and Human Services; 2004.

8. U.S. Institute of Medicine. *Dietary Reference Intakes for Calcium and Vitamin D.* National Academies Press; 2011.

9. Ross AC, Manson JE, Abrams SA, et al. Clarification of DRIs for calcium and vitamin D across age groups. *J Am Diet Assoc.* 2011;111(10):1467. doi:10.1016/j.jada.2011.08.022

10. Hoy M, Goldman J. *Calcium Intake of the U.S. Population: What We Eat in America, NHANES 2009-2010.* 2014. www.ars.usda.gov/SP2UserFiles/Place/80400530/pdf/DBrief/13_calcium_intake_0910.pdf

11. U.S. Department of Agriculture. USDA National Nutrient Database for Standard Reference, release 26. www.ars.usda.gov/ba/bhnrc/ndl

12. Yang J, Punshon T, Guerinot ML, Hirschi KD. Plant calcium content: Ready to remodel. *Nutrients.* 2012;4(8):1120-36. doi:10.3390/nu4081120

13. U.S. Food and Drug Administration. Guidance for industry: A food labeling guide. Center for Food Safety and Applied Nutrition (CFSAN). Updated August 20. Accessed March 25, 2016. www.fda.gov/Food/GuidanceRegulation/GuidanceDocumentsRegulatoryInformation/LabelingNutrition/ucm064928.htm

14. Christakos S, Dhawan P, Porta A, Mady LJ, Seth T. Vitamin D and intestinal calcium absorption. *Mol Cell Endocrinol.* 2011;347(1-2):25-29. doi:10.1016/j.mce.2011.05.038

15. Bakirhan H, Karabudak E. Effects of inulin on calcium metabolism and bone health. *Int J Vitam Nutr Res.* 2021:1-12. doi:10.1024/0300-9831/a000700

16. Rizzoli R, Biver E. Effects of fermented milk products on bone. *Calcif Tissue Int.* 2018;102(4):489-500. doi:10.1007/s00223-017-0317-9

17. Gupta RK, Gangoliya SS, Singh NK. Reduction of phytic acid and enhancement of bioavailable micronutrients in food grains. *J Food Sci Technol.* 2015;52(2):676-84. doi:10.1007/s13197-013-0978-y

18. Shkembi B, Huppertz T. Calcium absorption from food products: Food matrix effects. *Nutrients.* 2021;14(1):180. doi:10.3390/nu14010180

19. Heaney RP, Weaver CM, Recker RR. Calcium absorbability from spinach. *Am J Clin Nutr.* 1988;47(4):707-9. doi:10.1093/ajcn/47.4.707

20. Spencer H, Norris C, Osis D. Further studies of the effect of zinc on intestinal absorption of calcium in man. *J Am Coll Nutr.* 1992;11(5):561-6. doi:10.1080/07315724.1992.10718262
21. Fairweather-Tait SJ, Teucher B. Iron and calcium bioavailability of fortified foods and dietary supplements. *Nutr Rev.* 2002;60(11):360-7. doi:10.1301/00296640260385801
22. Massey LK, Whiting SJ. Caffeine, urinary calcium, calcium metabolism and bone. *J Nutr.* 1993;123(9):1611-4.
23. Barrett-Connor E, Chang JC, Edelstein SL. Coffee-associated osteoporosis offset by daily milk consumption: The Rancho Bernardo Study. *JAMA.* 1994;271(4):280-3.
24. Heaney RP, Rafferty K. Carbonated beverages and urinary calcium excretion. *Am J Clin Nutr.* 2001;74(3):343-7.
25. Heaney RP, Layman DK. Amount and type of protein influences bone health. *Am J Clin Nutr.* 2008;87(5):1567S-1570S.
26. Kerstetter JE, O'Brien KO, Caseria DM, Wall DE, Insogna KL. The impact of dietary protein on calcium absorption and kinetic measures of bone turnover in women. *J Clin Endocrinol Metab.* 2005;90(1):26-31. doi:10.1210/jc.2004-0179
27. Testa G, Pavone V, Mangano S, et al. Normal nutritional components and effects on bone metabolism in prevention of osteoporosis. *J Biol Regul Homeost Agents.* 2015;29(3):729-36.
28. Fenton TR, Lyon AW, Eliasziw M, Tough SC, Hanley DA. Meta-analysis of the effect of the acid-ash hypothesis of osteoporosis on calcium balance. *J Bone Miner Res.* 2009;24(11):1835-40. doi:10.1359/jbmr.090515
29. Dawson-Hughes B, Harris SS, Rasmussen H, Song L, Dallal GE. Effect of dietary protein supplements on calcium excretion in healthy older men and women. *J Clin Endocrinol Metab.* 2004;89(3):1169-73. doi:10.1210/jc.2003-031466
30. Cao JJ, Nielsen FH. Acid diet (high-meat protein) effects on calcium metabolism and bone health. *Curr Opin Clin Nutr Metab Care.* 2010;13(6):698-702. doi:10.1097/MCO.0b013e32833df691
31. Shams-White MM, Chung M, Du M, et al. Dietary protein and bone health: A systematic review and meta-analysis from the National Osteoporosis Foundation. *Am J Clin Nutr.* 2017;105(6):1528-1543. doi:10.3945/ajcn.116.145110
32. Straub DA. Calcium supplementation in clinical practice: A review of forms, doses, and indications. *Nutr Clin Pract.* 2007;22(3):286-96.
33. Tinawi M. Disorders of calcium metabolism: Hypocalcemia and hypercalcemia. *Cureus.* 2021;13(1):e12420. doi:10.7759/cureus.12420
34. Weaver CM, Gordon CM, Janz KF, et al. The National Osteoporosis Foundation's position statement on peak bone mass development and lifestyle factors: A systematic review and implementation recommendations. *Osteoporos Int.* 2016;27(4):1281-386. doi:10.1007/s00198-015-3440-3
35. National Institutes of Health. Osteoporosis: Peak bone mass in women. NIH Osteoporosis and Related Bone Diseases National Resource Center. www.niams.nih.gov/health_info/bone/osteoporosis/bone_mass.asp
36. Fulgoni VL, 3rd, Keast DR, Bailey RL, Dwyer J. Foods, fortificants, and supplements: Where do Americans get their nutrients? *J Nutr.* 2011;141(10):1847-54. doi:10.3945/jn.111.142257
37. Michaelsson K, Melhus H, Warensjo Lemming E, Wolk A, Byberg L. Long term calcium intake and rates of all cause and cardiovascular mortality: Community based prospective longitudinal cohort study. *BMJ.* 2013;346:f228. doi:10.1136/bmj.f228
38. Behrens SB, Deren ME, Matson A, Fadale PD, Monchik KO. Stress fractures of the pelvis and legs in athletes: A review. *Sports Health.* 2013;5(2):165-74. doi:10.1177/1941738112467423
39. De Souza MJ, Williams NI, Nattiv A, et al. Misunderstanding the female athlete triad: Refuting the IOC consensus statement on relative energy deficiency in sport (RED-S). *Br J Sports Med.* 2014;48(20):1461-5. doi:10.1136/bjsports-2014-093958
40. U.S. Institute of Medicine. *Dietary Reference Intakes for Calcium, Phosphorus, Magnesium, Vitamin D, and Fluoride.* National Academies Press; 1997.
41. Moser M, White K, Henry B, et al. Phosphorus content of popular beverages. *Am J Kidney Dis.* 2015;65(6):969-71. doi:10.1053/j.ajkd.2015.02.330
42. Moshfegh A, Goldman J, Ahuja J, Rhodes D, LaComb R. *Usual Intakes From Food and Water Compared to 1997 Dietary Reference Intakes for Vitamin D, Calcium, Phosphorus, and Magnesium: What We Eat in America, NHANES 2005-2006.* 2009.
43. Moshfegh A, Kovalchik AF, Clemens JC. *Phosphorus Intake of the U.S. Population: What We Eat in America, NHANES 2011-2012.* 2016. Dietary Data Brief No. 15.
44. Aoi W, Ogaya Y, Takami M, et al. Glutathione supplementation suppresses muscle fatigue induced by prolonged exercise via improved aerobic metabolism. *J Int Soc Sports Nutr.* 2015;12:7. doi:10.1186/s12970-015-0067-x
45. Sakaguchi Y, Hamano T, Isaka Y. Magnesium and progression of chronic kidney disease: Benefits beyond cardiovascular protection? *Adv Chronic Kidney Dis.* 2018;25(3):274-280. doi:10.1053/j.ackd.2017.11.001
46. Kass L, Weekes J, Carpenter L. Effect of magnesium supplementation on blood pressure: A meta-analysis. *Eur J Clin Nutr.* 2012;66(4):411-8. doi:10.1038/ejcn.2012.4
47. Zhang X, Li Y, Del Gobbo LC, et al. Effects of magnesium supplementation on blood pressure: A meta-analysis of randomized double-blind placebo-controlled trials. *Hypertension.* 2016;68(2):324-33. doi:10.1161/HYPERTENSIONAHA.116.07664
48. Song Y, Manson JE, Buring JE, Liu S. Dietary magnesium intake in relation to plasma insulin levels

and risk of type 2 diabetes in women. *Diabetes Care.* 2004;27(1):59-65.

49. Fung TT, Manson JE, Solomon CG, Liu S, Willett WC, Hu FB. The association between magnesium intake and fasting insulin concentration in healthy middle-aged women. *J Am Coll Nutr.* 2003;22(6):533-8.

50. Lopez-Ridaura R, Willett WC, Rimm EB, et al. Magnesium intake and risk of type 2 diabetes in men and women. *Diabetes Care.* 2004;27(1):134-40.

51. Huerta MG, Roemmich JN, Kington ML, et al. Magnesium deficiency is associated with insulin resistance in obese children. *Diabetes Care.* 2005;28(5):1175-81.

52. de Lordes Lima M, Cruz T, Pousada JC, Rodrigues LE, Barbosa K, Cangucu V. The effect of magnesium supplementation in increasing doses on the control of type 2 diabetes. *Diabetes Care.* 1998;21(5):682-6.

53. Rodriguez-Moran M, Guerrero-Romero F. Oral magnesium supplementation improves insulin sensitivity and metabolic control in type 2 diabetic subjects: A randomized double-blind controlled trial. *Diabetes Care.* 2003;26(4):1147-52.

54. Yokota K, Kato M, Lister F, et al. Clinical efficacy of magnesium supplementation in patients with type 2 diabetes. *J Am Coll Nutr.* 2004;23(5):506S-509S.

55. Paolisso G, Sgambato S, Gambardella A, et al. Daily magnesium supplements improve glucose handling in elderly subjects. *Am J Clin Nutr.* 1992;55(6):1161-7.

56. Guerrero-Romero F, Tamez-Perez HE, Gonzalez-Gonzalez G, et al. Oral magnesium supplementation improves insulin sensitivity in non-diabetic subjects with insulin resistance: A double-blind placebo-controlled randomized trial. *Diabetes Metab.* 2004;30(3):253-8.

57. de Valk HW, Verkaaik R, van Rijn HJ, Geerdink RA, Struyvenberg A. Oral magnesium supplementation in insulin-requiring type 2 diabetic patients. *Diabet Med.* 1998;15(6):503-7. doi:10.1002/(SICI)1096-9136(199806)15:6<503::AID-DIA596>3.0.CO;2-M

58. Paolisso G, Scheen A, Cozzolino D, et al. Changes in glucose turnover parameters and improvement of glucose oxidation after 4-week magnesium administration in elderly noninsulin-dependent (type II) diabetic patients. *J Clin Endocrinol Metab.* 1994;78(6):1510-4. doi:10.1210/jcem.78.6.8200955

59. Fang X, Wang K, Han D, et al. Dietary magnesium intake and the risk of cardiovascular disease, type 2 diabetes, and all-cause mortality: A dose-response meta-analysis of prospective cohort studies. *BMC Med.* 2016;14(1):210. doi:10.1186/s12916-016-0742-z

60. McCarty MF. Magnesium may mediate the favorable impact of whole grains on insulin sensitivity by acting as a mild calcium antagonist. *Med Hypotheses.* 2005;64(3):619-27. doi:10.1016/j.mehy.2003.10.034

61. Ranade VV, Somberg JC. Bioavailability and pharmacokinetics of magnesium after administration of magnesium salts to humans. *Am J Ther.* 2001;8(5):345-57.

62. Firoz M, Graber M. Bioavailability of US commercial magnesium preparations. *Magnes Res.* 2001;14(4):257-62.

63. Lindberg JS, Zobitz MM, Poindexter JR, Pak CY. Magnesium bioavailability from magnesium citrate and magnesium oxide. *J Am Coll Nutr.* 1990;9(1):48-55.

64. Walker AF, Marakis G, Christie S, Byng M. Mg citrate found more bioavailable than other Mg preparations in a randomised, double-blind study. *Magnes Res.* 2003;16(3):183-91.

65. Muhlbauer B, Schwenk M, Coram WM, et al. Magnesium-L-aspartate-HCl and magnesium-oxide: Bioavailability in healthy volunteers. *Eur J Clin Pharmacol.* 1991;40(4):437-8.

66. Ford ES, Mokdad AH. Dietary magnesium intake in a national sample of US adults. *J Nutr.* 2003;133(9):2879-82.

67. Galan P, Preziosi P, Durlach V, et al. Dietary magnesium intake in a French adult population. *Magnes Res.* 1997;10(4):321-8.

68. Vaquero MP. Magnesium and trace elements in the elderly: Intake, status and recommendations. *J Nutr Health Aging.* 2002;6(2):147-53.

69. Huang W, Ma X, Liang H, et al. Dietary magnesium intake affects the association between serum vitamin D and type 2 diabetes: A cross-sectional study. *Front Nutr.* 2021;8:763076. doi:10.3389/fnut.2021.763076

70. Zhang Y, Qiu H. Dietary magnesium intake and hyperuricemia among US adults. *Nutrients.* 2018;10(3):296. doi:10.3390/nu10030296

71. Jackson SE, Smith L, Grabovac I, et al. Ethnic differences in magnesium intake in U.S. older adults: Findings from NHANES 2005-2016. *Nutrients.* 2018;10(12):1901. doi:10.3390/nu10121901

72. Rosanoff A. Perspective: US adult magnesium requirements need updating: Impacts of rising body weights and data-derived variance. *Adv Nutr.* 2021;12(2):298-304. doi:10.1093/advances/nmaa140

73. U.S. Department of Agriculture. *Usual Nutrient Intake From Food and Beverages, by Gender and Age: What We Eat in America, NHANES 2015-2018.* 2021. www.ars.usda.gov/nea/bhnrc/fsrg

74. Bailey RL, Fulgoni VL, 3rd, Keast DR, Dwyer JT. Dietary supplement use is associated with higher intakes of minerals from food sources. *Am J Clin Nutr.* 2011;94(5):1376-81. doi:10.3945/ajcn.111.020289

75. Chaudhary DP, Sharma R, Bansal DD. Implications of magnesium deficiency in type 2 diabetes: A review. *Biol Trace Elem Res.* 2010;134(2):119-29. doi:10.1007/s12011-009-8465-z

76. Tosiello L. Hypomagnesemia and diabetes mellitus: A review of clinical implications. *Arch Intern Med.* 1996;156(11):1143-8.

77. Rivlin RS. Magnesium deficiency and alcohol intake: Mechanisms, clinical significance and possible relation to cancer development (a review). *J Am Coll Nutr.* 1994;13(5):416-23.

78. Musso CG. Magnesium metabolism in health and disease. *Int Urol Nephrol.* 2009;41(2):357-62. doi:10.1007/s11255-009-9548-7

79. Barbagallo M, Belvedere M, Dominguez LJ. Magnesium homeostasis and aging. *Magnes Res.* 2009;22(4):235-46. doi:10.1684/mrh.2009.0187

80. Garfinkel D, Garfinkel L. Magnesium and regulation of carbohydrate metabolism at the molecular level. *Magnesium.* 1988;7(5-6):249-61.
81. Chen HY, Cheng FC, Pan HC, Hsu JC, Wang MF. Magnesium enhances exercise performance via increasing glucose availability in the blood, muscle, and brain during exercise. *PLoS One.* 2014;9(1):e85486. doi:10.1371/journal.pone.0085486
82. Newhouse IJ, Finstad EW. The effects of magnesium supplementation on exercise performance. *Clin J Sport Med.* 2000;10(3):195-200.
83. Carvil P, Cronin J. Magnesium and implications on muscle function. *Strength Cond J.* 2010;32(1):48-54.
84. Santos DA, Matias CN, Monteiro CP, et al. Magnesium intake is associated with strength performance in elite basketball, handball and volleyball players. *Magnes Res.* 2011;24(4):215-9. doi:10.1684/mrh.2011.0290
85. Lukaski HC, Nielsen FH. Dietary magnesium depletion affects metabolic responses during submaximal exercise in postmenopausal women. *J Nutr.* 2002;132(5):930-5.
86. Kramer JH, Mak IT, Phillips TM, Weglicki WB. Dietary magnesium intake influences circulating pro-inflammatory neuropeptide levels and loss of myocardial tolerance to postischemic stress. *Exp Biol Med (Maywood).* 2003;228(6):665-73.
87. Weglicki WB, Dickens BF, Wagner TL, Chmielinska JJ, Phillips TM. Immunoregulation by neuropeptides in magnesium deficiency: Ex vivo effect of enhanced substance P production on circulating T lymphocytes from magnesium-deficient mice. *Magnes Res.* 1996;9(1):3-11.
88. Dickens BF, Weglicki WB, Li YS, Mak IT. Magnesium deficiency in vitro enhances free radical-induced intracellular oxidation and cytotoxicity in endothelial cells. *FEBS Lett.* 1992;311(3):187-91.
89. Freedman AM, Mak IT, Stafford RE, et al. Erythrocytes from magnesium-deficient hamsters display an enhanced susceptibility to oxidative stress. *Am J Physiol.* 1992;262(6 Pt 1):C1371-5.
90. Volpe SL. Magnesium and the athlete. *Curr Sports Med Rep.* 2015;14(4):279-83. doi:10.1249/JSR.0000000000000178
91. Zalcman I, Guarita HV, Juzwiak CR, et al. Nutritional status of adventure racers. *Nutrition.* 2007;23(5):404-11. doi:10.1016/j.nut.2007.01.001
92. Wierniuk A, Wlodarek D. Estimation of energy and nutritional intake of young men practicing aerobic sports. *Rocz Panstw Zakl Hig.* 2013;64(2):143-8.
93. Silva MR, Paiva T. Low energy availability and low body fat of female gymnasts before an international competition. *Eur J Sport Sci.* 2015;15(7):591-9. doi:10.1080/17461391.2014.969323
94. Noda Y, Iide K, Masuda R, et al. Nutrient intake and blood iron status of male collegiate soccer players. *Asia Pac J Clin Nutr.* 2009;18(3):344-50.
95. Heaney S, O'Connor H, Gifford J, Naughton G. Comparison of strategies for assessing nutritional adequacy in elite female athletes' dietary intake. *Int J Sport Nutr Exerc Metab.* 2010;20(3):245-56.
96. Juzwiak CR, Amancio OM, Vitalle MS, Pinheiro MM, Szejnfeld VL. Body composition and nutritional profile of male adolescent tennis players. *J Sports Sci.* 2008;26(11):1209-17. doi:10.1080/02640410801930192
97. Imamura H, Iide K, Yoshimura Y, et al. Nutrient intake, serum lipids and iron status of colligiate rugby players. *J Int Soc Sports Nutr.* 2013;10(1):9. doi:10.1186/1550-2783-10-9
98. de Sousa EF, Da Costa TH, Nogueira JA, Vivaldi LJ. Assessment of nutrient and water intake among adolescents from sports federations in the Federal District, Brazil. *Br J Nutr.* 2008;99(6):1275-83. doi:10.1017/S0007114507864841
99. Nielsen FH, Lukaski HC. Update on the relationship between magnesium and exercise. *Magnes Res.* 2006;19(3):180-9.
100. Brilla LR, Haley TF. Effect of magnesium supplementation on strength training in humans. *J Am Coll Nutr.* 1992;11(3):326-9.
101. Setaro L, Santos-Silva PR, Nakano EY, et al. Magnesium status and the physical performance of volleyball players: Effects of magnesium supplementation. *J Sports Sci.* 2014;32(5):438-45. doi:10.1080/02640414.2013.828847
102. Reno AM, Green M, Killen LG, O'Neal EK, Pritchett K, Hanson Z. Effects of magnesium supplementation on muscle soreness and performance. *J Strength Cond Res.* 2020;36(8):2198-2203. doi:10.1519/JSC.0000000000003827
103. Veronese N, Berton L, Carraro S, et al. Effect of oral magnesium supplementation on physical performance in healthy elderly women involved in a weekly exercise program: A randomized controlled trial. *Am J Clin Nutr.* 2014;100(3):974-81. doi:10.3945/ajcn.113.080168
104. Guerrera MP, Volpe SL, Mao JJ. Therapeutic uses of magnesium. *Am Fam Physician.* 2009;80(2):157-62.
105. U.S. Institute of Medicine. *Dietary Reference Intakes for Sodium and Potassium.* National Academies Press; 2019:594.
106. Hajjar IM, Grim CE, George V, Kotchen TA. Impact of diet on blood pressure and age-related changes in blood pressure in the US population: Analysis of NHANES III. *Arch Intern Med.* 2001;161(4):589-93.
107. Whelton PK, He J, Cutler JA, et al. Effects of oral potassium on blood pressure: Meta-analysis of randomized controlled clinical trials. *JAMA.* 1997;277(20):1624-32.
108. Morris RC, Jr., Sebastian A, Forman A, Tanaka M, Schmidlin O. Normotensive salt sensitivity: Effects of race and dietary potassium. *Hypertension.* 1999;33(1):18-23.
109. Poorolajal J, Zeraati F, Soltanian AR, Sheikh V, Hooshmand E, Maleki A. Oral potassium supplementation for management of essential hypertension: A meta-analysis of randomized controlled trials. *PLoS One.* 2017;12(4):e0174967. doi:10.1371/journal.pone.0174967

110. Filippini T, Violi F, D'Amico R, Vinceti M. The effect of potassium supplementation on blood pressure in hypertensive subjects: A systematic review and meta-analysis. *Int J Cardiol.* 2017;230:127-135. doi:10.1016/j.ijcard.2016.12.048

111. Haddy FJ, Vanhoutte PM, Feletou M. Role of potassium in regulating blood flow and blood pressure. *Am J Physiol Regul Integr Comp Physiol.* 2006;290(3):R546-R552. doi:10.1152/ajpregu.00491.2005

112. Hunter RW, Bailey MA. Hyperkalemia: Pathophysiology, risk factors and consequences. *Nephrol Dial Transplant.* 2019;34(Suppl 3):iii2-iii11. doi:10.1093/ndt/gfz206

113. Vinceti M, Filippini T, Crippa A, de Sesmaisons A, Wise LA, Orsini N. Meta-analysis of potassium intake and the risk of stroke. *J Am Heart Assoc.* 2016;5(10):e004210. doi:10.1161/JAHA.116.004210

114. Aburto NJ, Hanson S, Gutierrez H, Hooper L, Elliott P, Cappuccio FP. Effect of increased potassium intake on cardiovascular risk factors and disease: Systematic review and meta-analyses. *BMJ.* 2013;346:f1378. doi:10.1136/bmj.f1378

115. D'Elia L, Iannotta C, Sabino P, Ippolito R. Potassium-rich diet and risk of stroke: Updated meta-analysis. *Nutr Metab Cardiovasc Dis.* 2014;24(6):585-7. doi:10.1016/j.numecd.2014.03.001

116. Hoy M, Goldman J. *Potassium Intake of the U.S. Population: What We Eat in America, NHANES 2009-2010.* 2012. Accessed November 12, 2015. http://ars.usda.gov/Services/docs.htm?docid=19476

117. U.S. Institute of Medicine. *Dietary Reference Intakes for Water, Potassium, Sodium, Chloride, and Sulfate.* National Academies Press; 2005.

118. Seifter J. Potassium disorders. In: Goldman L, Schafer A, eds. *Goldman's Cecil Medicine.* Elsevier Saunders; 2016.

119. Luft FC, Weinberger MH, Grim CE. Sodium sensitivity and resistance in normotensive humans. *Am J Med.* 1982;72(5):726-36.

120. Sacks FM, Svetkey LP, Vollmer WM, et al. Effects on blood pressure of reduced dietary sodium and the Dietary Approaches to Stop Hypertension (DASH) diet. *N Engl J Med.* 2001;344(1):3-10. doi:10.1056/NEJM200101043440101

121. Mandal AK. Hypokalemia and hyperkalemia. *Med Clin North Am.* 1997;81(3):611-39.

122. Choi HY, Park HC, Ha SK. Salt sensitivity and hypertension: A paradigm shift from kidney malfunction to vascular endothelial dysfunction. *Electrolyte Blood Press.* 2015;13(1):7-16. doi:10.5049/EBP.2015.13.1.7

123. He J, Gu D, Chen J, et al. Gender difference in blood pressure responses to dietary sodium intervention in the GenSalt study. *J Hypertens.* 2009;27(1):48-54.

124. Schmidlin O, Forman A, Sebastian A, Morris RC, Jr. Sodium-selective salt sensitivity: Its occurrence in blacks. *Hypertension.* 2007;50(6):1085-92. doi:10.1161/HYPERTENSIONAHA.107.091694

125. Chen J, Gu D, Huang J, et al. Metabolic syndrome and salt sensitivity of blood pressure in non-diabetic people in China: A dietary intervention study. *Lancet.* 2009;373(9666):829-35. doi:10.1016/S0140-6736(09)60144-6

126. Gu D, Rice T, Wang S, et al. Heritability of blood pressure responses to dietary sodium and potassium intake in a Chinese population. *Hypertension.* 2007;50(1):116-22. doi:10.1161/HYPERTENSIONAHA.107.088310

127. Oh YS, Appel LJ, Galis ZS, et al. National Heart, Lung, and Blood Institute working group report on salt in human health and sickness: Building on the current scientific evidence. *Hypertension.* 2016;68(2):281-8. doi:10.1161/HYPERTENSIONAHA.116.07415

128. U.S. Department of Health and Human Services and U.S. Department of Agriculture. *Dietary Guidelines for Americans, 2020-2025.* 9th ed. 2020.

129. U.S. Institute of Medicine, Strom BL, Yaktine AL, Oria M. *Sodium Intake in Populations: Assessment of Evidence.* National Academies Press; 2013.

130. O'Donnell M, Mente A, Rangarajan S, et al. Urinary sodium and potassium excretion, mortality, and cardiovascular events. *N Engl J Med.* 2014;371(7):612-23. doi:10.1056/NEJMoa1311889

131. Tzemos N, Lim PO, Wong S, Struthers AD, MacDonald TM. Adverse cardiovascular effects of acute salt loading in young normotensive individuals. *Hypertension.* 2008;51(6):1525-30. doi:10.1161/HYPERTENSIONAHA.108.109868

132. Dickinson KM, Clifton PM, Keogh JB. Endothelial function is impaired after a high-salt meal in healthy subjects. *Am J Clin Nutr.* 2011;93(3):500-5. doi:10.3945/ajcn.110.006155

133. Dickinson KM, Keogh JB, Clifton PM. Effects of a low-salt diet on flow-mediated dilatation in humans. *Am J Clin Nutr.* 2009;89(2):485-90. doi:10.3945/ajcn.2008.26856

134. Farquhar WB, Edwards DG, Jurkovitz CT, Weintraub WS. Dietary sodium and health: More than just blood pressure. *J Am Coll Cardiol.* 2015;65(10):1042-50. doi:10.1016/j.jacc.2014.12.039

135. Maughan RJ, Leiper JB. Sodium intake and post-exercise rehydration in man. *Eur J Appl Physiol Occup Physiol.* 1995;71(4):311-9.

136. Levenhagen DK, Gresham JD, Carlson MG, Maron DJ, Borel MJ, Flakoll PJ. Postexercise nutrient intake timing in humans is critical to recovery of leg glucose and protein homeostasis. *Am J Physiol Endocrinol Metab.* 2001;280(6):E982-93.

137. Coris EE, Ramirez AM, Van Durme DJ. Heat illness in athletes: The dangerous combination of heat, humidity and exercise. *Sports Med.* 2004;34(1):9-16.

138. U.S. Food and Drug Administration. Title 21: Food and drugs—chapter 1: Food and Drug Administration—subchapter B: Food for human consumption—part 101: Food labeling. *Code of Federal Regulations.*

139. U.S. Institute of Medicine. *Dietary Reference Intakes for Thiamin, Riboflavin, Niacin, Vitamin B6, Folate, Vitamin B12, Pantothenic Acid, Biotin, and Choline.* National Academies Press; 1998.

140. U.S. Institute of Medicine. *Dietary Reference Intakes for Vitamin A, Vitamin K, Arsenic, Boron, Chromium, Copper, Iodine, Iron, Manganese, Molybdenum, Nickel, Silicon, Vanadium, and Zinc.* National Academies Press; 2001.

141. Allen L, de Benoist B, Dary O, Hurrell R. *Guidelines on Food Fortification With Micronutrients.* World Health Organization and Food and Agricultural Organization of the United Nations; 2006.

142. U.S. Department of Agriculture. FoodData Central. https://fdc.nal.usda.gov

143. Anderson RA, Bryden NA, Polansky MM. Dietary chromium intake: Freely chosen diets, institutional diet, and individual foods. *Biol Trace Elem Res.* 1992;32:117-21.

144. Linder MC, Hazegh-Azam M. Copper biochemistry and molecular biology. *Am J Clin Nutr.* 1996;63(5):797S-811S.

145. Brownlie T, Utermohlen V, Hinton PS, Giordano C, Haas JD. Marginal iron deficiency without anemia impairs aerobic adaptation among previously untrained women. *Am J Clin Nutr.* 2002;75(4):734-42.

146. Hinton PS, Giordano C, Brownlie T, Haas JD. Iron supplementation improves endurance after training in iron-depleted, nonanemic women. *J Appl Physiol.* 2000;88(3):1103-11.

147. Bermejo F, Garcia-Lopez S. A guide to diagnosis of iron deficiency and iron deficiency anemia in digestive diseases. *World J Gastroenterol.* 2009;15(37):4638-43.

148. Kamel K, Lin S, Yang S, Halperin M. Clinical disorders of hyperkalemia. In: Alpern R, Moe O, Caplan M, eds. *Seldin and Giebisch's The Kidney.* 5th ed. Elsevier; 2013.

149. Hagler L, Askew EW, Neville JR, Mellick PW, Coppes RI, Jr., Lowder JF, Jr. Influence of dietary iron deficiency on hemoglobin, myoglobin, their respective reductases, and skeletal muscle mitochondrial respiration. *Am J Clin Nutr.* 1981;34(10):2169-77.

150. Eftekhari MH, Keshavarz SA, Jalali M, Elguero E, Eshraghian MR, Simondon KB. The relationship between iron status and thyroid hormone concentration in iron-deficient adolescent Iranian girls. *Asia Pac J Clin Nutr.* 2006;15(1):50-55.

151. Krebs NF. Dietary zinc and iron sources, physical growth and cognitive development of breastfed infants. *J Nutr.* 2000;130(2S Suppl):358S-360S.

152. Galy B, Ferring-Appel D, Kaden S, Grone HJ, Hentze MW. Iron regulatory proteins are essential for intestinal function and control key iron absorption molecules in the duodenum. *Cell Metab.* 2008;7(1):79-85. doi:10.1016/j.cmet.2007.10.006

153. Fulgoni VL, 3rd, Keast DR, Auestad N, Quann EE. Nutrients from dairy foods are difficult to replace in diets of Americans: Food pattern modeling and an analyses of the National Health and Nutrition Examination Survey 2003-2006. *Nutr Res.* 2011;31(10):759-65. doi:10.1016/j.nutres.2011.09.017

154. Monsen ER. Iron nutrition and absorption: Dietary factors which impact iron bioavailability. *J Am Diet Assoc.* 1988;88(7):786-90.

155. Tapiero H, Gate L, Tew KD. Iron: Deficiencies and requirements. *Biomed Pharmacother.* 2001;55(6):324-32.

156. Hallberg L, Brune M, Rossander L. Iron absorption in man: Ascorbic acid and dose-dependent inhibition by phytate. *Am J Clin Nutr.* 1989;49(1):140-4.

157. Wallace KL, Curry SC, LoVecchio F, Raschke RA. Effect of magnesium hydroxide on iron absorption after ferrous sulfate. *Ann Emerg Med.* 1999;34(5):685-7.

158. Petry N, Egli I, Gahutu JB, Tugirimana PL, Boy E, Hurrell R. Phytic acid concentration influences iron bioavailability from biofortified beans in Rwandese women with low iron status. *J Nutr.* 2014;144(11):1681-7. doi:10.3945/jn.114.192989

159. Wierzejska R. Tea and health—a review of the current state of knowledge. *Przegl Epidemiol.* 2014;68(3):501-6, 595-9.

160. Muller MJ, Bosy-Westphal A, Klaus S, et al. World Health Organization equations have shortcomings for predicting resting energy expenditure in persons from a modern, affluent population: Generation of a new reference standard from a retrospective analysis of a German database of resting energy expenditure. *Am J Clin Nutr.* 2004;80(5):1379-90.

161. Risser WL, Lee EJ, Poindexter HB, et al. Iron deficiency in female athletes: Its prevalence and impact on performance. *Med Sci Sports Exerc.* 1988;20(2):116-21.

162. Malczewska J, Raczynski G, Stupnicki R. Iron status in female endurance athletes and in non-athletes. *Int J Sport Nutr Exerc Metab.* 2000;10(3):260-276.

163. Sim M, Garvican-Lewis LA, Cox GR, et al. Iron considerations for the athlete: A narrative review. *Eur J Appl Physiol.* 2019;119(7):1463-1478. doi:10.1007/s00421-019-04157-y

164. Peeling P, Dawson B, Goodman C, Landers G, Trinder D. Athletic induced iron deficiency: New insights into the role of inflammation, cytokines and hormones. *Eur J Appl Physiol.* 2008;103(4):381-91. doi:10.1007/s00421-008-0726-6

165. Toh SY, Zarshenas N, Jorgensen J. Prevalence of nutrient deficiencies in bariatric patients. *Nutrition.* 2009;25(11-12):1150-6. doi:10.1016/j.nut.2009.03.012

166. Hinton PS. Iron and the endurance athlete. *Appl Physiol Nutr Metab.* 2014:1-7. doi:10.1139/apnm-2014-0147

167. Naghii MR, Fouladi AI. Correct assessment of iron depletion and iron deficiency anemia. *Nutr Health.* 2006;18(2):133-9.

168. Kim SK, Kang HS, Kim CS, Kim YT. The prevalence of anemia and iron depletion in the population aged 10 years or older. *Korean J Hematol.* 2011;46(3):196-9. doi:10.5045/kjh.2011.46.3.196

169. Larson-Meyer DE, Woolf K, Burke L. Assessment of nutrient status in athletes and the need for supplementation. *Int J Sport Nutr Exerc Metab.* 2018;28(2):139-158. doi:10.1123/ijsnem.2017-0338

170. Lee EC, Fragala MS, Kavouras SA, Queen RM, Pryor JL, Casa DJ. Biomarkers in sports and exercise:

Tracking health, performance, and recovery in athletes. *J Strength Cond Res.* 2017;31(10):2920-2937. doi:10.1519/JSC.0000000000002122

171. Beard JL. Iron biology in immune function, muscle metabolism and neuronal functioning. *J Nutr.* 2001;131(2S-2):568S-579S.

172. Allison MC, Howatson AG, Torrance CJ, Lee FD, Russell RI. Gastrointestinal damage associated with the use of nonsteroidal antiinflammatory drugs. *N Engl J Med.* 1992;327(11):749-54. doi:10.1056/NEJM199209103271101

173. Park SC, Chun HJ, Kang CD, Sul D. Prevention and management of non-steroidal anti-inflammatory drugs-induced small intestinal injury. *World J Gastroenterol.* 2011;17(42):4647-53. doi:10.3748/wjg.v17.i42.4647

174. DellaValle DM, Haas JD. Impact of iron depletion without anemia on performance in trained endurance athletes at the beginning of a training season: A study of female collegiate rowers. *Int J Sport Nutr Exerc Metab.* 2011;21(6):501-6.

175. Brownlie T, Utermohlen V, Hinton PS, Haas JD. Tissue iron deficiency without anemia impairs adaptation in endurance capacity after aerobic training in previously untrained women. *Am J Clin Nutr.* 2004;79(3):437-43.

176. Scott SP, Murray-Kolb LE. Iron status is associated with performance on executive functioning tasks in nonanemic young women. *J Nutr.* 2016;146(1):30-37. doi:10.3945/jn.115.223586

177. Finley J, Davis C. Manganese deficiency and toxicity: Are high or low dietary amounts of manganese cause for concern? *BioFactors.* 1999;10:15-24.

178. O'Neal SL, Zheng W. Manganese toxicity upon overexposure: A decade in review. *Curr Environ Health Rep.* 2015;2(3):315-28. doi:10.1007/s40572-015-0056-x

179. U.S. House of Representatives. Title 21: Food and drugs—subchapter II: Definitions—chapter 9: Federal Food, Drug, and Cosmetic Act. *United States Code.* 2010. http://uscode.house.gov/view.xhtml?path=/prelim@title21/chapter9/subchapter2&edition=prelim

180. Rink L, Gabriel P. Zinc and the immune system. *Proc Nutr Soc.* 2000;59(4):541-52.

181. Caruso TJ, Prober CG, Gwaltney JM, Jr. Treatment of naturally acquired common colds with zinc: A structured review. *Clin Infect Dis.* 2007;45(5):569-74. doi:10.1086/520031

182. Prasad AS, Beck FW, Bao B, Snell D, Fitzgerald JT. Duration and severity of symptoms and levels of plasma interleukin-1 receptor antagonist, soluble tumor necrosis factor receptor, and adhesion molecules in patients with common cold treated with zinc acetate. *J Infect Dis.* 2008;197(6):795-802. doi:10.1086/528803

183. Turner RB, Cetnarowski WE. Effect of treatment with zinc gluconate or zinc acetate on experimental and natural colds. *Clin Infect Dis.* 2000;31(5):1202-8. doi:10.1086/317437

184. Eby GA, Halcomb WW. Ineffectiveness of zinc gluconate nasal spray and zinc orotate lozenges in common-cold treatment: A double-blind, placebo-controlled clinical trial. *Altern Ther Health Med.* 2006;12(1):34-38.

185. Singh M, Das RR. Zinc for the common cold. *Cochrane Database Syst Rev.* 2011;(2):CD001364. doi:10.1002/14651858.CD001364.pub3

186. Peake JM, Gerrard DF, Griffin JF. Plasma zinc and immune markers in runners in response to a moderate increase in training volume. *Int J Sports Med.* 2003;24(3):212-6. doi:10.1055/s-2003-39094

187. Haase H, Rink L. Multiple impacts of zinc on immune function. *Metallomics.* 2014;6(7):1175-80. doi:10.1039/c3mt00353a

188. Sandstead HH. Requirements and toxicity of essential trace elements, illustrated by zinc and copper. *Am J Clin Nutr.* 1995;61(3 Suppl):621S-624S.

189. Spencer H, Norris C, Williams D. Inhibitory effects of zinc on magnesium balance and magnesium absorption in man. *J Am Coll Nutr.* 1994;13(5):479-84.

190. Giolo De Carvalho F, Rosa FT, Marques Miguel Suen V, Freitas EC, Padovan GJ, Marchini JS. Evidence of zinc deficiency in competitive swimmers. *Nutrition.* 2012;28(11-12):1127-31. doi:10.1016/j.nut.2012.02.012

191. Ziegler PJ, Nelson JA, Jonnalagadda SS. Nutritional and physiological status of U.S. national figure skaters. *Int J Sport Nutr.* 1999;9(4):345-60.

192. Keith RE, O'Keeffe KA, Alt LA, Young KL. Dietary status of trained female cyclists. *J Am Diet Assoc.* 1989;89(11):1620-3.

193. Micheletti A, Rossi R, Rufini S. Zinc status in athletes: Relation to diet and exercise. *Sports Med.* 2001;31(8):577-82.

194. Hawley JA, Dennis SC, Lindsay FH, Noakes TD. Nutritional practices of athletes: Are they sub-optimal? *J Sports Sci.* 1995;13 Spec No:S75-S81. doi:10.1080/02640419508732280

195. Rossi L, Migliaccio S, Corsi A, et al. Reduced growth and skeletal changes in zinc-deficient growing rats are due to impaired growth plate activity and inanition. *J Nutr.* 2001;131(4):1142-6.

196. Krotkiewski M, Gudmundsson M, Backstrom P, Mandroukas K. Zinc and muscle strength and endurance. *Acta Physiol Scand.* 1982;116(3):309-11. doi:10.1111/j.1748-1716.1982.tb07146.x

197. Lukaski HC. Low dietary zinc decreases erythrocyte carbonic anhydrase activities and impairs cardiorespiratory function in men during exercise. *Am J Clin Nutr.* 2005;81(5):1045-51.

198. Brun JF, Dieu-Cambrezy C, Charpiat A, et al. Serum zinc in highly trained adolescent gymnasts. *Biol Trace Elem Res.* 1995;47(1-3):273-8. doi:10.1007/BF02790127

199. Nishlyama S, Inomoto T, Nakamura T, Higashi A, Matsuda I. Zinc status relates to hematological deficits in women endurance runners. *J Am Coll Nutr.* 1996;15(4):359-63.

200. Nishiyama S, Irisa K, Matsubasa T, Higashi A, Matsuda I. Zinc status relates to hematological deficits in middle-aged women. *J Am Coll Nutr.* 1998;17(3):291-5.

201. Heffernan SM, Horner K, De Vito G, Conway GE. The role of mineral and trace element supplementation in exercise and athletic performance: A systematic review. *Nutrients.* 2019;11(3):696. doi:10.3390/nu11030696

202. Jeejeebhoy KN, Chu RC, Marliss EB, Greenberg GR, Bruce-Robertson A. Chromium deficiency, glucose intolerance, and neuropathy reversed by chromium supplementation, in a patient receiving long-term total parenteral nutrition. *Am J Clin Nutr.* 1977;30(4):531-8.

203. Althuis MD, Jordan NE, Ludington EA, Wittes JT. Glucose and insulin responses to dietary chromium supplements: A meta-analysis. *Am J Clin Nutr.* 2002;76(1):148-55.

204. Wapnir RA. Copper absorption and bioavailability. *Am J Clin Nutr.* 1998;67(5 Suppl):1054S-1060S. doi:10.1093/ajcn/67.5.1054S

205. Betteridge DJ. What is oxidative stress? *Metabolism.* 2000;49(2 Suppl 1):3-8.

206. National Institutes of Health. Multivitamin/mineral supplements. U.S. Department of Health & Human Services. https://ods.od.nih.gov/factsheets/MVMS-Consumer

207. Misner B. Food alone may not provide sufficient micronutrients for preventing deficiency. *J Int Soc Sports Nutr.* 2006;3:51-55. doi:10.1186/1550-2783-3-1-51

208. Rodriguez NR, DiMarco NM, Langley S, et al. Position of the American Dietetic Association, Dietitians of Canada, and the American College of Sports Medicine: Nutrition and athletic performance. *J Am Diet Assoc.* 2009;109(3):509-27.

209. Calton JB. Prevalence of micronutrient deficiency in popular diet plans. *J Int Soc Sports Nutr.* 2010;7:24. doi:10.1186/1550-2783-7-24

Chapter 8

1. U.S. Institute of Medicine. *Dietary Reference Intakes for Water, Potassium, Sodium, Chloride, and Sulfate.* National Academies Press; 2005.

2. Jequier E, Constant F. Water as an essential nutrient: The physiological basis of hydration. *Eur J Clin Nutr.* 2010;64(2):115-23. doi:10.1038/ejcn.2009.111

3. Riebl SK, Davy BM. The hydration equation: Update on water balance and cognitive performance. *ACSMs Health Fit J.* 2013;17(6):21-28. doi:10.1249/FIT.0b013e3182a9570f

4. Maughan RJ, Watson P, Cordery PA, et al. A randomized trial to assess the potential of different beverages to affect hydration status: Development of a beverage hydration index. *Am J Clin Nutr.* 2016;103(3):717-23. doi:10.3945/ajcn.115.114769

5. Sollanek KJ, Tsurumoto M, Vidyasagar S, Kenefick RW, Cheuvront SN. Neither body mass nor sex influences beverage hydration index outcomes during randomized trial when comparing 3 commercial beverages. *Am J Clin Nutr.* 2018;107(4):544-549. doi:10.1093/ajcn/nqy005

6. Spaeth AM, Goel N, Dinges DF. Cumulative neurobehavioral and physiological effects of chronic caffeine intake: Individual differences and implications for the use of caffeinated energy products. *Nutr Rev.* 2014;72(Suppl 1):34-47. doi:10.1111/nure.12151

7. Maughan RJ, Watson P, Cordery PAA, et al. Sucrose and sodium but not caffeine content influence the retention of beverages in humans under euhydrated conditions. *Int J Sport Nutr Exerc Metab.* 2019;29(1):51-60. doi:10.1123/ijsnem.2018-0047

8. Zhang Y, Carter SJ, Schumacker RE, et al. Effect of caffeine ingestion on fluid balance during exercise in the heat and during recovery. *South African Journal of Sports Medicine.* 2014;26(2):43-47.

9. Zhang Y, Coca A, Casa DJ, Antonio J, Green JM, Bishop PA. Caffeine and diuresis during rest and exercise: A meta-analysis. *J Sci Med Sport.* 2015;18(5):569-74. doi:10.1016/j.jsams.2014.07.017

10. Rogers PJ, Heatherley SV, Mullings EL, Smith JE. Faster but not smarter: Effects of caffeine and caffeine withdrawal on alertness and performance. *Psychopharmacology (Berl).* 2013;226(2):229-40. doi:10.1007/s00213-012-2889-4

11. Yang A, Palmer AA, de Wit H. Genetics of caffeine consumption and responses to caffeine. *Psychopharmacology (Berl).* 2010;211(3):245-57. doi:10.1007/s00213-010-1900-1

12. U.S. Institute of Medicine. *Caffeine for the Sustainment of Mental Task Performance: Formulations for Military Operations.* National Academies Press. www.nap.edu/catalog/10219/caffeine-for-the-sustainment-of-mental-task-performance-formulations-for

13. Crawford C, Teo L, Lafferty L, et al. Caffeine to optimize cognitive function for military mission-readiness: A systematic review and recommendations for the field. *Nutr Rev.* 2017;75(Suppl 2):17-35. doi:10.1093/nutrit/nux007

14. Stepan ME, Altmann EM, Fenn KM. Caffeine selectively mitigates cognitive deficits caused by sleep deprivation. *J Exp Psychol Learn Mem Cogn.* 2021;47(9):1371-1382. doi:10.1037/xlm0001023

15. Popkin BM, D'Anci KE, Rosenberg IH. Water, hydration, and health. *Nutr Rev.* 2010;68(8):439-58. doi:10.1111/j.1753-4887.2010.00304.x

16. Oppliger RA, Magnes SA, Popowski LA, Gisolfi CV. Accuracy of urine specific gravity and osmolality as indicators of hydration status. *Int J Sport Nutr Exerc Metab.* 2005;15(3):236-51.

17. National Center for Complementary and Integrative Health. "Detoxes" and "Cleanses." National Institutes of Health. https://nccih.nih.gov/health/detoxes-cleanses

18. Thomas DT, Erdman KA, Burke LM. Position of the Academy of Nutrition and Dietetics, Dietitians of Canada, and the American College of Sports Medicine: Nutrition and athletic performance. *J*

Acad Nutr Diet. 2016;116(3):501-28. doi:10.1016/j.jand.2015.12.006

19. Coris EE, Ramirez AM, Van Durme DJ. Heat illness in athletes: The dangerous combination of heat, humidity and exercise. *Sports Med.* 2004;34(1):9-16.

20. Gonzalez-Alonso J, Calbet JA, Nielsen B. Muscle blood flow is reduced with dehydration during prolonged exercise in humans. *J Physiol.* 1998;513(Pt 3):895-905.

21. Sawka MN, Burke LM, Eichner ER, Maughan RJ, Montain SJ, Stachenfeld NS. American College of Sports Medicine position stand: Exercise and fluid replacement. *Med Sci Sports Exerc.* 2007;39(2):377-90. doi:10.1249/mss.0b013e31802ca597

22. Cheuvront SN, Montain SJ, Sawka MN. Fluid replacement and performance during the marathon. *Sports Med.* 2007;37(4-5):353-7.

23. Ganio MS, Armstrong LE, Casa DJ, et al. Mild dehydration impairs cognitive performance and mood of men. *Br J Nutr.* 2011;106(10):1535-43. doi:10.1017/S0007114511002005

24. Armstrong LE, Ganio MS, Casa DJ, et al. Mild dehydration affects mood in healthy young women. *J Nutr.* 2012;142(2):382-8. doi:10.3945/jn.111.142000

25. Rowland T. Fluid replacement requirements for child athletes. *Sports Med.* 2011;41(4):279-88. doi:10.2165/11584320-000000000-00000

26. Cheuvront SN, Carter R, 3rd, Castellani JW, Sawka MN. Hypohydration impairs endurance exercise performance in temperate but not cold air. *J Appl Physiol.* 2005;99(5):1972-6. doi:10.1152/japplphysiol.00329.2005

27. Maughan RJ, Watson P, Shirreffs SM. Heat and cold: What does the environment do to the marathon runner? *Sports Med.* 2007;37(4-5):396-9.

28. Nadel ER. Control of sweating rate while exercising in the heat. *Med Sci Sports.* 1979;11(1):31-35.

29. Bar-Or O, Blimkie CJ, Hay JA, MacDougall JD, Ward DS, Wilson WM. Voluntary dehydration and heat intolerance in cystic fibrosis. *Lancet.* 1992;339(8795):696-9.

30. Tripette J, Loko G, Samb A, et al. Effects of hydration and dehydration on blood rheology in sickle cell trait carriers during exercise. *Am J Physiol Heart Circ Physiol.* 2010;299(3):H908-H914. doi:10.1152/ajpheart.00298.2010

31. Dalbo VJ, Roberts MD, Stout JR, Kerksick CM. Putting to rest the myth of creatine supplementation leading to muscle cramps and dehydration. *Br J Sports Med.* 2008;42(7):567-73. doi:10.1136/bjsm.2007.042473

32. Greenwood M, Kreider RB, Melton C, et al. Creatine supplementation during college football training does not increase the incidence of cramping or injury. *Mol Cell Biochem.* 2003;244(1-2):83-88.

33. Tsuzuki-Hayakawa K, Tochihara Y, Ohnaka T. Thermoregulation during heat exposure of young children compared to their mothers. *Eur J Appl Physiol Occup Physiol.* 1995;72(1-2):12-17.

34. Davies CT. Thermal responses to exercise in children. *Ergonomics.* 1981;24(1):55-61. doi:10.1080/00140138108924830

35. Docherty D, Eckerson JD, Hayward JS. Physique and thermoregulation in prepubertal males during exercise in a warm, humid environment. *Am J Phys Anthropol.* 1986;70(1):19-23. doi:10.1002/ajpa.1330700105

36. Rivera-Brown AM, Gutierrez R, Gutierrez JC, Frontera WR, Bar-Or O. Drink composition, voluntary drinking, and fluid balance in exercising, trained, heat-acclimatized boys. *J Appl Physiol.* 1999;86(1):78-84.

37. Rowland T, Hagenbuch S, Pober D, Garrison A. Exercise tolerance and thermoregulatory responses during cycling in boys and men. *Med Sci Sports Exerc.* 2008;40(2):282-7. doi:10.1249/mss.0b013e31815a95a7

38. Bar-Or O, Dotan R, Inbar O, Rotshtein A, Zonder H. Voluntary hypohydration in 10- to 12-year-old boys. *J Appl Physiol Respir Environ Exerc Physiol.* 1980;48(1):104-8.

39. Bergeron MF, McLeod KS, Coyle JF. Core body temperature during competition in the heat: National Boys' 14s Junior Championships. *Br J Sports Med.* 2007;41(11):779-83. doi:10.1136/bjsm.2007.036905

40. Greenleaf JE. Problem: Thirst, drinking behavior, and involuntary dehydration. *Med Sci Sports Exerc.* 1992;24(6):645-56.

41. Wilk B, Bar-Or O. Effect of drink flavor and NaCl on voluntary drinking and hydration in boys exercising in the heat. *J Appl Physiol (1985).* 1996;80(4):1112-7.

42. Meyer F, Bar-Or O, MacDougall D, Heigenhauser GJ. Sweat electrolyte loss during exercise in the heat: Effects of gender and maturation. *Med Sci Sports Exerc.* 1992;24(7):776-81.

43. Binkley HM, Beckett J, Casa DJ, Kleiner DM, Plummer PE. National Athletic Trainers' Association position statement: Exertional heat illnesses. *J Athl Train.* 2002;37(3):329-343.

44. Penning R, van Nuland M, Fliervoet LA, Olivier B, Verster JC. The pathology of alcohol hangover. *Curr Drug Abuse Rev.* 2010;3(2):68-75.

45. Taivainen H, Laitinen K, Tahtela R, Kilanmaa K, Valimaki MJ. Role of plasma vasopressin in changes of water balance accompanying acute alcohol intoxication. *Alcohol Clin Exp Res.* 1995;19(3):759-62.

46. National Institute on Alcohol Abuse and Alcoholism. *Beyond Hangovers: Understanding Alcohol's Impact on Your Health.* National Institutes of Health; 2010. http://pubs.niaaa.nih.gov/publications/Hangovers/beyondHangovers.htm

47. Whitfield AH. Too much of a good thing? The danger of water intoxication in endurance sports. *Br J Gen Pract.* 2006;56(528):542-5.

48. Draper SB, Mori KJ, Lloyd-Owen S, Noakes T. Overdrinking-induced hyponatraemia in the 2007 London Marathon. *BMJ Case Rep.* 2009;doi:10.1136/bcr.09.2008.1002

49. Noakes TD, Sharwood K, Speedy D, et al. Three independent biological mechanisms cause exercise-associated hyponatremia: Evidence from 2,135 weighed competitive athletic performances. *Proc Natl Acad Sci U S A*. 2005;102(51):18550-5. doi:10.1073/pnas.0509096102

50. Almond CS, Shin AY, Fortescue EB, et al. Hyponatremia among runners in the Boston Marathon. *N Engl J Med*. 2005;352(15):1550-6. doi:10.1056/NEJMoa043901

51. Arieff AI, Llach F, Massry SG. Neurological manifestations and morbidity of hyponatremia: Correlation with brain water and electrolytes. *Medicine (Baltimore)*. 1976;55(2):121-9.

52. Urso C, Brucculeri S, Caimi G. Physiopathological, epidemiological, clinical and therapeutic aspects of exercise-associated hyponatremia. *J Clin Med*. 2014;3(4):1258-75. doi:10.3390/jcm3041258

53. Maughan RJ, Leiper JB. Sodium intake and post-exercise rehydration in man. *Eur J Appl Physiol Occup Physiol*. 1995;71(4):311-9.

54. Stofan JR, Zachwieja JJ, Horswill CA, Murray R, Anderson SA, Eichner ER. Sweat and sodium losses in NCAA football players: A precursor to heat cramps? *Int J Sport Nutr Exerc Metab*. 2005;15(6):641-52.

55. Bergeron MF. Heat cramps: Fluid and electrolyte challenges during tennis in the heat. *J Sci Med Sport*. 2003;6(1):19-27.

56. Osterberg KL, Horswill CA, Baker LB. Pregame urine specific gravity and fluid intake by National Basketball Association players during competition. *J Athl Train*. 2009;44(1):53-57. doi:10.4085/1062-6050-44.1.53

57. Conley SB. Hypernatremia. *Pediatr Clin North Am*. 1990;37(2):365-72.

58. Adeleye O, Faulkner M, Adeola T, ShuTangyie G. Hypernatremia in the elderly. *J Natl Med Assoc*. 2002;94(8):701-5.

59. Nielsen FH, Lukaski HC. Update on the relationship between magnesium and exercise. *Magnes Res*. 2006;19(3):180-9.

60. U.S. Institute of Medicine. *Dietary Reference Intakes for Calcium, Phosphorus, Magnesium, Vitamin D, and Fluoride*. National Academies Press; 1997.

61. Sawka MN. Physiological consequences of hypohydration: Exercise performance and thermoregulation. *Med Sci Sports Exerc*. 1992;24(6):657-70.

62. Fletcher GO, Dawes J, Spano M. The potential dangers of using rapid weight loss techniques. *Strength Cond J*. 2014;36(2):45-48.

63. Wenos DL, Amato HK. Weight cycling alters muscular strength and endurance, ratings of perceived exertion, and total body water in college wrestlers. *Percept Mot Skills*. 1998;87(3 Pt 1):975-8. doi:10.2466/pms.1998.87.3.975

64. Batchelder BC, Krause BA, Seegmiller JG, Starkey CA. Gastrointestinal temperature increases and hypohydration exists after collegiate men's ice hockey participation. *J Strength Cond Res*. 2010;24(1):68-73. doi:10.1519/JSC.0b013e3181c49114

65. Gibson JC, Stuart-Hill LA, Pethick W, Gaul CA. Hydration status and fluid and sodium balance in elite Canadian junior women's soccer players in a cool environment. *Appl Physiol Nutr Metab*. 2012;37(5):931-7. doi:10.1139/h2012-073

66. Godek SF, Peduzzi C, Burkholder R, Condon S, Dorshimer G, Bartolozzi AR. Sweat rates, sweat sodium concentrations, and sodium losses in 3 groups of professional football players. *J Athl Train*. 2010;45(4):364-71. doi:10.4085/1062-6050-45.4.364

67. Stover EA, Zachwieja J, Stofan J, Murray R, Horswill CA. Consistently high urine specific gravity in adolescent American football players and the impact of an acute drinking strategy. *Int J Sports Med*. 2006;27(4):330-5. doi:10.1055/s-2005-865667

68. Bergeron MF, Waller JL, Marinik EL. Voluntary fluid intake and core temperature responses in adolescent tennis players: Sports beverage versus water. *Br J Sports Med*. 2006;40(5):406-10. doi:10.1136/bjsm.2005.023333

69. Bardis CN, Kavouras SA, Kosti L, Markousi M, Sidossis LS. Mild hypohydration decreases cycling performance in the heat. *Med Sci Sports Exerc*. 2013;45(9):1782-9. doi:10.1249/MSS.0b013e31828e1e77

70. Distefano LJ, Casa DJ, Vansumeren MM, et al. Hypohydration and hyperthermia impair neuromuscular control after exercise. *Med Sci Sports Exerc*. 2013;45(6):1166-73. doi:10.1249/MSS.0b013e3182805b83

71. Hayes LD, Morse CI. The effects of progressive dehydration on strength and power: Is there a dose response? *Eur J Appl Physiol*. 2010;108(4):701-7. doi:10.1007/s00421-009-1288-y

72. Jones LC, Cleary MA, Lopez RM, Zuri RE, Lopez R. Active dehydration impairs upper and lower body anaerobic muscular power. *J Strength Cond Res*. 2008;22(2):455-63. doi:10.1519/JSC.0b013e3181635ba5

73. Judelson DA, Maresh CM, Farrell MJ, et al. Effect of hydration state on strength, power, and resistance exercise performance. *Med Sci Sports Exerc*. 2007;39(10):1817-24. doi:10.1249/mss.0b013e3180de5f22

74. Smith MF, Newell AJ, Baker MR. Effect of acute mild dehydration on cognitive-motor performance in golf. *J Strength Cond Res*. 2012;26(11):3075-80. doi:10.1519/JSC.0b013e318245bea7

75. Montain SJ, Coyle EF. Influence of graded dehydration on hyperthermia and cardiovascular drift during exercise. *J Appl Physiol (1985)*. 1992;73(4):1340-50.

76. Schoffstall JE, Branch JD, Leutholtz BC, Swain DE. Effects of dehydration and rehydration on the one-repetition maximum bench press of weight-trained males. *J Strength Cond Res*. 2001;15(1):102-8.

77. Adan A. Cognitive performance and dehydration. *J Am Coll Nutr*. 2012;31(2):71-78.

78. Davis JK, Laurent CM, Allen KE, et al. Influence of dehydration on intermittent sprint performance. *J Strength Cond Res*. 2015;29(9):2586-93. doi:10.1519/JSC.0000000000000907

79. Stover EA, Petrie HJ, Passe D, Horswill CA, Murray B, Wildman R. Urine specific gravity in exercisers prior to physical training. *Appl Physiol Nutr Metab*. 2006;31(3):320-7. doi:10.1139/h06-004

80. Casa DJ, Armstrong LE, Hillman SK, et al. National Athletic Trainers' Association position statement: Fluid replacement for athletes. *J Athl Train*. 2000;35(2):212-24.

81. Volpe SL, Poule KA, Bland EG. Estimation of pre-practice hydration status of National Collegiate Athletic Association Division I athletes. *J Athl Train*. 2009;44(6):624-9. doi:10.4085/1062-6050-44.6.624

82. Simerville JA, Maxted WC, Pahira JJ. Urinalysis: A comprehensive review. *Am Fam Physician*. 2005;71(6):1153-62.

83. Palmer MS, Spriet LL. Sweat rate, salt loss, and fluid intake during an intense on-ice practice in elite Canadian male junior hockey players. *Appl Physiol Nutr Metab*. 2008;33(2):263-71. doi:10.1139/H08-011

84. Baker LB, Barnes KA, Anderson ML, Passe DH, Stofan JR. Normative data for regional sweat sodium concentration and whole-body sweating rate in athletes. *J Sports Sci*. 2016;34(4):358-68. doi:10.1080/02640414.2015.1055291

85. Nuccio RP, Barnes KA, Carter JM, Baker LB. Fluid balance in team sport athletes and the effect of hypohydration on cognitive, technical, and physical performance. *Sports Med*. 2017;47(10):1951-1982. doi:10.1007/s40279-017-0738-7

86. Gamble ASD, Bigg JL, Vermeulen TF, et al. Estimated sweat loss, fluid and carbohydrate intake, and sodium balance of male major junior, AHL, and NHL players during on-ice practices. *Int J Sport Nutr Exerc Metab*. 2019;29(6):612-619. doi:10.1123/ijsnem.2019-0029

87. Engell DB, Maller O, Sawka MN, Francesconi RN, Drolet L, Young AJ. Thirst and fluid intake following graded hypohydration levels in humans. *Physiol Behav*. 1987;40(2):229-36.

88. Kostelnik SB, Davy KP, Hedrick VE, Thomas DT, Davy BM. The validity of urine color as a hydration biomarker within the general adult population and athletes: A systematic review. *J Am Coll Nutr*. 2021;40(2):172-179. doi:10.1080/07315724.2020.1750073

89. Armstrong LE. Assessing hydration status: The elusive gold standard. *J Am Coll Nutr*. 2007;26(5 Suppl):575S-584S.

90. Shirreffs SM, Taylor AJ, Leiper JB, Maughan RJ. Post-exercise rehydration in man: Effects of volume consumed and drink sodium content. *Med Sci Sports Exerc*. 1996;28(10):1260-71.

91. Kovacs EM, Senden JM, Brouns F. Urine color, osmolality and specific electrical conductance are not accurate measures of hydration status during postexercise rehydration. *J Sports Med Phys Fitness*. 1999;39(1):47-53.

92. Bottin JH, Lemetais G, Poupin M, Jimenez L, Perrier ET. Equivalence of afternoon spot and 24-h urinary hydration biomarkers in free-living healthy adults. *Eur J Clin Nutr*. 2016;70(8):904-7. doi:10.1038/ejcn.2015.217

93. McDermott BP, Anderson SA, Armstrong LE, et al. National Athletic Trainers' Association position statement: Fluid replacement for the physically active. *J Athl Train*. 2017;52(9):877-895. doi:10.4085/1062-6050-52.9.02

94. Tilkian S, Boudreau C, Tilkian A. *Clinical & Nursing Implications of Laboratory Tests*. 5th ed. Mosby; 1995.

95. Armstrong LE, Maresh CM, Castellani JW, et al. Urinary indices of hydration status. *Int J Sport Nutr*. 1994;4(3):265-79.

96. Shirreffs SM, Maughan RJ. Urine osmolality and conductivity as indices of hydration status in athletes in the heat. *Med Sci Sports Exerc*. 1998;30(11):1598-602.

97. O'Neal E, Boy T, Davis B, et al. Post-exercise sweat loss estimation accuracy of athletes and physically active adults: A review. *Sports (Basel)*. 2020;8(8) doi:10.3390/sports8080113

98. O'Brien C, Young AJ, Sawka MN. Bioelectrical impedance to estimate changes in hydration status. *Int J Sports Med*. 2002;23(5):361-6. doi:10.1055/s-2002-33145

99. Gerber G, Brendler C. Evaluation of the urologic patient: History, physical examination, and the urinalysis. In: AJ W, ed. *Campbell-Walsh Urology*. 10th ed. Saunders Elsevier; 2011:1-25.

100. U.S. Department of Agriculture. USDA National Nutrient Database for Standard Reference, release 26. www.ars.usda.gov/ba/bhnrc/ndl

101. Matias CN, Santos DA, Judice PB, et al. Estimation of total body water and extracellular water with bioimpedance in athletes: A need for athlete-specific prediction models. *Clin Nutr*. 2016;35(2):468-74. doi:10.1016/j.clnu.2015.03.013

102. Shanholtzer BA, Patterson SM. Use of bioelectrical impedance in hydration status assessment: Reliability of a new tool in psychophysiology research. *Int J Psychophysiol*. 2003;49(3):217-26.

103. Goulet ED. Dehydration and endurance performance in competitive athletes. *Nutr Rev*. 2012;70(Suppl 2):S132-6. doi:10.1111/j.1753-4887.2012.00530.x

104. Morris DM, Huot JR, Jetton AM, Collier SR, Utter AC. Acute sodium ingestion before exercise increases voluntary water consumption resulting in preexercise hyperhydration and improvement in exercise performance in the heat. *Int J Sport Nutr Exerc Metab*. 2015;25(5):456-62. doi:10.1123/ijsnem.2014-0212

105. Mitchell JB, Costill DL, Houmard JA, Fink WJ, Robergs RA, Davis JA. Gastric emptying: Influence of prolonged exercise and carbohydrate concentration. *Med Sci Sports Exerc*. 1989;21(3):269-74.

106. Wilson PB. Multiple transportable carbohydrates during exercise: Current limitations and directions for future research. *J Strength Cond Res*. 2015;29(7):2056-70. doi:10.1519/JSC.0000000000000835

107. Jentjens RL, Achten J, Jeukendrup AE. High oxidation rates from combined carbohydrates ingested during exercise. *Med Sci Sports Exerc*. 2004;36(9):1551-8.

108. Bergeron MF, Devore CD, Rice SG. Climatic heat stress and exercising children and adolescents. *Pediatrics*. 2011;128(3):e741-e747.

109. American Academy of Pediatrics. Climatic heat stress and the exercising child and adolescent. *Pediatrics*. 2000;106(1):158-9.

110. U.S. Institute of Medicine. *Fluid Replacement and Heat Stress*. 1994:254.

111. Kovacs MS. A review of fluid and hydration in competitive tennis. *Int J Sports Physiol Perform*. 2008;3(4):413-23.

112. Evans GH, James LJ, Shirreffs SM, Maughan RJ. Optimizing the restoration and maintenance of fluid balance after exercise-induced dehydration. *J Appl Physiol (1985)*. 2017;122(4):945-951. doi:10.1152/japplphysiol.00745.2016

113. Shirreffs SM, Maughan RJ. Volume repletion after exercise-induced volume depletion in humans: Replacement of water and sodium losses. *Am J Physiol*. 1998;274(5 Pt 2):F868-F875.

114. Kavouras SA, Arnaoutis G, Makrillos M, et al. Educational intervention on water intake improves hydration status and enhances exercise performance in athletic youth. *Scand J Med Sci Sports*. 2012;22(5):684-9. doi:10.1111/j.1600-0838.2011.01296.x

Chapter 9

1. Graham-Paulson TS, Perret C, Smith B, Crosland J, Goosey-Tolfrey VL. Nutritional supplement habits of athletes with an impairment and their sources of information. *Int J Sport Nutr Exerc Metab*. 2015;25(4):387-95. doi:10.1123/ijsnem.2014-0155

2. Maughan RJ, Burke LM, Dvorak J, et al. IOC consensus statement: Dietary supplements and the high-performance athlete. *British Journal of Sports Medicine*. 2018;52(7):439. doi:10.1136/bjsports-2018-099027

3. Thomas DT, Erdman KA, Burke LM. Position of the Academy of Nutrition and Dietetics, Dietitians of Canada, and the American College of Sports Medicine: Nutrition and athletic performance. *J Acad Nutr Diet*. 2016;116(3):501-28. doi:10.1016/j.jand.2015.12.006

4. Mora-Rodriguez R, Pallares JG. Performance outcomes and unwanted side effects associated with energy drinks. *Nutr Rev*. 2014;72(Suppl 1):108-20. doi:10.1111/nure.12132

5. Informed Choice. Accessed December 2022. www.informed-choice.org

6. National Center for Complementary and Integrative Health. National Institutes of Health, U.S. Department of Health and Human Services. Accessed December 2022. www.nccih.nih.gov

7. U.S. Food and Drug Administration. Tainted products marketed as dietary supplements. Accessed December 2022. www.accessdata.fda.gov/scripts/sda/sdNavigation.cfm?filter=&sortColumn=1d&sd=tainted_supplements_cder&page=1

8. Knapik JJ, Steelman RA, Hoedebecke SS, Austin KG, Farina EK, Lieberman HR. Prevalence of dietary supplement use by athletes: Systematic review and meta-analysis. *Sports Med*. 2016;46(1):103-23. doi:10.1007/s40279-015-0387-7

9. U.S. Food and Drug Administration. Guidance for industry: A food labeling guide. Accessed December 2022. www.fda.gov/food/guidanceregulation/guidancedocumentsregulatoryinformation/labelingnutrition/ucm2006828.htm

10. Mayo Clinic. Caffeine content for coffee, tea, soda and more. Accessed December 2022. www.mayoclinic.org/healthy-lifestyle/nutrition-and-healthy-eating/in-depth/caffeine/art-20049372

11. U.S. Food and Drug Administration. Spilling the beans: How much caffeine is too much? Accessed December 2022. www.fda.gov/AboutFDA/Transparency/Basics/ucm194317.htm

12. Gurley BJ, Steelman SC, Thomas SL. Multi-ingredient, caffeine-containing dietary supplements: History, safety, and efficacy. *Clin Ther*. 2015;37(2):275-301. doi:10.1016/j.clinthera.2014.08.012

13. U.S. Food and Drug Administration. Dietary supplements. Accessed December 2022. www.fda.gov/Food/DietarySupplements/default.htm

14. Federal Trade Commission. Accessed December 2022. www.ftc.gov

15. Office of Dietary Supplements. National Institutes of Health. Accessed December 2022. https://ods.od.nih.gov

16. U.S. Food and Drug Administration. Safety alerts and advisories. Accessed December 2022. www.fda.gov/Food/RecallsOutbreaksEmergencies/SafetyAlertsAdvisories

17. U.S. Food and Drug Administration. Label claims for conventional foods and dietary supplements. Accessed December 2022. www.fda.gov/food/food-labeling-nutrition/label-claims-food-dietary-supplements

18. International Organization for Standardization. ISO/IEC 17065:2012 Conformity assessment—requirements for bodies certifying products, processes and services. Accessed December 2022. www.iso.org/standard/46568.html

19. Eichner AK, Coyles J, Fedoruk M, et al. Essential features of third-party certification programs for dietary supplements: A consensus statement. *Curr Sports Med Rep*. 2019;18(5):178-182. doi:10.1249/jsr.0000000000000595

20. Banned Substances Control Group. Accessed October, 2022. www.bscg.org

21. Consumer Lab. Accessed December 2022. www.consumerlab.com

22. U.S. Anti-Doping Agency. Supplement risk and NSF Certified for Sport®. Updated May 20. Accessed December 2022. www.usada.org/athlete-advisory/supplement-risk-nsf-certified-for-sport

23. U.S. Pharmacopeial Convention. Quality supplements. Accessed December 2022. www.quality-supplements.org

24. Akabas SR, Vannice G, Atwater JB, Cooperman T, Cotter R, Thomas L. Quality certification programs for dietary supplements. *Journal of the Academy of Nutrition and Dietetics*. 2016;116(9):1378-1379. doi:10.1016/j.jand.2015.11.003

25. World Anti-Doping Agency. Accessed December 2022. www.wada-ama.org

26. U.S. Food and Drug Administration. Medication health fraud. Accessed December 2022. www.fda.gov/drugs/buying-using-medicine-safely/medication-health-fraud#:~:text=In%20general%2C%20health%20fraud%20drug,%E2%80%94and%20even%20fatal%E2%80%94injuries

27. Cohen PA. Hazards of hindsight—monitoring the safety of nutritional supplements. *N Engl J Med*. 2014;370(14):1277-80. doi:10.1056/NEJMp1315559

28. Cohen PA, Maller G, DeSouza R, Neal-Kababick J. Presence of banned drugs in dietary supplements following FDA recalls. *JAMA*. 2014;312(16):1691-3. doi:10.1001/jama.2014.10308

29. Drug Free Sport International. Accessed December 2022. www.drugfreesport.com

30. U.S. Anti-Doping Agency. Supplement connect. Accessed December 2022. www.usada.org/substances/supplement-411

31. U.S. Food and Drug Administration. "Natural" on food labeling. Accessed December 2022. www.fda.gov/Food/GuidanceRegulation/GuidanceDocumentsRegulatoryInformation/LabelingNutrition/ucm456090.htm

32. Pronsky Z, Crowe S. *Food Medication Interactions*. 18th ed. Food-Medication Interactions; 2015.

33. Australian Institute for Sport. The Australian Institute for Sport sports supplement framework. Accessed October, 2022. www.ais.gov.au/nutrition/supplements

34. National Institutes of Health. Dietary supplements for weight loss. Accessed December 2022. https://ods.od.nih.gov/factsheets/WeightLoss-HealthProfessional

35. U.S. Department of Agriculture. The caffeine content of dietary supplements commonly purchased in the U.S.: Analysis of 53 products having caffeine-containing ingredients. Accessed December 2022. www.ars.usda.gov/research/publications/publication/?seqNo115=213752

36. U.S. Food and Drug Administration. Food labeling guide. Accessed September 7, 2016. www.fda.gov/Food/GuidanceRegulation/GuidanceDocumentsRegulatoryInformation/LabelingNutrition/ucm2006828.htm

37. Astorino TA, Roberson DW. Efficacy of acute caffeine ingestion for short-term high-intensity exercise performance: A systematic review. *J Strength Cond Res*. 2010;24(1):257-65. doi:10.1519/JSC.0b013e3181c1f88a

38. Spriet LL. Exercise and sport performance with low doses of caffeine. *Sports Med*. 2014;44(Suppl 2):S175-84. doi:10.1007/s40279-014-0257-8

39. Tarnopolsky MA. Caffeine and creatine use in sport. *Annals of Nutrition and Metabolism*. 2010;57(Suppl 2):1-8.

40. Ruiz-Moreno C, Gutiérrez-Hellín J, Amaro-Gahete FJ, et al. Caffeine increases whole-body fat oxidation during 1 h of cycling at Fatmax. *Eur J Nutr*. 2020;doi:10.1007/s00394-020-02393-z

41. Sawka MN, Burke LM, Eichner ER, Maughan RJ, Montain SJ, Stachenfeld NS. American College of Sports Medicine position stand: Exercise and fluid replacement. *Med Sci Sports Exerc*. 2007;39(2):377-90. doi:10.1249/mss.0b013e31802ca597

42. Zhang Y, Coca A, Casa DJ, Antonio J, Green JM, Bishop PA. Caffeine and diuresis during rest and exercise: A meta-analysis. *J Sci Med Sport*. 2015;18(5):569-74. doi:10.1016/j.jsams.2014.07.017

43. Guest N, Corey P, Vescovi J, El-Sohemy A. Caffeine, CYP1A2 genotype, and endurance performance in athletes. *Med Sci Sports Exerc*. 2018;50(8):1570-1578. doi:10.1249/mss.0000000000001596

44. Burke LM. Practical considerations for bicarbonate loading and sports performance. *Nestle Nutr Inst Workshop Ser*. 2013;75:15-26. doi:10.1159/000345814

45. Sahlin K. Muscle energetics during explosive activities and potential effects of nutrition and training. *Sports Med*. 2014;44(Suppl 2):S167-73. doi:10.1007/s40279-014-0256-9

46. Hobson RM, Saunders B, Ball G, Harris RC, Sale C. Effects of beta-alanine supplementation on exercise performance: A meta-analysis. *Amino Acids*. 2012;43(1):25-37. doi:10.1007/s00726-011-1200-z

47. Quesnele JJ, Laframboise MA, Wong JJ, Kim P, Wells GD. The effects of beta-alanine supplementation on performance: A systematic review of the literature. *Int J Sport Nutr Exerc Metab*. 2014;24(1):14-27. doi:10.1123/ijsnem.2013-0007

48. Alhosin M, Anselm E, Rashid S, et al. Redox-sensitive up-regulation of eNOS by purple grape juice in endothelial cells: Role of PI3-kinase/Akt, p38 MAPK, JNK, FoxO1 and FoxO3a. *PLoS One*. 2013;8(3):e57883. doi:10.1371/journal.pone.0057883

49. Forstermann U, Munzel T. Endothelial nitric oxide synthase in vascular disease: From marvel to menace. *Circulation*. 2006;113(13):1708-14. doi:10.1161/circulationaha.105.602532

50. Clements WT, Lee SR, Bloomer RJ. Nitrate ingestion: A review of the health and physical performance effects. *Nutrients*. 2014;6(11):5224-64. doi:10.3390/nu6115224

51. Wruss J, Waldenberger G, Huemer S, et al. Compositional characteristics of commercial beetroot products and beetroot juice prepared from seven beetroot varieties grown in Upper Austria. *J Food Compost Anal*. 2015;42:46-55. doi:10.1016/j.jfca.2015.03.005

52. Bryan NS, Ivy JL. Inorganic nitrite and nitrate: Evidence to support consideration as dietary nutrients. *Nutr Res*. 2015;35(8):643-54. doi:10.1016/j.nutres.2015.06.001

53. Jones AM. Dietary nitrate supplementation and exercise performance. *Sports Med.* 2014;44(Suppl 1):35-45. doi:10.1007/s40279-014-0149-y
54. Sindelar JJ, Milkowski AL. Human safety controversies surrounding nitrate and nitrite in the diet. *Nitric Oxide.* 2012;26(4):259-66. doi:10.1016/j.niox.2012.03.011
55. Chorley JN, Anding RH. Performance-enhancing substances. *Adolesc Med State Art Rev.* 2015;26(1):174-88.
56. Bone JL, Ross ML, Tomcik KA, Jeacocke NA, Hopkins WG, Burke LM. Manipulation of muscle creatine and glycogen changes dual X-ray absorptiometry estimates of body composition. *Med Sci Sports Exerc.* 2017;49(5):1029-1035. doi:10.1249/mss.0000000000001174
57. Devries MC, Phillips SM. Creatine supplementation during resistance training in older adults: A meta-analysis. *Med Sci Sports Exerc.* 2014;46(6):1194-203. doi:10.1249/mss.0000000000000220
58. Persky AM, Rawson ES. Safety of creatine supplementation. *Subcell Biochem.* 2007;46:275-89.
59. Kim HJ, Kim CK, Carpentier A, Poortmans JR. Studies on the safety of creatine supplementation. *Amino Acids.* 2011;40(5):1409-18. doi:10.1007/s00726-011-0878-2
60. Tarnopolsky MA. Clinical use of creatine in neuromuscular and neurometabolic disorders. *Subcell Biochem.* 2007;46:183-204.
61. Tarnopolsky MA. Creatine as a therapeutic strategy for myopathies. *Amino Acids.* 2011;40(5):1397-407. doi:10.1007/s00726-011-0876-4
62. Kreider RB, Kalman DS, Antonio J, et al. International Society of Sports Nutrition position stand: Safety and efficacy of creatine supplementation in exercise, sport, and medicine. *Journal of the International Society of Sports Nutrition.* 2017;14(1):18. doi:10.1186/s12970-017-0173-z
63. Molfino A, Gioia G, Rossi Fanelli F, Muscaritoli M. Beta-hydroxy-beta-methylbutyrate supplementation in health and disease: A systematic review of randomized trials. *Amino Acids.* 2013;45(6):1273-92. doi:10.1007/s00726-013-1592-z
64. Wu H, Xia Y, Jiang J, et al. Effect of beta-hydroxy-beta-methylbutyrate supplementation on muscle loss in older adults: A systematic review and meta-analysis. *Arch Gerontol Geriatr.* 2015;61(2):168-75. doi:10.1016/j.archger.2015.06.020
65. Zanchi NE, Gerlinger-Romero F, Guimaraes-Ferreira L, et al. HMB supplementation: Clinical and athletic performance-related effects and mechanisms of action. *Amino Acids.* 2011;40(4):1015-25. doi:10.1007/s00726-010-0678-0
66. Jakubowski JS, Nunes EA, Teixeira FJ, et al. Supplementation with the leucine metabolite β-hydroxy-β-methylbutyrate (HMB) does not improve resistance exercise-induced changes in body composition or strength in young subjects: A systematic review and meta-analysis. *Nutrients.* 2020;12(5). doi:10.3390/nu12051523
67. Jakubowski JS, Wong EPT, Nunes EA, et al. Equivalent hypertrophy and strength gains in β-hydroxy-β-methylbutyrate- or leucine-supplemented men. *Med Sci Sports Exerc.* 2019;51(1):65-74. doi:10.1249/mss.0000000000001752
68. Gallagher B, Tjoumakaris FP, Harwood MI, Good RP, Ciccotti MG, Freedman KB. Chondroprotection and the prevention of osteoarthritis progression of the knee: A systematic review of treatment agents. *Am J Sports Med.* 2015;43(3):734-44. doi:10.1177/0363546514533777
69. Web MD. NSAIDs (nonsteroidal anti-inflammatory drugs) and arthritis. Accessed December 2022. www.webmd.com/osteoarthritis/guide/anti-inflammatory-drugs#1
70. James C-B, Uhl TL. A review of articular cartilage pathology and the use of glucosamine sulfate. *Journal of Athletic Training.* 2001;36(4):413-419.
71. National Institutes of Health. Glucosamine and chondroitin for osteoarthritis. Accessed December 2022. www.nccih.nih.gov/health/glucosamine-and-chondroitin-for-osteoarthritis
72. Hewlings SJ, Kalman DS. Curcumin: A review of its effects on human health. *Foods.* 2017;6(10):92. doi:10.3390/foods6100092
73. Philpott JD, Witard OC, Galloway SDR. Applications of omega-3 polyunsaturated fatty acid supplementation for sport performance. *Res Sports Med.* 2019;27(2):219-237. doi:10.1080/15438627.2018.1550401
74. Whitney E, Rady Rolfes S. *Understanding Nutrition.* 16th ed. Cengage; 2022.
75. Wall BT, Morton JP, van Loon LJC. Strategies to maintain skeletal muscle mass in the injured athlete: Nutritional considerations and exercise mimetics. *European Journal of Sport Science.* 2015;15(1):53-62. doi:10.1080/17461391.2014.936326
76. Gammone MA, Riccioni G, Parrinello G, D'Orazio N. Omega-3 polyunsaturated fatty acids: Benefits and endpoints in sport. *Nutrients.* 2018;11(1):46. doi:10.3390/nu11010046
77. Oliver JM, Anzalone AJ, Jones MT, et al. Nutritional supplements for the treatment and prevention of sports-related concussion—omega 3 fatty acids: Evidence still lacking? *Current Sports Medicine Reports.* 2018;17(3):103-104. doi:10.1249/jsr.0000000000000465
78. Koboziev I, Karlsson F, Grisham MB. Gut-associated lymphoid tissue, T cell trafficking, and chronic intestinal inflammation. *Ann N Y Acad Sci.* 2010;1207(Suppl 1):E86-E93. doi:10.1111/j.1749-6632.2010.05711.x
79. Jäger R, Mohr AE, Carpenter KC, et al. International Society of Sports Nutrition position stand: Probiotics. *Journal of the International Society of Sports Nutrition.* 2019;16(1):62. doi:10.1186/s12970-019-0329-0
80. Gleeson M, Siegler JC, Burke LM, Stear SJ, Castell LM. A-Z of nutritional supplements: Dietary supplements, sports nutrition foods and ergogenic aids for health and performance—Part 31. *Br J Sports Med.* 2012;46(5):377-8. doi:10.1136/bjsports-2012-090981

81. Pyne DB, West NP, Cox AJ, Cripps AW. Probiotics supplementation for athletes—clinical and physiological effects. *Eur J Sport Sci.* 2015;15(1):63-72. doi:10.1080/17461391.2014.971879

82. Sivamaruthi BS, Kesika P, Chaiyasut C. Effect of probiotics supplementations on health status of athletes. *Int J Environ Res Public Health.* 2019;16(22):4469. doi:10.3390/ijerph16224469

83. DiMarco NM, West NP, Burke LM, Stear SJ, Castell LM. A-Z of nutritional supplements: Dietary supplements, sports nutrition foods and ergogenic aids for health and performance—Part 30. *Br J Sports Med.* 2012;46(4):299-300. doi:10.1136/bjsports-2012-090933

84. Academy of Nutrition and Dietetics. *Sports Nutrition.* 6th ed. The Academy of Nutrition and Dietetics; 2017.

85. Manore MM. Weight management for athletes and active individuals: A brief review. *Sports Med.* 2015;45(Suppl 1):83-92. doi:10.1007/s40279-015-0401-0

86. Tabrizi R, Saneei P, Lankarani KB, et al. The effects of caffeine intake on weight loss: A systematic review and dose-response meta-analysis of randomized controlled trials. *Crit Rev Food Sci Nutr.* 2019;59(16):2688-2696. doi:10.1080/10408398.2018.1507996

87. Batsis JA, Apolzan JW, Bagley PJ, et al. A systematic review of dietary supplements and alternative therapies for weight loss. *Obesity (Silver Spring).* 2021;29(7):1102-1113. doi:10.1002/oby.23110

88. National Institutes of Health. Green tea. Accessed December 2022. https://nccih.nih.gov/health/greentea

89. U.S. Anti-Doping Agency. Effects of performance-enhancing drugs. Accessed December 2022. www.usada.org/athletes/substances/effects-of-performance-enhancing-drugs

90. National Institutes of Health. Raynaud's; also known as Raynauds phenomenon. 2022. www.nhlbi.nih.gov/health-topics/raynaudsRaynaud's

91. Hatton CK, Green GA, Ambrose PJ. Performance-enhancing drugs: Understanding the risks. *Phys Med Rehabil Clin N Am.* 2014;25(4):897-913. doi:10.1016/j.pmr.2014.06.013

92. American College of Sports Medicine. Anabolic-androgenic steroid use in sports, health and society: A new consensus statement from ACSM. Accessed December 2022. www.acsm.org/search-results/all-blog-posts/acsm-blog/acsm-blog/2021/08/31/anabolic-androgenic-steroid-use-sports-health-acsm-consensus-statement

93. National Center for Complementary and Integrative Health. Cannabis (marijuana) and cannabinoids: What you need to know. Accessed December 2022. www.nccih.nih.gov/health/cannabis-marijuana-and-cannabinoids-what-you-need-to-know

94. Ware MA, Jensen D, Barrette A, Vernec A, Derman W. Cannabis and the health and performance of the elite athlete. *Clin J Sport Med.* 2018;28(5):480-484. doi:10.1097/jsm.0000000000000650

95. McCartney D, Benson MJ, Desbrow B, Irwin C, Suraev A, McGregor IS. Cannabidiol and sports performance: A narrative review of relevant evidence and recommendations for future research. *Sports Medicine–Open.* 2020;6(1):27. doi:10.1186/s40798-020-00251-0

96. Zhou J, Heim D, Levy A. Sports participation and alcohol use: Associations with sports-related identities and well-being. *J Stud Alcohol Drugs.* 2016;77(1):170-9.

97. Barnes MJ. Alcohol: impact on sports performance and recovery in male athletes. *Sports Med.* 2014;44(7):909-19. doi:10.1007/s40279-014-0192-8

98. Parr EB, Camera DM, Areta JL, et al. Alcohol ingestion impairs maximal post-exercise rates of myofibrillar protein synthesis following a single bout of concurrent training. *PLoS ONE.* 2014;9(2):e88384. doi:10.1371/journal.pone.0088384

99. Burke LM, Collier GR, Broad EM, et al. Effect of alcohol intake on muscle glycogen storage after prolonged exercise. *J Appl Physiol (1985).* 2003;95(3):983-90. doi:10.1152/japplphysiol.00115.2003

100. National Institute on Alcohol Abuse and Alcoholism. College drinking. National Institutes of Health. Accessed December 2022. http://pubs.niaaa.nih.gov/publications/CollegeFactSheet/CollegeFactSheet.pdf

101. Lamis DA, Ellis JB, Chumney FL, Dula CS. Reasons for living and alcohol use among college students. *Death Stud.* 2009;33(3):277-86. doi:10.1080/07481180802672017

102. American College of Sports Medicine. Alcohol consumption and exercise performance. Accessed December 2022. www.acsm.org/search-results/all-blog posts/certification-blog/acsm-certified-blog/2022/05/19/alcohol-consumption-and-exercise-performance

Chapter 10

1. Opio J, Croker E, Odongo GS, Attia J, Wynne K, McEvoy M. Metabolically healthy overweight/obesity are associated with increased risk of cardiovascular disease in adults, even in the absence of metabolic risk factors: A systematic review and meta-analysis of prospective cohort studies. *Obesity Reviews.* 2020;21(12):e13127. doi:10.1111/obr.13127

2. Guh DP, Zhang W, Bansback N, Amarsi Z, Birmingham CL, Anis AH. The incidence of co-morbidities related to obesity and overweight: A systematic review and meta-analysis. *BMC Public Health.* 2009;9:88. doi:10.1186/1471-2458-9-88

3. Centers for Disease Control and Prevention. Adult obesity causes and consequences. Centers for Disease Control and Prevention. www.cdc.gov/obesity/adult/causes.html

4. Centers for Disease Control and Prevention. Assessing your weight. Centers for Disease Control and Prevention. www.cdc.gov/healthyweight/assessing/index.html

5. Centers for Disease Control and Prevention. Obesity and overweight. Updated September 6, 2022. www.cdc.gov/nchs/fastats/obesity-overweight.htm

6. Prevalence of obesity and severe obesity among adults: United States, 2017-2018. NCHS Data Brief; 2020.

7. Center for Disease Control and Prevention. Overweight and obesity, data and statistics. U.S. Department of Health and Human Services. Updated August 7, 2019. Accessed November 24, 2020, 2020. www.cdc.gov/obesity/data/index.html

8. American Medical Association. Is obesity a disease? (Resolution 115-A-12). The American Medical Association. Accessed February 20, 2017. www.ama-assn.org/sites/default/files/media-browser/public/about-ama/councils/Council%20Reports/council-on-science-public-health/a13csaph3.pdf

9. International Association for the Study of Obesity. Is obesity a disease? International Association for the Study of Obesity. Accessed February 19, 2017. www.worldobesity.org/site_media/uploads/Is_obesity_a_disease.pdf

10. Stoner L, Cornwall J. Did the American Medical Association make the correct decision classifying obesity as a disease? *Australas Med J*. 2014;7(11):462-464. doi:10.4066/AMJ.2014.2281

11. Aguilar-Valles A, Inoue W, Rummel C, Luheshi GN. Obesity, adipokines and neuroinflammation. *Neuropharmacology*. 2015;96(Pt A):124-34. doi:10.1016/j.neuropharm.2014.12.023

12. Thompson JL, Manore MM, Vaughan LA. *The Science of Nutrition*. vol 4. Pearson Education; 2017.

13. Thomas DT, Erdman KA, Burke LM. Position of the Academy of Nutrition and Dietetics, Dietitians of Canada, and the American College of Sports Medicine: Nutrition and athletic performance. *J Acad Nutr Diet*. 2016;116(3):501-28. doi:10.1016/j.jand.2015.12.006

14. Manore MM. Weight management for athletes and active individuals: A brief review. *Sports Med*. 2015;45(Suppl 1):83-92. doi:10.1007/s40279-015-0401-0

15. Centers for Disease Control and Prevention. About adult BMI. Centers for Disease Control and Prevention. www.cdc.gov/healthyweight/assessing/bmi/adult_bmi/index.html

16. Hoffman J. *Norms for Fitness, Performance, and Health*. Human Kinetics; 2006.

17. U.S. Food and Drug Administration. Medications target long-term weight control. U.S. Food and Drug Administration. www.fda.gov/downloads/ForConsumers/ConsumerUpdates/UCM312391.pdf

18. Hall DM, Cole TJ. What use is the BMI? *Arch Dis Child*. 2006;91(4):283-6. doi:10.1136/adc.2005.077339

19. Seidell JC, Perusse L, Despres JP, Bouchard C. Waist and hip circumferences have independent and opposite effects on cardiovascular disease risk factors: The Quebec Family Study. *Am J Clin Nutr*. 2001;74(3):315-21.

20. Etchison WC, Bloodgood EA, Minton CP, et al. Body mass index and percentage of body fat as indicators for obesity in an adolescent athletic population. *Sports Health*. 2011;3(3):249-52. doi:10.1177/1941738111404655

21. Wallner-Liebmann SJ, Kruschitz R, Hubler K, et al. A measure of obesity: BMI versus subcutaneous fat patterns in young athletes and nonathletes. *Coll Antropol*. 2013;37(2):351-7.

22. Jonnalagadda SS, Skinner R, Moore L. Overweight athlete: Fact or fiction? *Curr Sports Med Rep*. 2004;3(4):198-205.

23. Freedman DS, Sherry B. The validity of BMI as an indicator of body fatness and risk among children. *Pediatrics*. 2009;124 Suppl 1:S23-34. doi:10.1542/peds.2008-3586E

24. National Heart Lung and Blood Institute. Clinical guidelines on the identification, evaluation, and treatment of overweight and obesity in adults: The evidence report. National Heart, Lung, and Blood Institute. Accessed February 20, 2017. www.nhlbi.nih.gov/files/docs/guidelines/ob_gdlns.pdf

25. Ross CA, Caballero B, Cousins RJ, Tucker KL, Ziegler TR. *Modern Nutrition in Health and Disease*. 11th ed. Lippincott Williams & Wilkins; 2014.

26. Heyward VH, Wagner DR. *Applied Body Composition Assessment*. Human Kinetics; 2004.

27. Lohman TG, Going SB. Multicompartment models in body composition research. *Basic Life Sci*. 1993;60:53-58.

28. Jeukendrup AE, Gleeson M. *Sport Nutrition*. 2nd ed. Human Kinetics; 2010.

29. Siri WE. Body composition from fluid spaces and density: Analysis of methods. In: Brozek J, Henschel A, eds. *Techniques for Measuring Body Composition*. National Academy of Sciences; 1961:223-244.

30. American College of Sports Medicine. *ACSM's Resource Manual for Guidelines for Exercise Testing and Prescription*. 9th ed. Wolters Kluwer-Lippincott, Williams & Williams; 2014.

31. Radiological Society of North America. Bone densitometry. Radiological Society of North America, Inc. (RSNA). www.radiologyinfo.org/en/info.cfm?pg=dexa

32. van Marken Lichtenbelt WD, Hartgens F, Vollaard NB, Ebbing S, Kuipers H. Body composition changes in bodybuilders: A method comparison. *Med Sci Sports Exerc*. 2004;36(3):490-7. doi:10.1249/01.mss.0000117159.70295.73

33. Nattiv A, Loucks AB, Manore MM, Sanborn CF, Sundgot-Borgen J, Warren MP. American College of Sports Medicine position stand. The female athlete triad. *Med Sci Sports Exerc*. Oct 2007;39(10):1867-82. doi:10.1249/mss.0b013e318149f111

34. Durnin JVGA, Womersley J. Body fat assessed from total body density and its estimation from skinfold thickness: Measurements of 481 men and women aged from 17-72 years. *Br J Nutr*. 1974;32:77-97.

35. Jackson AS, Pollock ML. Practical assessment of body composition. *Phys Sportsmed*. 1985;13:76-90.

36. Lohman TG, Roche AF, Martorell R. *Anthropometric Standardization Reference Manual*. Human Kinetics; 1988.

37. Howley E, Thompson D. *Fitness Professional's Handbook*. 7th ed. Human Kinetics; 2017:592.
38. Bone JL, Ross ML, Tomcik KA, Jeacocke NA, Hopkins WG, Burke LM. Manipulation of muscle creatine and glycogen changes dual X-ray absorptiometry estimates of body composition. *Med Sci Sports Exerc*. 2017;49(5):1029. doi:10.1249/MSS.0000000000001174
39. Ackland TR, Lohman TG, Sundgot-Borgen J, et al. Current status of body composition assessment in sport: Review and position statement on behalf of the ad hoc research working group on body composition health and performance, under the auspices of the I.O.C. Medical Commission. *Sports Med*. 2012;42(3):227. doi:10.2165/11597140-000000000-00000
40. Santos DA, Dawson JA, Matias CN, et al. Reference values for body composition and anthropometric measurements in athletes. *PLoS ONE*. 2014;9(5):e97846. doi:10.1371/journal.pone.0097846
41. O'Connor H, Slater G. Losing, gaining and making weight for athletes. *Sport and Exercise Nutrition*. Wiley-Blackwell; 2011:210-232.
42. Sundgot-Borgen J, Garthe I. Elite athletes in aesthetic and Olympic weight-class sports and the challenge of body weight and body compositions. *J Sports Sci*. 2011;29(Suppl 1):S101. doi:10.1080/02640414.2011.565783

Chapter 11

1. Karpinski C, Rosenbloom C. *Sports Nutrition: A Handbook for Professionals*. 6th ed. Academy of Nutrition and Dietetics; 2017.
2. Kenney WL, Wilmore JH, Costill DL. *Physiology of Sport and Exercise*. 8th ed. Human Kinetics; 2022.
3. Brooks GA, Mercier J. Balance of carbohydrate and lipid utilization during exercise: The "crossover" concept. *J Appl Physiol*. 1985;76(6):2253-61.
4. Bergstrom J, Hermanssen L, Saltin B. Diet, muscle glycogen, and physical performance. *Acta Physiol*. 1967;71(2):140-150.
5. Brooks GA. Bioenergetics of exercising humans. *Compr Physiol*. 2012;2(1):537-62.
6. Shaw CS, Clark J, Wagenmakers AJ. The effect of exercise and nutrition on intramuscular fat metabolism and insulin sensitivity. *Annu Rev Nutr*. 2010;30:13-34. doi:10.1146/annurev.nutr.012809.104817
7. van Loon LJ. Use of intramuscular triacylglycerol as a substrate source during exercise in humans. *J Appl Physiol*. 2004;97(4):1170-87. doi:10.1152/japplphysiol.00368.2004
8. Romijn JA, Coyle EF, Sidossis LS, Zhang XJ, Wolfe RR. Relationship between fatty acid delivery and fatty acid oxidation during strenuous exercise. *J Appl Physiol*. 1995;79:1939-1945.
9. Spriet LL. New insights into the interaction of carbohydrate and fat metabolis, during exercise. *Sports Med*. 2014;44(Suppl 1):S87-S96.
10. Hawley JA, Burke LM. Carbohydrate availability and training adaptation: Effects on cell metabolism. *Exerc Sport Sci Rev*. 2010;38(4):152-160.
11. Manore MM. Weight management for athletes and active individuals: A brief review. *Sports Med*. 2015;45(Suppl 1):83-92. doi:10.1007/s40279-015-0401-0
12. Manore MM, Brown K, Houtkooper L, et al. Energy balance at a crossroads: Translating the science into action. *J Acad Nutr Diet*. 2014;114(7):1113-1119. doi:10.1016/j.jand.2014.03.012
13. Thomas DT, Erdman KA, Burke LM. Position of the Academy of Nutrition and Dietetics, Dietitians of Canada, and the American College of Sports Medicine: Nutrition and athletic performance. *J Acad Nutr Diet*. 2016;116(3):501-28. doi:10.1016/j.jand.2015.12.006
14. Mountjoy M, Sundgot-Borgen J, Burke L, et al. The IOC consensus statement: Beyond the female athlete triad—relative energy deficiency in sport (RED-S). *Br J Sports Med*. 2014;48(7):491-497. doi:10.1136/bjsports-2014-093502
15. National Academy of Sciences. *Dietary Reference Intakes for Energy, Carbohydrate, Fiber, Fat, Fatty Acids, Cholesterol, Protein, and Amino Acids (Macronutrients)*. 2005. www.nap.edu
16. National Institutes of Health. Nutrient recommendations: Dietary reference intakes. Accessed December 2022. https://ods.od.nih.gov/HealthInformation/Dietary_Reference_Intakes.aspx
17. Bandegan A, Courtney-Martin G, Rafii M, Pencharz PB, Lemon PWR. Indicator amino acid oxidation protein requirement estimate in endurance-trained men 24 h postexercise exceeds both the EAR and current athlete guidelines. *Am J Physiol Endocrinol Metab*. 2019;316(5):E741-E748. doi:10.1152/ajpendo.00174.2018
18. Jeukendrup AE, Gleeson, M. *Sport Nutrition*. 2nd ed. Human Kinetics; 2010.
19. Kreitzman SN, Coxon AY, Szaz KF. Glycogen storage: Illusions of easy weight loss, excessive weight regain, and distortions in estimates of body composition. *Am J Clin Nutr*. 1992;56(1 Suppl):292s-293s.
20. Coyle EF. Timing and method of increased carbohydrate intake to cope with heavy training, competition and recovery. *J Sports Sci*. 1991;9:29-51. doi:10.1080/02640419108729865
21. Burke LM. Nutrition strategies for the marathon: Fuel for training and racing. *Sports Med*. 2007;37(4-5):344-7.
22. Burke LM. Re-examining high-fat diets for sports performance: Did we call the "nail in the coffin" too soon? *Sports Med*. 2015;45(Suppl 1):S33-49. doi:10.1007/s40279-015-0393-9
23. Tarnopolsky LJ, MacDougall JD, Atkinson SA, Tarnopolsky MA, Sutton JR. Gender differences in substrate for endurance exercise. *J Appl Physiol*. 1990;68(1):302-8.
24. Tarnopolsky MA, Bosman M, Macdonald JR, Vandeputte D, Martin J, Roy BD. Postexercise protein-carbohydrate and carbohydrate supplements increase muscle glycogen in men and women. *J Appl Physiol*. 1997;83(6):1877-83.

25. Walker JL, Heigenhauser GJ, Hultman E, Spriet LL. Dietary carbohydrate, muscle glycogen content, and endurance performance in well-trained women. *J Appl Physiol.* 2000;88(6):2151-8.

26. Burke LM, Hawley JA, Wong SHS, Jeukendrup AE. Carbohydrates for training and competition. *J Sports Sci.* 2011;29(S1):S17-S27.

27. O'Reilly J, Wong S, Chen Y. Glycaemic index, glycaemic load, and exercise performance. *Sports Med.* 2010;40(1):27-39.

28. Burke LM, Hawley JA, Jeukendrup A, Morton JP, Stellingwerff T, Maughan RJ. Toward a common understanding of diet-exercise strategies to manipulate fuel availability for training and competition preparation in endurance sport. *Int J Sport Nutr Exerc Metab.* 2018;28(5):451-463. doi:10.1123/ijsnem.2018-0289

29. Cermak NM, van Loon LJC. The use of carbohydrates during exercise as an ergogenic aid. *Sports Med.* 2013;43:1139-1155.

30. Jeukendrup AE. Multiple transportable carbohydrates and their benefits. *Gatorade Sports Science Exchange.* 2013;26(108):1-5.

31. Jeukendrup AE. A step towards personalized sports nutrition: Carbohydrate intake during exercise. *Sports Med.* 2014;44(Suppl 1):S25-S33.

32. de Oliveira EP, Burini RC, Jeukendrup A. Gastrointestinal complaints during exercise: Prevalence, etiology, and nutritional recommendations. *Sports Med.* 2014;44(Suppl 1):S79-85. doi:10.1007/s40279-014-0153-2

33. Jeukendrup AE. Nutrition for endurance sports: Marathon, triathlon, and road cycling. *J Sports Sci.* 2011;29(S1):S91-S99.

34. Stellingwerff T, Maughan RJ, Burke LM. Nutrition for power sports: Middle-distance running, track cycling, rowing, canoeing/kayaking, and swimming. *J Sports Sci.* 2011;29(Suppl 1):S79-89. doi:10.1080/02640414.2011.589469

35. Burke LM, Kiens B, Ivy JL. Carbohydrates and fat for training and recovery. *J Sports Sci.* 2004;22:15-30.

36. Beelen M, Burke LM, Gibala MJ, van Loon LJC. Nutritional strategies to promote postexercise recovery. *J Phys Act Health.* 2010:1-17.

37. van Loon LJ. Is there a need for protein ingestion during exercise? *Sports Med.* 2014;44 (Suppl 1):S105-S111. doi:10.1007/s40279-014-0156-z

38. Burke LM, Loucks AB, Broad N. Energy and carbohydrates for training and recovery. *J Sports Sci.* 2006;24(7):675-685.

39. Jeukendrup AE. Performance and endurance in sport: Can it all be explained by metabolism and its manipulation? *Dialog Cardiovasc Med.* 2012;17(1):40-45.

40. Donaldson C, Perry T, Rose M. Glycemic index and endurance performance. *Int J Sport Nutr Exerc Metab.* 2010;20:154-165.

41. Phillips SM, Van Loon LJ. Dietary protein for athletes: From requirements to optimum adaptation. *J Sports Sci.* 2011;29(Suppl 1):S29-38. doi:10.1080/02640414.2011.619204

42. U.S. Food and Drug Administration. Guidance for industry: A food labeling guide. Accessed December 2022. www.fda.gov/food/guidanceregulation/guidancedocumentsregulatoryinformation/labelingnutrition/ucm2006828.htm

43. U.S. Food and Drug Administration. High intensity sweeteners. Accessed December 2022. www.fda.gov/Food/IngredientsPackagingLabeling/FoodAdditivesIngredients/ucm397716.htm

44. U.S. Food and Drug Administration. Additional information about high-intensity sweeteners permitted for use in food in the United States. Accessed December 2022. www.fda.gov/food/food-additives-petitions/additional-information-about-high-intensity-sweeteners-permitted-use-food-united-states#Advantame

45. U.S. Department of Agriculture. FoodData Central. Accessed December 2022. https://fdc.nal.usda.gov

46. Rong Y, Sillick M, Gregson CM. Determination of dextrose equivalent value and number average molecular weight of maltodextrin by osmometry. *J Food Sci.* 2009;74(1):C33-C40. doi:10.1111/j.1750-3841.2008.00993.x

47. Jozsi AC, Trappe TA, Starlling RD, et al. The influence of starch structure on glycogen resynthesis and subsequent cycling performance. *Int J Sports Med.* 1996;17(05):373-378. doi:10.1055/s-2007-972863

48. Roberts MD, Lockwood C, Dalbo VJ, Volek J, Kerksick CM. Ingestion of a high-molecular-weight hydrothermally modified waxy maize starch alters metabolic responses to prolonged exercise in trained cyclists. *Nutrition.* 2011;27(6):659-65. doi:10.1016/j.nut.2010.07.008

49. Sands AL, Leidy HJ, Hamaker BR, Maguire P, Campbell WW. Consumption of the slow-digesting waxy maize starch leads to blunted plasma glucose and insulin response but does not influence energy expenditure or appetite in humans. *Nutrition Research.* 29(6):383-390. doi:10.1016/j.nutres.2009.05.009

50. Stephens FB, Roig M, Armstrong G, Greenhaff PL. Post-exercise ingestion of a unique, high molecular weight glucose polymer solution improves performance during a subsequent bout of cycling exercise. *J Sports Sci.* 2008;26(2):149-154. doi:10.1080/02640410701361548

51. Jeukendrup AE, Rollo I, Carter JM. Carbohydrate mouth rinse: Performance effects and mechanisms. *Gatorade Sports Science Exchange.* 2013;26(118):1-8.

52. Brietzke C, Franco-Alvarenga PE, Coelho-Júnior HJ, Silveira R, Asano RY, Pires FO. Effects of carbohydrate mouth rinse on cycling time trial performance: A systematic review and meta-analysis. *Sports Medicine.* 2019;49(1):57-66. doi:10.1007/s40279-018-1029-7

53. Peart DJ. Quantifying the effect of carbohydrate mouth rinsing on exercise performance. *J Strength Cond Res.* 2017;31(6):1737-1743. doi:10.1519/jsc.0000000000001741

54. Heffernan SM, Horner K, De Vito G, Conway GE. The role of mineral and trace element supplementation

in exercise and athletic performance: A systematic review. *Nutrients*. 2019;11(3):696. doi:10.3390/nu11030696

55. National Institutes of Health. Dietary supplements for exercise and athletic performance. Accessed December 2022. https://ods.od.nih.gov/factsheets/ExerciseAndAthleticPerformance-HealthProfessional

56. Pfeiffer B, Stellingwerf T, Hodgson AB, et al. Nutritional intake and gastrointestinal problems during competitive endurance events. *Med Sci Sports Exerc*. 2012;44(2):344-351.

57. Prado de Oliveira E. Nutritional recommendations to avoid gastrointestinal complaints during exercise. *Gatorade Sports Science Exchange*. 2013;26(114):1-4.

58. Prado de Oliveira E, Burini RC, Jeukendrup AE. Gastrointestinal complaints during exercise: Prevalence, etiology, and nutritional recommendations. *Sports Med*. 2014;44(Suppl 1):S79-S85.

59. Baar K. Nutrition and the adaptation to endurance training. *Sports Medicine*. 2014;44(Suppl 1):S5-S12.

60. Bartlett JD, Hawley JA, Morton JP. Carbohydrate availability and exercise training adaptation: Too much of a good thing? *Eur J Sport Sci*. 2015;15(1):3-12. doi:10.1080/17461391.2014.920926

61. Burke LM. Fueling strategies to optimize performance: Training high or training low. *Scand J Med Sci Sports*. 2010;20(Suppl 2):48-58.

62. Ormsbee MJ, Bach CW, Baur DA. Pre-exercise nutrition: The role of macronutrients, modified starches and supplements on metabolism and endurance performance. *Nutrients*. 2014;6(5):1782-808. doi:10.3390/nu6051782

63. Burke LM, Castell LM, Casa DJ, et al. International Association of Athletics Federations consensus statement 2019: Nutrition for athletics. *Int J Sport Nutr Exerc Metab*. 2019;29(2):73-84. doi:10.1123/ijsnem.2019-0065

64. Lane SC, Camera DM, Lassiter DG, et al. Effects of sleeping with reduced carbohydrate availability on acute training responses. *J Appl Physiol (1985)*. 2015;119(6):643-55. doi:10.1152/japplphysiol.00857.2014

65. Ma S, Suzuki K. Keto-adaptation and endurance exercise capacity, fatigue recovery, and exercise-induced muscle and organ damage prevention: A narrative review. *Sports*. 2019;7(2):40. doi:10.3390/sports7020040

66. Harvey KL, Holcomb LE, Kolwicz SC, Jr. Ketogenic diets and exercise performance. *Nutrients*. 2019;11(10):2296. doi:10.3390/nu11102296

67. Bailey CP, Hennessy E. A review of the ketogenic diet for endurance athletes: Performance enhancer or placebo effect? *J Int Soc Sports Nutr*. 2020;17(1):33. doi:10.1186/s12970-020-00362-9

68. Kang J, Ratamess NA, Faigenbaum AD, Bush JA. Ergogenic properties of ketogenic diets in normal-weight individuals: A systematic review. *J Am Coll Nutr*. 2020;39(7):665-675. doi:10.1080/07315724.2020.1725686

69. Kaspar MB, Austin K, Huecker M, Sarav M. Ketogenic diet: From the historical records to use in elite athletes. *Curr Nutr Rep*. 2019;8(4):340-346. doi:10.1007/s13668-019-00294-0

70. McSwiney FT, Doyle L. Low-carbohydrate ketogenic diets in male endurance athletes demonstrate different micronutrient contents and changes in corpuscular haemoglobin over 12 weeks. *Sports*. 2019;7(9):201.

71. McSwiney FT, Wardrop B, Hyde PN, Lafountain RA, Volek JS, Doyle L. Keto-adaptation enhances exercise performance and body composition responses to training in endurance athletes. *Metabolism*. 2018;81:25-34. doi:10.1016/j.metabol.2017.10.010

72. Murphy NE, Carrigan CT, Margolis LM. High-fat ketogenic diets and physical performance: A systematic review. *Adv Nutr*. 2020:223-233. doi:10.1093/advances/nmaa101

73. Shaw DM, Merien F, Braakhuis A, Maunder E, Dulson DK. Exogenous ketone supplementation and keto-adaptation for endurance performance: Disentangling the effects of two distinct metabolic states. *Sports Medicine*. 2020;50(4):641-656. doi:10.1007/s40279-019-01246-y

74. Burke LM, Ross ML, Garvican-Lewis LA, et al. Low carbohydrate, high fat diet impairs exercise economy and negates the performance benefit from intensified training in elite race walkers. *The Journal of Physiology*. 2017;595(9):2785-2807. doi:10.1113/JP273230

75. Harvey C, Schofield GM, Williden M. The use of nutritional supplements to induce ketosis and reduce symptoms associated with keto-induction: A narrative review. *PeerJ*. 2018;6:e4488. doi:10.7717/peerj.4488

76. Sports and Human Performance Nutrition. CSSD. Academy of Nutrition & Dietetics. Accessed December 2022. www.shpndpg.org/shpn/professional-resources/cssd

77. Kellmann M, Bertollo M, Bosquet L, et al. Recovery and performance in sport: Consensus statement. *Int J Sports Physiol Perform*. 2018;13(2):240-245. doi:10.1123/ijspp.2017-0759

78. Kreher JB, Schwartz JB. Overtraining syndrome: A practical guide. *Sports Health*. 2012;4(2):128-138. doi:10.1177/1941738111434406

79. Meeusen R, Duclos M, Foster C, et al. Prevention, diagnosis, and treatment of the overtraining syndrome: Joint consensus statement of the European College of Sports Medicine and the American College of Sports Medicine. *Med Sci Sports Exerc*. 2013;45(1):186-205.

Chapter 12

1. Wolfe RR. The underappreciated role of muscle in health and disease. *Am J Clin Nutr*. 2006;84(3):475-82.

2. Judelson DA, Maresh CM, Anderson JM, et al. Hydration and muscular performance: Does fluid balance affect strength, power and high-intensity endurance? *Sports Med*. 2007;37(10):907-21.

3. Judelson DA, Maresh CM, Farrell MJ, et al. Effect of hydration state on strength, power, and resistance exercise performance. *Med Sci Sports Exerc.* 2007;39(10):1817-24. doi:10.1249/mss.0b013e-3180de5f22

4. Judelson DA, Maresh CM, Yamamoto LM, et al. Effect of hydration state on resistance exercise-induced endocrine markers of anabolism, catabolism, and metabolism. *J Appl Physiol (1985).* 2008;105(3):816-24. doi:10.1152/japplphysiol.01010.2007

5. Sekiguchi Y, Giersch GEW, Jordan DR, et al. Countermovement jump, handgrip, and balance performance change during euhydration, mild-dehydration, rehydration, and ad libitum drinking. *J Exerc Sci Fit.* 2022;20(4):335-339. doi:10.1016/j.jesf.2022.07.003

6. Sawka MN, Burke LM, Eichner ER, Maughan RJ, Montain SJ, Stachenfeld NS. American College of Sports Medicine position stand: Exercise and fluid replacement. *Med Sci Sports Exerc.* 2007;39(2):377-90. doi:10.1249/mss.0b013e31802ca597

7. Henselmans M, Bjornsen T, Hedderman R, Varvik FT. The effect of carbohydrate intake on strength and resistance training performance: A systematic review. *Nutrients.* 2022;14(4):856. doi:10.3390/nu14040856

8. de Moraes W, de Almeida FN, Dos Santos LEA, et al. Carbohydrate loading practice in bodybuilders: Effects on muscle thickness, photo silhouette scores, mood states and gastrointestinal symptoms. *J Sports Sci Med.* 2019;18(4):772-779.

9. Naharudin MN, Adams J, Richardson H, et al. Viscous placebo and carbohydrate breakfasts similarly decrease appetite and increase resistance exercise performance compared with a control breakfast in trained males. *Br J Nutr.* 2020:1-9. doi:10.1017/S0007114520001002

10. Reggiani C, Schiaffino S. Muscle hypertrophy and muscle strength: Dependent or independent variables? A provocative review. *Eur J Transl Myol.* 2020;30(3):9311. doi:10.4081/ejtm.2020.9311

11. Ahtiainen JP, Walker S, Peltonen H, et al. Heterogeneity in resistance training-induced muscle strength and mass responses in men and women of different ages. *Age (Dordr).* 2016;38(1):10. doi:10.1007/s11357-015-9870-1

12. Loenneke JP, Buckner SL, Dankel SJ, Abe T. Exercise-induced changes in muscle size do not contribute to exercise-induced changes in muscle strength. *Sports Med.* 2019;49(7):987-991. doi:10.1007/s40279-019-01106-9

13. Phillips SM, Tipton KD, Aarsland A, Wolf SE, Wolfe RR. Mixed muscle protein synthesis and breakdown after resistance exercise in humans. *Am J Physiol.* 1997;273(1 Pt 1):E99-E107.

14. Biolo G, Maggi SP, Williams BD, Tipton KD, Wolfe RR. Increased rates of muscle protein turnover and amino acid transport after resistance exercise in humans. *Am J Physiol.* 1995;268(3 Pt 1):E514-E520.

15. Haff GG, Koch AJ, Potteiger JA, et al. Carbohydrate supplementation attenuates muscle glycogen loss during acute bouts of resistance exercise. *Int J Sport Nutr Exerc Metab.* 2000;10(3):326-39.

16. Ivy JL. Regulation of muscle glycogen repletion, muscle protein synthesis and repair following exercise. *J Sports Sci Med.* 2004;3(3):131-8.

17. Pascoe DD, Costill DL, Fink WJ, Robergs RA, Zachwieja JJ. Glycogen resynthesis in skeletal muscle following resistive exercise. *Med Sci Sports Exerc.* 1993;25(3):349-54.

18. Parkin JA, Carey MF, Martin IK, Stojanovska L, Febbraio MA. Muscle glycogen storage following prolonged exercise: Effect of timing of ingestion of high glycemic index food. *Med Sci Sports Exerc.* 1997;29(2):220-4.

19. Glynn EL, Fry CS, Drummond MJ, et al. Muscle protein breakdown has a minor role in the protein anabolic response to essential amino acid and carbohydrate intake following resistance exercise. *Am J Physiol Regul Integr Comp Physiol.* 2010;299(2):R533-R540. doi:10.1152/ajpregu.00077.2010

20. Phillips SM. A brief review of critical processes in exercise-induced muscular hypertrophy. *Sports Med.* 2014;44 Suppl 1:71-7. doi:10.1007/s40279-014-0152-3

21. Cermak NM, Res PT, de Groot LC, Saris WH, van Loon LJ. Protein supplementation augments the adaptive response of skeletal muscle to resistance-type exercise training: A meta-analysis. *Am J Clin Nutr.* 2012;96(6):1454-64. doi:10.3945/ajcn.112.037556

22. Borsheim E, Cree MG, Tipton KD, Elliott TA, Aarsland A, Wolfe RR. Effect of carbohydrate intake on net muscle protein synthesis during recovery from resistance exercise. *J Appl Physiol (1985).* 2004;96(2):674-8. doi:10.1152/japplphysiol.00333.2003

23. Aragon AA, Schoenfeld BJ. Nutrient timing revisited: Is there a post-exercise anabolic window? *J Int Soc Sports Nutr.* 2013;10(1):5. doi:10.1186/1550-2783-10-5

24. Duplanty AA, Budnar RG, Luk HY, et al. Effect of acute alcohol ingestion on resistance exercise induced mTORC1 signaling in human muscle. *J Strength Cond Res.* 2017;31(1)doi:10.1519/JSC.0000000000001468

25. Boisseau N, Vermorel M, Rance M, Duche P, Patureau-Mirand P. Protein requirements in male adolescent soccer players. *Eur J Appl Physiol.* 2007;100(1):27-33. doi:10.1007/s00421-007-0400-4

26. Boisseau N, Delamarche P. Metabolic and hormonal responses to exercise in children and adolescents. *Sports Med.* 2000;30(6):405-22.

27. Folland JP, Williams AG. The adaptations to strength training: Morphological and neurological contributions to increased strength. *Sports Med.* 2007;37(2):145-68.

28. Hubal MJ, Gordish-Dressman H, Thompson PD, et al. Variability in muscle size and strength gain after unilateral resistance training. *Med Sci Sports Exerc.* 2005;37(6):964-72.

29. West DW, Phillips SM. Associations of exercise-induced hormone profiles and gains in strength and hypertrophy in a large cohort after weight training. *Eur J Appl Physiol.* 2012;112(7):2693-702. doi:10.1007/s00421-011-2246-z

30. Walsh S, Kelsey BK, Angelopoulos TJ, et al. CNTF 1357 G $\rightarrow$ A polymorphism and the muscle

strength response to resistance training. *J Appl Physiol.* 2009;107(4):1235-40. doi:10.1152/japplphysiol.90835.2008

31. Hulmi JJ, Laakso M, Mero AA, Hakkinen K, Ahtiainen JP, Peltonen H. The effects of whey protein with or without carbohydrates on resistance training adaptations. *J Int Soc Sports Nutr.* 2015;12:48. doi:10.1186/s12970-015-0109-4

32. Coffey VG, Hawley JA. Concurrent exercise training: Do opposites distract? *J Physiol.* 2017;595(9):2883-2896. doi:10.1113/JP272270

33. Camera DM, West DW, Phillips SM, et al. Protein ingestion increases myofibrillar protein synthesis after concurrent exercise. *Med Sci Sports Exerc.* 2015;47(1):82-91. doi:10.1249/MSS.0000000000000390

34. Donges CE, Burd NA, Duffield R, et al. Concurrent resistance and aerobic exercise stimulates both myofibrillar and mitochondrial protein synthesis in sedentary middle-aged men. *J Appl Physiol.* 2012;112(12):1992-2001. doi:10.1152/japplphysiol.00166.2012

35. Apro W, Wang L, Ponten M, Blomstrand E, Sahlin K. Resistance exercise induced mTORC1 signaling is not impaired by subsequent endurance exercise in human skeletal muscle. *Am J Physiol Endocrinol Metab.* 2013;305(1):E22-E32. doi:10.1152/ajpendo.00091.2013

36. Lundberg TR, Fernandez-Gonzalo R, Gustafsson T, Tesch PA. Aerobic exercise does not compromise muscle hypertrophy response to short-term resistance training. *J Appl Physiol (1985).* 2013;114(1):81-89. doi:10.1152/japplphysiol.01013.2012

37. Lundberg TR, Fernandez-Gonzalo R, Gustafsson T, Tesch PA. Aerobic exercise alters skeletal muscle molecular responses to resistance exercise. *Med Sci Sports Exerc.* 2012;44(9):1680-8. doi:10.1249/MSS.0b013e318256fbe8

38. Sabag A, Najafi A, Michael S, Esgin T, Halaki M, Hackett D. The compatibility of concurrent high intensity interval training and resistance training for muscular strength and hypertrophy: A systematic review and meta-analysis. *J Sports Sci.* 2018;36(21):2472-2483. doi:10.1080/02640414.2018.1464636

39. Kazior Z, Willis SJ, Moberg M, et al. Endurance exercise enhances the effect of strength training on muscle fiber size and protein expression of Akt and mTOR. *PLoS One.* 2016;11(2):e0149082. doi:10.1371/journal.pone.0149082

40. Shamim B, Devlin BL, Timmins RG, et al. Adaptations to concurrent training in combination with high protein availability: A comparative trial in healthy, recreationally active men. *Sports Med.* 2018;48(12):2869-2883. doi:10.1007/s40279-018-0999-9

41. Ribeiro N, Ugrinowitsch C, Panissa VLG, Tricoli V. Acute effects of aerobic exercise performed with different volumes on strength performance and neuromuscular parameters. *Eur J Sport Sci.* 2019;19(3):287-294. doi:10.1080/17461391.2018.1500643

42. Pugh JK, Faulkner SH, Jackson AP, King JA, Nimmo MA. Acute molecular responses to concurrent resistance and high-intensity interval exercise in untrained skeletal muscle. *Physiol Rep.* 2015;3(4)doi:10.14814/phy2.12364

43. Coffey VG, Jemiolo B, Edge J, Garnham AP, Trappe SW, Hawley JA. Effect of consecutive repeated sprint and resistance exercise bouts on acute adaptive responses in human skeletal muscle. *Am J Physiol Regul Integr Comp Physiol.* 2009;297(5):R1441-R1451. doi:10.1152/ajpregu.00351.2009

44. Fyfe JJ, Loenneke JP. Interpreting adaptation to concurrent compared with single-mode exercise training: Some methodological considerations. *Sports Med.* 2018;48(2):289-297. doi:10.1007/s40279-017-0812-1

45. Wilson JM, Marin PJ, Rhea MR, Wilson SM, Loenneke JP, Anderson JC. Concurrent training: A meta-analysis examining interference of aerobic and resistance exercises. *J Strength Cond Res.* 2012;26(8):2293-307. doi:10.1519/JSC.0b013e31823a3e2d

46. Baar K. Using molecular biology to maximize concurrent training. *Sports Med.* 2014;44 Suppl 2:S117-S125. doi:10.1007/s40279-014-0252-0

47. Perez-Schindler J, Hamilton DL, Moore DR, Baar K, Philp A. Nutritional strategies to support concurrent training. *Eur J Sport Sci.* 2014:1-12. doi:10.1080/17461391.2014.950345

48. Campbell B, Kreider RB, Ziegenfuss T, et al. International Society of Sports Nutrition position stand: Protein and exercise. *J Int Soc Sports Nutr.* 2007;4:8. doi:10.1186/1550-2783-4-8

49. Stokes T, Hector AJ, Morton RW, McGlory C, Phillips SM. Recent perspectives regarding the role of dietary protein for the promotion of muscle hypertrophy with resistance exercise training. *Nutrients.* 2018;10(2):180. doi:10.3390/nu10020180

50. Desbrow B, Burd NA, Tarnopolsky M, Moore DR, Elliott-Sale KJ. Nutrition for special populations: Young, female, and masters athletes. *Int J Sport Nutr Exerc Metab.* 2019;29(2):220-227. doi:10.1123/ijsnem.2018-0269

51. Rodriguez NR. Introduction to Protein Summit 2.0: Continued exploration of the impact of high-quality protein on optimal health. *Am J Clin Nutr.* 2015;doi:10.3945/ajcn.114.083980

52. Paddon-Jones D, Leidy H. Dietary protein and muscle in older persons. *Curr Opin Clin Nutr Metab Care.* 2014;17(1):5-11. doi:10.1097/MCO.0000000000000011

53. Churchward-Venne TA, Burd NA, Phillips SM. Nutritional regulation of muscle protein synthesis with resistance exercise: Strategies to enhance anabolism. *Nutr Metab (Lond).* 2012;9(1):40. doi:10.1186/1743-7075-9-40

54. Kimball SR, Jefferson LS. Regulation of protein synthesis by branched-chain amino acids. *Curr Opin Clin Nutr Metab Care.* 2001;4(1):39-43.

55. Norton LE, Layman DK, Bunpo P, Anthony TG, Brana DV, Garlick PJ. The leucine content of a complete meal directs peak activation but not duration of skeletal muscle protein synthesis and mammalian target of rapamycin signaling in rats. *J Nutr.* 2009;139(6):1103-9. doi:10.3945/jn.108.103853

56. Paddon-Jones D, Sheffield-Moore M, Zhang XJ, et al. Amino acid ingestion improves muscle protein synthesis in the young and elderly. *Am J Physiol Endocrinol Metab.* 2004;286(3):E321-E328.

57. Tipton KD, Ferrando AA, Phillips SM, Doyle D, Jr., Wolfe RR. Postexercise net protein synthesis in human muscle from orally administered amino acids. *Am J Physiol.* 1999;276(4 Pt 1):E628-E634.

58. Mai K, Cando P, Trasino SE. mTOR1c activation with the leucine "trigger" for prevention of sarcopenia in older adults during lockdown. *J Med Food.* 2022;25(2):117-120. doi:10.1089/jmf.2021.0094

59. Paddon-Jones D, Rasmussen BB. Dietary protein recommendations and the prevention of sarcopenia. *Curr Opin Clin Nutr Metab Care.* 2009;12(1):86-90. doi:10.1097/MCO.0b013e32831cef8b

60. Wilkinson DJ, Hossain T, Hill DS, et al. Effects of leucine and its metabolite beta-hydroxy-beta-methylbutyrate on human skeletal muscle protein metabolism. *J Physiol.* 2013;591(Pt 11):2911-23. doi:10.1113/jphysiol.2013.253203

61. Bohe J, Low JF, Wolfe RR, Rennie MJ. Latency and duration of stimulation of human muscle protein synthesis during continuous infusion of amino acids. *J Physiol.* 2001;532(Pt 2):575-9.

62. Atherton PJ, Etheridge T, Watt PW, et al. Muscle full effect after oral protein: Time-dependent concordance and discordance between human muscle protein synthesis and mTORC1 signaling. *Am J Clin Nutr.* 2010;92(5):1080-8. doi:10.3945/ajcn.2010.29819

63. Reidy PT, Walker DK, Dickinson JM, et al. Protein blend ingestion following resistance exercise promotes human muscle protein synthesis. *J Nutr.* 2013;143(4):410-6. doi:10.3945/jn.112.168021

64. Smeuninx B, Greig CA, Breen L. Amount, source and pattern of dietary protein intake across the adult lifespan: A cross-sectional study. *Front Nutr.* 2020;7:25. doi:10.3389/fnut.2020.00025

65. Deutz NE, Wolfe RR. Is there a maximal anabolic response to protein intake with a meal? *Clin Nutr.* 2013;32(2):309-13. doi:10.1016/j.clnu.2012.11.018

66. Symons TB, Sheffield-Moore M, Wolfe RR, Paddon-Jones D. A moderate serving of high-quality protein maximally stimulates skeletal muscle protein synthesis in young and elderly subjects. *J Am Diet Assoc.* 2009;109(9):1582-6. doi:10.1016/j.jada.2009.06.369

67. U.S. Department of Agriculture. Nutrient intakes from food: Mean amounts consumed per individual, by gender and age: What we eat in America, NHANES 2009-2010. www.ars.usda.gov/ba/bhnrc/fsrg

68. Rodriguez NR. Protein-centric meals for optimal protein utilization: Can it be that simple? *J Nutr.* 2014;144(6):797-8. doi:10.3945/jn.114.193615

69. Mamerow MM, Mettler JA, English KL, et al. Dietary protein distribution positively influences 24-h muscle protein synthesis in healthy adults. *J Nutr.* 2014;144(6):876-80. doi:10.3945/jn.113.185280

70. Schoenfeld BJ, Aragon AA. How much protein can the body use in a single meal for muscle-building? Implications for daily protein distribution. *J Int Soc Sports Nutr.* 2018;15:10. doi:10.1186/s12970-018-0215-1

71. Weijs PJM, Mogensen KM, Rawn JD, Christopher KB. Protein intake, nutritional status and outcomes in ICU survivors: A single center cohort study. *J Clin Med.* 2019;8(1):43. doi:10.3390/jcm8010043

72. Tipton KD. Nutritional support for exercise-induced injuries. *Sports Med.* 2015;45(Suppl 1):S93-104. doi:10.1007/s40279-015-0398-4

73. Bollwein J, Diekmann R, Kaiser MJ, et al. Distribution but not amount of protein intake is associated with frailty: A cross-sectional investigation in the region of Nurnberg. *Nutr J.* 2013;12:109. doi:10.1186/1475-2891-12-109

74. Rieu I, Balage M, Sornet C, et al. Leucine supplementation improves muscle protein synthesis in elderly men independently of hyperaminoacidaemia. *J Physiol.* 2006;575(Pt 1):305-15. doi:10.1113/jphysiol.2006.110742

75. Koopman R, Verdijk L, Manders RJ, et al. Co-ingestion of protein and leucine stimulates muscle protein synthesis rates to the same extent in young and elderly lean men. *Am J Clin Nutr.* 2006;84(3):623-32.

76. Verhoeven S, Vanschoonbeek K, Verdijk LB, et al. Long-term leucine supplementation does not increase muscle mass or strength in healthy elderly men. *Am J Clin Nutr.* 2009;89(5):1468-75. doi:10.3945/ajcn.2008.26668

77. Casperson SL, Sheffield-Moore M, Hewlings SJ, Paddon-Jones D. Leucine supplementation chronically improves muscle protein synthesis in older adults consuming the RDA for protein. *Clin Nutr.* 2012;31(4):512-9. doi:10.1016/j.clnu.2012.01.005

78. Leenders M, Verdijk LB, van der Hoeven L, et al. Prolonged leucine supplementation does not augment muscle mass or affect glycemic control in elderly type 2 diabetic men. *J Nutr.* 2011;141(6):1070-6. doi:10.3945/jn.111.138495

79. Loenneke JP, Loprinzi PD, Murphy CH, Phillips SM. Per meal dose and frequency of protein consumption is associated with lean mass and muscle performance. *Clin Nutr.* 2016;35(6):1506-1511. doi:10.1016/j.clnu.2016.04.002

80. Moore DR, Churchward-Venne TA, Witard O, et al. Protein ingestion to stimulate myofibrillar protein synthesis requires greater relative protein intakes in healthy older versus younger men. *J Gerontol A Biol Sci Med Sci.* 2015;70(1):57-62. doi:10.1093/gerona/glu103

81. Sarwar Gilani G, Wu Xiao C, Cockell KA. Impact of antinutritional factors in food proteins on the digestibility of protein and the bioavailability of amino acids and on protein quality. *Br J Nutr.* 2012;108 Suppl 2:S315-S332. doi:10.1017/S0007114512002371

82. Gilani GS, Cockell KA, Sepehr E. Effects of antinutritional factors on protein digestibility and amino acid availability in foods. *J AOAC Int.* 2005;88(3):967-87.

83. Antonio J, Peacock CA, Ellerbroek A, Fromhoff B, Silver T. The effects of consuming a high protein diet (4.4 g/kg/d) on body composition in resist-

ance-trained individuals. *J Int Soc Sports Nutr.* 2014;11:19. doi:10.1186/1550-2783-11-19

84. Pasiakos SM, Cao JJ, Margolis LM, et al. Effects of high-protein diets on fat-free mass and muscle protein synthesis following weight loss: A randomized controlled trial. *FASEB J.* 2013;27(9):3837-47. doi:10.1096/fj.13-230227

85. Pasiakos SM, Vislocky LM, Carbone JW, et al. Acute energy deprivation affects skeletal muscle protein synthesis and associated intracellular signaling proteins in physically active adults. *J Nutr.* 2010;140(4):745-51. doi:10.3945/jn.109.118372

86. Murray B, Rosenbloom C. Fundamentals of glycogen metabolism for coaches and athletes. *Nutr Rev.* 2018;76(4):243-259. doi:10.1093/nutrit/nuy001

87. Burke LM, van Loon LJC, Hawley JA. Postexercise muscle glycogen resynthesis in humans. *J Appl Physiol (1985).* 2017;122(5):1055-1067. doi:10.1152/japplphysiol.00860.2016

88. Kerksick C, Thomas A, Campbell B, et al. Effects of a popular exercise and weight loss program on weight loss, body composition, energy expenditure and health in obese women. *Nutr Metab (Lond).* 2009;6:23. doi:10.1186/1743-7075-6-23

89. Helms ER, Aragon AA, Fitschen PJ. Evidence-based recommendations for natural bodybuilding contest preparation: nutrition and supplementation. *J Int Soc Sports Nutr.* 2014;11:20. doi:10.1186/1550-2783-11-20

90. Dowis K, Banga S. The potential health benefits of the ketogenic diet: A narrative review. *Nutrients.* 2021;13(5):1654. doi:10.3390/nu13051654

91. Hall KD, Chen KY, Guo J, et al. Energy expenditure and body composition changes after an isocaloric ketogenic diet in overweight and obese men. *Am J Clin Nutr.* 2016;104(2):324-33. doi:10.3945/ajcn.116.133561

92. Volek JS, Noakes T, Phinney SD. Rethinking fat as a fuel for endurance exercise. *Eur J Sport Sci.* 2015;15(1):13-20. doi:10.1080/17461391.2014.959564

93. Paoli A, Grimaldi K, D'Agostino D, et al. Ketogenic diet does not affect strength performance in elite artistic gymnasts. *J Int Soc Sports Nutr.* 2012;9(1):34. doi:10.1186/1550-2783-9-34

94. Kapetanakis M, Liuba P, Odermarsky M, Lundgren J, Hallbook T. Effects of ketogenic diet on vascular function. *Eur J Paediatr Neurol.* 2014;18(4):489-94. doi:10.1016/j.ejpn.2014.03.006

95. Coppola G, Natale F, Torino A, et al. The impact of the ketogenic diet on arterial morphology and endothelial function in children and young adults with epilepsy: A case-control study. *Seizure.* 2014;23(4):260-5. doi:10.1016/j.seizure.2013.12.002

96. Cecelja M, Chowienczyk P. Role of arterial stiffness in cardiovascular disease. *JRSM Cardiovasc Dis.* 2012;1(4):1-10. doi:10.1258/cvd.2012.012016

97. Brown K, DeCoffe D, Molcan E, Gibson DL. Diet-induced dysbiosis of the intestinal microbiota and the effects on immunity and disease. *Nutrients.* 2012;4(8):1095-119. doi:10.3390/nu4081095

98. White AM, Johnston CS, Swan PD, Tjonn SL, Sears B. Blood ketones are directly related to fatigue and perceived effort during exercise in overweight adults adhering to low-carbohydrate diets for weight loss: A pilot study. *J Am Diet Assoc.* 2007;107(10):1792-6. doi:10.1016/j.jada.2007.07.009

99. Garfinkel D, Garfinkel L. Magnesium and regulation of carbohydrate metabolism at the molecular level. *Magnesium.* 1988;7(5-6):249-61.

100. Chen HY, Cheng FC, Pan HC, Hsu JC, Wang MF. Magnesium enhances exercise performance via increasing glucose availability in the blood, muscle, and brain during exercise. *PLoS One.* 2014;9(1):e85486. doi:10.1371/journal.pone.0085486

101. Schott GD, Wills MR. Muscle weakness in osteomalacia. *Lancet.* 1976;1(7960):626-9.

102. Hassan-Smith ZK, Jenkinson C, Smith DJ, et al. 25-hydroxyvitamin D3 and 1,25-dihydroxyvitamin D3 exert distinct effects on human skeletal muscle function and gene expression. *PLoS One.* 2017;12(2):e0170665. doi:10.1371/journal.pone.0170665

103. LeBlanc ES, Zakher B, Daeges M, Pappas M, Chou R. Screening for vitamin D deficiency: A systematic review for the U.S. Preventive Services Task Force. *Ann Intern Med.* 2015;162(2):109-22. doi:10.7326/M14-1659

104. Bischoff-Ferrari HA, Shao A, Dawson-Hughes B, Hathcock J, Giovannucci E, Willett WC. Benefit-risk assessment of vitamin D supplementation. *Osteoporos Int.* 2010;21(7):1121-32. doi:10.1007/s00198-009-1119-3

105. Beaudart C, Buckinx F, Rabenda V, et al. The effects of vitamin D on skeletal muscle strength, muscle mass, and muscle power: A systematic review and meta-analysis of randomized controlled trials. *J Clin Endocrinol Metab.* 2014;99(11):4336-45. doi:10.1210/jc.2014-1742

106. Han Q, Li X, Tan Q, Shao J, Yi M. Effects of vitamin D3 supplementation on serum 25(OH)D concentration and strength in athletes: A systematic review and meta-analysis of randomized controlled trials. *J Int Soc Sports Nutr.* 2019;16(1):55. doi:10.1186/s12970-019-0323-6

107. Krotkiewski M, Gudmundsson M, Backstrom P, Mandroukas K. Zinc and muscle strength and endurance. *Acta Physiol Scand.* 1982;116(3):309-11. doi:10.1111/j.1748-1716.1982.tb07146.x

108. Brun JF, Dieu-Cambrezy C, Charpiat A, et al. Serum zinc in highly trained adolescent gymnasts. *Biol Trace Elem Res.* 1995;47(1-3):273-8. doi:10.1007/BF02790127

109. Van Loan MD, Sutherland B, Lowe NM, Turnlund JR, King JC. The effects of zinc depletion on peak force and total work of knee and shoulder extensor and flexor muscles. *Int J Sport Nutr.* 1999;9(2):125-35.

110. Tarnopolsky M. Caffeine and creatine use in sport. *Ann Nutr Metab.* 2010;57(Suppl 2):1-8.

111. Cribb PJ, Williams AD, Hayes A. A creatine-protein-carbohydrate supplement enhances responses to resistance training. *Med Sci Sports Exerc.* 2007;39(11):1960-8. doi:10.1249/mss.0b013e31814fb52a

112. Kerksick CM, Wilborn CD, Campbell WI, et al. The effects of creatine monohydrate supplementation with and without D-pinitol on resistance training adaptations. *J Strength Cond Res.* 2009;23(9):2673-82. doi:10.1519/JSC.0b013e3181b3e0de

113. Devries MC, Phillips SM. Creatine supplementation during resistance training in older adults: A meta-analysis. *Med Sci Sports Exerc.* 2014;46(6):1194-203. doi:10.1249/MSS.0000000000000220

114. Van Koevering M, Nissen S. Oxidation of leucine and alpha-ketoisocaproate to beta-hydroxy-beta-methylbutyrate in vivo. *Am J Physiol.* 1992;262(1 Pt 1):E27-E31.

115. Deutz NE, Pereira SL, Hays NP, et al. Effect of beta-hydroxy-beta-methylbutyrate (HMB) on lean body mass during 10 days of bed rest in older adults. *Clin Nutr.* 2013;32(5):704-12. doi:10.1016/j.clnu.2013.02.011

116. Stout JR, Smith-Ryan AE, Fukuda DH, et al. Effect of calcium beta-hydroxy-beta-methylbutyrate (CaHMB) with and without resistance training in men and women 65+yrs: A randomized, double-blind pilot trial. *Exp Gerontol.* 2013;48(11):1303-10. doi:10.1016/j.exger.2013.08.007

117. Vukovich MD, Stubbs NB, Bohlken RM. Body composition in 70-year-old adults responds to dietary beta-hydroxy-beta-methylbutyrate similarly to that of young adults. *J Nutr.* 2001;131(7):2049-52.

118. Jakubowski JS, Wong EPT, Nunes EA, et al. Equivalent hypertrophy and strength gains in beta-hydroxy-beta-methylbutyrate- or leucine-supplemented men. *Med Sci Sports Exerc.* 2019;51(1):65-74. doi:10.1249/MSS.0000000000001752

119. Jakubowski JS, Nunes EA, Teixeira FJ, et al. Supplementation with the leucine metabolite beta-hydroxy-beta-methylbutyrate (HMB) does not improve resistance exercise-induced changes in body composition or strength in young subjects: A systematic review and meta-analysis. *Nutrients.* 2020;12(5) doi:10.3390/nu12051523

Chapter 13

1. Hall DM, Cole TJ. What use is the BMI? *Arch Dis Child.* 2006;91(4):283-6. doi:10.1136/adc.2005.077339

2. McArdle W, Katch F, Katch V. *Exercise Physiology, Energy, Nutrition, and Human Performance.* 6th ed. Lippincott Williams & Wilkins; 2007.

3. Lima MM, Pareja JC, Alegre SM, et al. Visceral fat resection in humans: Effect on insulin sensitivity, beta-cell function, adipokines, and inflammatory markers. *Obesity (Silver Spring).* 2013;21(3):E182-9. doi:10.1002/oby.20030

4. Gastaldelli A, Miyazaki Y, Pettiti M, et al. Metabolic effects of visceral fat accumulation in type 2 diabetes. *J Clin Endocrinol Metab.* 2002;87(11):5098-103. doi:10.1210/jc.2002-020696

5. Hardy OT, Czech MP, Corvera S. What causes the insulin resistance underlying obesity? *Curr Opin Endocrinol Diabetes Obes.* 2012;19(2):81-87. doi:10.1097/MED.0b013e3283514e13

6. Golan R, Shelef I, Rudich A, et al. Abdominal superficial subcutaneous fat: A putative distinct protective fat subdepot in type 2 diabetes. *Diabetes Care.* 2012;35(3):640-7. doi:10.2337/dc11-1583

7. Wang SC, Bednarski B, Patel S, et al. Increased depth of subcutaneous fat is protective against abdominal injuries in motor vehicle collisions. *Annu Proc Assoc Adv Automot Med.* 2003;47:545-59.

8. Thomas EL, Frost G, Taylor-Robinson SD, Bell JD. Excess body fat in obese and normal-weight subjects. *Nutr Res Rev.* 2012;25(1):150-61. doi:10.1017/S0954422412000054

9. Pi-Sunyer X. The medical risks of obesity. *Postgrad Med.* 2009;121(6):21-33. doi:10.3810/pgm.2009.11.2074

10. Fryar C, Carroll, MD, Afful, J. *Prevalence of Overweight, Obesity, and Severe Obesity Among Adults Aged 20 and Over: United States, 1960–1962 Through 2017–2018.* 2020. NCHS Health E-Stats. Accessed September 6, 2021. www.cdc.gov/nchs/data/hestat/obesity-adult-17-18/overweight-obesity-adults-H.pdf

11. Fryar C, Carroll M, Afful J. *Prevalence of Overweight, Obesity, and Severe Obesity Among Children and Adolescents Aged 2–19 Years: United States, 1963–1965 Through 2017–2018.* 2020. NCHS Health E-Stats.

12. Elsayed EF, Tighiouart H, Weiner DE, et al. Waist-to-hip ratio and body mass index as risk factors for cardiovascular events in CKD. *Am J Kidney Dis.* 2008;52(1):49-57. doi:10.1053/j.ajkd.2008.04.002

13. Pouliot MC, Despres JP, Lemieux S, et al. Waist circumference and abdominal sagittal diameter: Best simple anthropometric indexes of abdominal visceral adipose tissue accumulation and related cardiovascular risk in men and women. *Am J Cardiol.* 1994;73(7):460-8.

14. National Heart Lung and Blood Institute. What is cholesterol? Accessed May 1, 2016. www.nhlbi.nih.gov/health/health-topics/topics/hbc

15. Miller M, Stone NJ, Ballantyne C, et al. Triglycerides and cardiovascular disease: A scientific statement from the American Heart Association. *Circulation.* 2011;123(20):2292-333. doi:10.1161/CIR.0b013e3182160726

16. Nordestgaard BG, Varbo A. Triglycerides and cardiovascular disease. *Lancet.* 2014;384(9943):626-35. doi:10.1016/S0140-6736(14)61177-6

17. Schmieder RE, Messerli FH. Does obesity influence early target organ damage in hypertensive patients? *Circulation.* 1993;87(5):1482-8.

18. National Heart Lung and Blood Institute. Atherosclerosis. Accessed April 16, 2016. www.ncbi.nlm.nih.gov/pubmedhealth/PMH0062943

19. Wadei HM, Textor SC. The role of the kidney in regulating arterial blood pressure. *Nat Rev Nephrol.* 2012;8(10):602-9. doi:10.1038/nrneph.2012.191

20. Ye J. Mechanisms of insulin resistance in obesity. *Front Med.* 2013;7(1):14-24. doi:10.1007/s11684-013-0262-6

21. National Institute of Diabetes and Digestive and Kidney Diseases. *Insulin Resistance and Prediabetes.* 2014. Accessed April 17, 2016.

22. Whitmore C. Type 2 diabetes and obesity in adults. *Br J Nurs.* 2010;19(14):880, 882-6. doi:10.12968/bjon.2010.19.14.49041

23. Fox CS. Cardiovascular disease risk factors, type 2 diabetes mellitus, and the Framingham Heart Study. *Trends Cardiovasc Med.* 2010;20(3):90-95. doi:10.1016/j.tcm.2010.08.001

24. Vidal J. Updated review on the benefits of weight loss. *Int J Obes Relat Metab Disord.* 2002;26(Suppl 4):S25-8. doi:10.1038/sj.ijo.0802215

25. Djiogue S, Nwabo Kamdje AH, Vecchio L, et al. Insulin resistance and cancer: The role of insulin and IGFs. *Endocr Relat Cancer.* 2013;20(1):R1-R17. doi:10.1530/ERC-12-0324

26. Multhoff G, Molls M, Radons J. Chronic inflammation in cancer development. *Front Immunol.* 2011;2:98. doi:10.3389/fimmu.2011.00098

27. Roberts DL, Dive C, Renehan AG. Biological mechanisms linking obesity and cancer risk: New perspectives. *Annu Rev Med.* 2010;61:301-16. doi:10.1146/annurev.med.080708.082713

28. Schwab RJ, Pasirstein M, Pierson R, et al. Identification of upper airway anatomic risk factors for obstructive sleep apnea with volumetric magnetic resonance imaging. *Am J Respir Crit Care Med.* 2003;168(5):522-30. doi:10.1164/rccm.200208-866OC

29. Paschos P, Paletas K. Non alcoholic fatty liver disease and metabolic syndrome. *Hippokratia.* 2009;13(1):9-19.

30. King LK, March L, Anandacoomarasamy A. Obesity & osteoarthritis. *Indian J Med Res.* 2013;138:185-93.

31. Borchers JR, Clem KL, Habash DL, Nagaraja HN, Stokley LM, Best TM. Metabolic syndrome and insulin resistance in Division 1 collegiate football players. *Med Sci Sports Exerc.* 2009;41(12):2105-10. doi:10.1249/MSS.0b013e3181abdfec

32. Smith GI, Mittendorfer B, Klein S. Metabolically healthy obesity: Facts and fantasies. *J Clin Invest.* 2019;129(10):3978-3989. doi:10.1172/JCI129186

33. Ortega FB, Lee DC, Katzmarzyk PT, et al. The intriguing metabolically healthy but obese phenotype: Cardiovascular prognosis and role of fitness. *Eur Heart J.* 2013;34(5):389-97. doi:10.1093/eurheartj/ehs174

34. Ortega FB, Cadenas-Sanchez C, Migueles JH, et al. Role of physical activity and fitness in the characterization and prognosis of the metabolically healthy obesity phenotype: A systematic review and meta-analysis. *Prog Cardiovasc Dis.* 2018;61(2):190-205. doi:10.1016/j.pcad.2018.07.008

35. Duncan GE. The "fit but fat" concept revisited: Population-based estimates using NHANES. *Int J Behav Nutr Phys Act.* 2010;7:47. doi:10.1186/1479-5868-7-47

36. Yerrakalva D, Mullis R, Mant J. The associations of "fatness," "fitness," and physical activity with all-cause mortality in older adults: A systematic review. *Obesity (Silver Spring).* 2015;23(10):1944-56. doi:10.1002/oby.21181

37. Barry VW, Baruth M, Beets MW, Durstine JL, Liu J, Blair SN. Fitness vs. fatness on all-cause mortality: A meta-analysis. *Prog Cardiovasc Dis.* 2014;56(4):382-90. doi:10.1016/j.pcad.2013.09.002

38. Serodio PM, McKee M, Stuckler D. Coca-Cola: A model of transparency in research partnerships? A network analysis of Coca-Cola's research funding (2008–2016). *Public Health Nutr.* 2018;21(9):1594-1607. doi:10.1017/S136898001700307X

39. Bluher M. Metabolically healthy obesity. *Endocr Rev.* 2020;41(3):bnaa004. doi:10.1210/endrev/bnaa004

40. Mongraw-Chaffin M, Foster MC, Anderson CAM, et al. Metabolically healthy obesity, transition to metabolic syndrome, and cardiovascular risk. *J Am Coll Cardiol.* 2018;71(17):1857-1865. doi:10.1016/j.jacc.2018.02.055

41. Williams RL, Wood LG, Collins CE, Callister R. Effectiveness of weight loss interventions—is there a difference between men and women: A systematic review. *Obes Rev.* 2015;16(2):171-86. doi:10.1111/obr.12241

42. Chaston TB, Dixon JB, O'Brien PE. Changes in fat-free mass during significant weight loss: A systematic review. *Int J Obes (Lond).* 2007;31(5):743-50. doi:10.1038/sj.ijo.0803483

43. Garthe I, Raastad T, Refsnes PE, Koivisto A, Sundgot-Borgen J. Effect of two different weight-loss rates on body composition and strength and power-related performance in elite athletes. *Int J Sport Nutr Exerc Metab.* 2011;21(2):97-104.

44. Johannsen DL, Knuth ND, Huizenga R, Rood JC, Ravussin E, Hall KD. Metabolic slowing with massive weight loss despite preservation of fat-free mass. *J Clin Endocrinol Metab.* 2012;97(7):2489-96. doi:10.1210/jc.2012-1444

45. Turocy PS, DePalma BF, Horswill CA, et al. National Athletic Trainers' Association position statement: Safe weight loss and maintenance practices in sport and exercise. *J Athl Train.* 2011;46(3):322-36.

46. Zanker CL. Regulation of reproductive function in athletic women: An investigation of the roles of energy availability and body composition. *Br J Sports Med.* 2006;40(6):489-90; discussion 490. doi:10.1136/bjsm.2004.016758

47. Caronia LM, Martin C, Welt CK, et al. A genetic basis for functional hypothalamic amenorrhea. *N Engl J Med.* 2011;364(3):215-25. doi:10.1056/NEJMoa0911064

48. Manore MM. Weight management for athletes and active individuals: A brief review. *Sports Med.* 2015;45(Suppl 1):S83-S92. doi:10.1007/s40279-015-0401-0

49. Thompson J, Manore MM. Predicted and measured resting metabolic rate of male and female endur-

ance athletes. *J Am Diet Assoc.* 1996;96(1):30-34. doi:10.1016/S0002-8223(96)00010-7

50. Ainsworth BE, Haskell WL, Herrmann SD, et al. 2011 compendium of physical activities: A second update of codes and MET values. *Med Sci Sports Exerc.* 2011;43(8):1575-81. doi:10.1249/MSS.0b013e31821ece12

51. Harris J, Benedict F. *A Biometric Study of Basal Metabolism in Man.* 1919.

52. Levine JA. Non-exercise activity thermogenesis (NEAT). *Best Pract Res Clin Endocrinol Metab.* 2002;16(4):679-702.

53. Thompson J, Manore MM, Skinner JS. Resting metabolic rate and thermic effect of a meal in low- and adequate-energy intake male endurance athletes. *Int J Sport Nutr.* 1993;3(2):194-206.

54. Seagle HM, Strain GW, Makris A, Reeves RS, American Dietetic A. Position of the American Dietetic Association: Weight management. *J Am Diet Assoc.* 2009;109(2):330-46.

55. Murphy CH, Hector AJ, Phillips SM. Considerations for protein intake in managing weight loss in athletes. *Eur J Sport Sci.* 2014:1-8. doi:10.1080/17461391.2014.936325

56. Wishnofsky M. Caloric equivalents of gained or lost weight. *Am J Clin Nutr.* 1958;6(5):542-6.

57. Byrne NM, Wood RE, Schutz Y, Hills AP. Does metabolic compensation explain the majority of less-than-expected weight loss in obese adults during a short-term severe diet and exercise intervention? *Int J Obes (Lond).* 2012;36(11):1472-8. doi:10.1038/ijo.2012.109

58. Hall KD, Heymsfield SB, Kemnitz JW, Klein S, Schoeller DA, Speakman JR. Energy balance and its components: Implications for body weight regulation. *Am J Clin Nutr.* 2012;95(4):989-94. doi:10.3945/ajcn.112.036350

59. Thomas DM, Bouchard C, Church T, et al. Why do individuals not lose more weight from an exercise intervention at a defined dose? An energy balance analysis. *Obes Rev.* 2012;13(10):835-47. doi:10.1111/j.1467-789X.2012.01012.x

60. Hall KD, Sacks G, Chandramohan D, et al. Quantification of the effect of energy imbalance on bodyweight. *Lancet.* 2011;378(9793):826-37. doi:10.1016/S0140-6736(11)60812-X

61. Franz MJ, VanWormer JJ, Crain AL, et al. Weight-loss outcomes: A systematic review and meta-analysis of weight-loss clinical trials with a minimum 1-year follow-up. *J Am Diet Assoc.* 2007;107(10):1755-67. doi:10.1016/j.jada.2007.07.017

62. Hall KD, Kahan S. Maintenance of lost weight and long-term management of obesity. *Med Clin North Am.* 2018;102(1):183-197. doi:10.1016/j.mcna.2017.08.012

63. Anderson JW, Konz EC, Frederich RC, Wood CL. Long-term weight-loss maintenance: A meta-analysis of US studies. *Am J Clin Nutr.* 2001;74(5):579-84. doi:10.1093/ajcn/74.5.579

64. Astrup A, Gotzsche PC, van de Werken K, et al. Meta-analysis of resting metabolic rate in formerly obese subjects. *Am J Clin Nutr.* 1999;69(6):1117-22. doi:10.1093/ajcn/69.6.1117

65. Fothergill E, Guo J, Howard L, et al. Persistent metabolic adaptation 6 years after "The Biggest Loser" competition. *Obesity (Silver Spring).* 2016;24(8):1612-9. doi:10.1002/oby.21538

66. Weinheimer EM, Sands LP, Campbell WW. A systematic review of the separate and combined effects of energy restriction and exercise on fat-free mass in middle-aged and older adults: Implications for sarcopenic obesity. *Nutr Rev.* 2010;68(7):375-88. doi:10.1111/j.1753-4887.2010.00298.x

67. Deurenberg P, Weststrate JA, Hautvast JG. Changes in fat-free mass during weight loss measured by bioelectrical impedance and by densitometry. *Am J Clin Nutr.* 1989;49(1):33-36.

68. Stiegler P, Cunliffe A. The role of diet and exercise for the maintenance of fat-free mass and resting metabolic rate during weight loss. *Sports Med.* 2006;36(3):239-62.

69. Knuth ND, Johannsen DL, Tamboli RA, et al. Metabolic adaptation following massive weight loss is related to the degree of energy imbalance and changes in circulating leptin. *Obesity (Silver Spring).* 2014;22(12):2563-9. doi:10.1002/oby.20900

70. Mitchell BG, Gupta N. Roux-en-Y gastric bypass. *StatPearls.* 2022. www.ncbi.nlm.nih.gov/books/NBK430685

71. Polidori D, Sanghvi A, Seeley RJ, Hall KD. How strongly does appetite counter weight loss? Quantification of the feedback control of human energy intake. *Obesity (Silver Spring).* 2016;24(11):2289-2295. doi:10.1002/oby.21653

72. Zhou Y, Rui L. Leptin signaling and leptin resistance. *Front Med.* 2013;7(2):207-22. doi:10.1007/s11684-013-0263-5

73. Leibel RL, Rosenbaum M, Hirsch J. Changes in energy expenditure resulting from altered body weight. *N Engl J Med.* 1995;332(10):621-8. doi:10.1056/NEJM199503093321001

74. Silva AM, Judice PB, Carraca EV, King N, Teixeira PJ, Sardinha LB. What is the effect of diet and/or exercise interventions on behavioural compensation in non-exercise physical activity and related energy expenditure of free-living adults? A systematic review. *Br J Nutr.* 2018;119(12):1327-1345. doi:10.1017/S000711451800096X

75. Nakamura Y, Koike S. Association of disinhibited eating and trait of impulsivity with insula and amygdala responses to palatable liquid consumption. *Front Syst Neurosci.* 2021;15:647143. doi:10.3389/fnsys.2021.647143

76. Wing RR, Papandonatos G, Fava JL, et al. Maintaining large weight losses: The role of behavioral and psychological factors. *J Consult Clin Psychol.* 2008;76(6):1015-21. doi:10.1037/a0014159

77. Heymsfield SB, Gonzalez MC, Shen W, Redman L, Thomas D. Weight loss composition is one-fourth fat-free mass: A critical review and critique of this widely cited rule. *Obes Rev.* 2014;15(4):310-21. doi:10.1111/obr.12143

78. Johnston BC, Kanters S, Bandayrel K, et al. Comparison of weight loss among named diet programs in overweight and obese adults: A meta-analysis. *JAMA*. 2014;312(9):923-33. doi:10.1001/jama.2014.10397

79. Pasiakos SM, Cao JJ, Margolis LM, et al. Effects of high-protein diets on fat-free mass and muscle protein synthesis following weight loss: A randomized controlled trial. *FASEB J*. 2013;27(9):3837-47. doi:10.1096/fj.13-230227

80. Pasiakos SM, Vislocky LM, Carbone JW, et al. Acute energy deprivation affects skeletal muscle protein synthesis and associated intracellular signaling proteins in physically active adults. *J Nutr*. 2010;140(4):745-51. doi:10.3945/jn.109.118372

81. Churchward-Venne TA, Burd NA, Phillips SM. Nutritional regulation of muscle protein synthesis with resistance exercise: Strategies to enhance anabolism. *Nutr Metab (Lond)*. 2012;9(1):40. doi:10.1186/1743-7075-9-40

82. Hector AJ, Marcotte GR, Churchward-Venne TA, et al. Whey protein supplementation preserves postprandial myofibrillar protein synthesis during short-term energy restriction in overweight and obese adults. *J Nutr*. 2015;145(2):246-52. doi:10.3945/jn.114.200832

83. Murphy CH, Churchward-Venne TA, Mitchell CJ, et al. Hypoenergetic diet-induced reductions in myofibrillar protein synthesis are restored with resistance training and balanced daily protein ingestion in older men. *Am J Physiol Endocrinol Metab*. 2015;308(9):E734-E743. doi:10.1152/ajpendo.00550.2014

84. Jonnalagadda SS, Skinner R, Moore L. Overweight athlete: Fact or fiction? *Curr Sports Med Rep*. 2004;3(4):198-205.

85. Sundgot-Borgen J, Meyer NL, Lohman TG, et al. How to minimise the health risks to athletes who compete in weight-sensitive sports: Review and position statement on behalf of the Ad Hoc Research Working Group on Body Composition, Health and Performance, under the auspices of the IOC Medical Commission. *Br J Sports Med*. 2013;47(16):1012-22. doi:10.1136/bjsports-2013-092966

86. Mamerow MM, Mettler JA, English KL, et al. Dietary protein distribution positively influences 24-h muscle protein synthesis in healthy adults. *J Nutr*. 2014;144(6):876-80. doi:10.3945/jn.113.185280

87. de Graaf C, Blom WA, Smeets PA, Stafleu A, Hendriks HF. Biomarkers of satiation and satiety. *Am J Clin Nutr*. 2004;79(6):946-61.

88. Cummings DE, Overduin J. Gastrointestinal regulation of food intake. *J Clin Invest*. 2007;117(1):13-23. doi:10.1172/JCI30227

89. Valassi E, Scacchi M, Cavagnini F. Neuroendocrine control of food intake. *Nutr Metab Cardiovasc Dis*. 2008;18(2):158-68. doi:10.1016/j.numecd.2007.06.004

90. Brunstrom JM, Shakeshaft NG, Scott-Samuel NE. Measuring "expected satiety" in a range of common foods using a method of constant stimuli. *Appetite*. 2008;51(3):604-14. doi:10.1016/j.appet.2008.04.017

91. Paddon-Jones D, Leidy H. Dietary protein and muscle in older persons. *Curr Opin Clin Nutr Metab Care*. 2014;17(1):5-11. doi:10.1097/MCO.0000000000000011

92. Long SJ, Jeffcoat AR, Millward DJ. Effect of habitual dietary-protein intake on appetite and satiety. *Appetite*. 2000;35(1):79-88. doi:10.1006/appe.2000.0332

93. Leidy HJ, Bales-Voelker LI, Harris CT. A protein-rich beverage consumed as a breakfast meal leads to weaker appetitive and dietary responses v. a protein-rich solid breakfast meal in adolescents. *Br J Nutr*. 2011;106(1):37-41. doi:10.1017/S0007114511000122

94. Leidy HJ, Bossingham MJ, Mattes RD, Campbell WW. Increased dietary protein consumed at breakfast leads to an initial and sustained feeling of fullness during energy restriction compared to other meal times. *Br J Nutr*. 2009;101(6):798-803.

95. Peters HP, Boers HM, Haddeman E, Melnikov SM, Qvyjt F. No effect of added beta-glucan or of fructooligosaccharide on appetite or energy intake. *Am J Clin Nutr*. 2009;89(1):58-63. doi:10.3945/ajcn.2008.26701

96. Lowery LM. Dietary fat and sports nutrition: A primer. *J Sports Sci Med*. 2004;3(3):106-17.

97. Skarin F, Wastlund E, Gustafsson H. Maintaining or losing intervention-induced health-related behavior change: A mixed methods field study. *Front Psychol*. 2021;12:688192. doi:10.3389/fpsyg.2021.688192

98. Kelley CP, Sbrocco G, Sbrocco T. Behavioral modification for the management of obesity. *Prim Care*. 2016;43(1):159-75. doi:10.1016/j.pop.2015.10.004

99. Ilowiecka K, Glibowski P, Skrzypek M, Styk W. The long-term dietitian and psychological support of obese patients who have reduced their weight allows them to maintain the effects. *Nutrients*. 2021;13(6):2020. doi:10.3390/nu13062020

100. Howell S, Kones R. "Calories in, calories out" and macronutrient intake: the hope, hype, and science of calories. *Am J Physiol Endocrinol Metab*. 2017;313(5):E608-E612. doi:10.1152/ajpendo.00156.2017

101. Jensen MD, Ryan DH, Apovian CM, et al. 2013 AHA/ACC/TOS guideline for the management of overweight and obesity in adults: A report of the American College of Cardiology/American Heart Association Task Force on Practice Guidelines and The Obesity Society. *Circulation*. 2014;129(25 Suppl 2):S102-S138. doi:10.1161/01.cir.0000437739.71477.ee

102. Tsai AG, Wadden TA. Systematic review: An evaluation of major commercial weight loss programs in the United States. *Ann Intern Med*. 2005;142(1):56-66.

103. Ryan DH, Kushner R. The state of obesity and obesity research. *JAMA*. 2010;304(16):1835-6. doi:10.1001/jama.2010.1531

104. Ashtary-Larky D, Bagheri R, Bavi H, et al. Ketogenic diets, physical activity, and body composition: A review. *Br J Nutr*. 2021:1-68. doi:10.1017/S0007114521002609

105. Choi YJ, Jeon SM, Shin S. Impact of a ketogenic diet on metabolic parameters in patients with obesity or overweight and with or without type 2 diabetes: A meta-analysis of randomized controlled trials. *Nutrients*. 2020;12(7):2005. doi:10.3390/nu12072005

106. American Diabetes Association. 5. Lifestyle Management: *Standards of Medical Care in Diabetes—2019*. *Diabetes Care*. 2019;42(Suppl 1):S46-S60. doi:10.2337/dc19-S005

107. Hall KD, Chen KY, Guo J, et al. Energy expenditure and body composition changes after an isocaloric ketogenic diet in overweight and obese men. *Am J Clin Nutr*. 2016;104(2):324-33. doi:10.3945/ajcn.116.133561

108. Gibson AA, Seimon RV, Lee CM, et al. Do ketogenic diets really suppress appetite? A systematic review and meta-analysis. *Obes Rev*. 2015;16(1):64-76. doi:10.1111/obr.12230

109. Makris A, Foster GD. Dietary approaches to the treatment of obesity. *Psychiatr Clin North Am*. 2011;34(4):813-27. doi:10.1016/j.psc.2011.08.004

110. Conlin LA, Aguilar DT, Rogers GE, Campbell BI. Flexible vs. rigid dieting in resistance-trained individuals seeking to optimize their physiques: A randomized controlled trial. *J Int Soc Sports Nutr*. 2021;18(1):52. doi:10.1186/s12970-021-00452-2

111. Ismaeel A, Weems S, Willoughby DS. A comparison of the nutrient intakes of macronutrient-based dieting and strict dieting bodybuilders. *Int J Sport Nutr Exerc Metab*. 2018;28(5):502-508. doi:10.1123/ijsnem.2017-0323

112. Palascha A, van Kleef E, van Trijp HC. How does thinking in black and white terms relate to eating behavior and weight regain? *J Health Psychol*. 2015;20(5):638-48. doi:10.1177/1359105315573440

113. Stephens AM, Dean LL, Davis JP, Osborne JA, Sanders TH. Peanuts, peanut oil, and fat free peanut flour reduced cardiovascular disease risk factors and the development of atherosclerosis in Syrian golden hamsters. *J Food Sci*. 2010;75(4):H116-H122. doi:10.1111/j.1750-3841.2010.01569.x

114. Baer DJ, Gebauer SK, Novotny JA. Measured energy value of pistachios in the human diet. *Br J Nutr*. 2012;107(1):120-5. doi:10.1017/S0007114511002649

115. Novotny JA, Gebauer SK, Baer DJ. Discrepancy between the Atwater factor predicted and empirically measured energy values of almonds in human diets. *Am J Clin Nutr*. 2012;96(2):296-301. doi:10.3945/ajcn.112.035782

116. Traoret CJ, Lokko P, Cruz AC, et al. Peanut digestion and energy balance. *Int J Obes (Lond)*. 2008;32(2):322-8. doi:10.1038/sj.ijo.0803735

117. Barr SB, Wright JC. Postprandial energy expenditure in whole-food and processed-food meals: Implications for daily energy expenditure. *Food Nutr Res*. 2010;54. doi:10.3402/fnr.v54i0.5144 www.ncbi.nlm.nih.gov/pubmed/20613890

118. Thivel D, Aucouturier J, Metz L, Morio B, Duche P. Is there spontaneous energy expenditure compensation in response to intensive exercise in obese youth? *Pediatr Obes*. 2014;9(2):147-54. doi:10.1111/j.2047-6310.2013.00148.x

119. Paravidino VB, Mediano MF, Hoffman DJ, Sichieri R. Effect of exercise intensity on spontaneous physical activity energy expenditure in overweight boys: A crossover study. *PLoS One*. 2016;11(1):e0147141. doi:10.1371/journal.pone.0147141

120. Riou ME, Jomphe-Tremblay S, Lamothe G, et al. Energy compensation following a supervised exercise intervention in women living with overweight/obesity is accompanied by an early and sustained decrease in non-structured physical activity. *Front Physiol*. 2019;10:1048. doi:10.3389/fphys.2019.01048

121. Areta JL, Burke LM, Camera DM, et al. Reduced resting skeletal muscle protein synthesis is rescued by resistance exercise and protein ingestion following short-term energy deficit. *Am J Physiol Endocrinol Metab*. 2014;306(8):E989-E997. doi:10.1152/ajpendo.00590.2013

122. Vianna JM, Werneck FZ, Coelho EF, Damasceno VO, Reis VM. Oxygen uptake and heart rate kinetics after different types of resistance exercise. *J Hum Kinet*. 2014;42:235-44. doi:10.2478/hukin-2014-0077

123. Kelleher AR, Hackney KJ, Fairchild TJ, Keslacy S, Ploutz-Snyder LL. The metabolic costs of reciprocal supersets vs. traditional resistance exercise in young recreationally active adults. *J Strength Cond Res*. 2010;24(4):1043-51. doi:10.1519/JSC.0b013e3181d3e993

124. Wang Z, Ying Z, Bosy-Westphal A, et al. Evaluation of specific metabolic rates of major organs and tissues: Comparison between men and women. *Am J Hum Biol*. 2011;23(3):333-8. doi:10.1002/ajhb.21137

125. Heydari M, Freund J, Boutcher SH. The effect of high-intensity intermittent exercise on body composition of overweight young males. *J Obes*. 2012;2012:480467. doi:10.1155/2012/480467

126. Boutcher SH. High-intensity intermittent exercise and fat loss. *J Obes*. 2011;2011:868305. doi:10.1155/2011/868305

127. Greer BK, Sirithienthad P, Moffatt RJ, Marcello RT, Panton LB. EPOC comparison between isocaloric bouts of steady-state aerobic, intermittent aerobic, and resistance training. *Res Q Exerc Sport*. 2015;86(2):190-5. doi:10.1080/02701367.2014.999190

128. Kelly B, King JA, Goerlach J, Nimmo MA. The impact of high-intensity intermittent exercise on resting metabolic rate in healthy males. *Eur J Appl Physiol*. 2013;113(12):3039-47. doi:10.1007/s00421-013-2741-5

129. Shaw K, Gennat H, O'Rourke P, Del Mar C. Exercise for overweight or obesity. *Cochrane Database Syst Rev*. 2006;(4):CD003817. doi:10.1002/14651858.CD003817.pub3

130. Curioni CC, Lourenco PM. Long-term weight loss after diet and exercise: A systematic review. *Int J Obes (Lond)*. 2005;29(10):1168-74. doi:10.1038/sj.ijo.0803015

131. Schwingshackl L, Dias S, Hoffmann G. Impact of long-term lifestyle programmes on weight loss

and cardiovascular risk factors in overweight/obese participants: A systematic review and network meta-analysis. *Syst Rev.* 2014;3:130. doi:10.1186/2046-4053-3-130

132. Dhurandhar EJ, Kaiser KA, Dawson JA, Alcorn AS, Keating KD, Allison DB. Predicting adult weight change in the real world: A systematic review and meta-analysis accounting for compensatory changes in energy intake or expenditure. *Int J Obes (Lond).* 2015;39(8):1181-7. doi:10.1038/ijo.2014.184

133. Thompson W. *ACSM's Guidelines for Exercise Testing and Prescription.* Lippincott Williams & Wilkins.

134. Sundgot-Borgen J, Garthe I. Elite athletes in aesthetic and Olympic weight-class sports and the challenge of body weight and body compositions. *J Sports Sci.* 2011;29(Suppl 1):S101-S114. doi:10.1080/02640414.2011.565783

135. Sanfilippo J, Krueger D, Heiderscheit B, Binkley N. Dual-energy X-ray absorptiometry body composition in NCAA Division I athletes: Exploration of mass distribution. *Sports Health.* 2019;11(5):453-460. doi:10.1177/1941738119861572

136. Stark M, Lukaszuk J, Prawitz A, Salacinski A. Protein timing and its effects on muscular hypertrophy and strength in individuals engaged in weight-training. *J Int Soc Sports Nutr.* 2012;9(1):54. doi:10.1186/1550-2783-9-54

137. Bray GA, Smith SR, de Jonge L, et al. Effect of dietary protein content on weight gain, energy expenditure, and body composition during overeating: A randomized controlled trial. *JAMA.* 2012;307(1):47-55. doi:10.1001/jama.2011.1918

138. Frost E. Effect of dietary protein intake on diet-induced thermogenesis during overfeeding. Presented at Obesity Society Annual Meeting, November 2-7, 2014.

139. Bouchard C, Tchernof A, Tremblay A. Predictors of body composition and body energy changes in response to chronic overfeeding. *Int J Obes (Lond).* 2014;38(2):236-42. doi:10.1038/ijo.2013.77

140. Horton TJ, Drougas H, Brachey A, Reed GW, Peters JC, Hill JO. Fat and carbohydrate overfeeding in humans: Different effects on energy storage. *Am J Clin Nutr.* 1995;62(1):19-29.

141. Hertzler SR, Lieblein-Boff JC, Weiler M, Allgeier C. Plant proteins: Assessing their nutritional quality and effects on health and physical function. *Nutrients.* 2020;12(12):3704. doi:10.3390/nu12123704

142. Campbell B, Kreider RB, Ziegenfuss T, et al. International Society of Sports Nutrition position stand: Protein and exercise. *J Int Soc Sports Nutr.* 2007;4:8. doi:10.1186/1550-2783-4-8

143. Boisseau N, Vermorel M, Rance M, Duche P, Patureau-Mirand P. Protein requirements in male adolescent soccer players. *Eur J Appl Physiol.* 2007;100(1):27-33. doi:10.1007/s00421-007-0400-4

144. van Loon LJ, Greenhaff PL, Constantin-Teodosiu D, Saris WH, Wagenmakers AJ. The effects of increasing exercise intensity on muscle fuel utilisation in humans. *J Physiol.* 2001;536(Pt 1):295-304.

145. Tsintzas K, Williams C. Human muscle glycogen metabolism during exercise: Effect of carbohydrate supplementation. *Sports Med.* 1998;25(1):7-23.

146. Berg J, JL T, L S. Fuel choice during exercise is determined by intensity and duration of activity. *Biochemistr.* 5th ed. W.H. Freeman; 2002.

147. Spriet LL. New insights into the interaction of carbohydrate and fat metabolism during exercise. *Sports Med.* 2014;44(Suppl 1):S87-S96. doi:10.1007/s40279-014-0154-1

148. Ortenblad N, Nielsen J, Saltin B, Holmberg HC. Role of glycogen availability in sarcoplasmic reticulum Ca2+ kinetics in human skeletal muscle. *J Physiol.* 2011;589(Pt 3):711-25. doi:10.1113/jphysiol.2010.195982

149. Duhamel TA, Perco JG, Green HJ. Manipulation of dietary carbohydrates after prolonged effort modifies muscle sarcoplasmic reticulum responses in exercising males. *Am J Physiol Regul Integr Comp Physiol.* 2006;291(4):R1100-R1110. doi:10.1152/ajpregu.00858.2005

150. Ortenblad N, Westerblad H, Nielsen J. Muscle glycogen stores and fatigue. *J Physiol.* 2013;591(18):4405-13. doi:10.1113/jphysiol.2013.251629

151. MacDougall JD, Ray S, Sale DG, McCartney N, Lee P, Garner S. Muscle substrate utilization and lactate production. *Can J Appl Physiol.* 1999;24(3):209-15.

152. Burd NA, Beals JW, Martinez IG, Salvador AF, Skinner SK. Food-first approach to enhance the regulation of post-exercise skeletal muscle protein synthesis and remodeling. *Sports Med.* 2019;49(Suppl 1):59-68. doi:10.1007/s40279-018-1009-y

153. Cribb PJ, Williams AD, Hayes A. A creatine-protein-carbohydrate supplement enhances responses to resistance training. *Med Sci Sports Exerc.* 2007;39(11):1960-8. doi:10.1249/mss.0b013e-31814fb52a

154. Kerksick CM, Wilborn CD, Campbell WI, et al. The effects of creatine monohydrate supplementation with and without D-pinitol on resistance training adaptations. *J Strength Cond Res.* 2009;23(9):2673-82. doi:10.1519/JSC.0b013e3181b3e0de

155. Devries MC, Phillips SM. Creatine supplementation during resistance training in older adults: A meta-analysis. *Med Sci Sports Exerc.* 2014;46(6):1194-203. doi:10.1249/MSS.0000000000000220

156. Longland TM, Oikawa SY, Mitchell CJ, Devries MC, Phillips SM. Higher compared with lower dietary protein during an energy deficit combined with intense exercise promotes greater lean mass gain and fat mass loss: A randomized trial. *Am J Clin Nutr.* 2016;103(3):738-46. doi:10.3945/ajcn.115.119339

157. Phillips SM. A brief review of higher dietary protein diets in weight loss: A focus on athletes. *Sports Med.* 2014;44 Suppl 2:S149-S153. doi:10.1007/s40279-014-0254-y

158. Mojtahedi MC, Thorpe MP, Karampinos DC, et al. The effects of a higher protein intake during energy restriction on changes in body composition and physical function in older women. *J Gerontol A Biol Sci Med Sci.* 2011;66(11):1218-25. doi:10.1093/gerona/glr120

159. Falcone PH, Tai CY, Carson LR, et al. Caloric expenditure of aerobic, resistance, or combined high-intensity interval training using a hydraulic resistance system in healthy men. J Strength Cond Res. 2015;29(3):779-85. doi:10.1519/JSC.0000000000000661

Chapter 14

1. National Institute of Arthritis and Musculoskeletal and Skin Diseases. Preventing musculoskeletal sports injuries in youth: A guide for parents. National Institute of Arthritis and Musculoskeletal and Skin Diseases. www.niams.nih.gov/Health_Info/Sports_Injuries/child_sports_injuries.asp

2. Desbrow B, Burd NA, Tarnopolsky M, Moore DR, Elliott-Sale KJ. Nutrition for special populations: Young, female, and masters athletes. *Int J Sport Nutr Exerc Metab.* 2019;29:220-227. doi:10.1123/ijsnem.2018-0269

3. Arnold A, Thigpen CA, Beattie PF, Kissenberth MJ, Shanley E. Overuse physeal injuries in youth athletes. *Sports Health.* 2017;9(2):139-147. doi:10.1177/1941738117690847

4. Joy E, De Souza MJ, Nattiv A, et al. 2014 female athlete triad coalition consensus statement on treatment and return to play of the female athlete triad. *Curr Sports Med Rep.* 2014;13(4):219-32. doi:10.1249/jsr.0000000000000077

5. Merkel DL. Youth sport: Positive and negative impact on young athletes. *Open Access J Sports Med.* 2013;4:151-160. doi:10.2147/OAJSM.S33556

6. Torun B. Energy requirements of children and adolescents. *Public Health Nutr.* 2005;8(7a):968-93. doi:10.1079/phn2005791

7. Falk B, Dotan R. Children's thermoregulation during exercise in the heat—a revisit. *Applied Physiology, Nutrition, and Metabolism.* 2008;33(2):420-427. doi:10.1139/h07-185 %m 18347699

8. Desbrow B, McCormack J, Burke LM, et al. Sports Dietitians Australia position statement: Sports nutrition for the adolescent athlete. *Int J Sport Nutr Exerc Metab.* 2014;24(5):570-584. doi:10.1123/ijsnem.2014-0031

9. Kotnik K, Jurak G, Starc G, Golja P. Faster, stronger, healthier: Adolescent-stated reasons for dietary supplementation. *J Nutr Educ Behav.* 2017 49:817. doi:10.1016/j.jneb.2017.07.005

10. Edama M, Inaba H, Hoshino F, Natsui S, Maruyama S, Omori G. The relationship between the female athlete triad and injury rates in collegiate female athletes. *PeerJ.* 2021;9:e11092. doi:10.7717/peerj.11092

11. Thomas DT, Erdman KA, Burke LM. American College of Sports Medicine joint position statement: Nutrition and athletic performance. *Med Sci Sports Exerc.* 2016;48(3):543-68. doi:10.1249/mss.0000000000000852

12. Barnes HV. Physical growth and development during puberty. *Med Clin North Am.* 1975;59(6):1305-17. doi:10.1016/s0025-7125(16)31931-9

13. Frisch RE. Fatness, puberty, and fertility: The effects of nutrition and physical training on menarche and ovulation. In: Brooks-Gunn J, Petersen AC, eds. *Girls at Puberty: Biological and Psychosocial Perspectives.* Springer; 1983:29-49.

14. Rosenbloom CA, Coleman EJ, eds. *Sports Nutrition: A Practice Manual for Professionals.* 5th ed. Academy of Nutrition and Dietetics; 2012.

15. Hales CM, Carrol MD, Fryar CD, Ogden CL. Prevalence of obesity among adults and youth: United States, 2015–2016. National Center for Health Statistics. https://stacks.cdc.gov/view/cdc/49223

16. National Heart Lung Blood Institute. Expert panel on integrated guidelines for cardiovascular health and risk reduction in children and adolescents: Summary report. *Pediatrics.* 2011;128(Suppl 5):S213-56. doi:10.1542/peds.2009-2107C

17. National Institute of Diabetes and Digestive and Kidney Diseases. Helping your child who is overweight. National Institute of Diabetes and Digestive and Kidney Diseases. Accessed January 24, 2017. www.niddk.nih.gov/health-information/health-topics/weight-control/helping-overweight-child/Pages/helping-your-overweight-child.aspx

18. Schneider MB, Benjamin HJ. Sports drinks and energy drinks for children and adolescents: Are they appropriate? *Pediatrics.* 2011;127(6):1182-9. doi:10.1542/peds.2011-0965

19. U.S. Department of Agriculture and U.S. Department of Health & Human Services. Dietary Guidelines for Americans 2020-2025. October, 2022. www.DietaryGuidelines.gov

20. Casa D, Shirreffs S, Cheuvront SN, Galloway SR. Fluids needs for training, competition and recovery in track-and-field athletes. *Int J Sport Nutr Exerc Metab.* 2018;29(2):175. doi:10.1123/ijsnem.2018-0374

21. Liu J, Rehm C, Onopa J, D. M. Trends in diet quality among youth in the United States, 1999–2016. *JAMA.* 2020;323:1161.

22. Stang J, Story MT, Harnack L, Neumark-Sztainer D. Relationships between vitamin and mineral supplement use, dietary intake, and dietary adequacy among adolescents. *JADA.* 2000;100(905):905-10.

23. Slining M, Mathias KC, Popkin BM. Trends in food and beverage sources among US children and adolescents: 1989–2010. *J Acad Nutr Diet.* 2013;113:1683.

24. Tiwari K. Supplement (mis)use in adolescents. *Curr Opin Pediatrics.* 2020;32:471. doi:10.1097/MOP.0000000000000912

25. Institute of Medicine Subcommittee on the Interpretation and Uses of Dietary Reference Intakes. *Dietary Reference Intakes: Applications in Dietary Planning.* National Academies Press; 2003.

26. United Nations Department of Economic and Social Affairs Population Division. Population pyramids of the world from 1950 to 2100. https://populationpyramid.net/world/2040/

27. Stipanuk MH. *Biochemical and Physiological Aspects of Human Nutrition.* W.B. Saunders; 2000.

28. Tanaka H, Seals DR. Endurance exercise performance in masters athletes: Age-associated changes and underlying physiological mechanisms. *The Journal*

of Physiology. 2008;586(Pt 1):55-63. doi:10.1113/jphysiol.2007.141879

29. Bangsbo J, Blackwell J, Boraxbekk C, Caserotti Pea. Copenhagen consensus statement 2019: Physical activity and ageing. *Br J Sports Med.* 2019;53:856-858. doi:10.1136/bjsports-2018-100451

30. Barnes JN, Corkery AT. Exercise improves vascular function, but does this translate to the brain? *Brain Plasticity.* 2018;4:65-79. doi:10.3233/BPL-180075

31. Rosenbloom C, Bahns M. What can we learn about diet and physical activity from master athletes? *Holist Nurs Pract.* 2006;20(4):161-6.

32. Amanat S, Ghahri S, Dianatinasab A, Fararouei A, Dianatinasab M. Exercise and type 2 diabetes. In: Xiao J, ed. *Physical Exercise for Human Health Advances in Experimental Medicine and Biology.* Springer, Singapore; 2020:91-105.

33. Rizzoli R, Reginster JY, Arnal JF, et al. Quality of life in sarcopenia and frailty. *Calcif Tissue Int.* 2013;93(2):101-20. doi:10.1007/s00223-013-9758-y

34. von Haehling S, Morley JE, Anker SD. An overview of sarcopenia: Facts and numbers on prevalence and clinical impact. *J Cachexia Sarcopenia Muscle.* 2010;1(2):129-133. doi:10.1007/s13539-010-0014-2

35. Paddon-Jones D, Leidy H. Dietary protein and muscle in older persons. *Curr Opin Clin Nutr Metab Care.* 2014;17(1):5-11. doi:10.1097/mco.0000000000000011

36. Kim JS, Wilson JM, Lee SR. Dietary implications on mechanisms of sarcopenia: Roles of protein, amino acids and antioxidants. *J Nutr Biochem.* 2010;21(1):1-13. doi:10.1016/j.jnutbio.2009.06.014

37. Landi F, Liperoti R, Russo A, et al. Sarcopenia as a risk factor for falls in elderly individuals: Results from the ilSIRENTE study. *Clin Nutr.* 2012;31(5):652-8. doi:10.1016/j.clnu.2012.02.007

38. Sterling DA, O'Connor JA, Bonadies J. Geriatric falls: Injury severity is high and disproportionate to mechanism. *J Trauma.* 2001;50(1):116-9.

39. Jager TE, Weiss HB, Coben JH, Pepe PE. Traumatic brain injuries evaluated in U.S. emergency departments, 1992-1994. *Acad Emerg Med.* 2000;7(2):134-40.

40. Leenders M, Verdijk LB, van der Hoeven L, van Kranenburg J, Nilwik R, van Loon LJ. Elderly men and women benefit equally from prolonged resistance-type exercise training. *J Gerontol A Biol Sci Med Sci.* 2013;68(7):769-79. doi:10.1093/gerona/gls241

41. Churchward-Venne TA, Tieland M, Verdijk LB, et al. There are no nonresponders to resistance-type exercise training in older men and women. *J Am Med Dir Assoc.* 2015;16(5):400-11. doi:10.1016/j.jamda.2015.01.071

42. McGlory C, Vliet S, Stokes T, Mittendorfer B, Phillips SM. The impact of exercise and nutrition on the regulation of skeletal muscle mass. *J Physiol.* 2019;597(5):1251. doi:10.1113/JP275443

43. Cadore EL, Rodriguez-Manas L, Sinclair A, Izquierdo M. Effects of different exercise interventions on risk of falls, gait ability, and balance in physically frail older adults: A systematic review. *Rejuvenation Res.* 2013;16(2):105-14. doi:10.1089/rej.2012.1397

44. Mcleod JC, Stokes T, Phillips SM. Resistance exercise training as a primary countermeasure to age-related chronic disease. *Frontiers in Physiology.* 2019;10:645. doi:10.3389/fphys.2019.00645

45. Wilks DC, Winwood K, Gilliver SF, et al. Age-dependency in bone mass and geometry: A pQCT study on male and female master sprinters, middle and long distance runners, race-walkers and sedentary people. *J Musculoskelet Neuronal Interact.* 2009;9(4):236-46.

46. Velez NF, Zhang A, Stone B, Perera S, Miller M, Greenspan SL. The effect of moderate impact exercise on skeletal integrity in master athletes. *Osteoporos Int.* 2008;19(10):1457-64. doi:10.1007/s00198-008-0590-6

47. Szabo AN, Washburn RA, Sullivan DK, et al. The Midwest exercise trial for the prevention of weight regain: MET POWeR. *Contemp Clin Trials.* 2013;36(2):470-8. doi:10.1016/j.cct.2013.08.011

48. U.S. Department of Health and Human Services. *Physical Activity Guidelines for Americans.* 2nd ed. 2018.

49. Jakicic JM, Otto AD. Physical activity considerations for the treatment and prevention of obesity. *Am J Clin Nutr.* 2005;82(1 Suppl):226s-229s.

50. Tseng BY, Uh J, Rossetti HC, et al. Masters athletes exhibit larger regional brain volume and better cognitive performance than sedentary older adults. *J Magn Reson Imaging.* 2013;38(5):1169-76. doi:10.1002/jmri.24085

51. Johnson NF, Gold BT, Bailey AL, et al. Cardiorespiratory fitness modifies the relationship between myocardial function and cerebral blood flow in older adults. *Neuroimage.* 2016;131:126-32. doi:10.1016/j.neuroimage.2015.05.063

52. Bliss ES, Wong RH, Howe PR, Mills DE. Benefits of exercise training on cerebrovascular and cognitive function in ageing. *J Cereb Blood Flow Metab.* 2021;41(3):447-470. doi:10.11177/0271678X20957807

53. Quigley A, MacKay-Lyons M, G. E. Effects of exercise on cognitive performance in older adults: A narrative review of the evidence, possible biological mechanisms, and recommendations for exercise prescription. *Journal of Aging Research.* 2020:1407896. doi:10.1155/2020/1407896

54. Thompson J, Manore MM. Predicted and measured resting metabolic rate of male and female endurance athletes. *J Am Diet Assoc.* 1996;96(1):30-34. doi:10.1016/s0002-8223(96)00010-7

55. van den Brink AC, Brouwer-Brolsma EM, Berendsen A, van de Rest O. The Mediterranean, Dietary Approaches to Stop Hypertension (DASH), and Mediterranean-DASH Intervention for Neurodegenerative Delay (MIND) diets are associated with less cognitive decline and a lower risk of Alzheimer's disease—A review. *Adv Nutr.* 2019;10:1040-1065. doi:10.1093/advances/nmz054

56. Klimova B, Valis M. Nutritional interventions as beneficial strategies to delay cognitive decline in

healthy older individuals. *Nutrients*. 2018;10:905. doi:10.3390/nu10070905

57. Dominguez LJ, Barbagallo B. Nutritional prevention of cognitive decline and dementia. *Acta Biomed*. 2018;89:276-290. doi:10.23750/abm.v89i2.7401

58. Institute of Medicine. *Dietary Reference Intakes for Vitamin A, Vitamin K, Arsenic, Boron, Chromium, Copper, Iodine, Iron, Manganese, Molybdenum, Nickel, Silicon, Vanadium, and Zinc*. National Academies Press; 2001.

59. Ross AC, Manson JE, Abrams SA, et al. The 2011 Dietary Reference Intakes for calcium and vitamin D: What dietetics practitioners need to know. *J Am Diet Assoc*. 2011;111(4):524-7. doi:10.1016/j.jada.2011.01.004

60. Holick MF, Binkley NC, Bischoff-Ferrari HA, et al. Evaluation, treatment, and prevention of vitamin D deficiency: An Endocrine Society clinical practice guideline. *J Clin Endocrinol Metab*. 2011;96(7):1911-30. doi:10.1210/jc.2011-0385

61. Wicherts IS, van Schoor NM, Boeke AJ, et al. Vitamin D status predicts physical performance and its decline in older persons. *J Clin Endocrinol Metab*. 2007;92(6):2058-65. doi:10.1210/jc.2006-1525

62. Stalgis-Bilinski KL, Boyages J, Salisbury EL, Dunstan CR, Henderson SI, Talbot PL. Burning daylight: Balancing vitamin D requirements with sensible sun exposure. *Medical Journal of Australia*. 2011;194(7):345-348. doi:10.5694/j.1326-5377.2011.tb03003.x

63. Mallard SR, Howe AS, Houghton LA. Vitamin D status and weight loss: A systematic review and meta-analysis of randomized and nonrandomized controlled weight-loss trials. *The American Journal of Clinical Nutrition*. 2016;104(4):1151-1159. doi:10.3945/ajcn.116.136879

64. Adan A. Cognitive performance and dehydration. *J Am Coll Nutr*. 2012;31(2):71-78.

65. Savoie FA, Kenefick RW, Ely BR, Cheuvront SN, Goulet ED. Effect of hypohydration on muscle endurance, strength, anaerobic power and capacity and vertical jumping ability: A meta-analysis. *Sports Med*. 2015;45(8):1207-27. doi:10.1007/s40279-015-0349-0

66. National Diabetes Statistics Report, 2020. Estimates of Diabetes and Its Burden in the United States. U.S. Dept of Health and Human Services; 2020.

67. DeFronzo RA. Dysfunctional fat cells, lipotoxicity and type 2 diabetes. *Int J Clin Pract Suppl*. 2004;(143):9-21.

68. Yardley JE, Colberg SC. Update on Management of Type 1 Diabetes and Type 2 Diabetes in Athletes. *Curr Sports Med Rep*. 2017;16(1):38.

69. White SH, McDermott MM, Sufit RL, et al. Walking performance is positively correlated to calf muscle fiber size in peripheral artery disease subjects, but fibers show aberrant mitophagy: An observational study. *J Transl Med*. 2016;14(1):284. doi:10.1186/s12967-016-1030-6

70. Glenn DJ, Cardema MC, Gardner DG. Amplification of lipotoxic cardiomyopathy in the VDR gene knockout mouse. *J Steroid Biochem Mol Biol*. 2015:292-298. doi:10.1016/j.jsbmb.2015.09.034

71. Gallen I, Hume C, Lumb A. Fueling the athlete with type 1 diabetes. *Diabetes Obes Metab*. 2011;13:130-136.

72. Praet SF, van Loon LJ. Optimizing the therapeutic benefits of exercise in type 2 diabetes. *J Appl Physiol*. 2007;103(4):1113-20. doi:10.1152/japplphysiol.00566.2007

73. Praet SF, Manders RJ, Meex RC, et al. Glycaemic instability is an underestimated problem in type II diabetes. *Clin Sci (Lond)*. 2006;111(2):119-26. doi:10.1042/cs20060041

74. Jensen J. Nutritional concerns in the diabetic athlete. *Curr Sports Med Rep*. 2004;3(4):192-7.

75. American College of Obstetricians and Gynecologists. ACOG Committee opinion no. 650: Physical activity and exercise during pregnancy and the postpartum period. *Obstet Gynecol*. 2015;126(6):e135-e142. doi:10.1097/aog.0000000000001214

76. American College of Obstetricians and Gynecologists. Physical Activity and Exercise During Pregnancy and the Postpartum Period: ACOG Committee Opinion, Number 804. *Obstet Gynecol*. 2020;135(4):e178-e188. doi:10.1097/AOG.0000000000003772. PMID: 32217980

77. Kominiarek MA, Rajan P. Nutrition Recommendations in Pregnancy and Lactation. *Med Clin North Am*. 2016;100(6):1199–1215. doi:10.1016/j.mcna.2016.06.004.

78. Durham HA, Morey MC, Lovelady CA, Namenek Brouwer RJ, Krause KM, Ostbye T. Postpartum physical activity in overweight and obese women. *J Phys Act Health*. 2011;8(7):988-93.

79. American College of Obstetricians and Gynecologists. ACOG Committee opinion no. 548: Weight gain during pregnancy. *Obstet Gynecol*. 2013;121(1):210-212. doi:10.1097/01.AOG.0000425668.87506.4c

80. Institute of Medicine and National Research Council Committee to Reexamine Institute of Medicine Pregnancy Weight Guidelines. The National Academies Collection: Reports funded by National Institutes of Health. In: Rasmussen KM, Yaktine AL, eds. *Weight Gain During Pregnancy: Reexamining the Guidelines*. National Academies Press; 2009.

81. Institute of Medicine. *Dietary Reference Intakes for Energy, Carbohydrate, Fiber, Fat, Fatty Acids, Cholesterol, Protein, and Amino Acids (Macronutrients)*. National Academies Press; 2005:1357.

82. Mayo Clinic. Pregnancy weight gain: What's healthy. Mayo Clinic. www.mayoclinic.org/healthy-lifestyle/pregnancy-week-by-week/in-depth/pregnancy-weight-gain/art-20044360

83. Fink HH, Burgoon LA, Mikesky AE. *Practical Applications in Sports Nutrition*. 2nd ed. Jones and Bartlett; 2009.

84. Peternelj TT, Coombes JS. Antioxidant supplementation during exercise training: Beneficial or detrimental? *Sports Med*. 2011;41(12):1043-69. doi:10.2165/11594400-000000000-00000

85. Food and Nutrition Board. *Dietary Reference Intakes (DRIs): Recommended Dietary Allowances and Adequate Intakes, Vitamins*. National Academy of Sciences; 2011.
86. Fink HH, Mikesky AE, Burgoon LA. *Practical Applications in Sports Nutrition*. 3rd ed. Jones and Bartlett; 2012.
87. Bernhardt IB, Dorsey DJ. Hypervitaminosis A and congenital renal anomalies in a human infant. *Obstet Gynecol*. 1974;43(5):750-5.
88. Bui T, Christin-Maitre S. Vitamin D and pregnancy. *Ann Endocrinol (Paris)*. 2011;72(Suppl 1):S23-S28. Vitamine D et grossesse. doi:10.1016/s0003-4266(11)70006-3
89. Melina V, Craig W, Levin S. Position of the Academy of Nutrition and Dietetics: Vegetarian diets. *J Acad Nutr Diet*. 2016;116(12):1970-1980. doi:10.1016/j.jand.2016.09.025
90. Fuhrman J, Ferreri DM. Fueling the vegetarian (vegan) athlete. *Curr Sports Med Rep*. 2010;9(4):233-41. doi:10.1249/JSR.0b013e3181e93a6f
91. Craig WJ, Mangels AR. Position of the American Dietetic Association: Vegetarian diets. *J Am Diet Assoc*. 2009;109(7):1266-82.
92. Garner DM. *Eating Disorder Inventory-3: Professional Manual*. Psychological Assessment Resources; 2004.
93. Maughan RJ. *Sports Nutrition*. Wiley; 2013.
94. Venderley AM, Campbell WW. Vegetarian diets: Nutritional considerations for athletes. *Sports Med*. 2006;36(4):293-305.
95. Lynch H, Johnston C, Wharton C. Plant-based diets: Considerations for environmental impact, protein quality, and exercise performance. *Nutrients*. 2018;10(12):1841. doi:10.3390/nu10121841
96. Kushi LH, Doyle C, McCullough M, et al. American Cancer Society guidelines on nutrition and physical activity for cancer prevention: Reducing the risk of cancer with healthy food choices and physical activity. *CA Cancer J Clin*. 2012;62(1):30-67. doi:10.3322/caac.20140
97. Young VR, Pellett PL. Plant proteins in relation to human protein and amino acid nutrition. *Am J Clin Nutr*. 1994;59(5 Suppl):1203s-1212s.
98. Ciuris C, Lynch HM, Wharton C, Johnston CS. A comparison of dietary protein digestibility, based on DIAAS scoring, in vegetarian and non-vegetarian athletes. *Nutrients*. 2019;11(12):3016. doi:10.3390/nu11123016
99. Churchward-Venne TA, Burd NA, Mitchell CJ, et al. Supplementation of a suboptimal protein dose with leucine or essential amino acids: Effects on myofibrillar protein synthesis at rest and following resistance exercise in men. *J Physiol*. 2012;590(11):2751-65. doi:10.1113/jphysiol.2012.228833
100. Cowell BS, Rosenbloom CA, Skinner R, Summers SH. Policies on screening female athletes for iron deficiency in NCAA Division I-A institutions. *Int J Sport Nutr Exerc Metab*. 2003;13(3):277-85.
101. Driskell JA, Wolinsky I. *Sports Nutrition: Vitamins and Trace Elements*. 2nd ed. Nutrition in exercise and sport. Taylor & Francis; 2005.
102. DellaValle DM. Iron supplementation for female athletes: Effects on iron status and performance outcomes. *Curr Sports Med Rep*. 2013;12(4):234-9. doi:10.1249/JSR.0b013e31829a6f6b
103. Otten JJ, Hellwig JP, Meyers LD, Institute of Medicine, eds. *Dietary Reference Intakes: The essential guide to nutrient requirements*. National Academies Press; 2006.
104. Lukaski HC. Vitamin and mineral status: Effects on physical performance. *Nutrition*. 2004;20(7-8):632-644. doi:10.1016/j.nut.2004.04.001
105. Peeling P, Dawson B, Goodman C, Landers G, Trinder D. Athletic induced iron deficiency: New insights into the role of inflammation, cytokines and hormones. *Eur J Appl Physiol*. 2008;103(4):381-91. doi:10.1007/s00421-008-0726-6
106. Hunt JR. Bioavailability of iron, zinc, and other trace minerals from vegetarian diets. *Am J Clin Nutr*. 2003;78(3 Suppl):633s-639s.
107. Wentz L, Liu PY, Ilich JZ, Haymes EM. Dietary and training predictors of stress fractures in female runners. *Int J Sport Nutr Exerc Metab*. 2012;22(5):374-82.
108. Blancquaert L, Baguet A, Bex T, et al. Changing to a vegetarian diet reduces the body creatine pool in omnivorous women, but appears not to affect carnitine and carnosine homeostasis: A randomised trial. *Br J Nutr*. 2018;119(7):759-770. doi:10.1017/s000711451800017x
109. Lukaszuk JM, Robertson RJ, Arch JE, et al. Effect of creatine supplementation and a lacto-ovo-vegetarian diet on muscle creatine concentration. *Int J Sport Nutr Exerc Metab*. 2002;12(3):336-48.
110. Burke DG, Chilibeck PD, Parise G, Candow DG, Mahoney D, Tarnopolsky M. Effect of creatine and weight training on muscle creatine and performance in vegetarians. *Med Sci Sports Exerc*. 2003;35(11):1946-55. doi:10.1249/01.mss.0000093614.17517.79
111. Lukaszuk JM, Robertson RJ, Arch JE, Moyna NM. Effect of a defined lacto-ovo-vegetarian diet and oral creatine monohydrate supplementation on plasma creatine concentration. *J Strength Cond Res*. 2005;19(4):735-40. doi:10.1519/r-16224.1
112. Sundgot-Borgen J, Meyer NL, Lohman TG, et al. How to minimise the health risks to athletes who compete in weight-sensitive sports: Review and position statement on behalf of the Ad Hoc Research Working Group on Body Composition, Health and Performance, under the auspices of the IOC Medical Commission. *Br J Sports Med*. 2013;47(16):1012-22. doi:10.1136/bjsports-2013-092966
113. Wells KR, Jeacocke NA, Appaneal R, et al. The Australian Institute of Sport (AIS) and National Eating Disorders Collaboration (NEDC) position statement on disordered eating in high performance sport. *Br J Sports Med*. 2020;54:1247. doi:10.1136/bjsports-2019-101813

114. Sundgot-Borgen J, Torstveit MK. Aspects of disordered eating continuum in elite high-intensity sports. *Scand J Med Sci Sports.* 2010;20(Suppl 2):112-21. doi:10.1111/j.1600-0838.2010.01190.x
115. Nattiv A, Loucks AB, Manore MM, Sanborn CF, Sundgot-Borgen J, Warren MP. American College of Sports Medicine position stand: The female athlete triad. *Med Sci Sports Exerc.* 2007;39(10):1867-82. doi:10.1249/mss.0b013e318149f111
116. Mancine RP, Gusfa DW, Moshrefi A, Kennedy SF. Prevalence of disordered eating in athletes categorized by emphasis on leanness and activity type—a systematic review. *Journal of Eating Disorders.* 2020;8(47):1. doi:10.1186/s40337-020-00323-2
117. Sundgot-Borgen J. Prevalence of eating disorders in elite female athletes. *Int J Sport Nutr.* 1993;3(1):29-40.
118. Steiger H, Booij L. Eating disorders, heredity and environmental activation: Getting epigenetic concepts into practice. *J Clin Med.* 2020;9(5):1332. doi:10.3390/jcm9051332
119. American Psychiatric Association. *Anxiety Disorders: DSM-5 Selections.* American Psychiatric Association Publishing; 2016.
120. Sundgot-Borgen J, Torstveit MK. Prevalence of eating disorders in elite athletes is higher than in the general population. *Clin J Sport Med.* 2004;14(1):25-32.
121. Martinsen M, Sundgot-Borgen J. Higher prevalence of eating disorders among adolescent elite athletes than controls. *Med Sci Sports Exerc.* 2013;45(6):1188-97. doi:10.1249/MSS.0b013e318281a939
122. Aouad P, Hay P, Soh N, Touyz S. Chew and spit (CHSP): A systematic review. *Journal of Eating Disorders.* 2016;4(1):23. doi:10.1186/s40337-016-0115-1
123. Bennell KL, Malcolm SA, Wark JD, Brukner PD. Skeletal effects of menstrual disturbances in athletes. *Scand J Med Sci Sports.* 1997;7(5):261-73.
124. Melin AK, Heikura IA, Tenforde A, Mountjoy M. Energy availability in athletics: Health, performance, and physique. *International Journal of Sport Nutrition and Exercise Metabolism* 2019;29:152. doi:10.1123/ijsnem.2018-0201
125. Bratland-Sanda S, Martinsen EW, Sundgot-Borgen J. Changes in physical fitness, bone mineral density and body composition during inpatient treatment of underweight and normal weight females with longstanding eating disorders. *Int J Environ Res Public Health.* 2012;9(1):315-30. doi:10.3390/ijerph9010315
126. Statuta SM. The female athlete triad, relative energy deficiency in sport, and the male athlete triad: The exploration of low-energy syndromes in athletes. *Curr Sports Med Rep.* 2020;19(2):43.
127. Mountjoy M, Sundgot-Borgen J, Burke L, et al. The IOC consensus statement: Beyond the female athlete triad—relative energy deficiency in sport (RED-S). *Br J Sports Med.* 2014;48(7):491-7. doi:10.1136/bjsports-2014-093502

INDEX

Note: The italicized *f* and *t* following page numbers refer to figures and tables, respectively.

A

AAS (anabolic androgenic steroids) 259-260
absorption. *See* nutrient absorption
Academy of Nutrition and Dietetics 20, 21
accelerometers 59
acceptable daily intake (ADI) 88, 89*t*-90*t*
acceptable macronutrient distribution range (AMDR) 5
  athletes and 10-11, 145-146
  for carbohydrate 5, 77
  in diabetes 360
  for fat 6, 114, 286, 350
  for protein 6, 136, 145-146
acesulfame potassium (acesulfame-K) 88, 89*t*
acetyl-CoA
  in alcohol consumption 46
  in carbohydrate catabolism 39-40, 40*f*
  in fat catabolism 44-45
  in gluconeogenesis 51*f*
  in lipogenesis 51
  from protein catabolism 46, 121*f*
  pyruvate dehydrogenase complex 39
  in TCA cycle 27, 28, 40, 40*f*
acid–base balance 104, 125, 128, 129*t*
acidosis 104, 128
acromegaly 260
ACSM (American College of Sports Medicine) 19, 20
active transport. *See also* cell transporters
  of amino acids 131, 132*f*, 133
  ATP in 69, 129, 131, 132*f*
  competition in 133
  of fructose 69, 133, 290*f*
  of galactose 69, 290, 290*f*
  of glucose 71-72, 72*f*, 290, 290*f*, 357-358, 362*f*
  protein pumps in 129, 129*f*, 132*f*
activities of daily living 327, 328*t*, 336
activity factors 327, 328*t*
adenosine, caffeine and 248
adenosine diphosphate (ADP) 30, 30*f*
adenosine monophosphate (AMP) 30
adenosine triphosphate (ATP). *See* ATP (adenosine triphosphate)
adenosine triphosphate-phosphocreatine system (ATP-PC) 12, 31. *See also* anaerobic glycolysis
adequate intake (AI) 5, 5*f*, 114
ADH (antidiuretic hormone). *See* antidiuretic hormone (ADH)
ADI (acceptable daily intake) 88, 89*t*-90*t*
adipocytes 70, 266
adipokines 266
adipose tissue. *See also* body fat; obesity and overweight
  caffeine and 248, 259
  caloric value of 32-33
  in exercise 94, 95-96
  inflammation from 266
  storage in 6, 70, 70*f*, 94
  use of body fat 94-95
  white 266
adolescents
  bone health 188, 344, 352
  carbohydrate needs for 349, 349*t*
  creatine and 34, 254
  energy in 346
  fat needs 350
  folate in female 175
  growth and development in 346-348, 347*f*, 348*t*
  human growth hormone in 260
  hydration plans for 232-233, 350
  leucine and 312, 313*f*
  macronutrients 349-350, 349*t*
  micronutrients 193, 350
  obesity in 347, 348, 350
  protein needs in 135, 151, 312, 313*f*, 349-350
  secondary sexual characteristics 347, 348*f*
  sports drinks 232-233
  strategies for healthy eating 348
  supplements and ergogenic aids for 345-346, 350-351
  vitamin D and 165*t*
  water and fluid intake 217-218, 350
ADP (adenosine diphosphate) 30, 30*f*
ADP (air displacement plethysmography) 274
advantame 88, 90*t*
aerobic capacity ($\dot{V}O_2$max) 36-38, 37*f*, 40, 48-50
aerobic endurance training. *See* endurance sports
aerobic energy system
  chemical energy from carbohydrate 39-42, 40*f*, 41*f*, 42*f*, 42*t*
  endurance training and 38
  mechanism of 31-33, 32*f*, 36-38, 37*f*
aerobic glycolysis 12*f*
aerobic physical activity 11
aerobic power (aerobic capacity) 11-12
aesthetically judged sport 373
African Americans
  calcium in 189
  potassium in 195-196
  salt sensitivity in 198
  vitamin D in 163-164
aging. *See* older adults
AI (adequate intake) 5, 5*f*, 114
air displacement plethysmography (ADP) 274
ALA (alpha-linolenic acid) 98, 101*t*, 107, 107*f*, 114, 255
alanine 143, 143*f*
albumin 128, 128*f*
alcohol
  athletic performance and 261, 309
  chemical energy from 27, 28, 46-47, 47*f*, 51
  concentration of, in drinks 220*f*
  fluid balance and 214, 222, 355
  folate and 367
  hangovers from 220, 220*f*
  high iron levels and 203
  hormonal responses to 309
  resistance training and 309
aldosterone 197
all-cause mortality 322
allulose 88
alpha bonds 65
alpha-carotene 156, 158*f*, 159
alpha-linolenic acid (ALA) 98, 101*t*, 107, 107*f*, 114, 255
alpha-tocopherol 170. *See also* vitamin E
altitude, training at high 38, 217
AMA (American Medical Association) 266
AMDR (acceptable macronutrient distribution range). *See* acceptable macronutrient distribution range (AMDR)
amenorrhea 352, 377
American College of Sports Medicine (ACSM) 19, 20
American Medical Association (AMA) 266
amino acids. *See also* essential amino acids; proteins; *names of individual amino acids*
  absorption of 131, 133
  amino acid pool 122, 122*f*, 132-133
  aromatic 118, 119*f*
  branched chain 118, 143, 147, 254, 258, 308*f*
  carbon skeleton 46, 118, 120
  classification of 119*f*
  as energy source 120-121, 121*f*, 282
  in gluconeogenesis 51*f*
  limiting 139-140, 139*t*
  in metabolism 118-120
  nonessential 119, 120, 134, 138
  proteinogenic 118
  in protein powders 135, 139
  protein quality and 122-123, 137-142, 138*t*, 139*t*
  recycling of 118, 134
  in resistance training 306
  structure and classification of 118-119, 118*f*, 119*f*

449

amino acid scores 138, 138t, 139-142, 139t
amino groups 122
AMP (adenosine monophosphate) 30
amphetamines 259
amylopectin 66
amylose 66, 67f
anabolic androgenic steroids (AAC) 259-260
anabolism 26, 27f, 309-310
anaerobic activity 12, 12f, 359
anaerobic energy system 31-33, 32f, 34-36, 35f, 38
anaerobic glycolysis 12f, 34
anaerobic power or capacity 12
android body shape 270, 270f, 277
anemia
 hemolytic 170, 196, 230t
 iron-deficiency 22t, 202-204, 203f, 370
 megaloblastic 174-175, 177, 178, 367
 microcytic 177
 NSAIDs and 203
 pernicious 177-178
 in pregnancy with multiple babies 365, 367
 vitamins and 170, 174
angiogenesis 48
animal protein 111-112, 111t, 122, 137, 149, 349
anorexia nervosa 374-375, 375f, 376. See also disordered eating
antacids, iron and 203
antibodies 125, 126f, 127, 129t
anticoagulants 170, 171, 172
antidiuretic hormone (ADH)
 alcohol consumption and 47, 47f, 220
 mechanism of 197, 216
 stroke or head trauma and 231t
antioxidants. See also vitamin A; vitamin C; vitamin E
 in carotenoids 156
 in endurance athletes 296
 in foods 139, 169, 171, 369
 functions of 158-159, 241
 muscle soreness and 180
 in pregnancy 367
arachidonic acid (ARA) 101t, 106
L-arginine 133, 198, 252
artery stiffness 105, 199, 318
arthritis 109, 203, 255
ascorbic acid. See vitamin C
asparagine 46, 119, 120, 121f
aspartame 88, 89t
aspartic acid 119-120, 119f
atherosclerosis 324, 324f
atomic-level body composition model 273
ATP (adenosine triphosphate)
 in active transport 69, 129, 131, 132f
 adenosine triphosphate-phosphocreatine system 12, 31
 from the aerobic energy system 12, 32t, 33, 36-38, 37f
 from alcohol 46-47, 47f

 from the anaerobic energy system 12, 12f, 32t, 34-36, 35f
 in brain cells 72
 from breakdown of amino acids 120-121
 from carbohydrate 37, 37f, 38-42, 40f, 41f, 42t
 creatine and 252
 from dietary fat 42-46, 43f, 44f, 45f, 339
 dietary nitrate and 49
 in endurance activities 282-283, 283f
 in energy systems 26, 31-33, 32f
 energy transfer of 30-31, 30f
 exercise intensity and 49-50, 76, 76t, 143, 282-283, 283f
 from fat 42-46, 43f, 44f, 45f
 from glucose 70, 70f, 71
 in lipogenesis 51
 metabolic pathways to 26-27, 27f, 28-29, 29f, 282
 from the phosphagen system 33, 33f
 from protein 46
 rates of production 339-340
 in substrate fatigue 77
 in TCA cycle 28-29, 29f
ATPase 30f
ATP-PC (adenosine triphosphate-phosphocreatine system) 12, 31. See also anaerobic glycolysis
ATP synthase 41
atypical anorexia nervosa 374-375, 375f, 376. See also disordered eating
autoimmune diseases 83-85, 161, 172, 177, 296, 298
avidin 174

B
baking soda 250
Banned Substances Control Group (BSCG) 243
bariatric surgery 203
basal (resting) metabolic rate (BMR) 54-55, 327, 329, 335, 353
BCAAs (branched chain amino acids) 118, 143, 147, 254, 258, 308f
beetroot juice 198, 251-252
behavior strategies in weight loss 332, 332f, 337f
beriberi 176
beta-alanine 250-251
beta bonds 66
beta-carotene 99, 156, 158f, 159-160, 171
beta cells of the pancreas 71-72
beta-cryptoxanthin 156, 158f, 159, 166t
beta-glucan 83, 331
beta-hydroxy-beta-methylbutyrate (HMB) 254, 318
beta-oxidation 36, 38, 41f, 44-45, 44f, 47
BIA (bioelectrical impedance analysis) 226, 229, 231, 277
bile 82, 94
binge drinking 46-47
binge eating disorder 375-376. See also disordered eating

bioavailability 137, 186, 355, 370, 372. See also nutrient absorption
bioelectrical impedance analysis (BIA) 226, 229, 231, 277
biological value (BV) of proteins 138t, 140, 148, 150t
biosynthesis pathways 50-52, 51f, 52f. See also gluconeogenesis; lipogenesis
biotin 166t-167t, 174
blood. See also anemia; blood glucose; blood pressure
 cholesterol in 98, 100, 102f, 104-105, 318
 clotting 171-172, 199, 204
 donation of 203
 magnesium in 193
 osmolarity of 199, 214, 226
 platelets and vitamins 170, 172
 vitamin K and 171-172
blood glucose. See also diabetes mellitus; glucose
 in diabetes 71, 325
 exercise and 75-76, 358-359
 glycemic index and load and 74, 292
 hypohydration and 304
 impaired metabolism and 71
 insulin resistance and 325
 interesterified fats and 112-113
 management 359-360, 360t
 perception of fatigue and 294-295
 in pregnancy 364
 regulation of 39, 71-72, 72f, 73f, 73t
 superstarch and waxy maize 295
 transport into cells 71-72, 72f, 290, 290f, 357-358, 362f
 typical amount of 70t, 71
blood pressure
 dehydration and 214, 215
 EPA and DHA effect on 108
 hypertension in pregnancy 365
 magnesium and 191
 obesity and 322-323
 potassium and 195
 sodium and 197-199
BMI (body mass index) 266, 269-270, 269t
BMR (basal (resting) metabolic rate). See basal (resting) metabolic rate (BMR)
board certified specialist in sports dietetics (CSSD) 20-21, 22, 78, 300
bodybuilders 254, 268, 316, 334. See also resistance training
body composition 267-279. See also body fat; body weight; lean body mass; obesity and overweight; weight gain; weight loss
 of adolescents and children 346-347
 assessment methods 273-277, 275f, 276f
 body fat types 271, 322
 body water in 213-214
 cancer and 325-326

choosing assessment methods 273
classification of body fat percentages 272t
compartment models 271, 272-273
daily energy needs 26
definition of 12, 271, 322
diabetes and 325, 361
energy intake and 51
"fit and fat" 326
gaining muscle mass 338-341
genetics and environment in 267
health implications of excess body fat 322-326, 323f, 324f
health implications of low body fat 326
healthy weight goal 267, 326-328, 326f, 328t
implications for specific sports 268-269
interpreting estimations 277-279
ketogenic diets and 104-105, 299, 333
losing fat and gaining muscle 338-341
margin of error in 278
optimal, for performance 16
protein intake and 146, 149
sport training and 267-269
statistical methods 273
supplements to alter 258-259, 262
body fat. *See also* adipose tissue; body composition
  in adolescents 347
  in athletes 268
  body mass index and 266, 269-270, 269t
  cell hypertrophy in 270
  essential 271, 322
  health implications of 322-326, 323f, 324f
  healthy weight goal 267, 326-328, 326f, 328t
  ketogenic diets and 104-105, 299, 317, 333
  losing, while gaining muscle 338-341
  overfeeding food types and 94
  patterns of 270-271, 270f
  sport-specific goals for 268-269, 336-338, 338t
  storage fat 271
  subcutaneous fat 322
  supplements and decreasing 258–259
  training, for losing 335-336
  trans fatty acids and 111
  visceral fat 103, 322
body image, in athletes 268
body mass index (BMI) 266, 269-270, 269t
body temperature, sweating and 6, 212, 219f
body weight. *See also* body composition; obesity and overweight; weight gain; weight loss
  anorexia nervosa and 373
  body mass index 266, 269-270, 269t
  in children 346
  environmental factors in 267

estimating desired weight for athletes 270, 278
genetic factors in 267
healthy 326-328
hydration status and 228, 228f
in older adults 353
pregnancy and 364, 364t
resting metabolic rate and 327
sport-specific goals for 268-269, 336-338, 338t
training adaptations and 48-49
yo-yo dieting 268
bomb calorimeters 52-53, 53f
bones
  in bed rest 189
  bone mineral density 162, 163, 189, 275, 377
  calcium and 184
  in children and adolescents 188, 344, 352
  DXA and 275
  in female athlete triad 59, 377, 377f, 378f, 379f
  fluoride and 208
  in older adults 188, 275, 352-353
  osteoporosis 172, 187-188, 187f, 352
  peak bone mass 188, 347
  phosphorus and 187, 190, 190f
  remodeling 188
  stress fractures in 169
  types of 187, 187f
  in vegan and vegetarian athletes 372
  vitamin D and 162, 163, 169, 352, 367
  in women and girls 188-189, 275, 377
"bonking" 284
branched chain amino acids (BCAAs) 118, 143, 147, 254, 258, 308f
BSCG (Banned Substances Control Group) 243
buffers 128
bulimia nervosa 375, 376. *See also* disordered eating
buoyancy 274
B vitamins 173-178
  biotin 166t-167t, 174
  choline 174
  folic acid/folate 166t-167t, 174-175, 175f, 366-367
  niacin 166t-167t, 174, 175, 366
  in pregnancy 174-175, 366-367
  vitamin B$_1$ (thiamin) 7, 166t-167t, 174, 176-177, 177f, 366
  vitamin B$_2$ (riboflavin) 166t-167t, 174, 175-176, 176f, 366
  vitamin B$_5$ (pantothenic acid) 166t-167t, 174, 175
  vitamin B$_6$ (pyridoxine) 166t-167t, 174, 177, 354
  vitamin B$_{12}$ (cobalamin) 149, 166t-167t, 174, 177-178, 354, 370
BV (biological value) of proteins 138t, 140, 148, 150t

C

caffeine

adenosine and 248
calcium and 187
dehydration and 216, 250
in energy drinks 247, 248-250, 249f, 293
energy from 52
fat-burning and 248, 249f, 293
glycogen replacement and 293
labeling requirements for 238, 248
research on FFA release and 248
toxicity of 248-249, 259
vegetarian diets and 372
in weight loss 259
calcidiol 162
calciferol. *See* vitamin D
calcitriol 160. *See also* vitamin D
calcium 184-189
  absorption of 186-187, 186f, 189
  bioavailability 372
  in children and adolescents 350
  deficiency and inadequacy 187-189, 201t
  in endurance athletes 296
  excess intake 189
  exercise and 189, 221
  functions of 184-185, 352
  intake recommendations 184t, 185t, 186-187, 201t
  in older adults 189, 354-355
  protein and 187
  relative energy deficiency and 378
  sources of 185-187, 185f, 200t
  in sweat 221, 221f
  U.S. population intake of 189, 189t
  in vegan and vegetarian diets 372
  vitamin D and 163
  in women 189-190, 189t
calories 52
  in energy expenditure 54-58
  estimating, in foods 52-53, 53f
  estimating needs 327-328, 328t
  in fat 4
  fat gain and 94, 95
  incomplete energy absorption and 335
  in "light" foods 9
  on Nutrition Facts Panel 8f, 82f
  during pregnancy 365
  weight gain and 94
cancer. *See also* names of individual types of cancer
  beta-carotene and 160
  excess iron intake and 203
  fiber and 82
  obesity and 325-326
  tanning beds and 161
  vegetarian diets and 369
  vitamin D and 161, 164
  vitamin E and 170
cannabidiol (CBD) 261
carbohydrate-electrolyte beverages. *See* sports drinks
carbohydrate loading 287, 316
carbohydrates 64-91
  availability of 286

carbohydrates *(continued)*
  benefits of 81-82
  calories per gram 4
  celiac disease and 83-85, 296
  in cell membranes 71, 72*f*
  chemical energy from 38-42, 40*f*, 41*f*, 42*f*, 42*t*
  for children and adolescents 349, 349*t*
  cognitive function and 354
  complex 64, 65-67, 67*f*
  content in foods 81, 81*f*
  crossover concept 48-50, 48*f*, 282, 283*f*
  definition of 64
  diabetes and 360, 361-362
  digestion and absorption of 68-69, 69*t*, 289-290, 290*f*
  for endurance athletes 282-283, 283*f*, 294-295
  during endurance events 287, 288-291, 288*t*, 289*f*, 290*f*, 316
  excess calorie storage 94, 149
  during exercise 4, 5, 36-38, 37*f*, 76, 76*t*
  before exercising 232
  glycemic response 73-76, 75*t*
  habitual intake amounts 284-287, 285*t*
  in high altitude training 38
  high-fructose corn syrup 86-87
  inability to consume extra, during activity 295
  in intermittent sports 291
  lactose intolerance 82-83
  for losing fat and gaining muscle 340-341
  for masters athletes 354, 354*t*
  metabolism of 32, 37*f*, 70, 70*f*, 70*t*
  muscle mass and 339
  muscle protein breakdown and 27*f*
  nutrient density of 5
  nutritive sweeteners 85-87
  overfeeding 94
  in pregnancy 365-366, 366*t*
  recommendations for 77-80, 78*t*, 79*t*, 80*f*, 80*t*
  regulation of glucose metabolism 39
  in resistance training 305, 306-307, 307*f*, 309, 349
  simple 64, 65, 65*f*, 86
  in sports drinks 290
  superstarch and waxy maize 295
  training the gut for 290
  types of 289, 289*f*, 294-295
  in weight loss 332
carbon skeleton 46, 118, 120
carboxyl groups 123
cardiac output, in pregnancy 363
cardiovascular disease (CVD)
  alpha-linolenic acid and 107
  beta-carotene and 160
  body mass index and 269
  carnitine and 43
  creatine and 34
  dietary fatty acids and 96
  EPA and DHA effect on 106, 107, 109
  excess body fat and 324
  fiber and 78, 82
  LDL cholesterol and 98-99, 100-103, 318
  muscle mass and 304
  potassium and 196
  saturated fat and 100, 102
  sodium and 198
  sugar and 86
  trans fatty acids and 112
  vitamin D and 164
cardiovascular fitness, in older adults 351-352
carnitine 43
carnitine shuttle 43
carnosine 250
carotenoids 156, 158-159, 158*f*. *See also* names of individual carotenoids
cartilage 6, 171, 208, 254-255
casein protein 139, 141
catabolism 26-27
  carbohydrate 38-42, 40*f*, 41*f*, 42*f*, 42*t*
  fat 42-45, 43*f*, 44*f*, 45*f*
  protein 27*f*, 120-122, 121*f*, 134, 151
CBD (cannabidiol) 261
CCK (cholecystokinin) 131
CDE (certified diabetes educator) 361
celiac disease 83-85, 172, 296, 298
cell membranes
  amino acids in 122*f*
  fatty acids and 100, 106, 106*f*, 109
  glucose and 71, 72*f*
  LDL and 323
  phospholipids in 99
  sterols in 98
  vitamin E and 169, 170
cell transporters. *See also* active transport
  in amino acid absorption 131, 132*f*, 133
  facilitated transport 131, 132*f*, 290*f*
  for glucose and fructose 71-72, 72*f*, 290, 290*f*, 357-358, 362*f*
  hormones and 71-72, 72*f*, 308*f*
  proteins as channels in 128-129, 129*f*, 129*t*
  proteins as pumps in active transport 129, 132*f*
cellular edema 218
certifications in exercise science and fitness. *See* credentials and certifications
certified diabetes educator (CDE) 361
certified specialist in sports dietetics (CSSD) 20-21, 22, 78, 300
CHD (coronary heart disease) 100-102, 104, 105, 108-111, 136. *See also* cardiovascular disease (CVD)
cheilosis 159, 177
chelated minerals 206
chemical digestion 68
chemical energy 26-27
chemical score of proteins 138*t*, 139-140, 139*t*
chemiosmotic coupling 41-42, 42*f*
chew and spit (CHSP) 376
chewing food 171

children
  body weight in 346
  bone health 188, 344, 352
  calcium in 350
  carbohydrate needs 349, 349*t*
  dehydration in 217-218, 350
  energy needs 346, 347-348
  fat needs 350
  growth and development in 346
  hydration plans for 232-233, 350
  injuries in 344
  leucine in 312, 313*f*
  low energy availability in 344, 346
  metabolism in 344
  micronutrients in 350
  obesity in 86, 269
  physiological differences in 344-345
  protein needs 310, 312, 349-350
  risks and benefits of sport 344
  saturated fatty acids 344
  sport performance 345
  sports drinks 232-233
  strategies for healthy eating 348
  type 1 diabetes in 355-356
  vitamin D in 163, 350
chitosan 259
chloride 184*t*, 199, 224
chocolate 248
cholecalciferol (vitamin D$_3$) 161. *See also* vitamin D
cholecystokinin (CCK) 131
cholesterol
  anabolic androgenic steroids and 260
  in blood 98, 100, 102*f*, 104-105, 318
  from fat digestion 94
  fiber and 94
  food sources of 100, 104-105
  heart disease and 100
  high-density lipoprotein 100, 323-324
  in ketogenic diets 318
  low-density lipoprotein 98-99, 100, 105, 318, 323-324
  obesity and 322-323
  structure and functions of 98-99, 99*f*
  sugar and 86
choline 174
chondroitin sulfate 254-255
chromium 100*t*, 184*t*, 200*t*, 206
chromium picolinate 259
CHSP (chew and spit) 376
chylomicrons 94, 129, 129*f*
chyme 131
cis configuration 98, 98*f*, 101*t*
citric acid cycle. *See* TCA (tricarboxylic acid) cycle
CLA (conjugated linoleic acid) 111*t*, 112, 259
cleanses 194, 217, 218
cobalamin (vitamin B$_{12}$) 149, 166*t*-167*t*, 174, 177-178, 354, 370
coconut oil 97, 101*t*
coenzyme A 39, 43-44, 43*f*
coenzymes 28-29, 39, 43-44, 43*f*, 171, 175
coffee 187, 238, 249-250. *See also* caffeine

Index

cognitive function
  carbohydrates and 354
  CBD and 261
  creatine and 254
  diet and 354
  fitness and 353
  glucose demand for 66
  hydration status and 217, 218, 223, 227, 355, 357
  iodine and 204
  iron and 203
  in older adults 353
collagen 120, 125, 255
colon (large intestine) 83
colon cancer 82, 268
complete protein 118, 137, 147
complex carbohydrates 64, 65-67, 67f
concurrent training 311
concussion (traumatic brain injury) 34, 104, 109-110, 254, 256, 261
conditionally essential amino acids 119-120
Conformity Assessment (ISO) 242-243
conjugated linoleic acid (CLA) 111t, 112, 259
conservation of energy, law of 26
contractile fibers 125-126, 144
copper 200, 205, 206
Cori cycle 50, 51f, 72
coronary heart disease (CHD) 100-102, 104, 105, 108-111, 136. *See also* cardiovascular disease
cortisol 72, 147, 304
cramping 87, 96, 218, 221, 254, 318
creatine
  ATP and 12, 174
  choline and 174
  dehydration and 218, 254
  delayed onset muscle soreness and 254
  food sources 31
  for increasing muscle mass 253, 340
  performance and 252-253
  in protein powders 135
  for resistance training 318
  supplements 34, 238, 247, 252-254, 318, 373
  therapeutic uses of 34, 253
  in traumatic brain injury 34
  in vegetarian diets 31, 372-373
creatine monohydrate 318, 340
credentials and certifications 18-23
  certificates 21
  certified diabetes educator 361
  certified specialist in sports dietetics 20-21, 22, 78, 300
  exercise science and fitness certifications 18-20, 19f
  registered dietitian 18
  registered dietitian nutritionist 7, 18, 20-21, 84, 331, 361
crossover concept 48-50, 282, 283f
crossover studies 17
CSSD (certified specialist in sports dietetics) 20-21, 22, 78, 300

Cunningham equation 58, 327
curcumin 255
CVD (cardiovascular disease). *See* cardiovascular disease (CVD)
cysteine 119, 119f, 137, 199
cystic fibrosis 217
cytokines 86, 308
cytoplasm 28
cytosol 26, 28, 28f, 39, 134

D

daily value (DV) 8, 173f, 185t
dairy products
  blood cholesterol and 104
  calcium in 185, 188
  casein in 139, 141
  lactose intolerance 82-83
  leucine in 148, 149
  milk allergy 83
  in muscle protein synthesis 148, 149, 312f
  trans fats in 111-112, 111t
  vitamin D in 296
  whey protein 137, 139, 146, 148, 150
  yogurt 83, 100, 104, 257
DASH diet 354
deamination 46, 120, 134
dehydration. *See also* hydration status
  blood pressure and 214, 215
  body fluid regulation and 214, 216
  caffeine and 216, 250
  in children and adolescents 217-218, 350
  cognitive function and 355
  creatine and 218, 254
  excess protein and 151
  gastrointestinal distress in 296, 298
  hypernatremia in 221
  hypohydration versus 216
  in older adults 197, 217-218, 355
  performance and 222-226, 222f, 223f, 224f
  resistance training and 304-305
  risk factors for 222
delayed onset muscle soreness (DOMS) 76, 110, 170, 180, 254
denaturation 127
densitometry 273-274
deoxyribonucleic acid (DNA), protein synthesis and 133-134, 133f
detox cleanses 194, 217, 218
detraining principle 13-14, 48
DHA (docosahexaenoic acid). *See also* omega-3 polyunsaturated fatty acids
  dietary recommendation for 114
  food sources of 101t, 107-108, 108f, 255
  structure of 106, 107f
  traumatic brain injury and 109-110
DIAAS (digestible indispensable amino acid score) 138t, 141-142
diabetes mellitus 355-363. *See also* type 1 diabetes; type 2 diabetes
  aging and 352

blood glucose levels in 71
chronic diseases from 358
complications 357
diagnosis 359t
exercise and 352, 358-360, 360t
gestational 363-364
glucose absorption in 356-358, 356f, 358f
glucose excretion 70
high-fiber diets and 83
hypoglycemia in 71, 360-361
insulin in 72, 86, 355-359, 356f
management 359-360, 360t
metabolic impacts 357-358, 358f
muscles and 311-315, 312f, 361
nutrition in 360-362, 362f
obesity and 356
prevalence 355
preventing emergencies in sport 362-363
PUFAs and 103
sugar intake and 86
superstarch and waxy maize and 295
symptoms 358
treatment 357-358
dietary fat. *See* fat, dietary
dietary fiber. *See* fiber
Dietary Guidelines for Americans (2020–2025) 7
  on multivitamin supplements 208
  MyPlate and 9-10, 9f
  on sodium 198, 198f, 224
Dietary Reference Intake (DRI) 4-5, 5f, 77
  for carbohydrate 285
  for fiber 77-78
  for minerals 184t
Dietary Supplement Health and Education Act (DSHEA) 238-239
dietary supplements. *See* supplements
diets
  detox and cleansing diets 194, 217, 218
  energy-restricted 332-333
  FODMAP 84-85
  high-fat 96
  high-fiber 83
  ketogenic 45, 104-105, 299-300, 316-318, 333
  low-calorie 332-333
  low-carbohydrate. *See* low-carbohydrate diets
  low-carbohydrate, high fat 297-299
  low-fat 332
  low-glycemic index 74
  Mediterranean 105
  plant-based 61, 137
  processed foods in 205
  sample, for resistance training 307f
  training low, competing high 297-299
  vegan. *See* vegan diets
  vegetarian. *See* vegetarian diets
  very low-carbohydrate 317
  for weight loss 332-334
  yo-yo dieting 268

digestible indispensable amino acid score (DIAAS) 138t, 141-142
digestion 68. *See also* nutrient absorption
  of carbohydrate 70, 70f
  chemical 68
  digestive tract 68-69, 68f, 69f, 69t
  elimination in 68, 82
  enzymes in 68
  of fat 94-95
  mechanical 68
  of protein 130-131, 130f, 132f
digestive tract 68-69, 68f, 69f
dinucleotide phosphate (NADPH) 51
direct calorimetry 52-53, 53f, 55-56, 56f
disaccharides 65, 65f
disordered eating 373-380
  anorexia nervosa 374-375, 375f, 376
  binge eating disorder 375-376
  bulimia nervosa 375, 376
  disordered eating spectrum 373-374
  Eating Disorder Not Otherwise Specified 376
  etiology 374
  health impacts 376-377, 377f, 378f, 379f
  help for 379
  as mental illness 374
  night eating syndrome 376
  Other Specified Feeding or Eating Disorders 376
  performance problems 377-379, 378f
  prevalence of 374
  prevention and management 379-380, 380f
  purging disorder 375, 376
  rigidity in eating 16
  vegetarian diets in 368
diuretics, weight loss and 199, 217
diverticulitis 82
diverticulosis 82
DNA (deoxyribonucleic acid), protein synthesis and 133-134, 133f
docosahexaenoic acid. *See* DHA (docosahexaenoic acid)
docosapentaenoic acid (DPA) 101t
DOMS (delayed onset muscle soreness) 76, 110, 170, 180, 254
double-blind studies 112, 179, 194
doubly labeled water technique 56-57, 57f
DRI. *See* Dietary Reference Intake (DRI)
Drug Free Sport International 245
DSHEA (Dietary Supplement Health and Education Act) 238-239
drugs in sports 243, 245, 259-261
dual-energy x-ray absorptiometry (DXA) 274-275, 275f
duodenum 131
DV (daily value) 8, 173f, 185t
dyslipidemia 86, 100

E

EA (energy availability) 59-60, 286, 326, 346
EAA. *See* essential amino acids (EAAs)

EAR (estimated average requirement) 4, 5f
Eating Disorder Not Otherwise Specified (EDNOS) 376
eating disorders. *See* disordered eating
eccentric contractions 13
ectomorphs 270
EDNOS (Eating Disorder Not Otherwise Specified) 376
EE (energy expenditure). *See* energy expenditure (EE)
EEE (energy expenditure from exercise) 55, 58, 59
EER (estimated energy requirement) 5
egg protein 139, 141, 174
eicosanoids 105, 106, 107f
eicosapentaenoic acid (EPA) 101t, 106, 107-109, 107f, 114, 255. *See also* omega-3 polyunsaturated fatty acids
elaidic acid 110, 112
electrolytes
  in body fluid regulation 212, 214, 221, 221f
  exercise performance and 222-226, 222f, 223f, 224f
  minerals in 184
  salt for athletes 226
  sweating and 221, 221f
electron transport chain (ETC)
  in anaerobic energy system 35, 35f
  in beta-oxidation 44, 44f
  in carbohydrate breakdown 41-42, 41f
  in chemiosmotic coupling 41-42, 42f
  endurance training and 47-48
  in the TCA cycle 28-29, 40
elemental magnesium 191-192
endomorphs 270
endoplasmic reticulum 325
endurance sports
  aerobic capacity and 48-50
  alcohol and 261
  ATP production in 282-283, 283f
  caffeine in 293
  carbohydrate intake during events 288-291, 289f, 290f
  carbohydrate loading 287, 316
  carbohydrate types 289, 289f, 294-295
  concurrent resistance training as 311
  continuous versus intermittent activities 291
  energy requirements 285-286, 285f
  energy source utilization 48-50, 282-283, 283f
  on event day 287-288, 288t
  fatty acid oxidation 282-284, 283f, 296-297
  food selection 293-294, 293f, 294f
  gastrointestinal distress in 295-296, 298
  in a glycogen-depleted state 297-299
  glycogen repletion after events 291-293, 292f
  habitual intake of energy macronutrients 284-287, 285t

  hydration status and 218
  inability to consume extra carbohydrates 295
  iron in 202
  ketogenic diets in 299-300, 317
  metabolism adaptations 47-50, 48f, 301
  micronutrients 296
  mouth rinsing 295
  muscle protein synthesis in 286-287
  new foods 289
  protein in 142-143, 286-287, 291
  recovery from 300
  training in glycogen-depleted state 297-299
  training low 284
  ultraendurance athletes 96, 285, 317
energy. *See also* ATP (adenosine triphosphate); carbohydrates; energy expenditure (EE); energy systems
  from alcohol 4f, 46-47
  assessing intake in athletes 53
  backloading intake 146
  caffeine and 52, 247, 293
  from creatine 253, 373
  for endurance activities 285-286, 285f
  estimating calories in food 52-53, 53f
  estimating needs 347-348
  from fat 94, 96
  in gaining muscle mass 338-339
  inadequate intake 5-6
  for masters athletes 353
  metabolic pathways 26-27, 27f
  from protein 46
  TCA cycle 28-29, 29f, 40-41, 40f
  units of 4
energy availability (EA) 59-60, 286, 326, 346
energy-dense foods 4, 266
energy drinks 52, 247, 248-250, 249f. *See also* sports drinks
energy expenditure (EE) 54
  Cunningham equation 58
  direct calorimetry 52-53, 53f, 55-56, 56f
  estimating 54-55, 55t, 58-59
  Harris-Benedict equation 57
  indirect calorimetry 56-57, 57f
  prediction equations 58-59
  in pregnancy 365
  resting metabolic rate and 54-55
  thermic effect of activity and 54, 55
  thermic effect of feeding and 55, 55t
  wearable activity monitors 59
energy expenditure from exercise (EEE) 55, 58, 59
energy systems
  aerobic 31-33, 32f, 36-38, 37f
  anaerobic 31-33, 32f, 34-36, 35f
  exercise duration and 31
  food sources for 31
  phosphagen system 12, 31-32, 32f, 33-34, 33f, 36
  in sedentary people 36, 38, 45-46, 48

energy-yielding macronutrients 4. *See also* carbohydrate; fat, dietary; proteins
   in endurance events 282-284, 283f, 288-291, 289f, 290f
   function of 5-6
   habitual intake of 284-287, 285t
eNOS (nitric oxide synthase) 251
enrichment of food 66, 67, 162
enterocytes 69
enterokinases 131
enzymes. *See also names of individual enzymes*
   in absorption 68-69, 69t
   binding by 126f
   in carbohydrate digestion 65-66, 69, 69t
   coenzymes 28-29, 39, 43-44, 171, 175
   copper and 206
   in digestion 130-131, 130f
   in fat digestion 43-44, 43f, 94-95
   functions of 29, 125-127, 126f, 129t
   in lactose intolerance 82-83
   in protein metabolism 143-144
EPA (eicosapentaenoic acid) 101t, 106, 107-110, 107f, 114, 255. *See also* omega-3 polyunsaturated fatty acids
epilepsy, ketogenic diets and 105, 300, 318
epinephrine 72
epithelial cells 106
EPOC (excess postexercise oxygen consumption) 335-336
ergocalciferol (vitamin D_2) 161. *See also* vitamin D
ergogenic supplements 248. *See also* supplements, nutritional and sport
essential amino acids (EAAs)
   in complementary proteins 137-138
   listing of 119-120
   profile 137
   in protein synthesis 134, 312-314, 313f
   in resistance training 308f
   structure of 119f
   supplementing, in protein-poor meals 314-315
essential body fat 271, 322
essential fatty acids 96, 106, 114-115. *See also* alpha-linolenic acid (ALA); linoleic acid (LA)
estimated average requirement (EAR) 4, 5f
estimated energy requirement (EER) 5
estrogens 98, 325, 352
ETC (electron transport chain). *See* electron transport chain (ETC)
ethanol. *See* alcohol
euglycemia 71
euhydration 222
evidence-based practice 16
excess postexercise oxygen consumption (EPOC) 335-336
exercise. *See also* exercise intensity

alcohol and 46-47
average energy cost of 328t
blood glucose regulation in 75-76, 358-359
blood sugar testing and 359-360, 360t
caffeine and 52, 247
calcium and 189, 221
carbohydrate in 76, 76t
cognitive function and 328t, 353
in diabetes 358-359
diabetes management in 359-360, 360t
dietary fats and 96
energy systems and duration of 32f
fitness components 11-12
glycemic index in 75-76
health benefits of 11
high-impact 352
in hot, humid weather 222-223, 222f
hydration recommendations for 232-234
hydration status in 222-226, 222f, 223f, 224f
hypohydration at the start of 222-223, 232
insulin sensitivity and 361
iron and 204
magnesium and 193-195
maximal oxygen consumption and 11-12, 352
by older adults 11-12, 341, 351-352, 353
oxygen availability in 40-41, 45
phosphorus and 190-191
potassium and 197
pregnancy and 363, 364
protein metabolism in 142-144, 143f
pyridoxine and 177
recommendation for adults 11
riboflavin and 176
sodium and 199
sodium bicarbonate and 25
thiamin and 176-177
vitamin A and 160
vitamin C and 179
vitamin D and 165, 168
vitamin E and 170-171
weight-bearing 352
zinc and 206
exercise fatigue 76-77, 297
exercise intensity
   aerobic energy system and 37-38
   anaerobic energy system and 35-36
   ATP production and 282-283, 283f
   carbohydrate needs and 48, 48f, 78, 78t, 291, 298
   "fat burning zone" 336
   fat needs and 48-49
   glucose use and 76
   high-intensity interval training 311, 336
   increasing capacity for 49-50
   metabolic fatigue and 76-77
   phosphagen system and 33-34
   protein needs and 143, 144-146, 145t

   weight loss and 48-49, 48f, 336
exercise performance. *See* sport performance
exercise physiology 15
exercise science and fitness certifications 18-20, 19f
exercise training principles 12-15. *See also* training
extreme sports 344

F

facilitated diffusion 131, 132f, 290f
$FADH_2$ (flavin adenine dinucleotide) 29
fast-twitch muscle fibers 165
fat, body. *See* body fat
fat, dietary 94-115. *See also* fatty acids; triglycerides
   alcohol metabolism and 46
   calories per gram 4
   calorie storage from 5
   cell membranes and 106, 106f, 109
   chemical energy from 42-46, 43f, 44f, 45f
   for children and adolescents 350
   cis/trans 98, 98f, 101t
   classification of 96-97, 96f
   crossover concept 48-50, 282, 283f
   diabetes and 357, 360-361
   dietary recommendations 114
   digestion and metabolism 94-95
   for endurance athletes 5-6
   as energy source 4, 5-6, 94-96
   interesterified 112-114
   lipids and 96-99, 96f, 97f, 98f, 99f, 352
   for masters athletes 354t
   metabolic pathways 32, 37f
   overfeeding 94
   phospholipids 94, 99
   in pregnancy 366t
   saturation status of foods 100, 101t
   sterols 98-99, 99f
   in weight loss 332
"fat burning zone" 336
fat-free mass (FFM) 12, 57-58, 271, 322, 353
fatigue
   aerobic energy system and 38
   alcohol and 220
   anaerobic energy system and 36
   antioxidants and 180
   beta-alanine and 250
   blood glucose and perception of 294-295
   caffeine and 216
   carbohydrates and 297, 339, 366
   diabetes and 358, 363
   folate status and 174, 367
   hydration status and 222, 224
   iron and 200t, 203
   ketogenic diets and 104, 318
   magnesium and 191, 192, 193, 194, 201t, 318
   mental 300
   metabolic 76-77, 250, 283
   metabolic pathways and 36, 38, 50

fatigue (continued)
  overreaching and 14-15
  potassium and 201t
  substrate 76-77, 282, 283, 286
  training-induced, in muscles 13
  vitamin E and 170
fat loading 297
fat-soluble vitamins 6, 156-172. *See also names of individual vitamins*
fatty acids. *See also* polyunsaturated fatty acids (PUFA); saturated fatty acids; triglycerides; unsaturated fatty acids
  alcohol consumption and 46
  ATP production from 27, 282-283, 283f, 344
  caffeine and 248, 249f, 293
  cis and trans configurations 98, 98f, 101t
  content in oils 97, 99f
  enhancing oxidation of 296-297, 298
  essential 96, 106, 114-115
  free-fatty acids 94, 282-283
  from lipogenesis 27f, 51, 70
  metabolic pathways 26-27, 27f
  monounsaturated fatty acids 97-98, 97f, 101t, 105
  omega-3 fatty acids 97-98, 105, 106-110, 107f, 108f, 255-256
  omega-6 fatty acids 97-98, 97f, 105, 106, 107f
  polyunsaturated 97-98, 97f, 101t, 102-103, 105-110, 106f, 107f
  in training low 284, 297-298
  trans fatty acids 96f, 101t, 110-114, 111f, 111t
  types of, in foods 101f
fatty liver 46
FDA (U.S. Food and Drug Administration). *See* U.S. Food and Drug Administration (FDA)
Federal Trade Commission (FTC) 238
feedback inhibition 35
female athletes. *See* women and girls
female athlete triad 59, 377, 377f, 378f, 379f
fermentable olio-, di-, and monosaccharides and polyols (FODMAPs) 84-85
fermentation 66, 100
FFA (free-fatty acids) 94, 282-283
FFM (fat-free mass) 12, 57-58, 271, 322, 353
fiber
  classification of 66
  gastrointestinal distress and 296, 298
  health benefits of 66, 78, 81-82, 94
  in Nutrition Facts panel 8f
  in pregnancy 77
  recommendations for 77-78
  rule of five and 67
  satiety and 66, 331
  structure of 66
fish consumption 107-109, 108f, 114
fish oil 107-110, 108f, 115. *See also* omega-3 polyunsaturated fatty acids
"fit and fat" 326
fitness components 11-12
flavin adenine dinucleotide (FADH$_2$) 29
fluid balance. *See* hydration status
fluid maintenance 128, 128f
fluid retention 214, 234, 260
fluoride 184t, 208
FODMAPs (fermentable olio-, di-, and monosaccharides and polyols) 84-85
folic acid/folate 166t-167t, 174-175, 175f, 366-367
food composition tables 137, 294
Food Data Central (USDA) 294
food diaries 191
food exchange lists 137
food frequency questionnaires 100
food labels 7-9, 8f
  calories on 4
  Nutrition Facts panel 8, 82, 82f, 173, 293f
  protein on 135, 136-137
  required components on 7-9
  serving sizes 7-8, 8f
  supplement labels 242, 244
  verification and seal programs and 243-244
  Whole Grain Stamp 67
Food Safety and Inspection Service (USDA-FSIS) 7
football (American) players, hydration status of 224, 224f, 225f
foot strike hemolysis 202, 203
fortification of foods 162
four-compartment body composition model 271, 273
free-fatty acids (FFA) 94, 282-283
free radicals 156, 158f, 170, 180
fructans 84
fructooligosaccharides 65
fructose
  in endurance events 289-290, 290f
  gastrointestinal distress from 296, 298
  metabolism of 289-290, 290f
  structure of 65, 65f
FTC (Federal Trade Commission) 238
functional fiber 66. *See also* fiber

G
galactans 84
galactose 65, 65f
gallbladder 94, 266
gamma-linolenic acid (GLA) 101t
gas exchange method 56-57
gastrointestinal distress 84, 249, 250, 295-296, 298, 300
GDM (gestational diabetes mellitus) 363-364
gelatin 255
generally recognized as safe (GRAS) 88
genetic factors 12, 83, 267, 347, 374
gestational diabetes mellitus (GDM) 363-364
GI (glycemic index) 73-76, 75t, 292
GLA (gamma-linolenic acid) 101t
globulin 128
glucagon 72, 73f, 73t
glucomannan 259
gluconeogenesis
  alcohol and 261
  in exercise 76-77
  in glucose metabolism regulation 72, 73t
  process of 45, 50, 51f, 52f
  in protein catabolism 143, 143f
glucosamine 254-255
glucose. *See also* blood glucose; gluconeogenesis; glycolysis; sugars
  absorption of 69, 356-357
  in athletic training 358-360, 360t
  biosynthesis of 30
  in brain functioning 66
  from carbohydrates 26-27, 32, 69, 69t, 70, 70f
  from the Cori cycle 50, 51f, 72
  in diabetes 71, 355, 356-357
  in endurance events 282-283, 283f, 288-291, 289f, 290f
  excretion of 70
  fructose combined with 289-290, 290f
  from glycogenolysis 50
  in glycogen replenishment 292-293, 292f
  lipogenesis of 51
  lowered blood sugar after eating 75
  metabolic fates of 70, 70f
  metabolic fatigue and 76-77, 250, 283
  metabolism of 71-73, 72f, 73f
  from photosynthesis 64
  from protein 120, 143, 143f
  in starvation 45, 46, 143, 357
  structure of 65, 65f
  in type 2 diabetes 356-357, 356f
  typical body concentration of 70t
glucose–alanine cycle 50, 72, 143
glucose transport proteins 71-72, 72f, 290, 290f, 357-358, 362f
GLUT4 72, 292, 292f
glutamic acid 119-120
glutamine 119-120, 135
glutathione 119, 199
gluten sensitivity 83-84
glycemic index (GI) 73-76, 75t, 292
glycemic load 74-76, 75t
glycemic response 73-76, 75t
glycerol 43, 94, 98
glycine 135
glycogen
  in blood glucose regulation 71, 73f, 73t, 325
  in carbohydrate loading 287
  in concurrent resistance training 311
  in endurance events 283-284, 291-293, 292f, 297-299
  extreme depletion of 80, 284, 306
  glucose storage in 66
  from glycogenesis 39, 50-51

insulin and 292-293, 292f, 325
in low-carbohydrate, high-fat diets 297-299
in meat and poultry 66
in muscle tissue 32, 39, 76, 76t, 283
in resistance training 305, 306, 307f
structure of 67f
synthesis of 52, 292
training in a glycogen-depleted state 297-299
glycogenesis 39, 50-51
glycogenolysis 50
glycogen replenishment 291-293, 292f, 305, 306, 307f, 361
glycogen storage disease 295
glycogen synthase 292
glycolysis
 aerobic 12f, 34, 37f, 41f
 anaerobic 12f, 34-35, 38-39, 250
 cellular site of 28, 34
 cytosol and 28
 gluconeogenesis and 45, 50, 51f, 52f, 98
glycolytic activity 345, 347
goiter 204
good manufacturing practices (GMPs) 239
grains 10, 67, 81, 83, 104, 369. *See also* whole grains
GRAS (generally recognized as safe) 88
gravitational sports 373
green tea 259
growth charts, for children 346
growth hormones 147, 260, 308f
guanosine triphosphate (GTP) 40
gut flora 256-257, 266, 318
gut health supplements 256-257
gynecomastia 260
gynoid body shape 270, 270f, 277

H
hangovers 220, 220f
Harris–Benedict equation 58, 327
HDL (high-density lipoprotein). *See* high-density lipoprotein (HDL)
health claims, on food 8-9
heart. *See also* cardiovascular disease (CVD)
 coronary heart disease 100-102, 104, 105, 108-111, 136
 diet and 48, 86, 100, 103, 109
 endurance training and 48
 fish consumption and 107-109, 114
 in metabolic syndrome 356, 390
 obesity and 323
heat illness 218, 219f, 221, 222
heat index 222, 222f
heme iron 202
hemoglobin 125, 175, 199
hemolytic anemia 170, 196, 230t
HFCS (high-fructose corn syrup) 86-87
hGH (human growth hormone) 260
high altitude training 38, 217
high blood pressure 191, 195, 324, 364-365. *See also* blood pressure

high carbohydrate availability 286
high-density lipoprotein (HDL) 100, 323-324
high-fructose corn syrup (HFCS) 86-87
high-intensity interval training (HIIT) 311, 336
histidine 118, 119, 120, 250
"hitting the wall" 284
HMB (beta-hydroxy-beta-methylbutyrate) 254, 318
homeostasis, water and fluid intake in 212-213, 212f, 213f
hormones. *See also* names of individual hormones
 in blood sugar regulation 71-72, 72f, 73t
 cholesterol and 98
 in fluid balance 197, 216
 in glucose regulation 71-73, 72f, 73f, 73t
 in metabolic control 51-52, 52f
 in muscle protein synthesis 147
 peptide hormones 125, 127, 127f, 260
 in protein digestion 131
 in relative energy deficiency in sport 378, 378f
 stress 304
 thyroid 204
human energy metabolism. *See* metabolism
human growth hormone (hGH) 260
hunger 333, 357, 376
hydration status. *See also* dehydration; water and fluid intake
 alcohol and 47, 214, 222, 355
 antidiuretic hormone in 197, 216
 assessment of 226-231, 227f, 228f, 229f, 229t-230t, 231t
 blood glucose and 304
 in body composition estimation 272, 277, 278
 body fluid regulation 214-216, 215f
 caffeine and 216, 250
 in children and adolescents 217-218, 350
 cognition and 217, 218, 223, 227, 355, 357
 creatine and 218, 254
 in exercise 217-218, 222-226, 222f, 224f
 fluid needs 213-214
 heat illness and 218, 221
 homeostasis and 212-213, 212f, 213f
 hydration plans 225f, 232-234, 350
 hyperhydration 213, 218, 220-221
 hypohydration 216-218, 222, 223-224, 304-305, 350
 for masters athletes 197, 218, 355
 prehydrating 232
 regulation of fluid balance 214-216, 215f
 rehydrating after exercise 224, 226, 233-234
 in resistance training 304-305, 306
 sodium in 197

sport performance and 222-226, 222f, 224f
sports drinks 221, 232-233, 290
strategies to increase fluid intake 215, 215f
in studying 217
hydrochloric acid 130
hydrodensitometry 273-274
hydrogenation of fats 110, 111f
hydrometry 273
hydrostatic weighing 273-274
hydroxyapatite 184
25-hydroxyvitamin D (25(OH)D) 162. *See also* vitamin D
hypercalcemia 162t, 167t, 189
hyperglycemia 71, 128, 355-358, 356f, 363
hyperhydration 213, 218, 220-221. *See also* hydration status
hyperkalemia 196-197
hypernatremia 221, 231t
hyperparathyroidism 163, 165t, 189
hyperphosphatemia 190
hyperplasia 270
hypertension 191, 195, 324, 364-365. *See also* blood pressure
hypertrophy, muscle 309, 311, 312-314, 316, 338-339
hypoglycemia 71
 in athletes 358-360, 361
 body response to 72
 emergencies in sport 363
 exercise and 72-73, 143
 postprandial 75
 reactive 75
 regulation of 72, 143
 symptoms of 363
 in type 2 diabetes 71, 358-360, 360t
hypohydration 216-218, 222-224, 304-305, 350. *See also* dehydration; hydration status
hypokalemia 192, 196
hyponatremia 213, 218, 220-221, 224, 226
hypophosphatemia 190
hypothyroidism 204

I
IDGT (insulin-dependent glucose transport) 72
"If It Fits Your Macros" (IIFYM) diet 334
IGF-1 (insulin-like growth factor-1) 147, 206, 308f, 325-326
immune system
 alcohol consumption and 220
 antibodies in 125, 126f, 127, 129t
 in autoimmune diseases 83-84
 human gut and 256-257, 318
 inflammation and 147
 iron and 203
 minerals and 201t, 203, 205-206
 probiotics and prebiotics 256-257
 resistance training and 308f
 supplements and 247, 256-258
 in type 1 diabetes 355-356, 356f

immune system *(continued)*
  vaccines and 127
  vitamin A and 156, 159
  vitamin C and 171, 178-179, 257-258, 367
  vitamin D and 161, 165, 257, 296
  zinc and 205
inactivity 11
incomplete protein 134, 135, 141, 371
indirect calorimetry 56-57, 57*f*
industrial trans fatty acids 110-111, 114
infants and babies
  biotin and 174
  calcium and 187
  carbohydrate needs 77
  dietary fat needs 114
  feeding formulas for 138
  folic acid/folate and 167*t*, 174
  obesity risk in 364
  vitamin A and 159
  vitamin D and 160-161, 163, 165
  vitamin E and 170
  vitamin K and 172
inflammation
  arachidonic acid and 106
  carbohydrates and 86
  creatine and muscle soreness 254
  curcumin and 255
  DHA and EPA and 109-110
  fatty acids and 255
  fiber and 82
  magnesium and 193
  muscle protein breakdown and 147, 308*f*
  in obesity 266, 326
  omega-3 fatty acids 255-256
  omega-6 fatty acids and 107*f*
  refined carbohydrates and 86
  in resistance training 308
  trans fatty acids and 111
  visceral fat and 322
  vitamin D and 160
influenza vaccines 127
Informed Choice 243-244
injuries 147
inorganic phosphate 30, 165
insensible perspiration 212, 212*f*
insoluble fiber 66
Institute of Medicine 4-5, 198
insulin. *See also* insulin resistance; insulin sensitivity
  in blood sugar regulation 71-72, 72*f*, 73*f*, 73*t*, 325
  chromium and 206
  in diabetes mellitus 86, 355-359, 356*f*
  diet and 294-295, 361
  endurance sports performance and 294-295
  exercise and 352-353
  fatty acids and 98
  in glucose transport into cells 71-72, 72*f*, 357-358, 362*f*
  in glycogen replenishment 292-293, 292*f*
  glycogen storage and 70, 325
  injections of 359

interesterified fats and 113
magnesium and 191
metabolism and 52*f*
in muscle protein synthesis 147
in obesity 324-325
as peptide hormone 127, 127*f*
in pregnancy 363
sport emergencies and 362-363
insulin-dependent glucose transport (IDGT) 72
insulin-like growth factor-1 (IGF-1) 147, 206, 308*f*, 325-326
insulin resistance. *See also* diabetes mellitus
  exercise by older adults and 351, 352
  magnesium and 191
  obesity and 324-325
  in pregnancy 363-364
  in type 1 and 2 diabetes 355-356, 356*f*, 357
insulin sensitivity
  in athletes with diabetes 362
  caffeine and 293
  cellular transport and 71-72, 357-358
  endurance training and 361
  exercise and 361
  in glycogen replenishment 292
  magnesium and 191
  PUFAs and 103
interesterified fats 112-114
international units (IUs) 159
Internet, evaluating information on 18
inulin 186
iodine 162, 184*t*, 185*t*, 204
iron 202-204
  bioavailability of 372
  calcium and 189
  in children and adolescents 350
  daily value for 185
  dietary reference intake for 184*t*
  in endurance athletes 296
  excess intake 200*t*, 203, 204
  exercise and 204
  functions of 199
  inadequate intake 200*t*, 202-203, 203*f*
  in pregnancy 202, 367-368
  in relative energy deficiency 378
  sources of 200*t*, 202, 202*f*, 372
  in vegan and vegetarian diets 202
  vitamin C and 179
iron-deficiency anemia 22*t*, 202-204, 203*f*, 370
irritable bowel syndrome 296
isoleucine 119*f*, 120, 121*f*
isotopes 57
IUs (international units) 159

J

joint pain 109, 159, 171, 254-255, 260
journals, peer-reviewed 242
juice, gastrointestinal stress from 298

K

keratin 125
ketoacidosis 299, 359
ketogenesis 45, 45*f*, 134

ketogenic diets 45, 104-105, 299-300, 316-318
ketone bodies 45, 45*f*, 357
ketones, in LCHF diets 298-299
ketosis 317
kidneys
  blood pressure and 324
  in diabetes 357
  excess calcium intake and 189
  in filtering blood 214
  in gluconeogenesis 50
kilocalories 4, 52. *See also* calories
Krebs cycle. *See* TCA (tricarboxylic acid) cycle

L

LA (linolenic acid) 97*f*, 98, 106, 107*f*, 114
lactase 69, 69*t*, 82-83, 127
lactate 34, 35*f*, 50, 76, 194
lactate dehydrogenase (LDH) 35, 50
lactic acid 34-36, 76, 283
lacto-ovo-pesco vegetarians 149-150, 150*f*, 369*t*. *See also* vegetarian diets
lactose 65, 84, 84*f*
lactose intolerance 82-83
large intestine (colon) 83
LBM (lean body mass). *See* lean body mass (LBM)
LCHF (low-carbohydrate, high-fat) diet 297-299
LDH (lactate dehydrogenase) 35, 50
LDL (low-density lipoprotein) cholesterol. *See* low-density lipoprotein (LDL) cholesterol
LEA (low energy availability). *See* low energy availability (LEA)
lean body mass (LBM)
  in adolescence 347
  body composition and 271
  in compartment models 271, 272
  creatine and 253, 318, 373
  leucine and 148, 148*t*, 149, 258
  modified ketogenic diet and 317
  protein and 258, 339
  resting metabolic rate and 54-55
  supplements and 258-259, 340
lecithin (phosphatidylcholine) 99
"Leo the Lion Says 'Ger'" mnemonic 29
leptin 329
leucine
  beta-hydroxy-beta-methylbutyrate and 254, 318
  in children and adolescents 312, 313*f*
  in foods 149, 312, 312*f*
  in muscle protein synthesis 148, 148*t*, 258, 312, 313*f*, 314
  in older adults 312, 313*f*, 314
  structure and function of 118, 119*f*, 120, 254
  supplementing protein-poor meals with 137, 314-315
  in weight loss 331
licensure. *See* credentials and certifications
limiting amino acids 139-140, 139*t*

linoleic acid (LA) 97f, 98, 106, 107f, 114
lipases 94, 298
lipid peroxidation 114
lipids. *See also* cholesterol; fat, dietary; fatty acids; triglycerides
   in blood 113, 322, 332
   calories in 4
   classification and functions of 96-97, 96f
   exercising and 352
   oils 5-6, 97, 99f
   phospholipids 94, 96, 96f, 99, 174
   sterols 98-99, 99f
lipogenesis 27f, 51, 70
lipoprotein lipase 94
lipoproteins 129, 129f
"lite"/"light," meaning of 9
liver
   alcohol and 46, 47f
   amino acid cycling and 119, 122, 122f, 131
   in carbohydrate metabolism 39, 70, 70f
   Cori cycle and 50, 51f, 72
   in diabetes 357
   in fat metabolism 45-46
   in gluconeogenesis 50, 51f, 95, 120
   in glucose metabolism 71-72, 73f
   glycerol in 43
   in glycogenesis 50
   in glycogen storage 5, 50, 66, 70-71
   vitamins and 6, 159
low-carbohydrate, high-fat (LCHF) diet 297-299
low-carbohydrate diets 297-299, 316-317, 332-333. *See also* ketogenic diets
low-density lipoprotein (LDL) cholesterol
   anabolic androgenic steroids and 260
   fiber and 82
   functions of 323-324
   health risks from 97-99, 100, 102-102, 318, 323
   processed carbohydrates and 86
   saturated fat intake and 100, 101t, 102-105
   trans fatty acid intake and 101t, 111-112
low energy availability (LEA). *See also* disordered eating
   bone density and 189
   calcium needs in 372
   calculation of 346
   in children and adolescents 344, 346
   in disordered eating 377, 378-379, 378f, 379f, 380t
   in female athlete triad 59, 377, 377f, 378f, 379f
   low body fat and 326
   muscle protein breakdown in 147
low-fat diets 332
luminal brush border 131, 132f
luo han guo (monk fruit) 88, 90t
lupin kernel fiber 83, 331
lysine 133, 139t

M

macrocytic (megaloblastic) anemia 174, 364, 367
macrominerals 6, 184-199. *See also* names of individual macrominerals
macronutrients 4. *See also* carbohydrate; fat, dietary; proteins
magnesium 191-195
   elemental 191-192
   excess intake 193, 193f, 201t
   exercise and 193-195, 221
   functions of 191, 318
   inadequate intake 191, 192-193, 193f, 201t
   intake recommendations 184t
   in laxatives 194
   sources of 191-192, 192f, 201t
   in sweat 221, 221f
malabsorption syndromes
   in celiac disease 172
   pyridoxine and 177
   vitamin D and 163
   vitamin E and 170
   vitamin K and 172
male athletes. *See* men and boys
maltase 69, 69t
maltose 65, 69, 85
manganese 184t, 185t, 204
marathon runners 13, 38, 76, 179, 287, 338t
marijuana 260-261
masters athletes 351-355. *See also* older adults
   body weight in 353
   cardiovascular and metabolic health 351-352
   cognitive function 353
   definition of 351
   energy needs 352, 353
   exercise in 351
   high-impact exercise in 352
   musculoskeletal health 352-353
   nutrition needs 353-355, 354t
maximal oxygen consumption ($\dot{V}O_2$max) 11-12, 352
MCTs (medium-chain triglycerides) 94
mechanical digestion 68
medical nutrition therapy (MNT) 7, 360
Medication Health Fraud website 244-245
Mediterranean diet 105, 354
medium-chain triglycerides (MCTs) 94
megaloblastic (macrocytic) anemia 174-175, 177, 178, 367
melanin, vitamin D and 163
men and boys
   alcohol and 309
   body fat percentages for 272t
   fluid needs in 213
   growth spurts in adolescence 347
   minerals in 184t
   relative energy deficiency in sport 59
   resting metabolic rate in 54
menaquinones 171

mercury, in fish 108
mesomorphs 270
messenger RNA (mRNA) 133-134, 133f
metabolic adaptations
   protein and 148, 148t
   from training 47-50, 48f, 301
   from weight loss 329-330
metabolic fatigue 76-77, 250, 283
metabolic syndrome 87, 88, 355-356. *See also* diabetes mellitus
metabolism 26-60. *See also* energy systems
   advantages of training on 47-50, 48f
   of alcohol 27, 28, 46-47, 47f, 51
   biosynthesis and storage pathways 50-51, 51f
   of carbohydrate 38-42, 40f, 41f, 42f, 42t
   cell structures for ATP production 28, 28f
   in children 344
   definition 26
   in diabetes 356-358, 358f
   dietary nitrates and 49
   endurance training effects on 301
   energy availability 32-33, 286
   energy transfer of ATP 30-31, 30f
   of fats 32, 37f
   hormonal control of 51-52, 52f
   measuring energy intake and expenditure 52-60, 53f, 55t, 56f, 56t, 57f
   metabolic pathways 26-27, 27f
   of monosaccharides 65, 65f, 69, 69t
   in older adults 54-55, 353
   of omega-3 fatty acids 107f
   in pregnancy 365
   of protein in exercise 142-144, 143f
   regulation of glucose 71-73, 72f, 73f
   resting metabolic rate 54-55, 327, 329, 335, 353
   thermic effect of food 55, 353
D-methamphetamine 259
methionine 46, 119f, 120, 121f, 137
methylmercury 108, 108f
methylphenidate 259
microcytic (megaloblastic) anemia 174-175, 177, 178, 367
micronutrients. *See also* minerals; vitamins
   for children and adolescents 350
   in disordered eating 378
   for endurance athletes 4, 296
   on food labels 8, 1736
   for masters athletes 354-355
   in pregnancy 366
   recommendations on 6, 8, 354-355
   in vegetarian diets 370372
microvilli 69, 69f
Middle Eastern athletes 163
Mifflin–St. Jeor equation 327
milk. *See* dairy products
milk allergy 83
MIND diet 354
mindful eating 333

Index 459

minerals 184-209. *See also names of individual nutrients*
  chelated 206
  deficiencies 175f, 187-189
  on food labels 173, 173f
  functions 6, 184-185, 191, 352, 353
  ideal menus 207f
  intake recommendations 184t, 185t
  macrominerals 6, 184-199
  for masters athletes 354-355
  monitoring intake 191
  protein transporters of 125, 129t
  sources 67, 139, 162
  supplements 208, 238
  trace 199, 200t-201t, 202-208, 202f, 203f
  in vegan and vegetarian diets 207f, 372
  in vegetarian diets 149
mitochondria
  in aerobic system 35, 36, 45-46
  in anaerobic system 34-36
  athletic performance and 47-48, 48f
  in endurance exercise 142, 144, 286
  fat breakdown in 43-45, 43f
  at high altitude 38
  in metabolic pathways 26
  obesity and 325
  structure of 28, 28f, 42f
  TCA cycle in 40-41, 40f, 143
MNT (medical nutrition therapy) 7, 360
modeling, bone 188
molybdenum 184t
monosaccharides 65, 65f, 69, 69t
monounsaturated fatty acids (MUFA) 97-98, 97f, 101t, 105
mouth rinsing 295
MPB (muscle protein breakdown) 146-147, 308-309, 308f
MPS (muscle protein synthesis). *See* muscle protein synthesis (MPS)
mRNA (messenger RNA) 133-134, 133f
mTORC1 pathway 312
MUFA (monounsaturated fatty acids) 97-98, 97f, 101t, 105
multigrain foods 67
multivitamin supplements 177, 192, 204, 205, 208
muscle hypertrophy 309, 311, 312-314, 316, 338-339
muscle mass
  body composition measures 271-273
  carbohydrate needs 339-340
  in diabetes 361
  energy needs for 31-32, 79, 335, 338-339
  gaining 338-341
  glycogen storage and 71
  hydration status and 125, 213
  in older adults 304, 309, 312, 352, 353-354
  omega-3 fatty acids and 109-110
  protein and 142, 144, 258, 286-287, 312, 339
  sports supplements in 34, 260, 318, 340

  in weight loss 330-331, 336
muscle protein balance 308-310, 310f
muscle protein breakdown (MPB) 146-147, 308-309, 308f
muscle protein synthesis (MPS)
  alcohol and 261, 309
  amino acids in 122, 122f, 132-134
  branched chain amino acids in 118, 143, 147, 254, 258, 308f
  concurrent training and 311
  endurance training and 286-287
  factors affecting 146-148
  food-based protein sources and 137-139, 148, 149, 312f
  gene expression in 133-134, 133f
  in ketogenic diets 317
  leucine in 148, 148t, 258, 312, 313f, 314
  meal patterns and 312-314
  muscle protein breakdown in 309
  in protein-poor meals 314-315
  protein timing and 145-146, 149, 309-310, 312-314, 313f, 331
  protein type and 138
  in resistance exercise 146-147, 308-310, 308f, 310f, 335-336
  in restricted-calorie diets 315-318
muscles. *See also* muscle mass; skeletal muscle
  after endurance training 286-287
  after resistance training 308-310, 308f, 310f
  atrophy 304, 309
  Cori cycle and 50, 51f
  daily dietary intake and 311-315, 312f, 313f
  in diabetes 311-315, 312f, 361, 573f
  exercise fatigue in 76-77
  fast-twitch muscle fibers 165
  glucose in 32, 39, 76, 76t
  magnesium and 194, 318
  meal patterns and 312-314
  metabolic pathways and fatigue 36, 38, 50
  muscle hypertrophy 309, 311, 312-314, 316, 338-339
  net muscle protein balance 308-310, 310f
  nutrients that support 193f
  size of 306, 309
  soreness 76, 110, 170, 180, 254
  strength of 12, 168, 304, 306, 309, 318
  training-induced fatigue in 13
muscular dystrophy 253
muscular endurance 12
muscular flexibility 12
muscular power 12
myoglobin 199
MyPlate 9-10, 9f

N

NADH (nicotinamide adenine dinucleotide). *See* nicotinamide adenine dinucleotide (NADH)

National Commission for Certifying Agencies (NCCA) 20
National Strength and Conditioning Association (NSCA) 20
"natural," meaning of 86-87, 246, 258
NEAT (nonexercise activity thermogenesis) 55, 329, 335
neotame 88, 89t
net protein utilization (NPU) 138t, 141
niacin 166t-167t, 174, 175, 366
nicotinamide adenine dinucleotide (NADH)
  in ATP synthesis 29, 29f
  in energy from alcohol 47f
  in energy from carbohydrate 39-41, 40f, 41f, 42f
  in energy from fat 44, 44f
  in glycolysis 35, 35f, 39
  in lipogenesis 51
night eating syndrome 376. *See also* disordered eating
nitrates, dietary 49, 251, 252
nitric oxide 198, 251-252
nitric oxide synthase (eNOS) 251
nitrogen balance assessment 134-135
NNS (nonnutritive sweeteners) 87-88, 89t-90t
nonessential amino acids 119, 120, 134, 138
nonexercise activity thermogenesis (NEAT) 55, 329, 335
non-heme iron 179, 202
nonmedical nutrition therapy 21-23, 22t
nonnutritive sweeteners (NNS) 87-88, 89t-90t
nonproteinogenic amino acids 120
norepinephrine 72, 304
NPU (net protein utilization) 138t, 141
NSAIDs (nonsteroidal anti-inflammatory drugs) 175, 197, 203, 254
NSCA (National Strength and Conditioning Association) 20
NSF International 243
nucleus, cell 28, 28f
nutrient absorption 15-16. *See also* cell transporters; malabsorption syndromes
  of calcium 186-187, 186f, 189
  of carbohydrate 68-69, 69t, 289-290, 290f
  chewing and 171
  competition for 133
  facilitated diffusion 131, 132f, 290f
  of fat 94
  of glucose 69, 356-357
  of iron 372
  of protein 131, 132f
  of zinc 186-187
nutrient content claims 8, 240
nutrient density 365
nutrients, definition of 4
nutrigenomics 304
nutrition 4. *See also* sports nutrition
  credentials and certifications 18-23, 20f, 22t

evaluating sources of 17-18
evidence-based practice 16
on food labels 7-9, 8f
food safety and inspection 7
guidelines 6-11
ideal menus 207f
individualization in 300
medical nutrition therapy 7
MyPlate 9-10, 9f
nutrient groups 4
Nutrition Facts panel 8, 82, 82f, 173, 293f
nutritive sugars 85-87
for older adults 353-354, 354t
peer-reviewed journals 242
pregnancy and 364-366, 366t
scientific evidence in 16, 17f, 18
verification and seal programs and 243-244
Whole Grain Stamp 67
nutritional supplements. *See* supplements
nutrition education 9-10
Nutrition Facts panel 8, 8f, 82, 82f, 173, 293f
nutritionists. *See* credentials and certifications
nutrition periodization 16, 145, 300, 354, 360, 365
nutritive sweeteners 85-87
nuts 152t, 156, 170f, 191, 204, 335

O

obesity and overweight
  athletes and 335-336, 338
  body fat patterns 270-271, 270f
  in childhood and adolescence 7, 347, 348, 350
  definition of 266, 269-270, 269t, 272t
  diet and 86, 103, 136, 198, 317
  fitness and 326
  genetics and environment in 12
  health impacts of 105, 111, 266, 322, 325-326
  high-fructose corn syrup and 86-87
  inflammation and 266
  insulin resistance in 324-325
  in metabolic syndrome 87, 88, 355-356
  mortality and 322
  muscle mass and 331
  in older adults 353
  in pregnancy 364, 364t
  rise in prevalence of 322, 323f
  skinfold measurements and 275-277, 276f
  sodium and blood pressure in 198-199
  type 2 diabetes and 324-325, 356
  vitamin D and 163
  weight loss in 329, 332-335, 337f
OGTT (oral glucose tolerance test) 71
oils 5-6, 97, 99f. *See also* fat, dietary
older adults
  beta-hydroxy-beta-methylbutyrate and 254, 318
  body mass index of 269, 353
  bone density of 188, 275, 352-353
  calcium in 189, 354-355
  cardiovascular and metabolic health of 351-352
  cognitive function in 353
  creatine monohydrate in 318, 340
  dehydration in 197, 217-218, 355
  energy needs 353
  exercise benefits 11-12, 341, 351-352, 353
  fluid balance in 197, 355
  leucine needs 312, 313f, 314
  magnesium in 194.192
  metabolic syndrome in 198
  metabolism in 54-55, 353
  muscle mass in 304, 309, 312, 352, 353-354
  muscle protein synthesis in 312
  musculoskeletal health of 352-353
  nutrition needs 353-355, 354t
  obesity in 353
  omega-3 fatty acids in 109-110
  protein needs 6, 258, 312, 354
  resting metabolic rate in 54-55
  sarcopenia in 304, 309, 312, 352-353
  sodium in 197
  supplement use by 238
  thiamine in 176
  thirst response in 197, 218
  vitamin B_{12} in 178
  vitamin D in 163-164, 318, 355
oleic acid 101t, 105
oligomenorrhea 377
oligosaccharides 65
omega-3 polyunsaturated fatty acids. *See also* docosahexaenoic acid (DHA); eicosapentaenoic acid (EPA)
  food sources of 255
  functions of 105, 255-256
  health effects of 107-110, 108f
  metabolism of 107, 107f
  structure of 97-98, 97f, 106-107, 107f
  supplements 105, 110, 255-256
  traumatic brain injury and 110, 256
omega-6 polyunsaturated fatty acids 97-98, 97f, 105, 106, 107f
ORAC (oxygen radical absorbance capacity) 169
oral glucose tolerance test (OGTT) 71
organelles 38
ornithine 119f
OSFED (Other Specified Feeding or Eating Disorders) 376-377
osmolarity 199, 214, 226
osteoarthritis 171
osteoporosis 172, 187-188, 187f, 352
Other Specified Feeding or Eating Disorders (OSFED) 376-377
OTS (overtraining syndrome) 15, 15f, 300, 301
overhydration 218. *See also* hydration status
overload principle 13
overreaching 14-15, 300
overtraining 14-15, 15f
overtraining syndrome (OTS) 15, 15f, 300, 301
overweight. *See* obesity and overweight
oxalates/oxalic acid 149, 186, 186f
oxaloacetate 40, 45
oxidative decarboxylation 28-29, 29f, 38, 40
oxidative phosphorylation 28, 29f, 32f, 41, 42t
oxidative stress 159, 206, 208
oxygen availability
  in carbohydrate metabolism 33, 36, 37f, 38-39
  in fatty acid oxidation 45-46, 283
  in training 40-41, 45
oxygen radical absorbance capacity (ORAC) 169

P

palm kernel oil 97, 113, 156
PALs (physical activity levels) 7
pancreas 69, 69t, 72, 355-356
pancreatic amylase 69, 69t
pantothenic acid (vitamin B_5) 166t-167t, 174, 175
Parkinsonism, manganese-induced 204
Parkinson's disease 34
PCr (phosphocreatine) 31-32, 34
PDC (pyruvate dehydrogenase complex) 39
PDCAAS (protein digestibility corrected amino acid score) 138t, 141, 151
peak bone mass 188, 347
pea protein 312f
peer-reviewed journals 242
pellagra 175
pepsin 131
pepsinogen 131
peptide bonds 118, 123-125, 123f, 133
peptide hormones 127, 127f, 260
PER (protein efficiency ratio) 138t, 141
percent daily value (%DV) 8, 173f, 185t
performance. *See* sport performance
performance-enhancing supplements. *See* supplements, nutritional and sport
periodized training programs 13, 14f, 145, 338
peripheral neuropathy 170
pernicious anemia 177-178
personality, eating disorders and 16
perspiration, insensible 212, 213f, 232
pH, blood 128
phenylalanine 89t, 118, 119-120, 119f
phosphagen system (ATP-PC system) 12, 31-32, 32f, 33-34, 33f, 36
phosphocreatine (PCr) 31-32, 34
phospholipids 94, 96, 96f, 99, 174
phosphorus 163, 184t, 187, 190-191, 190f, 201t
photosynthesis 64
physical activity. *See* exercise
Physical Activity Guidelines for Americans 11

physical activity levels (PALs) 7
physical fitness components 11-12
phytates/phytic acid 149, 186, 202
pica 178
PINES (Professionals in Nutrition for Exercise and Sport) 20
piperine 255
plant-based diets 137. *See also* vegetarian diets
plant sterols 99
plaque in arteries 99, 114, 171, 324, 324f
plasma osmolarity 199, 214, 226
polydipsia 357, 358f
polyols 84, 87
polypeptides 123-125, 131
polyphagia 357, 358f
polyphenols 202, 251, 257
polysaccharides 65. *See also* fiber; glycogen; starch
polyunsaturated fatty acids (PUFA) 105-110. *See also* omega-3 polyunsaturated fatty acids
　cell membranes and 106, 106f
　food sources of 101t, 107-109
　functions of 105
　health effects of 102-103, 106-110
　omega-6 fatty acids 97-98, 97f, 105, 106, 107f
　structure of 97-98, 97f, 107f
polyuria 357, 358f
population-specific body composition methods 273
portal vein 130-131, 130f, 132f
portion sizes 8, 10
postprandial hypoglycemia 75
potassium 185t, 195-198, 199, 201t, 221, 223
practice exclusivity 21
prebiotics 257
preformed vitamin A 156, 159
pregnancy 363-368
　anemia in 365, 367
　B vitamins in 174-175, 366-367
　carbohydrate needs in 77
　DXA and 274-275
　exercise in 363, 364
　fish consumption in 108
　folate in 174-175
　gestational diabetes in 363-364
　iron in 202, 367-368
　minerals in 184t
　multiple babies 365, 367
　nutrient needs 364-366, 366t
　physiological changes in 363-364
　vitamins in 174-175, 208, 367
　water intake in 213
　weight distribution in 367
　weight gain in 364-365, 364t
primary protein structure 124, 124f
principle of detraining 13-14, 48
principle of periodization 13, 14f, 145
principle of specificity 13
probiotics 256-257
processed foods 205
proenzymes 131

Professionals in Nutrition for Exercise and Sport (PINES) 20
prolamins 83
proline 118-120, 119f, 121f
proprietary blends 246
prostate cancer 170, 266, 369
protease activation cascade 131
protein digestibility corrected amino acid score (PDCAAS) 138t, 141, 151
protein efficiency ratio (PER) 138t, 141
proteinogenic amino acids 118
protein powder 135, 139
protein pumps 129
proteins 118-152. *See also* amino acids; cell transporters; muscle protein synthesis (MPS); *names of individual proteins*
　absorption of 131, 132f
　amino acid pool 122, 122f, 132-122
　animal 111-112, 111t, 137, 149, 349
　as antibodies 125, 126f, 127, 129t
　in athletes 144-146, 145t
　in body structure 120, 125, 255
　calcium and 187
　calories per gram 4
　catabolism of 27f, 120-122, 121f, 134, 151
　as cell transporters. *See* cell transporters
　chemical energy from 46
　for children and adolescents 310, 312, 349-350
　complementary 137-138, 148, 370
　conformational changes in 124
　daily distribution of 146, 149
　deficiency and excess 151
　denaturation 127
　diabetes and 360-361
　dietary recommendations 6, 135-137
　digestion 130-131, 130f
　for endurance athletes 286-287, 291, 293
　as enzymes 125-127, 126f
　in fluid maintenance 128, 128f
　formation of 123-125, 124f
　functions 6, 125-130, 126f, 127f, 128f, 129f, 129t
　in ketogenic diets 317
　lipoproteins 129, 129f
　for losing fat and gaining muscle 340-341
　maximum usable amount 315
　metabolic fate of 132-135, 133f
　metabolism in exercise 32, 142-144, 143f
　muscle mass and 339-341
　muscle metabolic adaptation and 148, 148t
　nitrogen balance technique 134-135
　nutrients in sources of 152t
　older adults and 312, 354, 354t
　overfeeding 94
　oxidation of 143-144
　as peptide hormones 125, 127, 127f, 260

　periodization of 145, 354, 365
　in pregnancy 366, 366t
　quality of 122-123, 137-142, 138t, 139t
　recommended intake 145-146, 145t, 315
　in resistance training 304, 306, 309-310, 310f, 314-315
　satiety and 331
　sources of 6, 122-123, 123t, 149, 152t
　storage of 313
　structure of 123-125, 123f, 124f
　timing of 145-146, 149, 309-310, 312-314, 313f, 331
　vegetarian and vegan sources 122-123, 369-370
　in weight loss 315-318, 330-331
protein synthesis. *See* muscle protein synthesis
proton motive force 41
provitamin A carotenoids 156, 158-160, 158f
pubertal age 347
PUFA (polyunsaturated fatty acids). *See* polyunsaturated fatty acids (PUFA)
purging behavior/disorder 375, 376. *See also* disordered eating
pyridoxine (vitamin B_6) 166t-167t, 174, 177, 354
pyrophosphate 30
pyruvate
　in the aerobic system 37f, 38-39
　in amino acid breakdown 121f
　in the anaerobic system 34-35
　in ATP formation 28-29, 29f
　in carbohydrate breakdown 40-41, 40f, 41f
　in fat breakdown 43
　in gluconeogenesis 50, 51f, 143
　in protein catabolism 134
pyruvate dehydrogenase complex (PDC) 39

Q

quackery 17
quaternary protein structure 124f, 125

R

RAE (retinal activity equivalents) 159
Raynaud's phenomenon 259
RDN (registered dietitian nutritionist) 7, 18, 20-21, 84, 331, 361
reactive hypoglycemia 75
recommended dietary allowance (RDA) 5, 5f, 6
　for carbohydrate 77
　for fiber 77-78
　for protein 135-136
　for vitamin A 159
　for vitamin D 164
recovery from training
　alcohol and 47, 261
　antioxidants in 180, 296
　caffeine in 293
　cannabidiol in 261
　carbohydrates in 298, 349, 349t

creatine in 254
diabetes and 361-362, 363
gelatin plus vitamin C in 255
milk in 83
minerals in 193-194
multifaceted approach 300, 301
nitric oxide in 251
omega-3 fatty acids in 109-110, 256
protein in 360
vitamins in 156, 160, 168, 170
water in 234, 355
red blood cell magnesium 193f
RED-S (relative energy deficiency in sport) 59, 334, 377, 378f, 379f
REE (resting energy expenditure) 54-55
refined carbohydrates 86, 102, 136
registered dietitian nutritionist (RD or RDN) 7, 18, 20-21, 84, 331, 361
relative energy deficiency in sport (RED-S) 59, 334, 377, 378f, 379f
resistance training 303-319
   alcohol and 309
   carbohydrates in 305, 306-307, 307f, 309, 349
   concurrent training 311
   daily dietary intake 311-315, 312f, 313f
   glycogen replenishment 305, 306, 307f
   hydration 304-305
   ketogenic diets 316-318
   leucine in 308f, 311, 312, 312f, 313f, 314-315
   for losing fat and gaining muscle 340-341
   low-carbohydrate diets 316
   magnesium and 318
   muscle protein synthesis in 146-147, 308-310, 308f, 310f, 335-336
   nutrition after 306, 309-311
   nutrition before 304-306
   by older adults 352
   overload principle in 13
   protein in 308f, 309-310, 310f, 314-315
   protein oxidation in 142-144
   protein timing 146, 313-314, 313f
   recommendations for adults 11
   recovery from 300
   restricted-calorie diets and 315-316
   strength-training gains 309
   supplements for 253-254, 318, 340
   vitamin D and 318
   in weight loss 335-336
   zinc and 318
resorption, bone 188
resting cardiac output 363
resting energy expenditure (REE) 54-55
resting metabolic rate (RMR) 54-55, 327, 329, 335, 353
retinal activity equivalents (RAE) 159
retinoids 156, 159-160
retinol 156, 159, 367
reversibility principle 48
rhabdomyolysis 221, 230t
riboflavin (vitamin B$_2$) 166t-167t, 174, 175-176, 176f, 366
ribonucleic acid (RNA) 133, 133f

ribosomal RNA (rRNA) 134
ribosomes 133-134, 133f
rickets 163, 188, 190, 201, 367
RMR (resting metabolic rate) 54-55, 327, 329, 335, 353
RNA (ribonucleic acid) 133, 133f
rRNA (ribosomal RNA) 134
rule of five 67
ruminant trans fatty acids 111-112, 111t

S
saccharin 88, 89t
salivary amylase 68
salt 198-199, 204, 226. *See also* sodium
salt sensitivity 198
sarcopenia, age-related 304, 309, 312, 352-353
satiety 66, 83, 151, 315, 330-331
saturated fatty acids 100-105
   blood cholesterol and 102, 104-105
   in cell membranes 106, 106f
   children and adolescents and 344
   food sources of 100, 101t
   health effects of 98, 100-102, 356
   interesterified fats and 112-114
   LDL cholesterol and 100, 101t, 102-105
   replacement strategies 102-104, 102f, 103f
   structure of 97-98, 97f, 106f
   types of 101t
scientific method 16, 17f
scope of practice 21-23, 22t. *See also* credentials and certifications
SDA (stearidonic acid) 101t, 106-107
secondary protein structure 124, 124f
secondary sexual characteristics 347, 348f
secondhand smoke 324
secretin 131
SEE (standard error of the estimate) 274, 275, 277
selenium 184t, 206, 208
serine 99, 119-120, 119f, 121f
serum osmolality 226
serving sizes 7-8, 8f, 293
set point theory 267
sexual assaults, alcohol and 261
SHPN (Sports and Human Performance Nutrition) 20
sickle cell trait 217
significant scientific agreement (SSA) standard 240-241
simple carbohydrate 64, 65, 65f
simple sugars 65
six-compartment body composition model 273
skeletal muscle
   ATP in contraction of 38, 64
   breakdown and repair of 120, 134, 146
   in detraining 48
   dietary nitrate and 49
   dietary protein and 149
   fat breakdown by 94-95
   glucose uptake by 72, 77
   glycogen storage in 66, 70, 71

in older adults 304, 309, 312, 352-353
   in overtraining 15f
   rhabdomyolysis 221, 230t
skin cancer 161
skinfold thickness 275-277, 276f
sleep apnea 326
small intestine 68f
   carbohydrate digestion in 68-69, 69f, 69t
   fat digestion in 94, 127
   protein digestion in 130f, 131
smoking 103, 147, 158f, 220, 324
sodium
   blood pressure and 197-199
   exercise and 199, 221, 234
   hypernatremia 221, 231t
   hyponatremia 213, 218, 220-221, 224, 226
   intake recommendations 184t, 197-199
   in ketogenic diets 318
   potassium and 195
   sources of 198
   in sweat 221, 221f, 234
sodium bicarbonate 250
sodium nitrate 252
sodium–potassium pumps 129, 132f
soft drinks 85-86, 190, 349
soluble fibers 66
soy proteins 137, 141, 149, 201, 307
specificity principle 13, 47
sport performance. *See also* training
   alcohol use 47, 261, 309
   arginine 252
   BCAA 143
   benefits of training on 47-50, 48f
   body composition and 16, 267-268, 270, 271, 278-279
   body fat percentage and 326, 338, 338t
   B vitamins 173-178
   caffeine and energy drinks 248-249, 293
   calcium 191
   carbohydrate loading 287, 316
   carbohydrates 80, 80t, 284, 285t, 287-288, 291
   carbohydrate types 294-295
   by children and adolescents 347, 347f, 349-350, 349t
   concurrent training and 311
   creatine 252-253, 254
   diabetes and 359-360, 360t
   disordered eating and 373, 376-379, 378f, 379f
   electrolytes and 221, 222-226, 222f, 223f, 224f
   fat loading 297
   gastrointestinal distress and 296, 298, 376, 377-379, 379f
   glycogen replacement 306
   high-fat, low carbohydrate diet 95-96, 95f
   human growth hormone 260
   hydration status and 216, 222-226, 222f, 223f, 224f, 304-305

sport performance *(continued)*
　insulin and 294-295
　iron 200t, 203-204
　ketogenic diets 45, 104, 299-300, 316-317
　low-carbohydrate diets 316
　magnesium 192, 193-194
　marijuana 261
　in masters athletes 352, 354-355
　metabolic adaptations from training 47-50, 48f, 297
　minerals 184
　mouth rinsing 295
　muscle mass and 130, 340
　nitric oxide boosters 251
　omega-3 fatty acids 255-256
　overreaching and overtraining and 300-301
　in pregnancy 363-364, 367
　protein role in 129-130, 135-136, 142-146, 149, 315
　RED-S and 60, 334, 377, 379f
　sodium bicarbonate 250
　stimulants 294-295259
　vegetarian and vegan diets 151, 368-369, 370, 372-373
　vitamin A 160
　vitamin C 179, 180
　vitamin D 165, 169
　vitamin E 170-171
　vitamins and 156
　wearable activity monitors and 59
　zinc 206
Sports and Human Performance Nutrition (SHPN) 20
sports drinks 221, 232-233, 290. *See also* energy drinks
sports nutrition 15-18. *See also* nutrition; supplements, nutritional and sport
　credentials and certifications in 18-21
　diabetes and 360-362, 362f
　energy demands for different sports 285, 285t, 328t
　evidence-based practice in 16
　general principles in 15-16
　glycemic index and load 73-75, 75t
　guidelines for athletes 10-11
　for older adults 353-354, 354t
　periodization in 16, 145, 300, 354, 360, 365
　pregnancy and 364-366, 366t
　reputable information sources 17-18, 20
　scientific evidence in 16-17, 17f
　scope of practice 21-23, 22t
　third-party certification 242-244
sports-related concussions (traumatic brain injury) 34, 104, 109-110, 254, 256, 261
SSA (significant scientific agreement) standard 240-241
standard error of the estimate (SEE) 274, 275, 277
standard of identity 162
starch 65-66, 67f

starvation, glucose in 45, 46, 143, 357
stearidonic acid (SDA) 101t, 106-107
sterols 98-99, 99f. *See also* cholesterol
Stevia rebaudiana (Bertoni) 88, 90t
stimulants 52-53, 248, 259
St. John's wort 258
stomach 130-131, 130f
stress fractures 169
stress hormones 304
stroke 100, 108, 160, 195-196, 356
stroke volume 48, 216-217
structure/function claims 241
subcutaneous fat 322
substrate fatigue 76-77, 282, 283, 286
sucralose 88, 89t
sucrase 69, 69t
sucrose 65, 65f, 69, 87, 295
sugar alcohols 87
sugars 65, 65f, 85-86. *See also names of individual sugars*
suicide, alcohol and 261
sulfur 199, 255
sunscreens, vitamin D and 163
superstarch 295
supplements, nutritional and sport 247-259. *See also* drugs in sports
　adverse reaction reports 241
　alcohol use and 261, 309
　amphetamines 259
　anabolic androgenic steroids 259-260
　antioxidants 158-159, 296
　beetroot juice 198, 251-252
　beta-alanine 250-251
　beta-carotene 160
　beta-hydroxy-beta-methylbutyrate 254, 318
　biotin 174
　body composition and 16, 258-259
　branched chain amino acids 143, 254, 258
　caffeine and energy drinks 238, 239, 247-250, 249f, 293
　calcium 186, 372
　carnitine 43
　for children and adolescents 345-346, 350-351
　chitosan and glucomannan 259
　chondroitin sulfate 254-255
　choosing 245-246
　chromium 206
　claims for 240-241
　competitive athletes and 245
　conjugated linoleic acid 112, 259
　contraindications for 258
　creatine 34, 238, 247, 252-254, 318, 373
　creatine monohydrate 318, 340
　curcumin 255
　dehydration and 218
　DHA 109, 110
　dietary supplement definition 238-239
　disordered eating and 376, 377-379, 379f
　to enhance immunity 256-258
　EPA 109, 110

　evaluation of 241-246
　fish oil 117
　folic acid/folate 367
　glucosamine 254-255
　glycerol 43, 94, 98
　green tea 259
　insulin and 294-295
　iron 203-204
　labels for 242, 244
　leucine 258
　marketing 239
　metabolic adaptations and 47-50, 48f
　minerals as 184, 193-194, 203-204, 206
　mouth rinsing and 295
　multivitamins 208
　"natural" 86-87, 246, 258
　nitric oxide boosters 251-252
　omega-3 fatty acids 105, 110, 255-256
　for pain and inflammation 253-256
　phosphocreatine 34
　probiotics 256-257
　proprietary blends 246
　protein powder 135, 139
　quality assurance 242-245
　RED-S and 60
　regulation of 238-241
　for resistance training 253-254, 318, 340
　resources on 242-245
　safety of 239
　sodium bicarbonate 250
　stimulants 259
　superstarch or waxy maize 295
　Supplement Facts panel 240, 240f, 242
　vegetarian diets and 368-369
　vitamins and 156, 160, 165, 176
　vitamin A 160
　vitamin B$_{12}$ 179, 180
　vitamin C 179, 180, 255, 257-258
　vitamin D 161, 162, 165, 165t, 257-258, 318, 355
　vitamin E 170
　vitamin K 172
　zinc 186, 205, 257-258
sweating
　body temperature and 6, 212, 219f
　in children 218, 350
　cystic fibrosis and 199
　electrolytes and 197, 212, 221, 221f
　estimating water loss in 225f, 226, 228-229, 229f
　hydration status and 6, 216-218, 222-224
　loss during sports 221f, 223-224, 224f
　micronutrient loss in 296
　in pregnancy 363
sweat patches 226, 229

T

table sugar. *See* sucrose
TAC (total antioxidant capacity) 169
tanning beds, vitamin D and 161
taurine 135
TBW (total body water) 272-273

TCA (tricarboxylic acid) cycle
   anaerobic system and 34-36, 35f
   ATP production from 28-29, 29f
   carbohydrate catabolism and 40-41, 40f
   endurance training and 38
   fat catabolism and 44
   location of 28
   metabolic pathways 27f
   protein catabolism and 46, 120-121, 121f
TEA (thermic effect of activity) 54, 55
TEE (total energy expenditure) 54, 55-59, 56f, 56t, 57f, 353
TEF (thermic effect of food) 55, 353
tertiary protein structure 124, 124f
testosterone 147, 309
tetrahydrocannabinol (THC) 260
thermic effect of activity (TEA) 54, 55
thermic effect of food (TEF) 55, 353
thiamin (vitamin B_1) 7, 166t-167t, 174, 176-177, 177f, 366
third-party certification 242-244
thirst mechanism 197, 214-216, 218, 222, 355, 357
three-compartment body composition model 272-273
threonine 139t
thyroid, iodine and 204-295
tolerable upper intake level (UL) 5, 5f, 10
total antioxidant capacity (TAC) 169
total body water (TBW) 272-273
total energy expenditure (TEE) 54, 55-59, 56f, 56t, 57f, 353
trace minerals. *See also names of individual trace minerals*
training
   aerobic capacity and 48-50
   detraining 13-14, 48
   diabetes and 358-359
   at high altitudes 38, 217
   metabolic adaptations from 47-50, 48f, 301
   overload principle in 13
   overreaching 14, 300
   overtraining 14-15, 15f, 300, 301
   oxygen availability and 40-41, 45
   periodization principle in 13, 14f, 145
   in pregnancy 365-366
   principles of 12-15
   protein needs in 136, 306, 308f, 309-310, 310f, 314-315
   recovery from 109-110, 168-170, 180, 251, 254-255, 293, 300
   specificity principle in 13
   training load, in children 346
   training low 284, 297-299
   training the gut 290
training low, competing high diet 297-299
transamination 143
trans configuration 98, 98f
trans fatty acids 96f, 101t, 110-114, 111f, 111t
transfer RNA (tRNA) 133f, 134

traumatic brain injury (concussion) 34, 104, 109-110, 254, 256, 261
tricarboxylic cycle. *See* TCA (tricarboxylic acid) cycle
triglycerides. *See also* polyunsaturated fatty acids (PUFA); saturated fatty acids
   breakdown of 42-43, 44
   in chylomicrons 94
   classification of 96f
   EPA and DHA effect on 108
   in fat loading 207
   formation of 51-52, 52f, 70, 94
   health and 99-100
   interesterified fats and 112-113
   medium-chain 94
   obesity and 322-323
   sources of 96-97, 99, 99f
   structure of 97-98, 97f
   trans fatty acids and 96f, 101t, 110-114, 111f, 111t
   use of stored 94-95, 297
tRNA (transfer RNA) 133f, 134
trypsin 131
tryptophan 118, 119f, 120, 121f
turmeric 255
24-hour dietary recalls 100
two-compartment body composition model 272
type 1 diabetes mellitus. *See also* diabetes mellitus
   blood sugar regulation 359-360, 360t, 361
   carbohydrate availability in 45
   cause of 72
   hyperglycemia in 355-356, 356f
   nutrition for 360-362, 362f, 367
   symptoms and diagnosis of 358, 359t
   treatment for 357
type 2 diabetes mellitus 355-363. *See also* diabetes mellitus
   blood sugar management 356, 358-359
   body mass index and 269
   cause of 72
   chromium and 206
   exercise in 39, 352, 358-359
   high-fiber diets and 83
   hyperglycemia in 355
   hypoglycemia in 71, 358-360, 360t
   magnesium and 191-192
   metabolic syndrome and 355-358, 356f, 358f
   nutrition for 360-362, 362f
   obesity and 266, 324-325, 356
   in older adults 352
   polyunsaturated fatty acids and 103
   pregnancy and 363-364
   prevalence of 355, 356
   sugar intake and 87
   symptoms of 358
tyrosine 118-120, 119f, 120f

U

UL (tolerable upper intake level) 5, 5f, 10
ultraendurance athletes 96, 285, 317

ultraviolet light, vitamin D and 160, 160f, 161
underwater weighing 274
underweight, pregnancy and 365
United States Department of Agriculture (USDA) 4-5, 294
unsaturated fatty acids 97-98, 97f, 101t, 106, 106f. *See also* monounsaturated fatty acids; polyunsaturated fatty acids
Unspecified Feeding or Eating Disorder 374, 376. *See also* disordered eating
urea cycle 122
urine 214
urine color 228-229, 229f, 229t-230t, 350
urine osmolality (UOsmol) 226-227
urine specific gravity (USG) 223, 226-227, 227t
U.S. Anti-Doping Agency (USADA) 245
USDA (United States Department of Agriculture) 4-5, 294
U.S. Food and Drug Administration (FDA)
   on detoxes 217
   on hydrogenated oils 111
   on "light" or "lite" 9
   on "natural" 86-87, 246, 258
   on nonnutritive sweeteners 88
   nutrition labeling on foods 7-9, 173
   on PDCAAS 141
   on supplements 238-241, 242, 244-245
USG (urine specific gravity) 223, 226-227, 227t
U.S. Pharmacopeial Convention (USP) 244
UVA/UVB light, vitamin D and 160, 160f, 161, 186

V

vaccenic acid 110, 112
vaccines, influenza 127
valine 118-120, 119f, 121f
vegan diets 368t
   calcium in 372
   iron in 381
   phosphocreatine and 31
   protein sources in 139, 149-151, 150t, 369-370, 371f
   vitamins and minerals in 161, 168, 177, 370-372
vegetarian diets 149-151
   ATP generation and 31
   caffeine 372
   challenges in 150-151
   complementary proteins in 137-138, 148, 370, 371f
   creatine in 31, 372-373
   disordered eating and 368
   energy foods in 369
   health effects of 149, 151, 368-369
   ideal menus 207f
   iron in 202, 381
   nutrition needs in 369-370, 369f
   performance effects of 368-369
   protein in 139, 149-151, 150t, 370

vegetarian diets *(continued)*
  types of 368*t*
  vitamins and minerals in 168, 177, 205-206, 208, 370-372
very low-carbohydrate diets 317
villi, intestinal 68-69, 69*f*
visceral fat 103, 322
vitamins 156-180. *See also names of individual vitamins*
  deficiencies and toxicities 159-160, 166*t*-167*t*
  in diet 168, 207*f*
  fat-soluble 6, 156-172
  importance of 6, 156, 157*f*
  for masters athletes 354-355
  multivitamin supplements 208
  on Nutrition Facts Panel 173
  tolerable upper limits for 6, 10-11
  in vegan and vegetarian diets 207*f*
  water-soluble 6, 173-180
vitamin A 156-160, 158*f*, 159*t*, 166*t*-167*t*, 367
vitamin B_1 (thiamin) 7, 166*t*-167*t*, 174, 176-177, 177*f*, 366
vitamin B_2 (riboflavin) 166*t*-167*t*, 174, 175-176, 176*f*, 366
vitamin B_5 (pantothenic acid) 166*t*-167*t*, 174, 175
vitamin B_6 (pyridoxine) 166*t*-167*t*, 174, 177, 354
vitamin B_{12} (cobalamin) 149, 166*t*-167*t*, 174, 177-178, 354, 370
vitamin C (ascorbic acid)
  deficiency and excess 166*t*-167*t*
  food preparation and 179
  functions of 178-179, 255
  immune system and 171, 178-179, 257-258, 367
  iron absorption and 179
  muscle soreness and 190, 194
  in pregnancy 367
  sources of 179
vitamin D 160-169
  absorption of 186
  bone health and 162, 163, 169, 352, 367
  in children and adolescents 163, 350
  deficiency 162-165, 162*t*, 165*t*, 167*t*
  in endurance athletes 296
  exercise and 165, 168
  forms of 161-162, 318
  guidelines 162*t*, 164-165
  illness and 161, 165, 168, 257, 296
  injuries and 169
  muscle function and 318
  in older adults 163-164, 318, 355
  in pregnancy 367
  sources of 160, 166*t*
  toxicity of 162*t*, 165, 166*t*, 167*t*
  UV light and synthesis of 160, 160*f*
vitamin E 166*t*-167*t*, 169-171, 180

vitamin K 166*t*-167*t*, 171-172, 172*f*, 258
$\dot{V}O_2$max 11-12, 352

W

WADA (World Anti-Doping Agency) 243
waist circumference 270-271, 322, 323*f*
waist-to-hip ratio 322
WAT (white adipose tissue) 266
water and fluid intake 212-221. *See also* dehydration; hydration status
  in body composition 213
  by children and adolescents 217-218, 232-233
  in endurance events 218
  in exercise 232-234
  fiber and 66, 331
  fluid requirements 213-214
  functions of 6, 212, 212*f*
  homeostasis and 212-213, 212*f*, 213*f*
  hydration plans 225*f*, 232-234, 350
  hyperhydration 213, 218, 220-221
  by masters athletes 355
  rehydrating after exercise 224, 226, 233-234
  in resistance training 304-305
  sports drinks 221, 232-233, 290
  strategies to increase fluid intake 215, 215*f*
  water in foods and beverages 213-214, 214*t*
water-soluble vitamins 6, 173-180. *See also names of individual vitamins*
waxy maize 295
wearable activity monitors 59
websites, evaluating 16
weight-class sports 373
weight gain 325-326, 356, 362-365, 364*t*
weight loss
  by athletes 268-269, 336-338, 338*t*
  behavior therapy and strategies in 332, 332*f*, 337*f*
  caffeine in 259
  caloric deficit in 326*f*, 327, 337*f*
  in diabetes 325
  diets in 332-335
  diuretics, detoxes, and cleanses in 199, 217
  energy availability and 60, 326
  energy-yielding macronutrients in 330-332
  estimating energy needs 327
  exercise intensity and 48-49, 48*f*, 336
  flexible versus rigid dieting 333-334
  food type in 334-335
  metabolic adaptations from 329-330
  mindful eating 333
  muscle in 315-318, 330-331, 336
  nonnutritive sweeteners in 88
  in the off season 327
  plateaus and regaining weight 329-330
  protein in 315-318, 330-331

  satiation and satiety in 331
  sport-specific goals 268-269, 336-338, 338*t*
  training for losing body fat 48-49, 48*f*
  weight goals 267, 326-328, 326*f*, 328*t*
weight-loss calculators 328
wellness 6
Wernicke–Korsakoff syndrome 176
wheat allergy 84
whey protein 137, 139, 141, 148, 149, 312*f*
white adipose tissue (WAT) 266
white flour, enrichment of 66-67, 162
whole grains 9, 65-67, 81-83, 151, 152*t*, 307
Whole Grain Stamp 67
women and girls. *See also* pregnancy
  alcohol and 309
  amenorrhea 352, 377
  anabolic androgenic steroids and 260
  body composition in adolescence 347
  body fat percentages for 271-272, 272*t*
  bone density in 188-189, 275, 377
  calcium and 188-189, 189*t*
  carbohydrate loading 287
  energy availability 286
  female athlete triad 59, 377, 377*f*, 378*f*, 379*f*
  fluid needs in 213
  ideal menu 207*f*
  iron and 202
  low body fat in 326
  magnesium and 194
  minerals in 184*t*
  multivitamin supplements for 208
  postmenopausal 208
  relative energy deficiency in sport 59-60
  resistance training for 352
  resting metabolic rate in 327
World Anti-Doping Agency (WADA) 243

X

xerophthalmia 159

Y

yogurt 83, 100, 104, 257
yo-yo dieting 268

Z

zinc
  absorption of 186-187
  copper and 206
  exercise and 205-206
  functions of 205, 258
  muscles and 318
  recommended intake 184*t*, 201*t*, 205-206
  sources of 201*t*, 205
  supplements 186, 205, 257-258
  in vegan and vegetarian diets 206, 372
zinc gluconate lozenges 205

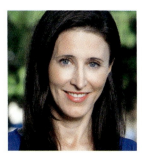

Marie A. Spano, MS, RD, CSCS, CSSD, is one of the country's leading sports nutritionists. She is the previous major league sports nutritionist for the Atlanta Braves (including the 2021 World Series champions), Atlanta Falcons, Atlanta Hawks, Atlanta Thrashers, Chicago Cubs, and Blackzilians (MMA). She combines science with practical experience to help athletes implement customized nutrition plans to maximize athletic performance, recovery, return to play, and career longevity. Also a nutrition communications expert, Spano has appeared on CNN; the Weather Channel; and NBC, ABC, Fox, and CBS affiliates. She has authored hundreds of magazine and trade publication articles in addition to book chapters in *NSCA's Essentials of Personal Training* and *Essentials of Strength Training and Conditioning*. She is coeditor of the first edition of *NSCA's Guide to Sport and Exercise Nutrition*.

A three-sport collegiate athlete, Spano earned her master's degree in nutrition from the University of Georgia, where she worked in the athletic department as a graduate assistant running the sports nutrition program. She earned her bachelor's degree in exercise and sports science from the University of North Carolina at Greensboro, where she also ran Division I cross country. Her experiences as a college athlete provide her an effective perspective when working with athletes of all levels, especially student athletes, by giving her a firsthand understanding of how the demands of athletics and the psychological aspects of injury, sleep, recovery, and nutrition can affect an athlete's overall well-being and performance.

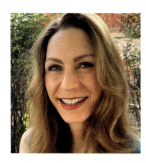

Laura J. Kruskall, PhD, RDN, CSSD, LD, FACSM, FAND, is an associate professor and program director in nutrition sciences at University of Nevada, Las Vegas (UNLV). She is also the director of the UNLV Nutrition Center. She has held numerous leadership positions at the local, state, and national levels, including serving on the board of trustees of the American College of Sports Medicine (ACSM) and as the cochair of the committee that authored "Standards of Practice and Standards of Professional Performance for Registered Dietitian Nutritionists (Competent, Proficient, and Expert) in Sports Nutrition and Dietetics," published in the *Journal of the Academy of Nutrition and Dietetics* in 2014. She is currently serving on the ACSM Publications Committee and is a member of the editorial board for *ACSM's Health & Fitness Journal*. She serves as the chair of the Dietitian Advisory Group for the Nevada Department of Health and Human Services, which leads governance of statute NRS.640E (licensure for dietitians in Nevada).

Kruskall earned her PhD in nutrition from Penn State University. She holds a certificate of training in Level 2 Adult Weight Management from the Commission on Dietetic Registration, is certified as an exercise physiologist by ACSM, holds the Exercise Is Medicine credential from ACSM, and has the Board-Certified Specialist in Sports Dietetics (CSSD) credential. She earned fellow status with both ACSM and the Academy of Nutrition and Dietetics for her leadership and contributions to the profession. Her areas of teaching and practice expertise are sports and human performance nutrition, weight management, and medical nutrition therapy. In addition to her academic duties at the university, she is a nutrition consultant for Canyon Ranch Spa Club in Las Vegas.

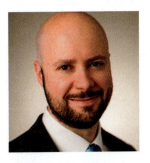

D. Travis Thomas, PhD, RDN, CSSD, LD, FAND, is an associate professor of clinical and sports nutrition and program director of the clinical nutrition masters program in the College of Health Sciences at the University of Kentucky. He teaches an advanced sports nutrition class for graduate students and a nutrition for injury prevention and rehabilitation class for undergraduate students. He also teaches and directs multiple clinical nutrition graduate courses and serves as director for the undergraduate certificate program in nutrition for human performance.

Thomas holds the Board-Certified Specialist in Sports Dietetics (CSSD) credential. He has held multiple volunteer and leadership positions with the Academy of Nutrition and Dietetics, Sports and Human Performance Nutrition practice group, and the Commission on Dietetic Registration. He served as lead author on the 2016 "Nutrition and Athletic Performance" position stand endorsed by the Academy of Nutrition and Dietetics, American College of Sports Medicine, and Dietitians of Canada. In 2016, he was inducted as a fellow of the Academy of Nutrition and Dietetics, and in 2020 he received the highest award from the Sports, Cardiovascular, and Wellness (SCAN) Practice Group: the National Career Achievement Award.

Thomas has 14 years of experience conducting human studies involving nutrition and exercise interventions across the life span. Since 2011, he has served as an investigator on funded research projects involving a wide range of nutrition issues associated with the preservation and enhancement of skeletal muscle function and performance. These studies have investigated the relationship between vitamin D and muscle metabolic function, nutrition, and physical function in aging and athletic populations; nutrition interventions to improve endothelial function and to reduce symptoms in patients with advanced heart failure; and nutritional strategies to preserve physical performance and lean body mass in patients with cancer.